WJ110 TEX.

TEXTBOOK IN PSYCHIATRIC EPIDEMIOLOGY

TEXTBOOK IN PSYCHIATRIC EPIDEMIOLOGY

Edited by

Ming T. Tsuang
Mauricio Tohen
Gwendolyn E.P. Zahner

Harvard Institute of Psychiatric
    Epidemiology and Genetics
Harvard Medical School
and
Harvard School of Public Health

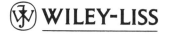 **WILEY-LISS**

A JOHN WILEY & SONS, INC. , PUBLICATION
New York • Chichester • Brisbane • Toronto • Singapore

Library of Congress Cataloging in Publication Data:

Textbook in psychiatric epidemiology / editors, Ming T. Tsuang,
   Mauricio Tohen, Gwendolyn E.P. Zahner.
       p.   cm.
    Includes index.
    ISBN 0–471–59375–3
    1. Psychiatric epidemiology.   I. Tsuang, Ming T., 1931–
II. Tohen, Mauricio.   III. Zahner, Gwendolyn E.P.
    [DNLM: 1. Mental Disorders—epidemiology. 2. Mental Disorders—
diagnosis. 3. Epidemiologic Methods. WM 100 T3545 1995]
RC455.2.E64T49   1995
614.5′989—dc20
DNLM/DLC
for Library of Congress   94–47953

Printed in the United States of America

10 9 8 7 6 5 4 3 2

CONTENTS

PART III ASSESSMENT

PART IV EPIDEMIOLOGY OF MAJOR PSYCHIATRIC DISORDERS

CONTRIBUTORS

James C. Anthony, Department of Mental Hygiene, School of Hygiene and Public Health, The Johns Hopkins University, Baltimore, MD 21205

Dan G. Blazer, Duke University Medical Center, School of Medicine, Durham, NC 27710

Evelyn J. Bromet, Department of Psychiatry and Behavioral Science, State University of New York at Stony Brook, Stony Brook, NY 11794

Jack D. Burke, Jr., Department of Psychiatry and Behavioral Science, Texas A&M University Health Science Center and Scott & White Clinic and Hospital, Temple, TX 76508

Nancy L. Day, Department of Psychiatry, University of Pittsburgh School of Medicine, Pittsburgh, PA 15260

Mary Amanda Dew, Department of Psychiatry, University of Pittsburgh, School of Medicine, Pittsburgh, PA 15260

Bruce P. Dohrenwend, Department of Social Psychiatry, New York State Psychiatric Institute, New York, NY 10032

William W. Eaton, Department of Mental Hygiene, School of Hygiene and Public Health, The Johns Hopkins University, Baltimore, MD 21205

Stephen V. Faraone, Harvard Medical School Department of Psychiatry at Massachusetts Mental Health Center and Brockton/West Roxbury VA Medical Center; Harvard Institute of Psychiatric Epidemiology and Genetics, Boston, MA 02115

Michael B. First, New York State Psychiatric Institute, New York, NY 10032

Jerome A. Fleming, Harvard Medical School Department of Psychiatry at Massachusetts Mental Health Center and Brockton/West Roxbury VA Medical Center; Harvard Institute of Psychiatric Epidemiology and Genetics, Boston, MA 02115

Steve Ford, Department of Psychiatry, Duke University Medical Center, Durham, NC 27710

Allen Frances, Department of Psychiatry, Duke University Medical Center, Durham, NC 27710

Jill M. Goldstein, Harvard Medical School Department of Psychiatry at Massachusetts

Mental Health Center and Brockton West/Roxbury VA Medical Center; Harvard Institute of Psychiatric Epidemiology and Genetics, Boston, MA 02115

Frederick K. Goodwin, The Center on Neuroscience Behavior and Society, George Washington University Medical Center, Washington, DC 20037

John E. Helzer, Department of Psychiatry, University of Vermont School of Medicine, Burlington, VT 05401

Stephen L. Hillis, Department of Statistics and Actuarial Science, University of Iowa, Iowa City, IA 52242

Leslie B. Hocking, Geropsychiatry Institute, John Umstead Hospital, Butner, NC 27509

Ewald Horwath, Washington Heights Community Service, New York State Psychiatric Institute, New York, NY 10032

Chung-Cheng Hsieh, Department of Epidemiology, Harvard School of Public Health, Boston, MA 02115

Charles T. Kaelber, Division of Epidemiology and Services Research, National Institute of Mental Health, NIH, Rockville, MD 20857

Ronald C. Kessler, Institute for Social Research, The University of Michigan, Ann Arbor, MI 48106

Harold G. Koenig, Center for Aging, Duke University Medical Center, Durham, NC 27710

Michael J. Lyons, Boston University Department of Psychology; Harvard Medical School Department of Psychiatry at Massachusetts Mental Health Center and Brockton/West Roxbury VA Medical Center; Harvard Institute of Psychiatric Epidemiology and Genetics, Boston, MA 02115

Avram H. Mack, Department of Psychiatry, Duke University Medical Center, Durham, NC 27710

Jane M. Murphy, Harvard Medical School Department of Psychiatry at Massachusetts General Hospital; Department of Epidemiology, Harvard School of Public Health; Harvard Institute of Psychiatric Epidemiology and Genetics, Boston, MA 02115

Darrel A. Regier, Division of Epidemiology and Services Research, National Institute of Mental Health, NIH, Rockville, MD 20857

Lee N. Robins, Department of Psychiatry, Washington University School of Medicine, St. Louis, MO 63110

Ruth Ross, Department of Psychiatry, Duke University Medical Center, Durham, NC 27710

Patrick E. Shrout, Department of Psychology, New York University, New York, NY 10003

John C. Simpson, Harvard Medical School Department of Psychiatry at Massachusetts Mental Health Center and Brockton/West Roxbury VA Medical Center, Boston, MA 02115

Mauricio Tohen, Harvard Medical School Department of Psychiatry at McLean Hospital; Department of Epidemiology, Harvard School of Public Health; Harvard Institute of Psychiatric Epidemiology and Genetics, Boston, MA 02115

Ming T. Tsuang, Harvard Medical School Department of Psychiatry at Massachusetts Mental Health Center and Brockton/West Roxbury VA Medical Center; Department of Epidemiology, Harvard School of Public Health; Harvard Institute of Psychiatric Epidemiology and Genetics, Boston, MA 02115

Nancy Vetterello, American Psychiatric Association, Washington, DC

Myrna M. Weissman, Division of Clinical and Genetic Epidemiology, New York State Psychiatric Institute, New York, NY 10032

Tom Widiger, Department of Psychology, University of Kentucky, Lexington, KY 40506

Robert F. Woolson, Department of Statistics and Actuarial Science, University of Iowa, Iowa City, IA 52242

Gwendolyn E.P. Zahner, Department of Epidemiology, Harvard School of Public Health; Harvard Institute of Psychiatric Epidemiology and Genetics, Boston, MA 02115

The impetus for this textbook arose from requests from our students in the Harvard Training Program in Psychiatric Epidemiology and Biostatistics. This program is supported by a training grant from the Epidemiology and Psychopathology Research Branch of the Division of Epidemiology and Services Research at the National Institute of Mental Health, and is one of 11 programs currently funded under these auspices nationally. In addition to courses in epidemiology and biostatistics offered to all graduate students at the Harvard School of Public Health, our program offers a series of seminars for pre- and postdoctoral fellows on the training grant and for mental health professionals enrolled in other degree and residency training programs at Harvard. These specialized courses attempt to introduce students to the types of epidemiologic research designs and biostatistical methods that are most frequently employed in studies of mental disorders. The curriculum also covers the complex issues in assessment and diagnosis in this field. Students are also offered courses that review the epidemiologic evidence for major psychiatric disorders and research strategies for studying genetic and environmental risk factors.

In our teaching endeavors, it became clear that there is no one textbook that encompasses the field of psychiatric epidemiology. Heretofore we have depended mostly on journal publications for reading materials in our courses. These publications are frequently not written at a level that is appropriate for graduate level training. Furthermore, many textbooks covering epidemiologic research designs and biostatistics do not describe psychiatric applications, leaving the student unclear as to how these methods have been previously used by psychiatric researchers, and uncertain as to how he or she might use them in future investigations in this area.

In preparing the textbook, we also wanted to consider the diversity of students who attend our courses. These students can be divided into two primary groups. First, there are students funded by the training program who, for the most part, are planning to become researchers in psychiatric epidemiology and biostatistics. The second group consists of psychiatric residents and junior faculty of the teaching hospitals who attend our courses to gain knowledge about the field as well as a grounding in research design. Our textbook has considered the needs of both types of students: those with little or no clinical training, and those with clinical training but little formal knowledge of quantitative research methods.

A final consideration was our choice of contributors to this textbook. We debated between developing a textbook from the lecture materials of Harvard faculty or soliciting chapters from nationally recognized experts in the field. The former approach has the advantage of presenting a coherent theoretical framework and consistent terminology; the latter offers students insights into contemporary thinking and expertise at different training centers. As we explored the possibility of engaging senior faculty at other NIMH-funded training programs as contributing authors, it became clear that other programs also saw the critical need for this textbook. The enthusiastic response from our colleagues at other training centers was the deciding factor in designing a textbook with multiple authors as contributors.

We have divided the textbook into four sections. The first section consists of a historical review. Section II is a review of study designs and methods. Section III covers assessment in psychiatric epidemiology, and Section IV includes the epidemiology of major psychiatric disorders, including prevalence and incidence data as well as risk factors for major disorders.

Our objective has been to provide a comprehensive yet understandable overview of methods and substantive information in psychiatric epidemiology. For purposes of manageability, however, we have limited the focus of this volume to basic research strategies and analytic methods. Not all psychiatric disorders are included, and in particular we have not attempted to cover the rapidly evolving area of child psychiatric epidemiology. Despite these limitations, we hope this textbook will meet the needs of students in the field of psychiatric epidemiology as well as the needs of psychiatric researchers in general.

As editors of this textbook, we would also like to acknowledge four individuals whose work does not appear directly in this book, but is present through the writings of others whose careers in psychiatric epidemiology they have fostered. Although our field is indebted to many such mentors, because we are based at Harvard we would like to name four who have been most instrumental in our own program: Dr. Alexander Leighton, who first brought research in psychiatric epidemiology to Harvard; Dr. Gerald Klerman, who laid the foundation for the current training program; Dr. Brian MacMahon, who integrated our training program into the Department of Epidemiology at the Harvard School of Public Health; and Ben Z. Locke, the former Chief of the Epidemiology and Psychopathology Research Branch at NIMH, who maintained training in psychiatric epidemiology as a priority area throughout his 16-year tenure.

MING T. TSUANG
MAURICIO TOHEN
GWENDOLYN E.P. ZAHNER

PART I

HISTORICAL OVERVIEW

CHAPTER 1

"The Problem of Validity in Field Studies of Psychological Disorders" Revisited

BRUCE P. DOHRENWEND

New York State Psychiatric Institute and Columbia University,
New York, NY 10032

INTRODUCTION

It is over 20 years since Barbara Dohrenwend and I published an article titled, "The problem of validity in field studies of psychological disorders" (Dohrenwend and Dohrenwend, 1965). We had occasions to update this review in 1974 (Dohrenwend and Dohrenwend, 1974), in 1980 with other colleagues (Dohrenwend et al., 1980a), and in 1982 (Dohrenwend and Dohrenwend, 1982). In these publications, we were concerned with what we came to term the "first generation" of pre-World War II studies and the post-war "second generation" in which research workers attempted to investigate the true prevalence of psychiatric disorders in communities all over the world (Dohrenwend and Dohrenwend, 1982). For the most part, these studies focused on prevalence within periods of a few months to a year. There were too few longitudinal studies to permit an examination of investigations of true incidence as well.

Epidemiologic research is dependent on the accuracy of diagnostic methods which is in turn dependent on the progress of laboratory and clinical research. Each of the first- and second-generation studies tended to pioneer its own unique methods and procedures for counting cases, with very little attention in any of them to problems of validity. This anarchy reflected the state of diagnostic affairs in the wider mental health community. However, a number of developments were under way that have brought about a rather different situation.

By 1980, with the appearance of DSM-III, and the changes in epidemiologic research

This paper was presented at the 1988 Annual Meeting of the American Psychopathological Association and first published in *The Validity of Psychiatric Diagnosis* (ed. L. N. Robins and J. E. Barrett), American Psychopathological Association Series, Raven Press: New York, 1989. It was subsequently updated and reprinted in *Psychological Medicine* 20:195–208, 1990. It is reprinted here with permission of Raven Press and Cambridge University Press and includes some minor stylistic revision.

procedures coincident with it, it has become meaningful, I think, to talk about the beginnings of a new, third generation of studies in psychiatric epidemiology. My purposes in this paper are to describe briefly as background the first- and second-generation studies and the problems of validity with their procedures for case identification and diagnosis; to consider some of the newer developments with regard to diagnostic instruments that either are or should be influencing third-generation studies; to discuss some of the problems of validity in third-generation studies completed so far; and to offer some suggestions for the future.

FIRST-GENERATION STUDIES

Sixteen studies, all of which took place between the turn of the century and World War II, comprise the first generation. Investigators in these studies tended to rely on key informants and agency records to supply the information that would enable them to identify cases. Such procedures tend to underestimate untreated cases of disorders that are characterized mainly by subjective distress that would be more likely to be revealed in direct interviews. Direct interviews were used in only six of these studies. Nevertheless, even in these six interview studies, where rates tended to be higher than in studies using key informants and agency records, the median for all types of disorders combined was only 3.6% as compared to a median of close to 20% in the second generation of studies conducted after World War II (Dohrenwend and Dohrenwend, 1974). The difference is a dramatic illustration of the effects of the tremendous expansion of psychiatric nomenclatures following World War II on rates of psychiatric disorders counted in community studies. The expansion itself reflected the experiences of the mental health professions with psychiatric screening for selective service and with subsequent psychiatric casualties in World War II (Raines, 1952). It marked the transition from the first to the second generation of epidemiologic studies.

SECOND-GENERATION STUDIES

Unlike the research workers in the first generation of studies, most of the investigators in more than 60 second-generation studies conducted after World War II and up to about 1980 relied on direct interviews with all subjects. Only rarely in these studies were the interviews supplemented systematically by data from key informants and official records, although such information is extremely useful for identifying or confirming some types of psychopathology such as substance abuse and antisocial behaviour. Two different types of interview were used.

First, in most of the European and Asian research, a single psychiatrist or a small team headed by a psychiatrist personally interviewed community residents and recorded diagnostic judgements on the basis of these interviews. As a rule, the interview procedures were not made explicit in this type of approach.

In the second type, by contrast, standard and explicit data-collection procedures were used. Although the interviews were sometimes done by psychiatrists and clinical psychologists and sometimes by lay interviewers, in all instances case identification depended on psychiatrists' evaluations of protocols compiled from the interview responses and, sometimes, from ancillary data from key informants, official records, and interviewers' observations. The Midtown study and the Stirling County study (Srole et al., 1962; Leighton et al., 1963) pioneered this approach, and some others adopted their procedures (e.g., Gillis et al., 1965; Rin et al., 1966; Shore et al., 1973). The resulting classifications were made not in terms of diagnostic types but rather in terms of ratings of "caseness" and "impairment."

Even more economical than having clinicians rate protocols constructed from data collected by lay interviewers is dispensing with clinical judgements altogether and using objectively scored measures of psychopathology. A number of the investigators in this second generation of studies took this route. The objective measure used most often is a 22-item screening instrument developed by Langner (1962) in the Midtown study on a purely actuarial basis to provide an approximation of their Mental Health Rating of psychiatric impairment. A similar, although less widely used, measure consisting of 20 Health Opinion Survey questions, was constructed by the Stirling County study research workers as well (Macmillan, 1957). Both have as their core a portion of the items from the Psychosomatic Scale of the Neuropsychiatric Screening Adjunct, developed as an aid to Selective Service screening during World War II (Star, 1950).

There exists by now a small family of these brief screening scales that appear highly similar in content and have been used in between a fourth and a third of the second generation of epidemiologic studies to measure such things as "mental health," "mental illness," "psychiatric disorders," "emotional adjustment," "symptoms of stress," and "psychophysiological symptoms" (Seiler, 1973, p. 257).

PROBLEM OF VALIDITY IN FIRST- AND SECOND-GENERATION STUDIES

There is little evidence of any of the usual types of validity in the first- and second-generation studies. Content validity was precluded because there was little consensus at any of the times these studies were done about the population of signs and symptoms to be sampled. Different nomenclatures were used by different investigators, and some investigators tended to bypass nomenclatures, substituting "caseness" (Leighton et al., 1963) and "impairment" (Srole et al., 1962) ratings. Nor is the picture much better for criterion-orientated or construct validity. Except for studies using the brief screening scales for case identification, no attempts were made to test the ability of the diagnostic procedures to identify and classify known cases of important types or to test whether the main measures agreed with very different measures of the same types of disorders.

There has been much more methodologic research on the brief screening scales used in these studies. They show good internal consistency (typically between 0.80 and 0.85) and tend to correlate with each other as highly as their reliabilities permit (Link and Dohrenwend, 1980). They are all measures of much the same thing. It is not readily apparent, however, from their content (symptoms of depressed mood, anxiety, and psychophysiologic disturbance) what this is. They certainly do not, for example, contain symptoms of all varieties of "mental illness" or "psychiatric disorders"; nor are they limited to "psychophysiologic symptoms"; nor do they exhaust the variety of stress reactions. Moreover, while whatever they measure frequently is accompanied by diagnosable mental disorders, it occurs with at least equal frequency in the absence of such disorders (Link and Dohrenwend, 1980). It is intriguing to enquire, therefore, into what it is that they are in fact measuring.

We have found that these brief screening scales have an extremely high correlation with measures of self-esteem, helplessness-hopelessness, dread, anxiety, sadness, and confused thinking (Dohrenwend et al., 1980b) all of which are major facets of what Frank (1973) has called "demoralization." In Frank's theoretical formulation, as well as in relevant research that we have reviewed with regard to the screening scales (Dohrenwend et al., 1979), this type of nonspecific psychological distress is likely to occur in response to a variety of predicaments: severe physical illnesses, especially those that are chronic; a build up of recent stressful life events; attempts to cope with psychotic symptoms; and being low in social class position. It is something like physical temperature in that you know something is wrong when it is elevated, but you do not know what is wrong until you learn more about the context. Thus, while these measures of nonspecific distress that I prefer to call "demoralization" are interesting in their own right, they are often very imperfectly related to diagnosable mental disorders.

BEGINNINGS OF A THIRD GENERATION

Epidemiologic studies are expensive and time consuming. It is unlikely that there have been more than a dozen since around 1980. There is lack of unanimity about the diagnostic procedures to be used. However, the procedures have tended to be very different from those used in the first- and second-generation studies.

There have been a number of developments in psychiatry and related sciences here and abroad that have changed the context of these studies. Concern with systematizing and refining diagnostic systems is no longer concentrated abroad, but, spear-headed by the Washington University group (Robins and Guze, 1970; Woodruff ct al., 1974), it has spread in the United States. Its embodiment is DSM-III. Semistructured diagnostic interview and rating examinations such as the PSE (Wing et al., 1974) and SADS (Endicott and Spitzer, 1978), developed for clinical research with patients and designed to be used by skilled clinicians, have been adapted for epidemiologic research. Psychometric instruments such as the SCL-90 (Derogatis, 1977) and the GHQ (Goldberg, 1972), also developed for clinical research and research with general practice patients, have been used in epidemiologic studies. In addition, there have been attempts to build instruments specifically for epidemiologic studies. These include psychometric instruments such as the CES-D scale (Center for Epidemiological Studies–Depression scale) (Radloff, 1977) and the set of screening scales from the Psychiatric Epidemiology Research Interview (PERI) (Shrout et al., 1986). They include the most influential of all and the most directly related to the new DMS-III, the NIMH Diagnostic Interview Schedule or DIS (Robins et al., 1981); the DIS is a fully structured diagnostic interview designed to be administered by lay interviewers.

PROBLEM OF VALIDITY IN THE BEGINNINGS
OF THE THIRD GENERATION

There has already been more research on the validity of third-generation case identification procedures than on those used in the first and second generation. This is, however, an instance of a little being a lot by comparison. I will start with the methodologic research on semistructured clinical examinations, move on to the more recently developed psychometric screening scales, and then the DIS.

Semistructured Clinical Examination

In the semistructured clinical interview, main reliance is placed on the experience and skill of the clinician to reduce measurement error. A degree of structure is introduced to increase reliability. Wing et al. (1974) describe the interviewing and rating procedure for one of the most prominent of these semistructured instruments, the PSE, as follows:

> Each of the items or symptoms is defined in greater or lesser detail (in a glossary of definitions of symptoms). For most of the items or symptoms, a form of questioning is suggested, so that it would be possible to carry out the whole of the interview without deviating from the schedule at all. In practice, this would never happen since no two interviewees are alike and the examiner must be able to adapt his technique to the situation. The wording of each question depends on the answer to the previous one. . . .

> A symptom should not be rated as present simply because the patient says 'yes.' A further description should be asked for, in the patient's own words, and further specific questions asked as necessary. Following this process of cross examination . . . the examiner should make up his own mind as to how the symptom should be rated. Similarly, the fact that the patient says 'no' to the standard question does not mean that the symptom should be rated as absent. All available cues, in behaviour and case record, and from all parts of the interview, should be used to determine whether a particular line of examination should proceed further.

There has been very little investigation of the validity of semistructured clinical interviews in third-generation epidemiologic research. By and large, they have been assumed to bring their credentials with them from their development with psychiatric patients and their use in clinical research, even when administered by pre-doctoral-level clinicians, as has been the case in some epidemiologic studies (Weissman and Myers, 1978; Vernon and Roberts, 1982). Such validity is by no means assured in field studies of psychiatric disorders in general populations where the conditions under which diagnoses are made are very different from those that obtain in research with patient samples and where the boundaries between normal and abnormal are an underexplored frontier.

Much of what I have learned about the matter comes from two methodologic studies. One is my own previous research with a DSM-II era forerunner of SADS called the Psychiatric Status Schedule (PSS) developed by Spitzer et al. (1970) and used by my colleagues and me in New York City (Dohrenwend et al., 1978); the second is a study by Wing and his colleagues (1978) with a shortened version of the PSE scored on their "Index of Definition" to assess whether a respondent is a case in whom more detailed criteria of specific syndromes should be investigated. It is interesting to note that this type of case–noncase determination, used again by Brown and Harris (1978), harks back to the Stirling County study "caseness" rating (Leighton et al., 1963) and has much in common with the Midtown Study mental health rating of impairment as well (Srole et al., 1962).

The PSS was an attempt to standardize interviews of the kinds used for intake and diagnosis in clinical settings and was designed to provide DMS-II diagnoses of each subject through the application of a computer program called DIAGNO (Spitzer and Endicott, 1968). The PSS consists of fixed questions, many of them open ended, together with suggested probes. The actual responses to these questions and probes, however, are not recorded. Rather, they form the basis for judgements by the interviewer as to whether each of the several hundred carefully described symptoms is "true" or "false" of the subject. These clinical judgements then become the basic data resulting from the interview.

A number of years ago, we chose to investigate the PSS on grounds that it was likely to have much in common with the less explicit and less reproducible types of clinical interviews used by a number of first- and second-generation epidemiologic investigators, especially those working in Europe and Asia rather than in North America (e.g., Bash, 1967; Hagnell, 1966; Lin, 1953). It is similar in type to the PSE and SADS, which I noted above have only recently been used with samples from the general population. Like these instruments it was developed on the assumption that its users had clinical experience and would undergo intensive training in making the clinical judgements required. Thus, the interviewer of choice with such instruments is an experienced psychiatrist, clinical psychologist, or psychiatric social worker. In our own research, the interviewers who used it were psychiatrists.

Fortunately, the items in the PSS, unlike the PSE and SADS, were not contingent on each other. It is thus possible to test their internal consistency reliabilities and make direct comparisons on this basis with measures from such self-report interviews as PERI. In our research, we were able to test a large number of PSS scales—those developed by its authors as well as our own a priori symptom groups—on a small sample from the general population as well as on a sample of psychiatric patients (Dohrenwend et al., 1978). The most striking finding was the contrast in internal consistency reliabilities of the scales for psychiatric patient and nonpatient samples. For example, we were able to replicate the findings of Spitzer and his colleagues (1970) that a large number of PSS scales they developed showed good internal consistency reliability in psychiatric patients; we found, however, that most of the same PSS scales proved unreliable in the general population.

This lack of internal consistency reliability of the PSS scales in samples from the general population is accompanied by problems of validity. For example, we found that the computer program DIAGNO, developed on the basis of research using the PSS with psychiatric patients, tended to grossly over diagnose "schizophrenia" in the community sample that we studied; the errors were most likely to occur among respondents who were black or Puerto Rican (Dohrenwend et al., 1980c). We found earlier that scores on the PSS can be misleading about rates of mental disorder in different social classes (Dohrenwend et al., 1971).

To illustrate, DIAGNO diagnosed 10 of the 133 community sample respondents as currently being schizophrenic. This rate of 7.5% is far higher than average prevalence rates of under 1% reported for a similar period of time in samples of adults from the general population. It is also considerably higher than rates of 4.5% diagnosed by the psychiatrists who interviewed the respondents and 3% by a psychiatrist who independently reviewed the transcripts of the interviews. Even the last rate of 3% seems high and may reflect the use of relatively broad pre-DSM-III definitions of schizophrenia. In any case, of the 10 DIAGNO schizophrenics only three were also diagnosed as schizophrenic by psychiatrists who interviewed them, and only two of these three were diagnosed as schizophrenic by both the psychiatrists who interviewed them and a second psychiatrist who independently reviewed the transcripts of the tape recordings of the original interviews. Moreover, the psychiatrists who interviewed the community sample subjects diagnosed three respondents as schizophrenic who were not classified as schizophrenic by DIAGNO, and two of these were independently confirmed by the second psychiatrist who reviewed the transcripts. If we take as the most conservative identification of schizophrenia those instances where there was a consensus between the psychiatrist who interviewed the subject and the psychiatrist who reviewed the transcript, then DIAGNO converged with this clinical consensus in only two of its 10 schizophrenic diagnoses.

I believe that these problems of reliability and validity of the PSS for use in the general population are not specific to this instrument but extend to other instruments modeled on the clinical examination and developed primarily on the basis of research with psychiatric patients. Consider in this regard some results reported by Wing and his colleagues (Wing et al., 1978). They come from a study in which the Present State Examination (PSE) was used by trained psychiatrists to investigate mental disorders among women sampled from the general population of a district in London. Like the PSS, the PSE data can also be reduced by a computer program, this one called "CATEGO" (Wing et al., 1974). The results of the PSE for each subject are summarized first in terms of an Index of Definition and, if the subject is above a cut-off on this index, into one or more psychiatric syndromes that correspond to diagnostic groupings of the mental disorders contained in the International Classification of Diseases (ICD-9). Of the 123 women in this sample, 22 were cases of "depressive disorders" on the basis of their identification as being above the threshold on the Index of Definition and their categorization as depressive disorders by CATEGO. However, when Wing and his colleagues (1978) examined the PSE scores in terms of widely used criteria for depressive disorders developed by Feighner et al. (1972) for this sample and for a sample of inpatients and outpatients, the results were as follows.

> One of the 22 'depressive disorders' in the general population series meets the standard, while two are probable. On the other hand, 16 of the 23 above threshold depressive disorders found in the in-patient series are definite and three are probable, while one patient with severe depressive retardation could not be rated on the subjective symptoms. Of the 14 above threshold depressive disorders in the out-patient series, seven are definite, five are probable, and two show only three of the Feighner et al. (1972) criteria (Wing et al., 1978, p. 213).

So far as the depressive disorders are concerned, the PSE and its Index of Definition and CATEGO system of case identification and classification are clearly not measuring the same thing in this general population sample as they are in samples of psychiatric patients.

Psychometric Screening Scales

It has been evident for some time that the unidimensional screening scales of nonspecific distress developed in the second generation of epidemiologic studies are very imperfectly related to clinical psychiatric disorders. Results that Bruce Link and I analyzed from three studies showed, for example, that at least half of those registering distress as severe as that of psychiatric outpatients did not have diagnosable disorders (Link and Dohrenwend, 1980). Later studies with the more recently developed CES-D also show very imperfect correspondence between the scale cut offs and diagnosable disorder (Myers and Weissman, 1980; Roberts and Vernon, 1983; Breslau, 1985). Thus, while these scales are brief, easily administered, and highly reliable in contrasting sex, class, and ethnic groups, they do not converge closely with diagnoses based on clinical interviews and ratings.

However, we have shown that it is possible to develop symptom scales that measure not only nonspecific psychological distress, but also a variety of other meaningful dimensions of psychopathology. These are the symptom scales in the Psychiatric Epidemiology Research Interview (PERI) (Dohrenwend et al., 1980b). We have also shown that subsets of seven or eight of these scales can discriminate cases from noncases with much higher sensitivity and specificity than a unidimensional scale of nonspecific distress (Shrout et al., 1986). However, the scales are not very precise in screening individual cases of particular disorders (Dohrenwend et al., 1986). The best they can do so far as individual disorders are concerned is isolate subsamples with much higher rates than the general population sample as a whole. Thus, while very economical of time and money to administer (about 15 minutes for all the items in seven or eight scales by a lay interviewer or even in self-administered format if comprehension and motivation can be assumed) and very reliable in different gender, class, and ethnic groups, the symptom scales cannot provide precise rates of particular disorders in the general population.

The Diagnostic Interview Schedule (DIS)

The DIS was developed as "a response to the desire to have an instrument that will, as closely as possible, replicate a psychiatrist's diagnoses for situations when the use of psychiatrists is impractical or impossible" (Helzer et al., 1985, p. 666). Large-scale epidemiologic studies are assumed to be such situations by its developers. The DIS is not a psychometric measure, nor is it a clinical examination. It is a fully structured interview administered by lay interviewers and designed to provide current and lifetime diagnoses of many DSM-III disorders, with adaptations that make it relevant to other nomenclatures as well. Unlike the other instruments that have been used for individual investigations, the DIS has been used in the ECA collaborative program that, in terms of number of settings and cumulative sample sizes, is the largest undertaking at any time or place in psychiatric epidemiology to date (Regier et al., 1984). Moreover, the influence of the DIS has spread. Now, translated into many languages, it is undoubtedly the most widely used procedure for case identification and classification in psychiatric epidemiology in the United States, and it is being adopted by a number of investigators abroad.

More research has been done on the validity of the DIS than on the validity of the semistructured clinical interviews used in third-generation studies. Conducted concurrently with or following the ECA studies, these methodologic investigations have usually taken the form of diagnostic follow-up interviews. A number have focused on patient samples. However, the most important of the investigations have been done with general population samples.

Some of these checks have involved closely spaced test–retest designs that varied the type of interview and/or the type of interviewer. For example, in a study reported by Helzer and his colleagues (1985) of a subsample of ECA respondents in the St Louis site, psychiatrists using the DIS and a DSM-III checklist were compared with lay interviewers using the DIS (Helzer et al., 1985). This study contrasts with a study reported by Anthony and his colleagues (1985) in which the follow-up of the lay interview DIS with a subsample of respondents in the Baltimore site was done by psychiatrists using a semistructured clinical interview and other information. Other studies have been 1 year or more follow-ups with lay-administered DIS interviews that permit checks on the accuracy of diagnoses of past disorders, essential to the DIS goal of estimating lifetime as well as current prevalence (Pulver and Carpenter, 1983; Anthony and Dryman, 1987).

The studies reported by Helzer et al. (1985) and Anthony et al. (1985) are particularly instructive. In these studies, the subsamples of ECA respondents designated for follow-up after the initial DIS lay interviews were drawn to over-represent cases. Although the sub-sample selection procedures were different, in each report the investigators present kappas for agreement (Cohen, 1960) between the initial DIS and the follow ups based, for most findings, on subsample data suitably weighted to represent the population sampled. For the Baltimore study reported by Anthony et al. (1985), only the kappas based on weighted data are provided. In the St Louis study reported by Helzer et al. (1985), kappas for both weighted data and unweighted data are given for most of the results. The kappas for the unweighted data are usually somewhat higher due to the oversampling of cases and consequent higher rates of disorders.

In my discussion of the two studies, I will refer for the most part to the weighted results, using unweighted results only when weighted data are not provided, as is the case with some of the St Louis findings. Given the differing designs of the follow-up subsamples in the two studies, the weighted results are more comparable. In addition, the weighted results are the only ones that can be generalized to the populations studied.

In the Helzer et al. (1985) study in St Louis, the subsample of respondents with various types of DIS lifetime diagnoses (including no disorder) based on lay interviews in the St Louis ECA site were reinterviewed within a few weeks to a few months after the initial interview. The second interview was done by psychiatrists using the DIS. However, after they made a DIS-alone diagnosis, they also made a diagnosis based on a DSM-III checklist that could be based on additional questions and observations. The first finding to note is that the psychiatrists agreed quite well with themselves, with a kappa of 0.73 with unweighted data for diagnoses combined versus none (kappas for weighted data were not provided for all versus none comparisons) and over 0.60 with weighted data for most individual diagnoses. For example, the kappa for major depression was 0.70 with weighted data. When the psychiatrists' DIS diagnoses were compared with the initial lay interviewers' diagnoses, agreement was considerably less, although overall agreement for any lifetime diagnosis versus no disorder remained reasonably good, as indicated by a kappa of 0.63 with unweighted data. It decreased only slightly, to 0.59, with unweighted data, when the initial DIS diagnoses by lay interviewers were compared with the checklist diagnoses these psychiatrists were permitted to make following the psychiatrists' DIS interviews. The kappas for individual diagnoses based on unweighted data tend to be much lower and, with weighted data, satisfactory to good only for alcohol abuse, drug abuse and, possibly, antisocial personality. For major depression, with weighted data, for example, they are only 0.33 when the DIS is compared with itself and only 0.28 when the checklist diagnosis is substituted for the DIS diagnosis. Kappas for most of the remaining disorders are even lower.

In the study by Anthony and his colleagues (1985), previous-month prevalence on DIS–DSM-III lay diagnoses were compared with previous-month prevalence diagnoses made on the basis of clinical examinations of a subsample of ECA cases from the Baltimore site. Two-thirds of the follow-up examinations took place within 3 weeks of the initial DIS interviews, 75% within 4 weeks, and 93% within 90 days. The results indicate that agreement is considerably worse than in the study by Helzer et al. (1985). Here, for example, alcohol abuse again does relatively well, but the kappa is only 0.35 in this comparison based on weighted data.

Robins has pointed out (personal communication of 31 May 1988) that a positive diagnosis according to the clinical examination used in Baltimore requires meeting full criteria for a particular disorder in the last month; by contrast, the DIS definition of 1 month prevalence requires that the criteria have been met in one's lifetime and that there was at least one relevant symptom in the last month. These definitions are different, and it is hard to know how much they would overlap in practice if the same instrument were used to operationalize each definition. Moreover, no methodologic study has yet been conducted with a semistructured research diagnostic interview designed for making DSM-III diagnoses—an interview such as the SCID, which is only now being developed by Spitzer et al. (1987). The PSE portion of the examination described by Anthony et al. (1985) that was used to cross-check the DIS was designed for making diagnoses other than DSM-III and had to be adapted for that purpose. It may have been too much to expect that DIS diagnoses would converge well with this particular clinical examination, especially with the added problems of differing approaches to defining 1 month prevalence and a time lag of 3 weeks to 3 months for the clinical follow-up after the initial interview.

By the same logic, however, it would have been very reasonable to expect the Helzer study to show strong convergence for *lifetime* diagnoses in re-tests done with the *DIS itself*, which, although the type of interviewer was varied, is more a test of reliability than validity. If the goal of the DIS, as Robins and colleagues (1981) have stated it, is to "enable lay interviewers to obtain psychiatric diagnoses comparable to those a psychiatrist would obtain" (Robins et al., 1981, p. 386), then these results from the St Louis and Baltimore ECA studies cannot be considered reassuring. Where the problem lies, however, and what should be done about it, are other matters.

Robins, I think, is having second thoughts about the appropriateness of the goal itself as described above. She has argued in a remarkable paper that the tests so far conducted are flawed, that we cannot assess the accuracy of the lay-administered DIS with a test–retest design using clinician examiners (Robins, 1985). She gives three reasons:

> The research diagnosis by the clinician is not a gold standard.
>
> There are problems of time-gap or order effects in the design.
>
> Available statistical methods for testing accuracy are inadequate (the base-rate problem).

Note that a test using the more appropriate SCID would not solve any of these problems.

Robins argues further that we do not need all that much accuracy for two of the important purposes of epidemiologic studies, estimating prevalence and investigating correlates of disorders in risk-factor studies. She notes that analyses of the St Louis data show that the discrepancies are most frequent for respondents whose DIS scores fall just short of meeting criteria or just barely meet the criteria—that is, are close to the cut point between the presence and absence of the disorder—and that these errors tend to be balanced among false positives and false negatives. She points out that unbiased estimates of rates require that there be equal numbers of false-positive and false-negative cases so that they cancel each other out. When rates are low, as with most disorders, and you have good specificity, a modest sensitivity can bring you nearer this goal than a very high sensitivity, as she illustrates.

However, there is no assurance that error with an instrument such as the DIS is itself randomly distributed among subgroups of the population defined by such factors as age, sex, and class. Perhaps most sobering in this regard is a comparison of initial DIS lifetime diagnoses made in four ECA sites with 1 year follow-up diagnoses made again by lay interviewers using the DIS. In analysing these data, Anthony and Dryman (1987) defined as a discrepancy a positive lifetime diagnosis for a particular disorder at Time 1 that disappeared altogether at Time 2. On the basis of this measure, 69% of baseline cases were discrepant (2,456 out of 3,572 cases). For example, 61% or 322 out of 529 respondents who had a lifetime DIS diagnosis of major depression at baseline did not have a lifetime diagnosis of major depression on the basis of the 1 year follow-up DIS.

Some of the marked discrepancies are due to the decreased reporting of positive diagnoses in general in the follow-up interview. This often occurs in repeated interviews over time with instruments of imperfect reliability and has been described as regression effects. The tendency appears to be particularly marked with the lay-interviewer-administered DIS; it did not occur in the test–retest designs used in St Louis and Baltimore, where some diagnoses were more frequent and some less frequent upon follow-up. More important with regard to the present issue, however, is the fact that the discrepancies are not randomly distributed according to age, gender, education, and ethnic status. As Robins (1985) pointed out, if you are interested in studying risk factors for particular types of disorder, you need high sensitivity to ensure an adequate sample of cases. There is, it seems to me, no way around the need for highly accurate measures that can do the job of unbiased measurement in the diverse social and cultural groups that make up the United States and many other modern societies. In the absence of biologic tests and under the circumstances where interviews and observations of behavior remain the tools available to us, how do we obtain such measures?

MULTIMETHODS APPROACHES

There are two very different ways of handling measurement error in interview approaches. One involves psychometric theory and method to develop and evaluate strong threads of truth in scales composed of self-report items, which, taken individually, are error prone. The second involves cross-examination by expert clinicians and application of their clinical judgement to rating signs and symptoms. Each of these procedures was used in rather primitive forms in some of the first- and second-generation studies.

As I reported earlier, the two approaches have different strengths and weaknesses even in their more sophisticated forms. For example, an instrument like the Psychiatric Epidemiology Research Interview (PERI), which is in the psychometric tradition and was developed through research with samples from the general population, can yield scales with high internal consistency reliabilities in contrasting subgroups and cover a wide variety of dimensions of psychopathology; but PERI does not provide psychiatric diagnoses on an individual basis. By contrast, we have diagnostic interviews such as the Psychiatric Status Schedule (PSS), SADS, and the Present State Examination (PSE) that were developed with psychiatric patients and yield reliable diagnoses for such patients but are unlikely to provide reliable measures of symptoms that differ widely in severity on diagnostically important dimensions of psychopathology in samples from the general population, and can yield misleading results in such samples (Dohrenwend et al., 1971, 1978, 1980c). A possible reason is that the expertise of the clinician that helps reduce measurement error in the use of such instruments as the PSS and PSE with patients is more limited than has been recognized. It may not extend to the full range and variety of symptomatology that are found in groups from contrasting social and cultural background in the general population.

There are strategies, however, in which the strengths and weaknesses of the two approaches can be used symbiotically to complement and cross-check each other. For example, a self-report interview like the PERI, based on a psychometric approach to measuring dimensions of psychopathology, can be used to economically screen samples from the general population. Such screening can be designed to yield subsamples of individuals with various types of severe symptomatology. Individuals screened by high scores on the screening scale can then be followed up in a second stage of the research and interviewed by experienced clinicians with diagnostic instruments like the Schedule for Affective Disorder and Schizophrenia (SADS) or the Present State Examination (PSE) to provide rates for particular types of disorder. Results with the PERI from a study in Israel lend credence to the possibility that it could with no more than seven of the 25 symptom scales, with a total of only 73 items, perform the first-stage screening function (Dohrenwend et al., 1986). Such a two-stage procedure capitalizes on the ability of a psychometric instrument to provide reliable measurement over the full range of important dimensions of psychopathology and on the ability of a clinical examination to provide reliable diagnoses in groups where the types of symptomatology involved are not rare.

While the potential practical advantages of two-stage procedures such as this have long been evident (cf. Cooper and Morgan, 1973), there have been only a handful of systematic attempts to use them for case identification and classification in psychiatric epidemiology. Duncan-Jones and Henderson (1978) have speculated that use of two-stage procedures is so rare because of fear of loss of respondents between the first screening stage and the follow-up diagnostic interview. They themselves found, however, that with careful planning, they were able to conduct interviews with 91% of the respondents designated for follow-up on the basis of initial screening. My colleagues and I are using this type of two-stage approach in an epidemiologic study in Israel. Let me summarize the field operation in Israel to provide a further example.

Our choice of Israel as the setting for the epidemiologic research was based mainly on two considerations. First, we needed an open-class, highly stratified urban society that contained a set of advantaged and disadvantaged ethnic groups to test theoretical issues having to do with class distributions of various types of disorder (Dohrenwend and Dohrenwend, 1981). Second, we needed a place with a Population Register that would make it possible to draw samples of birth cohorts from such ethnic groups.

Within this setting, we have focused on a full probability sample of 5,200 Israelis born in Israel between 1949, just after it became a state, and 1958. The goal was to contrast Israelis of European background with Israelis of North African background, when both were born in Israel during the same period. Our aim has been to identify and define cases of schizophrenia, major depression, alcoholism, substance abuse, antisocial personality, and severe nonspecific psychological distress or "demoralization." The first step was to draw a random sample of 19,000 Israel-born adults in the desired age range from the Population Register. Demographic prescreening of 98% of those 19,000 was completed to obtain information that would permit appropriate stratification into the 5,200 member target sample on the basis of gender, educational level, and ethnic background. Once selected into the stratified sample, respondents were given screening scales from the PERI (Shrout et al., 1986; Dohrenwend et al., 1986). Developed in the United States, these had been recalibrated in a previous pilot study in Israel (Shrout et al., 1986). Excluding the respondents who died or who are abroad who are being studied separately, we obtained the relevant PERI screening data from 94.5% of our target sample, as Figure 1 shows.

All of the screened positives (about half of the sample) and a subsample of over 15% of the negatives were given follow-up interviews by psychiatrists trained to administer a modification of the shorter version (SADS-L) of the Schedule for Affective Disorders and Schizophrenia (SADS) (Endicott and Spitzer, 1978) and to make diagnoses according to

Research Diagnostic Criteria (RDC) (Spitzer et al., 1978). Since this instrument was modified to provide more introductory history and to permit the dating of onsets of episodes, we call it SADS-I (for Israel). The 64 psychiatrists involved in the research were intensively trained by Itzhak Levav, who was himself trained at the NY State Psychiatric Institute, where SADS was developed. Their diagnostic interviews were tape recorded, permitting extensive quality and reliability checks. Our completion rate for this diagnostic follow up is 91%, as can be seen in Figure 1.

From these diagnosed respondents, it was possible to select and re-interview a sub-

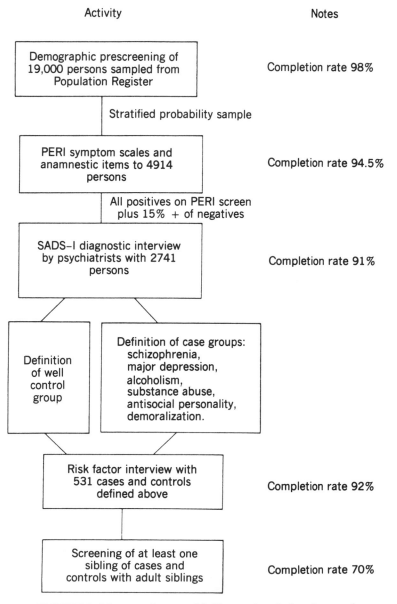

FIGURE 1. Nature and status of field operations in Israel research.

sample of 531 persons for an intensive case–control study of risk factors for various types of disorder; most of the cases were chosen to have had a recent onset of the disorder. From those persons who were not screened as possible cases in the first stage, a stratified random subsample of about 400 has also been chosen for diagnostic follow up. This follow up of screened negatives serves two purposes: 1) it provides a check on the number of false negatives from the first-stage screening interview; and 2) it provides a control group for use in the case–control study. As Figure 1 shows, completion rates were again excellent. It has also been possible to screen at least one sibling of the majority of cases and controls.

The two-stage procedure that we used in this research is, however, an economy. It would be best achieved following methodologic research employing a multimethod strategy in which both types of interview were conducted with all subjects, along, perhaps, with a third method based on reports from family members or other key informants. In such a multimethod investigation, there would be two means of establishing validity.

One would be by testing the convergence of the three methods. This is illustrated in Figure 2. The first method might consist of screening scales with the screened positives followed up at stage 2 by a clinical examination. When there is a divergence, categorization by a third method—perhaps informant reports—would be sought. The approach would be similar for screened negatives. 'Truth' in Figure 2 would be defined as a convergence across at least two out of three different methods of measuring the same thing—in the instance above, the diagnoses or other classifications dictated by the

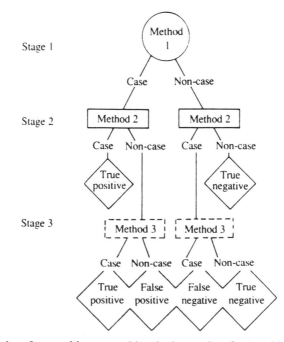

FIGURE 2. Flow chart for a multistage–multimethod procedure for case identification and classification. [From Dohrenwend, B. P. & Dohrenwend, B. S. (1982). Perspectives on the past and future of psychiatric epidemiology. American Journal of Public Health 72, 1271–1279.]

nomenclature or other theoretical constructs being used. Other things equal, the majority would rule.

However, other things are not likely to be equal in a situation where the different methods have different strengths and weaknesses. Thus, a second procedure would be to establish, not a gold standard of validity but rather what has been called by Leckman et al. (1982) a "best estimate" diagnosis in which the information from all three methods is assessed by two or more experts to arrive independently and then by consensus at a criterion diagnosis. It is something like the LEAD (Longitudinal, Expert, All Data) standard formulated by Spitzer (1983) for testing SCID and would be better with the longitudinal component Spitzer requires. The relative contributions of the separate methods to these best-estimate diagnoses can then be assessed for different diagnostic types and in different subgroups of the population as a basis for designing more economical two-stage procedures.

The validity achieved by such multimethod procedures would be relative to the validity of the particular diagnostic or classification system that dictates how the data on symptoms and signs are to be combined. Further tests of the validity of each of these systems are in order; as advocated by Robins and Guze (1970), these could include longitudinal studies to test stability of particular classes or types of psychopathology, family studies to test whether the disorders "breed true" as a function of genetic and/or environmental transmission, and outcome studies of the effectiveness of therapeutic trials.

Such tests can help those of us involved in epidemiologic enterprises to use the more promising classification systems and even contribute to their selection. Whatever system is selected for a particular epidemiologic study, however, epidemiologists will face the problem of how to validly classify people according to it. Perhaps some day there will be biologic markers to provide gold standards. Meanwhile, I shall be quite happy to settle for a combination of the democratic rule of the majority among methods and/or the authoritarian LEAD where a divergent minority method is too strong to be ignored.

ACKNOWLEDGMENTS

This work was supported by grants K05-MH14663 and MH30710 from the US National Institute of Mental Health.

REFERENCES

Anthony JC, Dryman A (1987): Analysis of discrepancy in lifetime diagnosis of mental disorders: results from the NIMH epidemiologic catchment area program. Presented at the September 1987 meeting of the World Psychiatric Association: Section on Epidemiology and Community Psychiatry, Reykjavik: Iceland.

Anthony JC, Folstein M, Romanoski AJ, Von Korff MR, Nestadt GR, Chahal R, Merchant A, Hendricks Brown C, Shapiro S, Kramer M, Gruenberg E (1985): Comparison of the lay diagnostic interview schedule and a standardized psychiatric diagnosis: Experience in Eastern Baltimore. Arch Gen Psychiatry 42:667–675.

Bash KW (1967): Untersuchungen über die Epidemiologie neuropsychiatrischer Erkrankungen unter der Landbevölkerung der Provinz Fars, Iran. Aktuelle Fragen Psychiatrie Neurol 5:162–178.

Breslau N (1985): Depressive symptoms, major depression and generalized anxiety: A comparison of self-reports on CES-D and results from diagnostic interviews. Psychiatry Res 15:219–229.

Brown GW, Harris T (1978): "Social Origins of Depression." New York: Free Press.

Cohen J (1960): A coefficient of agreement for nominal scales. Educ Psychol Measurement 20:37–46.

Cooper B, Morgan HG (1973): "Epidemiological Psychiatry." Springfield, IL: CC Thomas.

Derogatis LR (1977): "SCL-90R. (revised) Manual I." Baltimore, MD: Clinical Psychometrics Research Unit, Johns Hopkins University School of Medicine.

Dohrenwend BP, Dohrenwend BS (1965): The problem of validity in field studies of psychological disorder. J Abnorm Psychol 70:52–69.

Dohrenwend BP, Dohrenwend BS (1974): Social and cultural influences on psychopathology. Annu Rev Psychol 25:417–452.

Dohrenwend BP, Dohrenwend BS (1981): Socioenvironmental factors, stress, and psychopathology—Part 1: Quasi-experimental evidence on the social causation-social selection issue posed by class differences. Am J Community Psychol 9:146–159.

Dohrenwend BP, Dohrenwend BS (1982): Perspectives on the past and future of psychiatric epidemiology. Am J Public Health 72:1271–1279.

Dohrenwend BP, Egri G, Mendelsohn FS (1971): Psychiatric disorder in general populations: A study of the problem of clinical judgment. Am J Psychiatry 127:1304–1312.

Dohrenwend BP, Yager TJ, Egri G, Mendelsohn FS (1978): The psychiatric status schedule (PSS) as a measure of dimensions of psychopathology in the general population. Arch Gen Psychiatry 35:731–739.

Dohrenwend BP, Oksenberg L, Shrout PE, Dohrenwend BS, Cook D (1979): What brief psychiatric screening scales measure. In "Health Survey Research Methods: Third Biennial Research Conference." Washington DC: National Center for Health Services Research. US Department of Health and Human Services. DHHS pub. no. (PHS) 81-3268, pp 188–198.

Dohrenwend BP, Dohrenwend BS, Gould MS, Link B, Neugebauer R, Wunsch-Hitzig R (1980a): "Mental illness in the United States: Epidemiologic Estimates." Praeger: New York.

Dohrenwend BP, Shrout PE, Egri G, Mendelsohn FS (1980b): Nonspecific psychological distress and other dimensions of psychopathology: Measures for use in the general population. Arch Gen Psychiatry 37:1229–1236.

Dohrenwend BP, Yager TJ, Egri G, Mendelsohn FS (1980c): Some problems of validity with the Psychiatric Status Schedule as an instrument for case identification and classification in the general population (letter to the editor). Arch Gen Psychiatry 37:720–721.

Dohrenwend BP, Levav I, Shrout PE (1986): Screening scales from the Psychiatric Epidemiology Research Interview (PERI). In Weissman MM, Myers JK, Ross C (eds): "Community Surveys of Psychiatric Disorders." Brunswick, NJ: Rutgers University Press, pp 349–375.

Duncan-Jones P, Henderson S (1978): The use of a two-phase design in a prevalence survey. Social Psychiatry 13:231–237.

Endicott J, Spitzer RL (1978): A diagnostic interview: The schedule for affective disorders and schizophrenia. Arch Gen Psychiatry 35:837–844.

Feighner JP, Robins E, Guze SB, Woodruff RA, Winokur G, Munoz R (1972): Diagnostic criteria for use in psychiatric research. Arch Gen Psychiatry 26:57–63.

Frank JD (1973): "Persuasion and Healing." Baltimore, MD: Johns Hopkins University Press.

Gillis LS, Lewis JB, Slabbert M (1965): "Psychiatric Disturbance and Alcoholism in the Coloured People of the Cape Peninsula." Cape Town, South Africa: University of Cape Town Department of Psychiatry.

Goldberg DP (1972): "The Detection of Psychiatric Illness by Questionnaire." London: Oxford University Press.

Hagnell O (1966): "A Prospective Study of the Incidence of Mental Disorder." Stockholm: Svenska Bokforlaget Norstedts-Bonniers.

Helzer JE, Robins LN, McEnvoy LT, Spitznagel EL, Stoltzman RK, Farmer A, Brockington IF (1985): A comparison of clinical and diagnostic interview schedule diagnoses: Physician reexamination of lay-interviewed cases in the general population. Arch Gen Psychiatry 42:657–666.

Langner TS (1962): A twenty-two item screening score of psychiatric symptoms indicating impairment. J Health Hum Behav 3:269–276.

Leckman JF, Sholomskas D, Thompson DW, Belanger A, Weissman MM (1982): Best estimate of lifetime psychiatric diagnosis: A methodological study. Arch Gen Psychiatry 39:879–883.

Leighton DC, Harding JS, Macklin DB, Macmillan AM, Leighton AH (1963): "The Character of Danger." New York: Basic Books.

Lin T (1953): A study of the incidence of mental disorder in Chinese and other cultures. Psychiatry 16:313–336.

Link B, Dohrenwend BP (1980): Formulation of hypotheses about the true prevalence of demoralization in the United States. In Dohrenwend BP, Dohrenwend BS, Gould MS, Link B, Neugebauer R, Wunsch-Hitzig R (eds): "Mental Illness in the United States: Epidemiological Estimates." New York: Praeger, pp 114–132.

Macmillan AM (1957): The health opinion survey: Technique for estimating prevalence of psychoneurotic and related types of disorder in communities. Psychol Rep 3:325–329.

Myers JK, Weissman MM (1980): Use of a self-report symptom scale to detect the depressive syndrome. Am J Psychiatry 137:1081–1084.

Pulver AE, Carpenter WT (1983): Lifetime psychotic symptoms assessed with the DIS. Schiz Bull 9:377–382.

Radloff LS (1977): The CES-D scale: A self-report depression scale for research in the general population. Appl Psychol Measurement 1:385–401.

Raines GN (1952): Foreword in Committee on Nomenclature and Statistics of the American Psychiatric Association. In "Diagnostic and Statistical Manual: Mental Disorders." Washington, DC: American Psychiatric Association, pp V–XI.

Regier DA, Myers JK, Kramer M, Robins LN, Blazer DG, Hough RI, Eaton WW, Locke BZ (1984): The NIMH epidemiologic catchment area program. Arch Gen Psychiatry 41:934–941.

Rin H, Chu H, Lin T (1966): Psychological reactions of a rural and suburban population in Taiwan. Acta Psychiatr Scand 42:410–470.

Roberts RE, Vernon SW (1983): The center for epidemiologic studies depression scale: its use in a community sample. Am J Psychiatry 140:41–46.

Robins E, Guze SB (1970): Establishment of diagnostic validity in psychiatric illness: Its application to schizophrenia. Am J Psychiatry 126:983–987.

Robins LN (1985): Epidemiology: Reflections on testing the validity of psychiatric interviews. Arch Gen Psychiatry 42:918–924.

Robins LN, Helzer JE, Croughan J, Ratcliff KS (1981): National Institute of Mental Health Diagnostic Interview Schedule: Its history, characteristics, and validity. Arch Gen Psychiatry 38:381–389.

Seiler LH (1973): The 22-item scale used in field studies of mental illness: A question of method, a question of substance, and a question of theory. J Health Social Behav 14:252–264.

Shore JH, Kinzie JD, Hampson JL, Pattison EM (1973): Psychiatric epidemiology of an Indian village. Psychiatry 36:70–81.

Shrout PE, Dohrenwend BP, Levav I (1986): A discriminant rule for screening cases of diverse diagnostic types: Preliminary results. J Consult Clin Psychol 54:314–319.

Spitzer RL (1983): Psychiatric diagnosis: Are clinicians still necessary? Comp Psychiatry 24:399–411.

Spitzer RL, Endicott J (1968): DIAGNO: A computer program for psychiatric diagnosis utilizing the differential diagnostic procedure. Arch Gen Psychiatry 18:746–756.

Spitzer RL, Endicott J, Fleiss JL, Cohen J (1970): The psychiatric status schedule: A technique for evaluating psychopathology and impairment in role functioning. Arch Gen Psychiatry 23:41–55.

Spitzer RL, Endicott J, Robins E (1978): Research diagnostic criteria: rationale and reliability. Arch Gen Psychiatry 35:773–782.

Spitzer RL, Williams JBW, Gibbon M, First M (1987): "Structured Clinical Interview for DSM-III-R (SCID)." New York: Biometrics Research Department, New York State Psychiatric Institute.

Srole L, Langner TS, Michael ST, Opler MK, Rennie TAC (1962): "Mental Health in the Metropolis." New York: McGraw-Hill.

Star SA (1950): The screening of psychoneurotics in the army: Technical developments of tests. In Stouffer SA, Guttman L, Suchman EA, Lazarsfeld PF, Star SA, Clausen JA (eds): "Measurement and Prediction." vol 4. Princeton, NJ: Princeton University Press, pp 486–547.

Vernon SV, Roberts RE (1982): Use of the SADS-RDC in a tri-ethnic community sample. Arch Gen Psychiatry 39:47–52.

Weissman MM, Myers JK (1978): Affective disorders in a US urban community: The use of research diagnostic criteria in an epidemiological survey. Arch Gen Psychiatry 35:1304–1311.

Wing JK, Cooper JE, Sartorius N (1974): "The Measurement and Classification of Psychiatric Symptoms." London: Cambridge University Press.

Wing JK, Mann SA, Leff JP, Nixon JM (1978): The concept of a "case" in psychiatric population surveys. Psychol Med 8:203–217.

Woodruff RS, Goodwin DW, Guze SB (1974): "Psychiatric Diagnosis." New York: Oxford University Press.

PART II

STUDY DESIGNS AND METHODS

CHAPTER 2

Introduction to Epidemiologic Research Methods

GWENDOLYN E.P. ZAHNER, CHUNG-CHENG HSIEH, and
JEROME A. FLEMING

Department of Epidemiology, Harvard School of Public Health, Boston, MA 02115 (G.E.P.Z., C -C.H.);
Harvard Medical School Department of Psychiatry at Brockton/West Roxbury Veterans Administration
Medical Center, Psychiatry Service, Brockton, MA 02401 (J.A.F.)

INTRODUCTION

Epidemiology is the study of the distribution and determinants of disease frequency in humans (MacMahon and Pugh, 1970). Classic epidemiologic research designs developed to study chronic diseases are being used increasingly in investigations of psychiatric disorders. In turn, efforts to study psychiatric conditions have introduced new methodologic challenges for epidemiologists. Despite many advances in psychiatric classification in the last two decades, case definition, the sine qua non of many facets of epidemiologic research, remains an area of controversy in psychiatry. The complex manifestations and courses of psychiatric syndromes are often difficult to capture in basic epidemiologic study designs involving data collection at one or two points in time. In addition, risk factors for psychiatric conditions can be as difficult to conceptualize and assess as psychiatric outcomes.

Notwithstanding these methodologic challenges, epidemiology offers some of the best available research strategies for addressing critical questions in psychiatry concerning the nature, etiology, and prognosis of mental disorders. Psychiatric cases seen in treatment represent a small, highly self-selected segment of the full spectrum of psychopathology found in the general population. Epidemiologic study designs enable inferences to be made about the total population at risk, even when study subjects are drawn from treatment settings. Also, many putative determinants of mental disorders, such as gender, marital status, social class, and stress, cannot be randomly assigned to study groups for ethical or practical reasons. Experimental methods used in medicine and psychology that rely on randomization therefore cannot be used to study these types of risk factors. In comparison, observational epidemiologic designs are fully appropriate.

Textbook in Psychiatric Epidemiology, Edited by Tsuang, Tohen, and Zahner
ISBN 0-471-59375-3 © 1995 Wiley-Liss, Inc.

In this chapter, we review some of the common approaches to quantifying the occurrence of psychiatric outcomes in a population and will present basic epidemiologic research designs used to identify the determinants of psychiatric conditions. Biases associated with observational epidemiologic study designs, and factors to consider in interpreting findings from these studies, are discussed. Attention is also given to the special problems faced in the application of these methods to the study of psychiatric conditions.

EPIDEMIOLOGIC MEASURES OF OUTCOME OCCURRENCE IN POPULATION GROUPS

The frequency of outcome occurrence in a population group can be measured several ways. The two principal approaches involve measures of proportions and measures of densities ("rates"). The distinction and relation between these two types of measurements have been discussed in detail in the context of psychiatric research (Kramer, 1957). They are described briefly here.

Incidence Density (Force of Morbidity or Mortality)

Incidence refers to new events (outcomes) occurring over time among members of the population who are candidates for such events. There are two commonly employed incidence measures: incidence density and cumulative incidence.

An *incidence density* quantifies the number of events occurring per unit of population per unit of time. It is not dimensionless because time is retained in the unit of measurement. In estimating incidence density, the population under study should exclude all individuals with the health outcome at the start of the period of observation. This candidate population is often referred to as the *population at risk*. In practice, when the number of cases in the population under study is very small, such as in studies of rare diseases in general population samples, the total population can be used for the population at risk. In small study cohorts, however, it is important to remove all current cases from the baseline sample before calculating incidence.

Incidence density can be assessed for an instantaneous time point by the slope of a curve measuring change in disease-free population size over time. This instantaneous rate of change is often referred to as the *hazard rate* or the *force of morbidity*. Incidence density is also often expressed as an average rate of change over a time interval. For example, if a group of 300 manic-depressive patients is followed for an average of 10 years with 12 deaths (the outcome event) occurring during the follow-up, the numerator of the average incidence density of death (the "mortality rate") would be 12 deaths, and the denominator would be 300 patients times 10 years, or 3,000 person-years. After division, the mortality rate would be reported as 4 per 1,000 persons per year (or 4 per 1,000 person-years).

A density-type measure is usually referred to as a *rate*. However, in common usage, rates can also refer to proportions, such as "unemployment rate," "tax rate," and "prevalence rate." To avoid confusion, it is important to know the context in which *rate* is being used and to specify the method by which it has been calculated (Elandt-Johnson, 1975).

Cumulative Incidence, Risk, and Survival

Cumulative incidence, risk, and survival rates are estimates of the probability of the occurrence of an outcome event over a specified period of time. *Cumulative incidence* is usually used to describe the probability of outcome occurrence among a group or population. *Risk* is usually used to predict an individual's chance of such an event. Risk is also commonly expressed by its mathematical complement, the probability of surviving or the *survival rate*. Cumulative incidence, risk, and the survival rate are dimensionless measures.

Cumulative incidence can be either an observed probability or a theoretical quantity estimated from the incidence density function. The observed cumulative incidence is a simple proportion and is calculated as the number of health outcomes occurring over a time interval divided by the size of the population at risk. If the outcomes of all members of a candidate population are observed without any loss to follow-up from causes other than the event under study, cumulative incidence can be used as an estimate of individual "risk" for the time interval under study (e.g., 5 year risk of dying) or, in a complementary fashion, as the survival rate.

In practice, however, loss to follow up or "censoring" through subject drop-outs or death by other causes is common. The interpretability of the observed cumulative incidence measure when such loss occurs is seriously compromised. For example, an observed 5 year survival rate for a group of manic-depressive study subjects can be distorted by censoring, even if those who were lost had the same probability of surviving as the remaining study participants. This distortion will take place because outcomes occurring among subjects lost to follow up are excluded from the numerator of the observed cumulative incidence calculation. Cases lost to follow up are still retained in the denominator, however, which equals the total size of the candidate population at the start of the study with no adjustment for reduction in the size of the study cohort over the observation period. Consequently, observed cumulative incidence—and risk and survival estimates based on it—is only appropriate for studies in which there is negligible loss to follow up over the course of the study. The types of studies for which these observed measures are best suited involve "closed" or "fixed" cohorts (that is, cohorts in which the disease course of each subject in the study is individually monitored over the period of observation) in which there is no loss to follow up and the follow-up interval is short.

When loss-to-follow-up occurs, or when incidence is estimated for a "dynamic" community population (i.e., where the disease experience of each individual is not monitored), a more appropriate measure of the probability of disease occurrence is derived from the observed incidence density function (Chiang, 1968). The estimate of the observed incidence density is not affected by the competing causes of subject removal (e.g., loss to follow up) from a candidate population since those who are lost will no longer be among the candidates for the occurrence of the next outcome event. For the prognosis of an individual patient in this study, the complement of a 5 year survival rate derived from the incidence density can be appropriately interpreted as the risk of dying in 5 years.

Prevalence

Simply put, a prevalence or *prevalence rate* is that proportion of a population who have a particular health condition at a point or period in time. For example, the point prevalence of major depression in a community is the number of persons fulfilling diagnostic criteria for depression at a stated point in time divided by the number of persons in the community. As a proportion, prevalence is a dimensionless quantity; that is, it is not expressed in units of another characteristic, such as time.

Both newly onset cases and cases that begin prior to the study period contribute to prevalence. In a community population in which the numbers of entries and exits (from births, deaths, migrations, and so forth) are balanced and the disease rates are stable (a "steady state"), prevalence is proportional to the frequency of development of new cases of the condition (the incidence density) multiplied by the average duration of the condition. Exact relationships between prevalence, incidence, and duration have been presented by Freeman and Hutchison (1980, 1986).

Prevalence rates are frequently reported for population subgroups, such as age- or sex-specific rates. In these stratum-specific estimates, the numerator of the prevalence is formed by the number of cases within the population subgroup, and the denominator is the total size of the subgroup.

In psychiatric studies, "period" prevalence rates are also often reported. A period prevalence rate uses the same denominator as a point prevalence rate, but expands the numerator to include all cases present during a selected time period, such as 1 month, 6 months, 1 year, or a lifetime. Period prevalence has gained popularity in psychiatric epidemiology because of the complex, episodic course of many psychiatric conditions. Use of a period prevalence allows individuals with chronic psychiatric conditions who are temporarily in remission to be included in prevalence counts. Also, the diagnostic criteria for many psychiatric disorders requires the occurrence of clusters of symptoms over extended time intervals, such as 1 month (e.g., generalized anxiety) or 1 year (e.g., dysthymic disorder). A time period is therefore implicit in any prevalence measure involving these conditions, even a point prevalence.

Although period prevalence has several practical advantages, there are a number of limitations associated with this hybrid measure. In extended time periods, patients who remit early in the time interval without recurrence are likely to be missed in the period prevalence counts, especially when the information by disease status is gathered by recall (Aneshensel et al., 1987). In addition, empirical estimates of lifetime prevalence frequently exhibit a counter-intuitive age distribution. Over the age distribution of a population, lifetime prevalence should increase during age intervals associated with disease onset and remain constant at other ages. However, lifetime prevalences of many psychiatric disorders have been observed in several population surveys (Weissman and Myers, 1978; Robins et al., 1984) to decrease sharply in the older age groups. Several explanations have been offered for this artifact. In addition to recall bias, high case fatality rates (i.e., patients do not survive until older ages), increasing rates of psychopathology in recent cohorts, and changing diagnostic practices have been suggested as explanatory factors (Robins, 1985; Klerman, 1988).

Measures of Association and Impact: Relative Risk, Odds Ratio, and Attributable Risk

If there is an association between a study factor and a psychiatric disorder, the frequency with which the disorder occurs will differ in groups that vary on the study factor, such as groups who are "exposed" and "not exposed" to an environmental agent or a trait. Therefore, a measure of the association can be obtained by comparing the rates of disease occurrence in "exposed" and "unexposed" groups. Group comparisons can be expressed as a difference or as a ratio of rates. The magnitude of the difference or ratio is an indicator of the strength of association between the study factor and psychiatric outcome. In psychiatric epidemiology, ratios of disease rates are typically used to express the strength of the association. The ratio between two rates (or "rate ratio") is often referred to as the *relative risk*. Since "relative risk" can also be a risk ratio and rates and risks are different measures of disease occurrence (see Cumulative Incidence, Risk, and Survival, above), it is important to know the context in which "relative risk" is used.

To illustrate, suppose an investigator is interested in comparing the mortality rates of adults with and without a psychotic disorder in a community of 120,000. In this population, 1,200 persons (1%) meet diagnostic criteria for a psychotic disorder, and 118,800 do not. Over a 1 year period, 312 deaths occur, including 15 individuals with a diagnosis of psychosis and 297 without. The rate (density) of dying for the group with psychosis (15 of 1,200 psychotics) and without this disorder (297 of 118,800) expressed as a mortality rate ratio (relative risk of dying) would be 5 (15/1,200 divided by 297/118,800).

Certain types of epidemiologic studies do not directly assess the disease experience in a population and compare estimated disease rates for individuals with and without exposure. Instead, the *exposure histories* of samples of individuals with (cases) and without (controls) the disease from the population are compared. This type of subject selection is commonly referred to as *retrospective* or *case–control sampling*. It is possible, nevertheless, to estimate the rate ratio of disease occurrence among cases and controls in these studies if certain conditions are met.

Suppose in the example above that available resources do not allow the investigator to determine the mental health status for each of the 120,000 residents in the community. With a retrospective (case–control) sampling approach, cases would be the complete or partial sample of the 312 subjects with the outcome event (death), and controls would be a sample of the 120,000 residents who were candidates of the outcome event. If the available resources allowed for sampling approximately two times the number of controls as cases, an investigator might decide to select 600 subjects as the controls. With a random sample of the population, the distribution of the exposure (the psychotic disorder) among these 600 controls would be proportional to the distribution in the original population. Therefore, 6 controls (1%) would be expected to have a psychotic disorder and 594 would not after an examination of their mental health status. Table 1 displays the cross-tabulation of the outcome and exposure status from this sampling design.

To estimate the relative risk of dying among those with and without a psychotic disorder in this case–control study, the *odds* of exposure among the cases (12/297) is contrasted to the *odds* of exposure among the controls (6/594). The result of the division of these two odds, known as an *odds ratio*, is 5. Note that the odds ratio computed from the case–control study in this example yields the same result as the mortality rate ratio among psychotics and nonpsychotics in the total population. An odds ratio is frequently

TABLE 1. Results of a Case–Control Study of Relative Risk of Mortality Among Psychotics and Nonpsychotic Adults

Exposure Status	Cases	Controls
With psychotic disorder	15	6
Without psychotic disorder	297	594
Total	312	600

computed as an estimate of relative risk or incidence rate ratios in case–control studies. The accuracy of this approximation depends on a number of factors, including the nature of the source population (i.e., whether it is a dynamic population with a "steady state" of in- and out-migration), the rarity of the outcome, the use of incident versus prevalent cases, and the length of the risk period between exposure and disease occurrence. The reader is referred to Chapter 3 (this volume) and to Kleinbaum et al. (1982) for a detailed description of the conditions under which an odds ratio equals or approximates a rate ratio or relative risk in the retrospective sampling schemes used in case–control studies. For the most common types of case–control studies involving incident cases, the odds ratio estimates the rate ratio exactly.

Another commonly employed epidemiologic measure is *attributable risk* (AR), which is also known as the *etiologic fraction* or *population attributable risk percent* (Kleinbaum et al., 1982). The AR describes the proportion (or percent) of new cases arising in a population that are attributable to the exposure under study. The AR depends on the prevalence of the exposure in the population and on the strength of the association between the exposure and outcome. The AR can be estimated by the following formula:

$$AR = \frac{p_e (RR - 1)}{p_e (RR - 1) + 1}$$

where p_e is the proportion of the source population that is exposed and RR is the relative risk estimate. The AR ranges in value from 0 (none of the outcome occurrence is attributable to the exposure) to 1 (all occurrences take place in the presence of the exposure, i.e., the exposure is a "necessary" cause). The accuracy of this measure depends on the extent to which component measures used to calculate AR reflect current population characteristics. This index is useful for planning and policy purposes because it describes the potential impact of removing an exposure upon the frequency of disease occurrence.

Attributable risk can also be calculated specifically for individuals who have a positive history of exposure. This estimate, known as the *attributable risk among the exposed* (AR_e) or *attributable risk percent*, is computed as

$$AR_e = \frac{RR - 1}{RR}$$

The AR_e can be interpreted as the probability that an exposed case developed the condition as a result of the exposure. As a hypothetical example, in a study where exposure is family history and the outcome is schizophrenia, an AR_e of 0.75 would indicate that 75% of the schizophrenic cases with a positive family history for this disorder developed their condition because of their familial loading.

OVERVIEW OF STUDY DESIGNS

Epidemiologic research in its most elementary form involves studying the relationship between a risk factor and a health outcome. The risk factor is often referred to as the "exposure" or "treatment." To learn about its relationship to a health outcome, a comparative study is undertaken in which the experience of disease occurrence in a group of individuals with one characteristic (e.g., "exposed") of the risk factor is contrasted with that of another group differing on the characteristic ("not exposed").

Although the epidemiologic approach focuses on comparisons of the relative magnitudes of rates of disease occurrence between two groups, in practice a variety of research designs can be invoked. These designs can be distinguished by a number of characteristics. The most important distinctions involve the timing of data collection in relation to risk factors and disease occurrence, the separation between risk factor and disease occurrence in time, and the methods used in sampling study subjects (Miettinen, 1985a). In addition, studies vary in cost, feasibility, and quality of information gathered. The study designs listed below are in common use in psychiatric epidemiology, although there is some variation in the terminology employed at different research centers. We briefly describe each type of the study in turn and provide examples of studies examining psychiatric outcomes.

Experimental
Nonexperimental (observational)
  Cross-sectional
  Cohort
    Prospective
    Retrospective
  Case–control
  Hybrid studies
    Repeated cross-sectional
    Multistage
    Panel
  Ecologic studies
    Spatial distribution
    Time trend

In addition to these basic epidemiologic study designs, the reader is referred to Chapters 4 through 8 (this volume) for reviews and illustrations of other research designs currently employed in psychiatric epidemiology.

Experimental Studies

In an experimental study, the investigator controls the allocation of subjects to different comparison groups and also regulates the experimental conditions of each group. Study subjects are randomly assigned to comparison groups and followed up over time to record the outcome event of interest, such as the recurrence of a psychiatric illness or the occurrence of death. Clinical trials and intervention studies are the most common forms of experimental studies in human populations. To ensure the comparability between groups and obtain valid results, an experimental study employs three basic research strategies: randomization, placebo, and blinding.

Randomization. When an investigator randomly assigns subjects to different experimental conditions, differences between groups are determined by chance. If the randomization is carried out properly and the sample sizes are sufficiently large, the groups are likely to be similar in all regards other than the conditions under study. Consequently, if the experimental conditions have no effect the rates of disease occurrence are expected to be the same in the comparison groups.

Even with random allocation it is possible that the groups will be imbalanced with respect to extraneous factors that may influence the rates of disease occurrence, particularly if the sample sizes are small. Before analyzing the results of randomized experiments, it is generally recommended that investigators test whether the groups are balanced on all known or suspected determinants of the outcome under study. If an imbalance is detected, the investigator can use statistical methods to adjust for the effects of these factors on the distribution of disease occurrence across groups. For unknown determinants, it is usually assumed that randomization will achieve a balanced distribution on these factors in the long run over hypothetical repetitions of the same study. The confidence in this assumption increases if the number of study subjects is adequate.

Placebo. One complication of experimental studies is that extraneous aspects of the treatment procedure may influence the outcome under study. For example, psychiatric patients who are given a new medication may show improvements because they receive special attention from study staff monitoring the treatment trial. Participating in an experiment in and of itself can also influence outcomes, an artifact that is commonly known as the *Hawthorne effect.* To control for these unwanted effects, one comparison group is usually administered a placebo that, under optimal conditions, mimics the extraneous features of the experimental condition or treatment under study but does not otherwise influence the rates of disease occurrence. Differences in disease rates between the placebo and experimental groups can be attributed to the effect of treatment per se rather than to the effect of other aspects of the procedure, activity, or environment associated with the treatment. Differences between placebo groups and groups that are not assigned to any experimental condition are also measured in some randomized trials, and these differences are referred to as *placebo effects.*

Blinding. For many of the reasons discussed above with placebo treatments, it is important that participants in a randomized trial be unaware of the group to which they are is assigned. It is equally important to withhold this information from the investigator and other professionals who manage the trial. Knowledge that an individual has been assigned to the experimental treatment may influence the handling, treatment, and measurements of participants in the randomized trial. Standardization of the study procedures are also easier to enforce when both the investigator and the patient are unaware of the group assignments. The process of "double blinding," in which neither investigators nor study participants are given information about the group assignment, helps to ensure that group conditions are similar and that identical study procedures are followed with every study subject. Although double blinding is desirable in every randomized experiment, it is not always feasible, especially when the treatment produces other effects that are observable or require monitoring to protect participants, such as changes in blood pressure.

Even though experimental studies are considered a paradigm in many research fields, the randomized trial has several shortcomings for use in studying human populations. Ethical considerations dictate that experimental studies involving human subjects can only be used to study exposures (treatments or medications) that are likely to be beneficial. It is unethical to randomize human subjects to harmful exposures. Furthermore, constitutional characteristics such as inherited or congenital traits cannot be randomized. It is also not feasible to randomize groups into many other sociodemographic conditions that may influence mental health outcomes, such as marital status or religious denomination. Therefore, the effect of many putative risk factors for major psychiatric disorders cannot be evaluated by an experimental study. Also, if the follow-up period for the ascertainment of outcomes of an experimental procedure is long, the treatment assessed may be obsolete by the time the results are available (Elwood, 1988).

A Randomized Clinical Trial in Psychiatry. Gibbons et al. (1993) present results from a longitudinal analysis of a randomized clinical trial of two forms of psychotherapy using the NIMH Treatment of Depression Collaborative Research Program Dataset. The objectives of this clinical trial were to evaluate and compare the effectiveness of cognitive behavior therapy (CBT) and interpersonal psychotherapy (IPT) in comparison to a standard reference treatment, imipramine plus clinical management group (IMI-CM). A placebo plus clinical management group was also enrolled to control for effects of standard treatment (PLA-CM). Subjects (n = 250) were randomized into each of these four experimental conditions; 239 subjects entered treatment and 219 received measures after baseline. Depressive symptoms were assessed over 16 weeks with a modified Hamilton (1960) rating scale completed by clinical evaluators who were "blind" to treatment conditions. Contrasts between the experimental groups were made to test three main null hypotheses: 1) no difference between the two psychotherapies (IPT compared with CBT); 2) no difference between psychotherapy (IPT and CBT combined) and the standard treatment (IMI-CM); and 3) no difference between the standard treatment (IMI-CM) and the placebo (PLA-CM). No significant differences were found between the two psychotherapies (Hypothesis 1) or between psychotherapy and standard treatment (Hypothesis 2); but rate of improvement for the standard treatment (IMI-CM) was significantly greater than for the placebo. This detailed report also describes methods taken to control for potential bias introduced by attrition after randomization, missing data, differences between collaborating research sites, and assumptions in statistical modeling.

Nonexperimental (Observational) Studies

In a nonexperimental study, the investigator has no control over the group designation of each study subject. The investigator generally selects subjects for the different exposure conditions from previously existing groups and then observes the resulting health outcomes. Hence, epidemiologic nonexperimental studies are sometimes called *observational studies*. The three most common epidemiologic observational studies designs are cross-sectional, cohort, and case–control studies. Our discussion of observational designs begins with these classic methodologies.

Cross-Sectional Studies. In a cross-sectional study, the data on exposure and outcome are obtained at the same point in time, and both usually relate to the current period. The information is typically gathered through sample surveys of geographically defined populations. The current disease status of groups with and without the exposure, expressed as prevalence rates, are compared in analysis. By providing a "snapshot" of the current levels of illness in the total population and in different exposure groups, this design has been found to be useful for describing the health care needs of different populations.

Cross-sectional studies have enjoyed considerable popularity in psychiatric epidemiology for a number of reasons. A population survey allows investigators to gather information on all cases of disorder occurring in a defined area, including syndromes in an asymptomatic phase and conditions for which treatment is not routinely sought. Because current diagnostic procedures in psychiatry rely heavily upon the verbal report of symptoms, the interview methods used in most surveys can be used to obtain some of the basic information commonly used in formulating diagnoses. Also, prevalence rates obtained by cross-sectional surveys are widely used in psychiatry because onset (incidence) is difficult to demarcate. The chronicity of many psychiatric disorders also facilitates prevalence estimation, which, as it will be recalled, is proportional to the product of incidence times duration. Therefore, even though the incidence rates for most psychiatric disorders are believed to be very low, the number of prevalent cases detected in a cross-sectional survey of moderate size is often sufficient to obtain precise estimates of rates and measures of association.

For an illustration of a major cross-sectional study in psychiatric epidemiology, the reader is referred to Chapter 5 (this volume) on the Epidemiologic Catchment Area study.

Cross-Sectional Survey Sampling. A study sample that is representative of the target population is an essential feature of cross-sectional surveys. To achieve representativeness, subjects are selected as probability samples of the population using sample survey methods (Kish, 1965; Cochran, 1977). A variety of different sampling methods are in current use that vary in complexity. Before designing a cross-sectional survey, it is important to consult a statistician about the appropriate method to employ. The sampling method will influence the number of subjects required for the survey, and certain sampling designs will also require special data analytic procedures such as weighted data and variance adjustments. Although a comprehensive overview of sampling methods is beyond the scope of this text, we will mention some of the major approaches and highlight some of the major factors that influence selection of one method over another.

Before describing the sampling methods, some terminology must be defined. The *target population* is the group to which results are to be generalized. This may be inclusive of all individuals in a geographic area or may exclude certain groups, such as individuals above or below a certain age or institutionalized individuals. *Elementary units* are the elements or members of the target population to be studied. Individuals are usually the elementary units in epidemiologic studies, but examples of other elementary units include households, neighborhoods, or hospitals. A list of all of the units in the target population used to draw the sample is known as the *sampling frame*, and the entries (e.g., names or addresses) on the sampling frame are called *enumeration* or *listing units*. Examples of sampling frames include telephone directories, voter registration or tax lists, town censuses, and utility listings.

Before selecting a sampling scheme, the investigator should examine the available sampling frames. Ideally, there should be a one-to-one correspondence between the enumeration units on the sampling frame and the elementary units in the target population. In practice, this is rarely the case. Some frames only contain clusters or groupings of elementary units. For example, an investigator may wish to survey all individuals in a town, but only has access to a frame (e.g., utility listings) that enumerates households. Examples of other problems with sampling frames include *missing elements* (failing to provide coverage of all individuals in the target population), *duplicate entries*, and *blanks or foreign elements* (e.g., out-of-date lists that include individuals who have died or emigrated;

or overly inclusive lists, containing individuals outside the target population or individuals whose primary residence is outside the geographic area under study). Before the sample is drawn, the investigator should review and correct errors in the list. The list may need to be updated by contacting current residents in the survey area, a process referred to as *enumeration*.

There are several types of sampling plans used in cross-sectional surveys. Choice of a sampling plan depends on a number of issues, including the information contained in the sampling frame, the rarity of the characteristic under study, the desired precision of the prevalence estimates or prevalence ratios, the size of the area to be studied, and the cost of the study.

One of the most commonly cited sampling methods—but infrequently employed in actual practice—is simple random sampling. This method requires the availability of a complete listing of the population to use as a sampling frame. The usual method of drawing a simple random sample is to number each element on the sampling frame from 1 to N, where N is the size of the target population, assuming that the frame is completely accurate. A set of n unique random numbers, where n is the desired number of elements to be contacted for the survey, is then obtained either from a random number generator on a calculator or computer or from a published table of random numbers. The frame is then searched for elements whose numbers correspond to each of the n random numbers. These elements are chosen to be the study sample. If random numbers are not available, a lottery method can also be used by preparing N cards or tokens representing enumeration elements on the frame and drawing the desired n number of tokens at random.

In simple random sampling, the probability that any individual element is chosen is the ratio of the sample size to the size of the population: n divided by N. Although this sampling method is intuitively easy to understand, a complete listing of the population is not always available. In addition, it is possible that rare characteristics will not be represented in a simple random sample. This method is also very expensive for large study areas because interviewers will be required to travel throughout the survey region.

A modification of simple random sampling is known as *stratified random sampling*. In this method, the sampling frame is divided into different strata (such as age, sex, and ethnic–race groups), and simple random samples are drawn within each stratum. This approach ensures adequate representation of different groups under study. Under most conditions, it will also improve the precision of prevalence estimates. To carry out stratified random sampling, as with simple random sampling, a listing of the population is required. In addition, the characteristics to be used in stratification must also be available on the frame.

When a list of the population is not available, two commonly employed sampling methods are *systematic sampling* and *cluster sampling*. Systematic sampling is one of the most widely used methods in practice and has the advantage of being easily taught to individuals who have little knowledge of survey methods. It can also be used for samples that accrue over time, such as patient enrollments. In this method, sample members are drawn at fixed intervals, as, for example, every fifth household or every seventh name on a class enrollment list. The sampling interval, k, can be calculated by dividing the projected total population size (N) by the desired sample size (n). For example, if it is estimated that there will be 100 houses in a community and a sample of 25 is desired, the sampling interval is 100/25 or 4, and interviewers can be instructed to go to every fourth household. Despite its simplicity, an investigator should consult with a statistician before using this method, because it may yield biased, imprecise prevalence estimates. If the population (*N*) and sample size (*n*) are reasonably large and the elements randomly ordered, the estimates can be assumed to be unbiased with variances approximating simple random sampling.

Cluster sampling is the most complex survey sampling procedure of the four methods described here. As previously described, a *cluster* is a listing element that may contain more than one elementary unit. Examples of clusters of individuals include hospitals, classrooms and households. Geographic areas, such as states, counties, cities, or blocks, also represent clusters in many sampling schemes. In cluster sampling, a probability sample of "clusters" is drawn. In a single-stage cluster sample design, information is then gathered on all elements in each sampled cluster. Alternatively, multistage sampling may take place, in which probability samples of elements are drawn at each stage until a sample of the desired elementary units is obtained. To illustrate the multistage cluster sampling process, consider the following example of a five-stage design for a probability sample of adults in the United States: In stage 1, a random sample of counties is drawn; stage 2 consists of a random sample of towns within each selected county; in stage 3, a random sample of blocks is drawn from each selected town; stage 4 consists of a random sample of households in each sampled town; and the process concludes with a random selection of one adult from each household (stage 5).

There are several advantages to this approach. First, the investigator does not need a list of all of the elementary units (e.g., all adults in the United States) in order to sample. Second, data collection is concentrated in small areas, decreasing the fieldwork costs. These potential benefits have to be weighed against two principal disadvantages. First, there is frequently a loss in precision of the population estimates obtained by cluster sampling, which is reflected by larger standard errors, broader confidence intervals, or a decreased statistical power to detect differences between groups in the sample compared with simple random sampling. This loss in precision is commonly measured by a *design effect*, which is the ratio of variances obtained under cluster sampling versus simple random sampling. Another related disadvantage of cluster sampling is that special statistical software for complex survey samples may be needed in order to obtain correct variance estimates.

Measures of Disease and Exposure Status in a Cross-Sectional Survey. Study participants in a cross-sectional survey are not enrolled on the basis of their exposure or disease status. All information regarding these factors is obtained during the investigation and is usually limited to survey interview information. There are three common methods of conducting surveys: mail surveys, telephone surveys, and face-to-face interviews. These methods vary in expense and quality. Dr. Robins reviews the relative merits of these approaches in Chapter 11 (this volume).

We limit our discussion of measurement in cross-sectional studies to one problem concerning the time frame for information obtained in survey interviews. Cross-sectional surveys are conventionally viewed as assessing both disease and exposure data at the current point in time. Cause and effect cannot be distinguished for true cross-sectional data of this type. However, many cross-sectional surveys also attempt to obtain some information about events predating the current point in time. This historical information is usually based on the respondent's recollection and may be subject to considerable error (Neugebauer, 1981). Severe or salient events that are not embarrassing to report, such as death of a parent, birth of a child, or marriage, may be recalled with reasonable accuracy (Funch and Marshall, 1984; Kessler and Wethington, 1991). However, past emotions or behaviors are difficult to recall accurately, and historical reports of psychiatric symptoms may be biased by the current mental health of the respondent (Anehensel et al., 1987; Schrader et al., 1990). A researcher should exercise considerable caution in attempting to assess life history information through respondent recall. Time lines, visual cues such as medication charts, or organization of questions around concrete events or by social contexts (e.g., home, work, school) may be used as memory aides (Kessler and Wethington, 1991).

Cohort Studies. Cohort studies in epidemiology have two essential features. First, study subjects are defined by characteristics present *before* disease occurrence, and these individuals form the study cohort. This is in contrast to case–control studies, where subjects are selected according to their disease status, and to cross-sectional studies, where subjects are selected by neither disease nor exposure status, but, instead, are selected to be representative of a target population.

The second characteristic of a cohort study is that real time is allowed to elapse before disease status is ascertained. Cohort members are followed through time to determine the frequency of new outcomes or events in each group. Measures of exposures and outcomes thus are both gathered at the time of their occurrence. This type of study design thereby offers the greatest potential of the epidemiologic observational studies to separate cause and effect. However, if the time elapsing between exposure and disease onset is long, and if the exposure levels vary over time, this type of study can be extremely costly and difficult to undertake.

There are two types of cohort studies that differ primarily in regard to the timing of study in relation to the occurrence of exposure and disease outcomes. The experience of a cohort can be studied prospectively or retrospectively, as is described below.

Prospective Cohort Studies. In prospective cohort studies, groups of initially disease free people are classified in terms of their exposure and are then followed forward in time. It should be noted that *disease free* is a relative term. For disorders with a poorly defined onset, such as psychiatric disorders, it may be difficult to guarantee that all members of the cohort are truly disease free at the outset of the investigation. This issue is explored in greater detail in Chapter 6 (this volume) on studying the natural history of psychopathology. Also, in practice, some retrospective information on exposure history may also be collected at baseline in addition to assessing current exposure levels.

Prospective cohort studies can be further subdivided into two study types based on whether the cohort is selected with or without regard to exposure status. Selection without regard to exposure status is frequently undertaken by following a study cohort sampled in a cross-sectional population survey over time. Three major cross-sectional study samples that have formed longitudinal cohorts in psychiatric epidemiology include the U.S. Epidemiologic Catchment Area study (Eaton et al., 1989), the Stirling County study in Canada (Murphy et al., 1988), and the Lundby study in Sweden (Hagnell et al., 1982). Eaton details the methodologic problems encountered in assessing the course of psychiatric disorders in these studies in Chapter 6 (this volume).

The other major form of prospective cohort study involves stratification on exposure, that is, selection of an exposed cohort and appropriate comparison series. There have been several different types of exposure groups that have been studied in relation to psychiatric and psychosocial outcomes, including occupational groups such as workers in plants that are closing (Cobb and Kasl, 1977) or nuclear plant workers (Kasl et al., 1981); veterans exposed to combat stress (Helzer, 1981; Decoufle et al., 1992); and population-wide environmental exposures, such as the nuclear accident at Three Mile Island (Cleary and Houts, 1984). In a prospective cohort study stratified on exposure, an appropriate comparison group of "unexposed" individuals must be identified for follow up, such as other occupational groups that are not under stress, or workers who are not at risk of losing their jobs, or community samples drawn from an area with low rates of exposures. Published incidence rates for the general population that are available for comparisons with exposed cohorts for many chronic diseases are not routinely available for psychiatric disorders.

Prospective cohort studies, although appealing because exposure and disease onset are monitored in real time, are not without methodologic problems. Comparability of exposed and unexposed groups may present a problem, particularly if subject selection involves stratification by exposure. It is also difficult to obtain pre-exposure (baseline) measures on confounding factors.

Procedures for follow up and ascertainment of disease status over time may also be complicated in prospective studies. It is essential that the time frame for follow-up closely mirrors the disease induction period. For diseases with long latency periods, a follow-up interval spanning several decades may be required. Extended follow-up periods are costly from both a financial and a professional perspective. Additionally, as a study cohort ages over time it may not be representative of younger cohorts in the population. Changing knowledge of disease over time may identify new risk factors that were not measured at baseline. Definitions of *disease* and *disease free*, influenced largely by the American Psychiatric Association's Diagnostic and Statistical Manuals and the World Health Organization International Classification of Disease, are also subject to change over time. Furthermore, if risk factors vary over time and/or if cumulative exposure to risk factors influences the rates of outcome occurrence, prospective investigations have the added complication — and expense — of monitoring the exposures as well as the disease occurrence prospectively. There may also be artifactual testing effects introduced by frequent reassessment of study group.

A final, but not inconsequential, problem in prospective designs is that loss to follow-up may be significant. Certain types of high-risk populations of interest to psychiatric epidemiologists, such as residents of inner cities, are especially difficult to trace. It is essential that careful subject tracking systems be built into prospective studies at baseline. If the pattern of loss to follow up is related to exposure or length of observation, these factors must be taken into account in analysis in order to prevent bias in estimates of association.

Retrospective Cohort Studies. The previous section highlighted some of the difficulties in gathering longitudinal data on exposure and outcomes prospectively over time. A cost-effective alternative, known as the *retrospective cohort* study, is sometimes available to investigators. In a retrospective cohort study, information on disease status is obtained at the time of the study, or shortly before. Information on risk factors is available from records collected in the past at the actual time of the exposure. Thus, as in a prospective cohort study, measures of exposure and disease status are collected at the point in chronologic time during which these events took place, thereby permitting cause and effect to be distinguished. This cost-effective design is not readily accessible to researchers in every situation and depends on the availability of cohorts with good, complete exposure information.

Researchers should take advantage of opportunities for conducting retrospective cohort studies because of the enormous costs associated with prospective designs. Investigators contemplating a retrospective cohort study should be aware of several common limitations associated with this type of study, however, and should attempt to minimize the impact of these potential problems in their proposed investigations. First, quality of data regarding exposure may be of lower quality than information collected in a prospective fashion because the investigator has no control over data collection and relies on extant record information. Second, the information available for potential confounding variables may be limited. A third problem resides in the difficulties in tracing cohort members, which increase as the time interval between exposure and first attempt to follow up widens. An additional problem is that the cohort membership assembled by the investigator may depend on the outcome status; in such instances the cohort that is formed for a study may not represent the total population experience, leading to bias. Last, for episodic or treatable conditions it may be necessary to gather retrospective information on past episodes of illness occurring over an extended time interval as well as the current outcome status of the study subject. As discussed previously with cross-sectional studies, the quality of data on psychiatric outcomes will be compromised if the investigation depends extensively on recall data.

The Iowa 500 study represents an application of the retrospective cohort design in psychiatric epidemiology (Morrison et al., 1972; Tsuang et al., 1979a, b). One goal was to study the long-term outcomes of schizophrenia, mania, and depression. The study was conducted in the 1970s, and cohorts were identified from psychiatric hospital admission records of all patients admitted to the state psychiatric hospital in Iowa between 1934 and 1945, approximately 30–40 years before the study began. This investigation was possible because detailed symptom information had been gathered at the Iowa hospital. In addition, this hospital was the single treatment facility for all serious cases of mental disorders in the state. Using the Feigner et al. criteria (1972), records of 3,800 cases were reviewed, and subjects for three diagnostic study groups were assembled: schizophrenia (n = 200), mania (n = 100), and depression (n = 225). A nonpsychiatric surgical group was also selected using records of patients treated for appendectomy or herniorrhaphy during the same time period, matched to the psychiatric groups for sex, socioeconomic status, and age range. The members of the four study groups and their first-degree relatives were then located and interviewed between 1975 and 1979. The interview assessed the physical and psychiatric treatment history, family history, and long-term psychosocial outcomes. The principal outcomes assessed were marital, occupational, residential and psychiatric status, which included schizophrenic, affective, and neurotic symptomatologies. Interviewers were blind to the study group membership. The outcome measures, along with family data, were compared among the four different study groups.

Case–Control Studies. MacMahon and Pugh's definition of a case–control study in their classic 1970 textbook (p 241) remains one of most concise descriptions to date of the basic procedures of this study design: "A case control study is an inquiry in which groups of individuals are selected in terms of whether they do (the cases) or do not (the controls) have the disease of which the etiology is to be studied, and the groups are then compared with respect to existing or past characteristics judged to be of possible relevance to the etiology of the disease."

Conceptually, the case–control study differs from other epidemiologic designs primarily by the approach taken in sampling study subjects, which is on the basis of disease status. Contemporary epidemiologists regard case–control studies as a method of sampling the population experience of exposures and disease onsets from closed or open cohorts

(Walker, 1991). Cases are members of the population who have developed the disease outcome. Controls are sampled from the population from which the cases arise. Because the subjects are initially selected on the basis of disease status and information on exposures is subsequently obtained retrospectively, subject selection in case–control designs is often referred to as *retrospective sampling.*

The case–control design is advantageous for the study of rare diseases, and it is a relatively rapid and inexpensive method of inquiry. Case–control studies are usually restricted to a single outcome of interest, but they can accommodate a range of independent or interacting exposures. Case–control studies are not efficient for studying rare exposures, however, unless a rare exposure is a cause of a high proportion of cases for a particular outcome. Another limitation of many types of case–control studies is that they cannot be used to compute rates of disease occurrence in the population at risk, but only the *relative* rates between the exposed and unexposed (with a notable exception being the population-based case–control study). Case–control studies are also highly susceptible to bias, that is, the association between exposure and outcome occurrence measured in the study may be different from the true magnitude. Sources and control of bias are discussed in the concluding section of this chapter.

Selection of Cases. A case–control study requires a clear and reproducible set of criteria by which cases are identified, including both inclusion and exclusion rules. If diagnostic criteria for the outcome under study are controversial (which is the case for most psychiatric disorders), a case–control study should ideally be designed to include multiple case groups based on variously defined criteria. "Representativeness" is not the ultimate goal in a case definition. Instead, the investigator should seek to define a case group that reflects a *homogeneous etiologic entity.* Thus, for example, in a study of schizophrenia, an investigator would not seek to enroll a representative sample of all schizophrenics in the region under study. Instead, a subgroup believed to share a common etiologic pathway should be explicitly defined and enrolled as a case group.

Although most studies of psychiatric disorders currently focus on prevalent (i.e., existing) cases, incident (newly onset) cases are generally considered preferable in case–control studies. Prevalent cases may be enrolled at different stages of the disease process, complicating the interpretation of relationships between exposures and outcomes. Prevalent cases may also be "exposed" to etiologic agents both before and after the onset of disease, further clouding the interpretations of study results. An additional problem with prevalent cases is that individuals may alter their exposure levels after disease onset. For example, depressed persons may change their socialization patterns, diets, or activity levels. The relative risk measured after exposure levels have been altered in response to the disease may be different from measures based on exposure levels assessed before disease onset. This type of error in relative risk is sometimes referred to as *protopathic bias.* In general, use of prevalent cases can blur the distinction between factors related to *onset* versus *course* of disease, even for exposures occurring exclusively before disease incidence.

To select cases, a sampling protocol must be established. Features of this protocol should include 1) inclusion and exclusion criteria (e.g., age, sex, race); 2) the sampling frame (e.g., admissions records, registry data); and 3) sampling procedures (e.g., a total population census or random, systematic, stratified samples). The number of cases omitted by inclusion and exclusion criteria should be reported. In addition, the number of subjects who met inclusion criteria but were lost to study should be reported along with reasons for loss.

The usual *sources* of cases include 1) all individuals with disease onset in a specified period of time; 2) a representative subset of all population cases obtained by probability sampling; and 3) all cases seen at a particular medical care facility or group of facilities in a specified period of time. Although community-based cases (1 and 2) are preferred for studies of psychiatric conditions, they are not without limitations. A common problem associated with community-based cases concerns "caseness" definitions that incorporate history of prior treatment or diagnoses by health care professionals. Such "community" case series may in fact be restricted to individuals who use services, who may differ from all cases in the population in terms of socioeconomic status, education, and other potential risk factors. Also, community cases often have lower rates of cooperation than cases currently in medical care, and these refusals lead to increased bias.

Cases identified in inpatient (hospital) settings, although a cost-effective source of study subjects, are highly likely to introduce serious methodological problems in studies of psychiatric disorders. Treated cases usually differ from cases in the population on a broad range of social and demographic characteristics that may increase the difficulty of locating a comparable control group. Hospitals are often selective as to the type of patients whom they will treat (e.g., chronic cases may be served in state institutions, whereas first admission cases may be treated in private institutions), and it is unlikely that cases identified in these centers will be comparable to all cases of disorder arising in the population either in exposure or disease characteristics. When the probability for hospitalization differs for cases, noncases, and individuals with the exposure characteristic under study (a common result of high co-morbidity in hospitalized cases), a spurious association may be detected. This well-known limitation of hospital-based case–control studies was first described by Berkson (1946).

Lastly, a major impediment for psychiatric research in the United States is the virtual absence of comprehensive population registries covering a broad range of psychiatric disorders. In exceptional instances, communities may have systems of care providing comprehensive coverage all members of the population and maintaining linked medical records of all treatment contacts. The Monroe County, New York, registry is an example of a population-wide registry for psychiatric disorders. In such instances, treatment records can be used to assemble a case series for severe disorders that are usually seen in a treatment facility at some point in time (e.g.; schizophrenia). However, for other conditions in which only a small portion of cases are seen in treatment, such as depression and anxiety disorders, even a coordinated treatment system or treatment registry is an inadequate source of cases. For these disorders, a true population-based case series can only be identified through investigator-initiated population screening or assessment, which may be comparable to a population survey in total costs and level of effort.

Selection of Controls. Controls are used to evaluate whether the frequency or level of past exposures among the cases is different from that among *comparable* persons in the source population who do not have the disease under consideration. The selection of controls in a case–control study has been a subject of considerable controversy (Miettinen, 1985a). Nevertheless, theoretical and practical guidelines for selecting a valid control group have been proposed in the epidemiologic literature (Miettinen, 1985b). Controls should be representative of the population from which the cases arise in terms of their exposure distribution. This translates into three fundamental principles: 1) the cases and controls should come from a shared population source; 2) the selection of controls should be independent of the exposure or risk factor under study; and 3) exclusion criteria should be applied in a standardized ("symmetric") fashion for both cases and controls in regard to ancillary factors (such as age), secondary diagnoses, or co-morbid conditions (Schwartz and Link, 1989).

If it can be established that all cases are drawn from a defined geographic area, then controls should be selected from the same area so that their exposure distribution represents the source population for cases. Controls are frequently drawn from the same neighborhoods as cases in order to increase the likelihood that the two groups share a similar source population.

In selecting a source of controls, another consideration is the feasibility of obtaining information on study factors that can be collected in a comparable fashion as in the case group. This comparability should extend to records (quality and completeness); diagnostic procedures; response rates; and recall of exposure and knowledge of disease. Using hospitalized controls (such as surgical patients) in a case–control study in which cases are enrolled from an inpatient setting may increase comparability between groups in terms of the respondent's willingness to participate and other characteristics that may have influenced help-seeking. The interviews would also be conducted in a similar environment, which would increase comparability in terms of selective recall of health and exposure histories. However, it may be difficult to ascertain whether hospitalized controls have been selected independently of exposure so that their exposure distribution is representative of the population experience from which the cases arise.

Controls may also be selected as being similar to cases with respect to extraneous (confounding) factors, that is, variables that may lead to differences between cases and controls that do *not* reflect differences in risk factors under study. This procedure is referred to as *matching*. Usually, matching is limited to age, sex, and race. It is not cost-effective to employ matching in control selection unless information on matching factor is available before subject selection begins.

Two common forms of matching are individual (or pairwise) matching and group (or frequency) matching. In individual matching, one or more controls are selected for each case, and controls are identical to the case on the matched characteristics. In group matching, controls are selected in a manner that ensures that the proportions of the matching characteristics within the control group are the same as the case group. For continuous variables, such as age, the variable can be either categorized for purposes of matching or a "caliper" or tolerance limit for the match can be defined (e.g., age within 5 years of the case).

There are several limitations of matching. The costs may increase substantially as the number of matching variables increases. If individual matching involves multiple variables, it may be difficult to locate a control who matches a case on all characteristics, and many potential controls may be lost to the study because they share some, but not all, of the characteristics of a member of the case group. In addition, the pursuit of comparability between controls and cases in matching can go too far. If cases and controls are matched on a risk factor or on a measure of the disease process, no differences between cases and controls may be observed on that risk factor or some exposures or characteristics that are true causes. This problem is referred to as *overmatching*. It should be noted that control of effects of confounding factors can also be handled in *data analysis*, and this approach to achieving a balance between case and control groups is preferred in most contemporary studies.

Cost and feasibility enter into control group selection regardless of whether matching is employed. Different sources of controls vary in cost and feasibility. Two cost-effective sources of controls discussed earlier include 1) (for a hospital-based case series) a control group consisting of patients suffering from an illness unrelated to the disease under study and 2) neighbors. Economic constraints also dictate the *number* of controls to be drawn from a given source. The control group is characteristically of equal or larger size than the case group and generally should not exceed the case group by more than a factor of 4 or 5 (Rothman, 1986). Controls are easier to identify than cases, and increasing the size of the control group may be an economical approach to enhancing statistical power in data analysis.

When the process of selecting control subjects is undertaken, the cases usually have already been identified. Controls may be selected in a pairwise fashion with each case (e.g., next admission with certain diagnosis, neighbor, sibling), or controls may be selected as a group according to a sampling protocol. Examples of this latter approach include a community probability sample or a systematic sample of all traffic accident admissions (or patients) in given period. As with cases, an explicit protocol for selection procedures should be prepared *and* adhered to. Exclusion rules for specific individuals should also be clarified (e.g., exclusion of individuals with other psychiatric disorders).

If each source of controls is not an optimal reference group for the exposure likelihood of the case series, multiple control groups can be employed. Differences in magnitude of association between exposure and disease occurrence using alternate control groups may be helpful in assessing causality and sources of bias.

Measures of Exposure Status in a Case–Control Study. In a case–control study, disease status is determined at the time of subject selection. Therefore, measures obtained on study subjects focus on exposure histories. Measurement of exposure history in a case–control study should be made using well-defined and relevant variables. Timing of exposure, both current and past, must be ascertained. Comparable methods of collecting information on exposure must be used for cases and controls. Controls are less likely to be thinking about exposures related to disease than cases, and efforts must be made to minimize selective recall in the comparison groups. Whenever possible, records of exposure levels made before disease onset should be used, but, regardless of the types of measures that are employed, information sources must be the same for cases and controls.

Investigators gathering data on cases and controls should be blind to the case/control status. Additionally, checks on the comparability of exposure information should be made. For example, nonresponse rates for key exposure variables should be contrasted and found to be comparable for cases and controls. Frequency of reporting characteristics that are *not* of etiologic relevance should also be comparable between case and control groups.

Uses of Case–Control Studies in Psychiatric Research. An exemplary case–control study in psychiatric research is Brown and Harris' study of depression among women in the Camberwell district of London, described in their 1978 book *Social Origins of Depression*. These investigators hypothesized that onset of a depressive episode was precipitated by two stages of stress: 1) a underlying susceptibility to depression induced by exposure to certain social conditions or stressors with sustained psychological sequelae ("vulnerability factors") and 2) triggering of the episode among vulnerable women by a recent life stress or major difficulty ("provoking agents"). A third set of factors, principally including past loss, were hypothesized to influence the severity and shape of pathology and were labeled *symptom formation* factors.

Brown and Harris enrolled multiple case groups in their study, including groups of both treated and community cases. Each case group was subdivided by severity and onset (incident vs. chronic prevalent cases). The first case series consisted of patients (73 inpatients, 41 outpatients) aged 18–65 who made visits to Camberwell district psychiatrists during the study period and who were given a diagnosis of primary depression without underlying alcoholism or organic causes. An urban community case series was obtained from two random samples of women aged 18–65 in the Camberwell district conducted 4 years apart. A rural community case series was also assembled from surveying women who lived on an island in the Outer Hebrides. Interview data were used to subdivide the case groups further on the basis of meeting borderline or full case criteria or representing onset or chronic cases.

The primary source of controls were 295 women in the Camberwell community survey who were interviewed and found to be without depression. Nondepressives in the rural survey were also available as a control series. All cases and controls were interviewed about their histories of vulnerability and provoking factors. Stresses described in the interview were rated by panels of judges to control for biased reporting of the impact of events by depressed respondents.

The principal finding of this study was that risk of depression in community women was increased when a provoking agent occurred in the presence of three vulnerability factors (loss of a mother before age 11, presence of three or more children under age 14 at home, absence of a confiding relationship with husband or boyfriend). This model was re-evaluated for different case groups (severe vs. borderline cases, treated vs. untreated, chronic vs. recent onset cases). One important finding was that no association was observed for treated cases of depression and certain vulnerability factors, notably the presence of three or more children under 14 years at home. This vulnerability factor was observed to be negatively associated with help-seeking, possibly cancelling any observable elevated risk in treated cases. This elegant case–control study illustrates the importance of employing multiple case groups in studies of psychiatric disorders and the significance of using population-based samples to investigate the etiology of psychopathology.

Hybrid Studies. Each of the three basic observational epidemiologic study designs described thus far—cross-sectional, case–control, and cohort—can be developed further by adding special design features to permit estimation of additional parameters and/or to handle complex exposure or disease courses. In psychiatric epidemiology, various features of sociological studies have been invoked to handle the variable course of risk factors and disease outcomes. Using the terminology of Kleinbaum et al. (1982), we are referring to these derivative studies as *hybrid* designs. We do not attempt to catalog each possible hybrid design, but, rather, will select examples that illustrate some of the influential hybrid studies in psychiatric epidemiology. The interested reader is referred to the textbook by Kleinbaum et al. (1982) for a more formal presentation of these and other hybrid studies.

Repeated Cross-Sectional Survey. A hybrid study design that is based on the cross-sectional survey is the "repeated cross-sectional survey." In this type of study, independent, representative samples of a target population are drawn at two or more time periods and assessed separately. It is important to note that in a repeated cross-sectional survey, unlike a cohort study, different study samples are assessed at each time period. This type of hybrid study permits analysis of changing levels of disease rates in a population over time and of changing levels of association between exposure and disease when follow ups of a single study cohort are not feasible. This hybrid design was employed in the U.S. National Sample Surveys (Gurin et al., 1960; Veroff et al., 1981), in which two cross-sectional mental health and service use surveys involving separate national probability samples of the entire U.S. adult population were conducted in 1957 and 1976. To estimate changes in the mental health status over time, the data from the 1957 and 1976 national surveys were pooled into one database. Tests for differences in measures by year of survey were used to identify whether the mental health of Americans had changed over the decades between the surveys. Another major study in psychiatric epidemiology, the Stirling County study, included repeated cross-sectional surveys as well as cohort follow ups at each major assessment period in order to be able to examine secular population changes that would not be represented adequately in the prospective study cohort as it aged over time (Murphy et al., 1984).

Multistage Studies. A type of hybrid design known as a two (or multiple) stage study combines features of case–control and cross-sectional survey methodologies. In these studies, a cross-sectional survey employing a brief and inexpensive mental health screening instrument is conducted in the first stage of inquiry. Using the results of the screening information, a smaller sample of "cases" (screen positives) and "controls" (screen negatives) are selected with known probability from the cross-sectional survey sample. More extensive information is obtained on these case and control subjects in a second (and sometimes third) stage of data collection. Population prevalence estimates can be obtained from second-stage data by assigning weights to the study data reflecting the probability of selection at each stage and by adjusting for disease classification errors in the screening instrument. Variance adjustments may also be required to represent the underlying sampling scheme in analysis (Cain and Breslow, 1988). The accuracy of estimation in multistage studies depends on several factors, most notably on the quality of the screening instrument used in the first stage to identify cases and controls (Shrout et al., 1986; Newman et al., 1990). Also, because subjects are re-interviewed in multiple waves within a very short time span, there may be loss to follow up from subjects who consider multiple stages of assessment too burdensome. Retest "practice" effects may also occur if similar questions are repeated in both stages.

Two-stage studies have been used in a number of child mental health studies where data collection costs can be large because information is gathered from multiple informants. The Rutter et al. (1975) Isle of Wight and Inner London Borough studies of child psychiatric disorders in 8-year-old children and the Bird et al. (1988) Puerto Rican study of children are examples of two-stage studies in child psychiatric epidemiology. Another example of a multistage study is the Dohrenwend et al. (1992) study of socioeconomic status and psychiatric disorders in a birth cohort of 4,914 Israel-born adults of European and North African background, also described in Chapter 1 (this volume).

Panel Studies. An example of a hybrid study based on a cohort design is a "panel" study. In a panel study, repeated measures are taken on *both* exposure and disease characteristics of the cohort at each follow-up period. This type of design permits flexible handling of changing exposure levels and variable disease course over the study period. The 22 year follow up of a Midtown Manhattan study (Srole and Fisher, 1989) is an example of a major longitudinal study in psychiatric epidemiology that has utilized the "panel study" design. In the Midtown Manhattan study, a probability sample of 1,660 adults aged 20–59 residing in a predominantly white residential area of central Manhattan, ranging in social character from "Gold Coast to Slum," was assessed by household interviews. Two decades later, a total of 858 survivors were located, and interviews were completed with 695 individuals, or "panelists." This study found no significant net change in general mental health ratings over time after 22 years of exposure to residential living in or near Manhattan.

Ecologic Studies

Geographic Distribution Studies. In this last section on epidemiologic study designs we turn to the historical roots of psychiatric epidemiology and describe the ecologic study, which was commonplace during the first half of the twentieth century. An ecologic study is part of a larger class of "incomplete" study designs in which assessments of *both* exposure and disease statuses are not obtained for each individual subject (Kleinbaum et al., 1982).

In an ecologic study, measures of disease rates are ascertained for defined population groups (e.g., population data for different geographic areas or time periods) and compared with aggregate exposure measurements (e.g., mean exposure level or proportion exposed) for the groups in question. To illustrate the ecologic design, we briefly describe a classic ecologic study in psychiatric epidemiology by Faris and Dunham (1939) that examined geographic (areal) differences in rates of schizophrenia and other psychoses in an urban area. These investigators gathered hospital admission data and other statistical information for the city of Chicago in the 1930s. In this study, the units of data analysis were city zones that formed concentric circles spanning outward from the city center. Psychiatric hospital admission rates for the zones were contrasted with other aggregated statistical information for these areas, including the zone's average distance from the city center and seven indices of social disorganization. Two findings of this study were that rates of hospital admissions for schizophrenia were higher in zones close to the city center and in areas with high rates of foreign-born residents. Although information on mental health and place of birth were not obtained from individual residents in this study, the findings have stimulated hypotheses about relationships between urban social disorganization and schizophrenia among individuals (e.g., foreign-born individuals are more likely to develop schizophrenia). Faris and Dunham were cautious about making fallacious inferences about *individuals* living within city zones from the associations between aggregate characteristics of the zones. For example, they explored the possibility that high rates of hospital admissions in areas with foreign-born residents primarily resulted from higher risk among the native born persons who resided in these areas. Rates of hospitalized schizophrenics who were foreign or native born were compared for residential areas with high and low areas of foreign born, and no differences were observed.

An erroneous inference made about the associations between measures on an individual level based on relationships observed on group level is known as the *ecologic fallacy* or *cross-level bias*. Morgenstern (1982) has demonstrated that cross-level bias can be seen as a combination of "aggregation bias" and "specification bias." Aggregation bias is a mathematical artifact that results from grouping individuals in a manner that alters the "within group" and "between group" variances used in computing correlations coefficients, and the impact of this bias on ecologic data was first attributed to Robinson (1950). Aggregation bias is a particular problem for *correlations* computed between two grouped variables (e.g., rates of foreign born in census tracts correlated with hospital admissions rates for census tracts). Ecologic correlation coefficients tend to be spuriously inflated. Use of regression coefficients to describe associations between ecologic rates of exposures and outcomes is recommended as a means of avoiding this statistical artifact.

Morgenstern describes *specification bias* as confounding of the individual-level risk factor–disease outcome association by the group used as the unit of analysis. This may occur under a number of conditions. Extraneous exposures ("confounding factors") differentially distributed across the groups may lead to biased estimates of association. Also, the "group" may contain an inherent property influencing rates of disease above and beyond the individual risk factor(s) comprised in the group, that is, the whole may be more than the sum of its parts. For example, a residential area labeled as a "slum" may exert an unmeasurable influence of social stigma on the well being of residents above and beyond the component measures of poverty, limited education, high crime, poor leadership, and so forth. A related form of specification bias may also occur if individuals are placed at greater risk for mental disorders when they differ from average characteristics of the "group" or have a poor "person–environment fit" (Wechsler and Pugh, 1972). Faris and Dunham attempted to explore this problem in their 1939 ecologic study by contrasting, among other characteristics, admissions rates of foreign-born schizophrenics for areas with high and low percentages of foreign-born residents. A more definitive test of "person–environment fit" would combine and compare individual level data on risk factors with characteristics of the social or residential areas and would also give consideration to group properties, such as heterogeneity and size, that might mitigate the impact of poor "person–environment fit."

There are other problems associated with ecologic studies that should be briefly mentioned. These studies are susceptible to the problems associated with analysis of multicolinear data because exposures are often highly correlated within groups. Consequently, the unique effects of individual exposures frequently cannot be disentangled, and correlations of exposure rates with aggregate group outcome rates may also be spuriously inflated. Measures of many exposures are often not available in census or other large population surveys, and these variables cannot be studied as risk factors or controlled as confounding effects. Direction of cause and effect in ecologic associations is difficult to discern, even if incident disease data are employed. Also, the level of measurement error may be different at the ecologic versus the individual level, which may lead to differences in findings.

Despite these limitations, ecologic analyses continue to be undertaken. Interest in these studies persists in part because statistical information on rates of in- and outpatient psychiatric service contacts, delinquency, crime, and substance abuse gathered to meet other reporting requirements are often available to researchers at little or no cost. Ecologic analyses of these data are very appropriate to use for policy applications or for examining other hypotheses about socioenvironmental characteristics where inferences remain on the population group or "macro" level.

Time Trend Studies. Our illustration of ecologic studies has focused on geographic variation. Another form of ecologic study that has received considerable attention in contemporary psychiatric literature examines variations in rates over time, or time trend analysis. The general method of ecologic time trend studies is to examine aggregate rates of disease in a population at different points in time. Comparisons to changing exposure over time are made either directly (when exposure data have also been collected at each point in time) or indirectly (by inferring changing levels that have occurred over time or at different periods in time, as in war or peace time).

A well-known time trend study in psychiatric epidemiology is Brenner's study (1973) linking hospital admissions rates to fluctuations in the economy. This type of study is susceptible to a number of methodologic problems (Kasl, 1979). The impact of changing exposure levels on health outcomes may not be instantaneous, but it may be difficult to determine the appropriate time lag between exposure and disease trends. By altering the time lags in a study of mental health and the economy, fiscal upturns can be shown to be associated with increasing or decreasing hospital admissions rates. Also, changing diagnostic and statistical data collection procedures over time can lead to artifactual trends in the data. Changing treatment efficacy will also influence prevalence and mortality trends.

One of the most complicated areas of ecologic time trend analysis concerns the roles that age, period, and cohort effects may play in explaining time trends. Different trends in disease rates arrayed by year of birth, age of subject, and chronologic time can be used to suggest alternative etiologic hypotheses. In an *age effect*, disease rates are observed to vary with age, and factors associated with the aging process are usually considered to be the principal etiologic agents. If an age effect exists and the age structure of the population used for the time trend study has changed over chronologic time (e.g., more older persons in recent decades), variations in secular trends of disease rates may reflect factors associated with aging process rather than changes in the environment per se. A *period effect* is a fluctuation of disease rates during a discrete period of time, possibly related to a significant population exposure. For example, low suicide rates during the First and Second World Wars can be considered to be period effects. In a *cohort effect*, disease rates vary by birth year or by other significant life history events, such as cohorts defined by high school graduation class. Changing levels of socioenvironmental exposures during critical developmental periods are usually invoked as an explanation for changes in disease rates for different cohorts. One important methodologic issue in studying age, period, and cohort effects is that information on two of these effects will perfectly predict the third. This problem is known as "indeterminacy" in statistical modeling.

Findings from the Epidemiologic Catchment Area study and from family genetics studies stimulated interest in the study of age, period, and cohort effects in mental disorders, notably major depression. Klerman et al. (1988) reviewed several studies suggesting that an apparent decrease in lifetime prevalence of Major Depression with age (an age effect) may in fact be due to lower rates of depression reported by individuals born prior to War II (a cohort effect). The reader is referred to the review of Klerman et al. (1988) for a discussion of the empirical evidence and of some of the statistical techniques that have been employed to disentangle the influences of age and cohort effects for this disorder.

It should be noted that the usual sources of time series data used to study age, period, and cohort effects in epidemiology do not exist for most major psychiatric disorders, including depression. In most age–period–cohort analyses conducted to date, empirical data on rates of major depression occurring among young adults from early birth cohorts have been reconstructed through retrospective recall of older subjects. Even in studies that have supplemented recall data with medical records from the early periods and retrospective information provided by relatives, estimates of rates of major depression in the early part of this century used to explore age and cohort effects may contain substantial misclassification errors. Results derived from these retrospective data should be interpreted cautiously.

VALID GROUP COMPARISONS IN OBSERVATIONAL STUDIES

When two groups are compared in an observational study, the estimate of relative risk measuring the association between an exposure and disease outcome can be distorted by a number of factors that compromise the validity of the estimate. Factors contributing to noncomparability of groups include 1) the population composition of the groups; 2) the information obtained from each group; and 3) extraneous attributes unevenly distributed between the groups that may explain the difference in rates of disease occurrence (Miettinen, 1985). Noncomparability from any of these sources results in a "biased" relative risk estimate, that is, the relative risk observed in the study data differs from the true value. The bias may be negative (i.e., the observed estimate falls closer to the null value than the true relative risk) or positive (i.e., the observed estimate is farther from the null value). There are three broad classes of biases frequently encountered in epidemiologic studies: biases of selection, information, and confounding (Monson, 1990).

Selection Bias

Selection bias is most likely to occur in studies where the outcome status is known at the start of the study and is used to select subjects, as in case–control or retrospective cohort studies. If enrollment of exposed and nonexposed individuals is influenced by the disease status, selection bias will occur. For example, in a retrospective cohort study designed to study the association between occupational exposures and onset of Alzheimer's disease, if health records of individuals with Alzheimer's have been removed for any purpose related to the outcome status, such as for processing worker compensation, the disease experience in the study group will be underestimated. Consequently, the relationships between exposure and disease outcome will be biased.

Considerable attention has been given to sources of selection bias in case–control studies. To avoid selection bias in a case–control design, the distribution of the exposures in the control group should be representative of the population at risk. The sample of individuals enrolled into the control group may be systematically nonrepresentative for a number of reasons (Lewis and Pelosi, 1990). For example, individuals may refuse to cooperate in interviews, and this noncooperation may be systematically associated with the exposure under study. In a hospital-based case–control study, admission into a hospital may be determined by factors such as co-morbidity that is related to the exposures under study, a source of bias described earlier in this chapter as *Berkson's bias*. If the true source population of the case group is difficult to identify, the potential for selection bias increases because control subjects may not be sampled from the true "population at risk." Methods described earlier for control selection (shared population sources for cases and controls; selection of control subjects independently of exposure status; symmetric exclusion criteria for cases and controls) can effectively minimize selection bias in these studies.

Information Bias

Information bias refers to invalid estimates of the relationship between exposure and disease outcomes resulting from information obtained on study subjects. One form of information bias occurs when the data gathered for the different study groups is not comparable ("observation bias"). For example, observation bias can occur in a prospective cohort study when there is attrition because subjects are lost to follow up. When subject loss occurs, incomplete information is obtained about disease development on subjects who are not followed over time. If subjects who are lost to follow up from the exposed and unexposed cohorts have a different disease experience than the study participants in their respective cohorts, estimates of relative risk made from the available study data may be biased. Greenland (1977) provides a detailed account of the conditions in which nonresponse can lead to biased estimates in cohort studies.

Information bias can also occur when the comparison groups give information with varying levels of accuracy ("recall bias"). For example, mothers giving birth to mentally retarded children might recall medications taken during pregnancy with greater accuracy than mothers delivering healthy children.

Misclassification of a subject's exposure or disease status because of measurement error is another form of information bias. For dichotomous exposures and outcomes the direction of bias in the estimate of relative risk will be toward the null if misclassification is "nondifferential," that is, it occurs with the same magnitude and direction within the different study groups being compared (e.g., similar exposure misclassification rates for cases and controls in a case–control study; similar disease misclassification rates for exposed and nonexposed subjects in a cohort study). However, if misclassification occurs differentially for the comparison groups, the direction of bias can be in any direction. Even small amounts of misclassification error can lead to substantial bias in estimates in relative risk (Kleinbaum et al., 1982), and it is important to use measurement methods and data collection procedures that will ensure the highest degree of accuracy in classifying study subjects. The impact of measurement error on study estimates can be examined by recomputing estimates that adjust for error rates either through sensitivity analyses or by modeling measurement error (Rosner et al., 1989; Armstrong, 1990).

Confounding Bias

Confounding bias occurs when the study samples in the comparison groups are imbalanced with respect to other characteristics that are independent determinants of the disease under study. These ancillary characteristics, known as *confounders*, will be found to be associated with both the exposure and the disease in the study sample. Table 2 illustrates a hypothetical situation in which confounding bias could occur in a psychiatric research context.

In Table 2, it can be observed that age is a predictor of the outcome under study because mortality density is higher among the older subjects. In addition, age is unevenly distributed between the comparison groups: The schizophrenic group has more person-years contributed by younger subjects. Even though the true mortality rate ratio should be 3.0 comparing schizophrenia with bipolar disorder, the relative risk estimated in the total study sample is only 1.5. Hence, unless adjustments are made for differences in age distributions between the study groups, the observed relative risk will be biased.

Bias from confounding variables can be handled at two stages of a study: either in the

TABLE 2. Confounding in a Comparative Study of the Mortality Rate (Density) of Schizophrenia and Bipolar Disorder

	Deaths	Person-Years	Mortality Rate (per 1,000 Person-Years)
Young subjects (<45 years of age)			
Schizophrenia	18	6,000	3.0
Bipolar disorder	2	2,000	1.0
Relative risk = 3.0			
Old subjects (45+ years of age)			
Schizophrenia	30	2,000	15.0
Bipolar disorder	30	6,000	5.0
Relative risk = 3.0			
All subjects (young and old)			
Schizophrenia	48	8,000	6.0
Bipolar disorder	32	8,000	4.0
Relative risk = 1.5			

subject selection phase or in the data analysis stage. In the subject selection stage, confounding can be minimized by *restriction* or *matching*. In restriction, subject selection is limited to certain categories of a confounding variable. For example, in the example of age and mortality density, confounding by age could be controlled by restricting the age range of all subjects in the study to one age group, such as selecting all study subjects with schizophrenia and bipolar disorder to be under age 45. Alternatively, confounding could be controlled by matching schizophrenic and bipolar study groups on age during subject selection using the procedures described in the section on case–control studies. Matching will ensure that the groups are balanced with respect to the confounding factor. However, as discussed earlier in the overview of case–control studies, there are several drawbacks to matching. The association between age and the outcome cannot be directly estimated if matching is employed in subject selection. Also, matching can be inefficient and expensive compared with methods of controlling confounding in data analysis.

In the analysis phase, confounding is commonly controlled by use of stratified analyses or multivariable regression models. These procedures are described in Chapter 3 (this volume) and are only briefly summarized here. In stratified analyses, the study sample is grouped by the categories of the confounding variables. Relative risk estimates can be calculated within each group of the confounding variable. If the stratum-specific estimates do not differ from each other (usually evaluated by a chi-squared test of heterogeneity or determined a priori), a summary estimate of relative risk can be calculated by computing a weighted average of the stratum-specific relative risks. A variety of weighting schemes can be employed (Kleinbaum et al., 1982), and the most common method, suggested by Mantel and Haenzsel (1959), uses a weight that is inversely proportional to the variance in each stratum.

In the example provided in Table 2, the stratum-specific estimates of relative risk are identical to each other, equalling three in both older and younger patients. A summary measure of relative risk would also equal 3. However, if the relative risks differ for different levels of a confounder, "interaction" is said to exist between the confounder and the exposure under study with respect to the disease outcome. In this case, summary estimates of relative risk will not represent the true nature of the relationship between the exposure and the disease outcome because the value of the estimate depends on the subject's status on the confounding variable. If an interaction exists, the separate stratum-specific estimates of relative risk should be reported for separate categories of the confounding variables, for example, for older and for younger subjects.

Multivariable regression models can also be used to adjust for the influence of confounding variables on the exposure and disease outcome by introducing confounders as "covariate" independent terms in these models. Multivariable models can also be used to evaluate interactions. For a more detailed discussion of control of confounding, the interested reader is referred to basic texts in epidemiology (Kleinbaum et al., 1982; Monson, 1990; Rothman, 1986; Walker, 1991). Maldanado and Greenland (1993) discuss alternative analytic approaches to evaluating and controlling confounding in an epidemiologic investigation.

ACKNOWLEDGMENTS

This chapter was written while G.E.P.Z. was supported by an NIMH Scientist Development Award (1-K01-MH00745-05). The authors are members of the Harvard Training Program in Psychiatric Epidemiology and Biostatistics, which is funded in part by NIMH training grant 5-T32-MH17119-11.

REFERENCES

Aneshensel CS, Estrada AL, Hansell MJ, Clark VA (1987): Social psychological aspects of reporting behavior: Lifetime depressive episode reports. J Health Social Behav 28:232–246.

Armstrong BG (1990): The effects of measurement errors on relative risk regressions. Am J Epidemiol 132:1176–1184.

Berkson J (1946): Limitation of the application of fourfold table analysis to hospital data. Biom Bull 2:47–53.

Bird HR, Canino G, Rubio-Stipec M, et al. (1988): Estimates of the prevalence of childhood maladjustment in a community survey in Puerto Rico. Arch Gen Psychiatry 45:1120–1126.

Brenner MH (1973): "Mental Illness and the Economy." Cambridge, Harvard University Press.

Brown GW, Harris T (1978): "Social Origins of Depression." New York: Free Press.

Cain KC, Breslow NE (1988): Logistic regression analysis and efficient design for two-stage studies. Am J Epidemiol 128:1198–1206.

Chiang CL (1968): "Introduction to Stochastic Processes in Biostatistics." New York: John Wiley & Sons.

Cleary PD, Houts PS (1984): The psychological impact of the Three Mile Island accident. J Hum Stress 10:28–34.

Cobb S, Kasl SV (1977): Termination: The Consequences of Job Loss." DHEW(NIOSH) Publication No. 77-224.

Cochran WG (1977): "Sampling techniques," 3rd ed. New York: Wiley.

Decoufle P, Holmgreen P, Boyle CA, Stroup NE (1992): Self-reported health status of Vietnam veterans in relation to perceived exposure to herbicides and combat. Am J Epidemiol 135:312–323.

Dohrenwend BP, Levav I, Shrout PE et al. (1992): Socioeconomic status and psychiatric disorders: The causation-selection issue. Science 255:946–952.

Eaton WW, Kramer M, Anthony JC et al. (1989): The incidence of specific DIS/DSM-III mental disorders: Data from the NIMH Epidemiologic Catchment Area Program. Acta Psychiatr Scand 79:163–178.

Elandt-Johnson RC (1975): Definition of rates: Some remarks on their use and misuse. Am J Epidemiol 102:267–271.

Elwood JM (1988): "Causal Relationships in Medicine: A Practical System for Critical Appraisal." New York: Oxford University Press.

Faris RL, Dunham HW (1939): "Mental Disorders in Urban Areas." Chicago: University of Chicago Press.

Feighner JP, Robins E, Guze SM, et al. (1972): Diagnostic criteria for use in psychiatric research. Arch Gen Psychiatry 26:57–63.

Freeman J, Hutchison GB (1980): Prevalence, incidence, and duration. Am J Epidemiol 112:707–723.

Freeman J, Hutchison GB (1986): Duration of disease, duration indicators, and estimation of the risk ratio. Am J Epidemiol 124:134–149.

Funch DP, Marshall JR (1984): Measuring life stress: Factors affecting fall-off in the reporting of life events. J Health Social Behav 25:453–464.

Gibbons RD, Hedeker D, Elkin I, et al. (1993): Some conceptual and statistical issues in analysis of longitudinal psychiatric data: Application to the NIMH Treatment of Depression Collaborative Research Program Dataset. Arch Gen Psychiatry 50:739–750.

Greenland S (1977): Response and follow-up bias in cohort studies. Am J Epidemiol 106:184–187.

Gurin G, Veroff J, Feld S (1960): "Americans View Their Mental Health." New York: Basic Books.

Hagnell O, Lanke J, Rorsman B, Ojesjo L (1982): Are we entering and age of melancholy: Depressive illnesses in a prospective epidemiological study of over 25 years: The Lundby Study, Sweden. Psychol Med 12:279–289.

Hamilton M (1960): A rating scale for depression. J Neurol Neurosurg Psychiatry 23:56–62.

Helzer J (1981): Methodological issues in the interpretations of the consequences of extreme situations. In Dohrenwend BS, Dohrenwend BP (eds): "Stressful Life Events and Their Contexts." New York: Prodist, pp 108–129.

Kasl SV (1979): Mortality and the business cycle. Some questions about research strategies when utilizing macro-social and ecological data. Am J Public Health 69:784–788.

Kasl SV, Chisholm RF, Eskenazi B (1981): The impact of the accident at the Three Mile Island on the behavior and well-being of nuclear workers. Part II. Job tension, psychophysiological symptoms, and indices of distress. Am J Public Health 71:484–495.

Kessler RC, Wethington RC (1991): The reliability of life event reports in a community survey. Psychol Med 21:723–738.

Kish L (1965): "Survey Sampling." New York: Wiley.

Kleinbaum DG, Kupper LL, Morgenstern H (1982): "Epidemiologic Research: Principles and Quantitiative Methods." Belmont CA: Lifetime Learning Publications.

Klerman GL (1988): The current age of youthful melancholia: Evidence for increase in depression among adolescents and young adults. Br J Psychiatry 152:4–14.

Kramer M (1957): A discussion of the concepts of incidence and prevalence as related to epidemiologic studies of mental disorders. Am J Public Health 47:826–840.

Lewis G, Pelosi AJ (1990): The case-control study in psychiatry. Br J Psychiatry 157:197–207.

MacMahon B, Pugh TF (1970): "Epidemiology: Principles and Methods." Boston: Little Brown.

Maldanado G, Greenland S (1993): Simulation study of confounder selection strategies. Am J Epidemiol 138:923–936.

Mantel N, Haenszel W (1959): Statistical aspects of the analysis of data from retrospective studies of disease. JNCI 22:719–748.

Miettinen OS (1985a): "Theoretical Epidemiology." New York: John Wiley & Sons.

Miettinen OS (1985b): The "case–control" study: Valid selection of subjects (with discussions). J Chronic Dis 38:543–558.

Monson RR (1990): "Occupational Epidemiology," 2nd ed. Boca Raton: CRC Press.

Morgenstern H (1982): Uses of ecologic analysis in epidemiologic research. Am J Public Health 72:1336–1344.

Morrison J, Clancy J, Crowe R, Winokur G (1972): The Iowa 500: I. Diagnostic validity in mania, depression and schizophrenia. Arch Gen Psychiatry 27:457–461.

Murphy JM, Oliver DC, Monson RR, et al. (1988): Incidence of depression and anxiety: The Stirling County Study. Am J Public Health 78:534–540.

Murphy JM, Sobol AM, Neff RK, et al. (1984): Stability of prevalence: Depression and anxiety disorders. Arch Gen Psychiatry 41:990–997.

Neugebauer R (1981): The reliability of life event reports. In Dohrenwend BS, Dohrenwend BP (ed): "Stressful Life Events and Their Contexts." New York: Prodist, pp 85–107.

Newman SC, Shrout PE, Bland RC (1990): The efficiency of two-phase designs in prevalence surveys of mental disorders. Psychol Med 20:183–193.

Robins LN (1985): Epidemiology: Reflections on testing the validity of psychiatric interviews. Arch Gen Psychiatry 42:918–924.

Robins LN, Helzer JE, Weissman MM, et al. (1984): Lifetime prevalence of psychiatric disorders in three sites. Arch Gen Psychiatry 41:949–948.

Robinson WS (1950): Ecological correlations and the behavior of individuals. Am Sociol Rev 15:351–357.

Rosner B, Willet W, Spiegelman D (1989): Correction of logistic regression relative risk estimates and confience intervals for systematic within-person measurement error. Stat Med 8:1051–1070.

Rothman KJ (1986): "Modern Epidemiology." Boston: Little Brown.

Rutter M, Cox A, Tupling C, Berger M, Yule W (1975): Attainment and adjustment in two geographical areas: I. The prevalence of psychiatric disorder. Br J Psychiatry 126:493–509.

Schlesselman JJ (1982): "Case–control Studies: Design, Conduct, Analysis." New York: Oxford University Press.

Schrader G, Davis A, Stefanovic S, Christie P (1990): The recollection of affect. Psychol Med 20:105–109.

Schwartz S, Link BG (1989): The "well control" artefact in case/control studies of specific psychiatric disorders. Psychol Med 19:737–742.

Shrout PE, Dohrenwend BP, Levav I (1986): A discriminant rule for screening cases of diverse diagnostic types: Preliminary results. J Consult Clin Psychol 54:314–319.

Srole L, Fischer AK (1989): Changing lives and well-being: The Midtown Manhattan panel study, 1954–1976. Acta Psychiatr Scand 79(Suppl 348):35–44.

Tsuang MT, Woolson RF, Fleming JA (1979a): Long term outcome of major psychoses: I "Schizophrenia and affective disorders compared with psychiatrically symptom-free surgical conditions. Arch Gen Psychiatry 36:1295–1301.

Tsuang MT, Dempsey GM (1979b): Long term outcome of major psychoses: II "Schizoaffective" disorder compared with schizophrenia, affective disorders, and a surgical control group. Arch Gen Psychiatry 36:1302–1304.

Walker AM (1991): "Observation and Inference. An Introduction to the Methods of Epidemiology." Chestnut Hill: Epidemiology Resources, Inc.

Wechsler H, Pugh TF (1967): Fit of individual and community characteristics and rates of psychiatric hospitalization. Am J Sociol 73:331–338.

Weissman MM, Myers JK (1978): Affective disorders in a United States urban community: The use of Research Diagnostic Criteria in an epidemiologic survey. Arch Gen Psychiatry 35:1304–1311.

Veroff J, Douvan E, Kulka RA (1981): "The Inner American: A Self Portrait From 1957 to 1976." New York: Basic Books.

CHAPTER 3

Analysis of Categorized Data: Use of the Odds Ratio as a Measure of Association

STEPHEN L. HILLIS and ROBERT F. WOOLSON

Division of Biostatistics and Department of Statistics and Actuarial Science,University of Iowa, Iowa City, IA 52242

INTRODUCTION

In this chapter we discuss the use of the odds ratio as a measure of association between two dichotomous variables that typically indicate the presence or absence of a specific characteristic. For instance, in a clinical trial that randomly assigns subjects with a particular disease to either a drug group or a control group, the researcher is interested in the association between the dichotomous variables outcome status (improvement or no improvement) and treatment status (drug or control).

We consider the general situation where the data can be summarized by the familiar 2×2 contingency table presented in Table 1. For example, suppose that in a randomized study designed to assess the effect of lithium on manic-depression in males, 30 manic-depressive male patients are treated with lithium and 40 are given a placebo. In the first 3 months, 8 of the patients treated with lithium have manic-depressive episodes while 28 of the patients given the placebo have episodes. Table 2 presents these data.

In practice, the data for Table 1 are usually generated from one of three possible sampling methods: the *cross-sectional study,* the *prospective study,* or the *retrospective study.* We now briefly discuss these methods; a more detailed discussion of the methods and their advantages and disadvantages can be found in an epidemiologic methods textbook such as that of Kleinbaum et al. (1982) or Miettinen (1985).

In a *cross-sectional study* a random sample of size N is selected from the population of interest, and then the presence or absence of the characteristics corresponding to variables 1 and 2 is determined for each subject. For example, to study the association between sex (male or female) and psychosis (present or absent) in a community, a random sample could be drawn from the community, followed by the classification of each subject with respect to sex and psychosis. Of course, the psychosis classification would be determined by an appropriate diagnostic instrument.

In prospective and restrospective studies, two random samples are selected. Let vari-

---

Textbook in Psychiatric Epidemiology, Edited by Tsuang, Tohen, and Zahner
ISBN 0-471-59375-3 © 1995 Wiley-Liss, Inc.

TABLE 1. Data Layout for a 2 × 2 Contingency Table

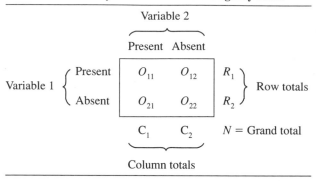

able 1 be the *antecedent variable*—that is, the subject can be classified in terms of the presence or absence of the variable 1 characteristic before a similar classification is possible for variable 2. For example, in clinical trials, treatment status (drug or placebo) is assigned before the outcome status (improvement or no improvement) is known, and hence treatment status is the antecedent variable. In studying the association between a risk factor variable, such as family history of psychiatric disease (present or absent), and a disease, such as depression, clearly the risk factor variable is antecedent.

In a *prospective study*, random samples of size R_1 and R_2 (see Table 1) are selected from the two populations corresponding to the two possibilities (called *levels*) of variable 1. The subjects are then followed over a specified period of time, after which subjects are classified according to variable 2. The study of the effect of lithium on manic-depression described above is a *randomized* prospective study, since the subjects are randomly assigned to the two levels of variable 1. As an example of a nonrandomized prospective study, one could study the association between family history of alcoholism and a particular psychiatric disorder by following two samples selected from populations of subjects with and without a family history of alcoholism over a period of, say, 20 years, and then recording the presence or absence of the disorder.

In a *retrospective study*, two random samples of size C_1 and C_2 (see Table 1) are selected from the two populations corresponding to the two levels for variable 2. For example, in a restrospective study of the association between family history of alcoholism and a psychiatric disorder, samples would be taken from populations with and without the

TABLE 2. Data Layout for a Hypothetical Randomized Study of the Effect of Lithium on Manic-Depression in Males

		Episodes within 3 months		
		Present	Absent	
Treatment	Lithium	8	22	30
	Placebo	28	12	40
		36	34	70

TABLE 3. Data Layout for a Hypothetical Retrospective Study of the Association Between Family History of Alcoholism and a Particular Psychiatric Disorder

		Disorder		
		Present	Absent	
Family history of alcoholism	Yes	20	5	25
	No	30	55	85
		50	60	110

disorder. A determination of family history status could then be ascertained by a combination of methods, such as examining medical records and interviewing subjects and relatives. Hypothetical data for such a study are given in Table 3; here the samples are selected from subjects having the disorder and from a control group of subjects without the disorder.

Each type of study has its advantages and disadvantages in terms of possible biases, expense, time consumption, and population parameters that can be estimated; again, the reader is referred to an epidemiologic methods textbook for a discussion of the pros and cons of each study design. Our purpose is to discuss a measure of association—the odds ratio—that can be estimated from all three studies. However, before discussing the odds ratio, we first review the most frequently used statistical tests of association.

TESTS OF ASSOCIATION

For all three sampling methods, the null hypothesis of no association between variable 1 and variable 2 can be tested using the familiar *chi-squared statistic*

$$\chi^2 = \frac{(O_{11} - E_{11})^2}{E_{11}} + \frac{(O_{12} - E_{12})^2}{E_{12}} + \frac{(O_{21} - E_{21})^2}{E_{21}} + \frac{(O_{22} - E_{22})^2}{E_{22}},$$

where $E_{ij} = R_i C_j / N$ is the expected frequency for the ijth cell under the null hypothesis of no association. For the lithium study data in Table 2 we have $E_{11} = (30)(36/70) = 30(0.514) = 15.429$; that is, since 51.4% of the subjects had episodes, then under the hypothesis of no association between episodes and treatment we expect that 51.4% of the 30 subjects assigned to the lithium group would have episodes.

If the chi-squared statistic exceeds the $(1 - \alpha)100$th percentile of a chi-squared distribution with 1 degree of freedom, denoted by $\chi^2_{\alpha;1}$, then the null hypothesis of no association is rejected and one concludes that there is an association between variables 1 and 2 (at a significance level equal to α). For example, at a significance level of 0.05, we conclude that there is an association if the calculated χ^2 exceeds $\chi^2_{0.05;1} = 3.84$. This test is intuitive since the chi-squared statistic increases as the observed frequencies deviate more from the expected frequencies. This test is called the *chi-squared test*.

TABLE 4. Data Summary for a Prospective Study

Variable 1	Sample Size	Proportion With Variable 2 Characteristic
Sample 1	R_1	$\hat{p}_1 = O_{11}/R_1$
Sample 2	R_2	$\hat{p}_2 = O_{21}/R_2$

For a prospective study, an alternative to the 2×2 contingency table for summarizing the data is a presentation of the proportion of subjects in the two samples having the variable 2 characteristic, as shown in Table 4. This format is illustrated in Table 5 for the prospective lithium study data given in Table 2. Thus we see that 27% of the subjects taking lithium had episodes within the 3 month period, whereas 70% of subjects not taking lithium had episodes. These sample proportions estimate the corresponding population proportions; that is, for the population of male manic-depressive patients that the subjects in this study were sampled from, we estimate that 27% would not suffer episodes within 3 months if treated with lithium, while 70% would have episodes within 3 months if not treated with lithium.

Similarly, for a retrospective study, we can tabulate the proportion of subjects in the two samples having the variable 1 characteristic, as shown in Table 6. This format is illustrated in Table 7 for the restrospective study data given in Table 3. We see that 40% of the subjects with the psychiatric disorder have a positive family history of alcoholism compared with only 8.3% of the control subjects. The proportions serve as estimates of the corresponding population proportions. Thus, we estimate that 40% of the disorder population have a positive family history of alcoholism compared with 8.3% of the control population.

Let n_1 and n_2 denote the sample sizes (thus for a prospective study $n_1 = R_1$ and $n_2 = R_2$, while for a retrospective study $n_1 = C_1$ and $n_2 = C_2$) and define

$$\bar{p} = (n_1\hat{p}_1 + n_2\hat{p}_2)/(n_1 + n_2).$$

For a prospective study $\bar{p}$ is the overall proportion of observations in the combined samples having the variable 2 characteristic, while for a retrospective study $\bar{p}$ is the proportion of observations in the combined samples having the variable 1 characteristic.

Consider the test statistic

$$z = \frac{\hat{p}_1 - \hat{p}_2}{\hat{\sigma}_{(\hat{p}_1 - \hat{p}_2)}},$$

TABLE 5. Data Summary for the Data in Table 2, Treated as a Prospective Study

Treatment	Sample Size	Proportion Having Episodes Within 3 Mo
Lithium	30	$\hat{p}_1 = 8/30 = 0.27$
Placebo	40	$\hat{p}_2 = 28/40 = 0.70$

TABLE 6. Data Summary for a Retrospective Study

Variable 2	Sample Size	Proportion With Variable 1 Characteristic
Sample 1	C_1	$\hat{p}_1 = O_{11}/C_1$
Sample 2	C_2	$\hat{p}_2 = O_{12}/C_2$

where

$$\hat{\sigma}_{(\hat{p}_1 - \hat{p}_2)} = \sqrt{\bar{p}(1 - \bar{p})\left(\frac{1}{n_1} + \frac{1}{n_2}\right)}$$

is the estimated standard deviation of $\hat{p}_1 - \hat{p}_2$ under the null hypothesis of no association. If $z > z_{\alpha/2}$ or if $z < -z_{\alpha/2}$, where z_α is the $(1 - \alpha)100th$ percentile of the standard normal distribution, then the null hypothesis of no association is rejected at a significance level equal to α. For the usual significance level of $\alpha = 0.05$, we use $z_{0.025} = 1.96$. Under the null hypothesis of no association the population proportions are equal, and hence their difference is zero. Thus this test is intuitive, since it rejects the null hypothesis if the difference of the sample proportions is statistically different from zero. We refer to this test as the *two-sample binomial test*.

It can be shown that $z^2 = \chi^2$ and $(z_{\alpha/2})^2 = \chi^2_{\alpha;1}$. Since rejecting the null hypothesis of no association if $z > z_{\alpha/2}$ or $z < -z_{\alpha/2}$ is equivalent to rejecting the null hypothesis if $z^2 > (z_{\alpha/2})^2$, that is, if $\chi^2 > \chi^2_{\alpha;1}$, we see that the chi-squared test and the two-sample binomial test always agree in terms of rejecting or accepting the null hypothesis. Also, both tests yield the same p value.

The two-sample binomial and chi-squared test should not be used unless the sample sizes are adequate. A conservative rule often given is that all of the expected cell frequencies (the E_{ij} in the chi-squared test) should be at least 5. The reason for this sample size requirement is that, under the null hypothesis, the z statistic has an *approximate* normal distribution and the χ^2 statistics has an *approximate* chi-squared distribution, with the approximations improving as the sample sizes increase. For small sample sizes the approximations are not acceptable.

An alternative to the chi-squared and two-sample binomial tests is *Fisher's exact test*. This test can be used with any sample size. Given specific values for the row and column totals, under the assumption of no association between variables 1 and 2 it is possible to compute the exact probability for each possible 2×2 table. For an observed 2×2 table, a p value can then be calculated by summing the probabilities of all possible tables having the same row and column totals as the observed table and that deviate at least as much as the observed table from the hypothesis of no association. For a stated significance level, the null hypothesis of no association will be rejected if the p value is less

TABLE 7. Data Summary for the Data in Table 3, Treated as a Retrospective Study

Disorder	Sample Size	Proportion With Family History of Alcoholism
Present	50	$\hat{p}_1 = 20/50 = 0.40$
Absent	60	$\hat{p}_2 = 5/60 = 0.08333$

than or equal to the significance level. The computations required for Fisher's exact test are such that this test is almost always performed by using either a table or a computer.

Since Fisher's exact test requires considerably more computer time than the chi-squared (or two-sample binomial) test, especially for large samples, Fisher's exact test has generally been used for small sample sizes with the chi-squared test being used for moderate or large samples sizes. However, as computers have become increasingly faster, Fisher's exact test has been used more frequently for larger sample sizes.

Usually the two tests give similar p values for large sample sizes. In Example 1 (below) we find that the p values for the data for Table 3 resulting from Fisher's exact test and the chi-squared test are both approximately zero.

Although Fisher's exact test has the advantage of yielding exact inference results for any sample size, its disadvantage is that it requires a computer or table to use and is not based on a simple intuitive statistic. The advantage of the chi-squared and two-sample binomial tests is that they are based on intuitive statistics and can easily be performed using a pocket calculator. Thus, although increasing computer speed will lead to more frequent use of Fisher's exact test for large sample sizes, we expect that the chi-squared and two-sample binomial tests will remain important for historical and pedagogical reasons.

Example 1. For the data in Table 3 we perform the chi-squared and two-sample binomial tests using a 0.05 significance level. For the chi-squared test the expected values are $E_{11} = 50(25)/110 = 11.3636$, $E_{12} = 60(25)/110 = 13.6364$, $E_{21} = 50(85)/110 = 38.6364$, and $E_{22} = 60(85)/110 = 46.3636$. Thus

$$\chi^2 = \frac{(20 - 11.3636)^2}{11.3636} + \frac{(5 - 13.6364)^2}{13.6364} +$$

$$\frac{(30 - 38.6364)^2}{38.6364} + \frac{(55 - 46.3636)^2}{46.3636} = 15.573.$$

Since $\chi^2 = 15.573 > \chi^2_{0.05;1} = 3.84$, we reject the null hypothesis of no association and conclude that there is an association between treatment and episodes.

For the two-sample binomial test we have from Table 7 $\hat{p}_1 = 0.4$ and $\hat{p}_2 = 0.08333$. Thus $\bar{p} = (n_1 \hat{p}_1 + n_2 \hat{p}_2)/(n_1 + n_2) = [50(0.4) + 60(0.08333)]/(50 + 60) = 0.22727$. Alternatively, since $\bar{p}$ is the proportion of subjects in the combined samples with a positive family history, we could have computed $\bar{p} = R_1/N = 25/110 = 0.22727$. Our test statistic is given by

$$z = \frac{\hat{p}_1 - \hat{p}_2}{\hat{\sigma}_{\hat{p}_1 - \hat{p}_2}} = \frac{0.4 - 0.08333}{\sqrt{0.22727(0.77273)\left(\frac{1}{50} + \frac{1}{60}\right)}} = 3.9463.$$

Since $z = 3.9463 > z_{0.025} = 1.96$, we reject the null hypothesis of no association and conclude that there is an association between treatment and episodes.

Note that $z^2 = (3.9463)^2 = 15.573 = \chi^2$ and that $z^2_{0.025} = (1.96)^2 = 3.84 = \chi^2_{0.05;1}$, and thus these tests are equivalent.

In Table 8 is a computer program and partial output from a computer analysis of these data using the SAS (Statistical Analysis System) statistical package. The numbers 1 and 2 are used to indicate the two possibilities for each of the dichotomous variables; of course, any two distinct numbers could have been used and the test results would have been the same. The result for the chi-squared and Fisher's exact test are marked by an arrow. The p

TABLE 8. SAS Statements and Partial SAS Output for Example 1

SAS Statements

```
data data1;
    input family disorder count;
cards;
    1  1  20
    1  2  5
    2  1  30
    2  2  55
;
proc freq; weight count;
    table family*disorder  /  chisq cmh;
run;
```

Partial SAS output

Statistics for Table of Family by Disorder			
Statistic	DF	Value	Prob
→ Chi-squared	1	15.573	0.000
Likelihood ratio chi-square	1	16.190	0.000
Continuity adj. chi-square	1	13.822	0.000
Mantel-Haenszel chi-square	1	15.431	0.000
Fisher's exact test (left)			1.000
(right)			8.07E-05
→ (2-tail)			8.91E-05

Estimates of the Common Relative Risk (Row1/Row2)				
			95%	
Type of Study	Method	Value	Confidence	Bounds
→ Case–Control	Mantel-Haenszel	7.333	2.714	19.817
→ (Odds ratio)	Logit	7.333	2.500	21.513
Cohort	Mantel-Haenszel	2.267	1.507	3.410
(Col1 risk)	Logit	2.267	1.600	3.211
Cohort	Mantel-Haenszel	0.309	0.172	0.555
(Col2 risk)	Logit	0.309	0.139	0.688

The confidence bounds for the M-H estimates are test based. Total sample size = 110.

value is the smallest significance level such that we can still reject the null hypothesis, given the data. Thus for the chi-squared test it is that value of α such that $\chi^2_{\alpha;1} = 15.573$, which from the computer output is 0.000 (it is in the column labeled "Prob.") Note that for Fisher's exact test there is no test statistic but just a p value, which in this case is 8.91E-05 = 0.0000891. We see that this p value is in agreement with the p value of 0.000 for the chi-squared test.

Several other measures of association are included in the SAS output: the likelihood ratio chi-squared, the continuity adjusted chi-squared, and the Mantel-Haenszel chi-squared, in addition to one-tailed p values for Fisher's exact test. The continuity adjusted chi-squared is similar to the chi-squared statistic except that it is adjusted slightly with the intent to improve the chi-squared approximation. A brief discussion with references for the likelihood ratio chi-squared and the Mantel-Haenszel chi-squared is included in the *SAS/STAT User's Guide*. For large sample sizes these statistics usually are similar.

The output under "Estimates of the Common Relative Risk (Row1/Row2)" in Table 8 is discussed later in Inference for the Odds Ratio for a Single 2 × 2 Table.

THE ODDS RATIO AS A MEASURE OF ASSOCIATION

Reporting the test of association result is only a first step in an analysis and by itself can be misleading. For example, in many situations one can argue that there must be some, although perhaps not much, association between the two dichotomous variables of interest. For example, males and females may respond somewhat differently to treatments. Thus what we are often interested in is not whether there is an association, but rather the degree of the association.

Furthermore, the result of a hypothesis test is related to the sample size. If there is a true association, then as the sample size increases the probability increases that the hypothesis test will reject the null hypothesis of no association—in statistical terms, the power of the test increases as the sample size increases. Since there is usually some underlying association (although perhaps of not much magnitude) we expect to have a significant test result when very large samples are used. However, finding a statistically significant association means only that we can conclude that there is some association and does not imply that the degree of the association is of practical importance, even if the p value is quite small.

Consider the data for the randomized prospective study of the effect of lithium on manic-depression in males given in Tables 2 and 5. Let p_1 denote the probability (or *risk*) that a male manic-depressive (selected from the same population as the study sample) treated with lithium will have an episode within 3 months, and let p_2 denote the probability that a male manic-depressive given the placebo will have an episode within 3 months. Since $\hat{p}_1 = 0.27$ of the lithium patients had episodes within 3 months compared with $\hat{p}_1 = 0.7$ of the placebo patients (see Table 5), we estimate p_1 and p_2 to be 0.27 and 0.7, respectively.

There are three common ways of estimating the magnitude of the association between the treatment and episodes variables: the *risk difference,* the *relative risk,* and the *odds ratio.* The *risk difference* is the difference of the probabilities, $p_1 - p_2$; the *relative risk* is the ratio of the probabilities, p_1/p_2; and the *odds ratio* is the ratio of the odds for each population, that is, $[p_1/(1 - p_1)]/[p_2/(1 - p_2)]$. These quantities can be estimated by replacing the population probabilities p_1 and p_2 by their sample estimates $\hat{p}_1$ and $\hat{p}_2$. Thus the sample estimate for the risk difference is $0.27 - 0.7 = -0.43$, the sample estimate for the relative risk is $0.27/0.7 = 0.39$, and the sample estimate for the odds ratio is $[0.27/0.73)]/[0.7/0.3] = 0.37/2.33 = 0.16$.

Often it is of interest to compare the degree of association between two dichotomous variables for different populations. For example, suppose that data similar to the lithium study data given in Table 3 for male manic-depressives have been collected for placebo and lithium groups of female manic-depressive patients. Furthermore, suppose that 33% of the female placebo group subjects had episodes within 3 months. What proportion of the female lithium group would we expect to find having episodes after 3 months if the association between treatment and episodes is the same for females as it is for males?

The easy answer is that it just depends on which measure of association that we are using. However, we quickly discover some problems. Since the estimated risk for the male lithium sample is 0.43 less than for the male control sample, then correspondingly the estimated risk for the female lithium sample should be 0.43 less than the estimated risk (0.33) for the female control sample using the risk difference measure, giving us an answer of $0.33 - 0.43 = -0.10$! This clearly is an unsatisfactory answer. Even if the answer had not been negative, it seems clear that the risk difference can be an unsatisfactory measure of association when comparing different populations; for example, a risk difference of 0.10 resulting from proportions of 0.01 and 0.11 intuitively represents a much stronger association than does a risk difference of 0.10 resulting from proportions of 0.50 and 0.60.

Now consider the relative risk measure. Since for the males the estimated risk for the lithium sample is 0.39 of the estimated risk for the control sample, then correspondingly for the females the proportion in the lithium sample having episodes should be 0.39 times the proportion (0.33) in the control sample having episodes, giving us an answer of $0.39(0.33) = 0.13$. There is also a problem with this answer. Suppose that 13% of the females in the lithium sample had an episode. If we alternatively define the risk to be the probability of not having an episode, instead of the probability of having an episode, then for the males the estimated relative risk is $(1 - 0.27)/(1 - 0.7) = 0.73/0.3 = 2.43$, while for the females it is $(1 - 0.13)/(1 - 0.33) = 1.30$. We see that although the sample relative risks are the same for males and females if risk is defined as the probability of having an episode, the sample relative risks are quite different if we define the risk as the probability of not having an episode. For this reason the relative risk can also be problematic when comparing different populations.

Before discussing the odds ratio, let us say a few words about odds in general. If the probability for an event, such as winning a game, is denoted by p, then the odds of the event is defined as the fraction $p/(1 - p)$. Thus, for example, if the probability of winning when playing a slot machine is 0.4, then the odds of winning is $0.4/0.6 = 2/3$ or 0.67. We say that the odds of winning "are 2 to 3," written as 2:3, because, on average, for every 2 wins there are 3 losses. This is a sensible measure for a gambler, because if his odds somehow double, then he is doing twice as well as before, since he is winning twice as many games for each game lost on average as before.

Similarly, the odds is a useful measure for medical data. For the lithium study data for male manic-depressives in Table 2 the population odds of a male patient on lithium having an episode is defined by $p_1/(1 - p_1)$. An estimate for the population odds is the sample odds $\hat{p}_1/(1 - \hat{p}_1) = (8/30)/(22/30) = 8/22 = 0.37$. Thus, for the population of patients given lithium, we estimate that, on average, for every 22 patients not having episodes, 8 will have episodes. Note that the sample odds can be estimated by the number in the sample having the characteristic divided by the number not having it. The sample odds of a male patient on placebo having an episode is $28/12 = 2.67$. The sample odds ratio, $(8/22)/(28/12) = .37/2.33 = 0.16$, compares the odds of having an episode for the lithium sample with the odds of having an episode for the placebo sample and is an estimate of the population odds ratio $[p_1/(1 - p_1)]/[p_2/(1 - p_2)]$. No association between the treatment and episode variables implies that $p_1 = p_2$; that is, male manic-depressives in the placebo and lithium populations have the same probability of having an episode within 3 months. Thus no association also implies that the population odds ratio is equal to 1.

Let us return to the question of what proportion of females on lithium we would expect to have episodes if 33% of the female placebo group had episodes and the association (measured by the odds ratio) between treatment and episodes is the same for males and females. Since the sample odds ratio for the males was 0.16 and the odds of an episode for females in the placebo sample is $0.33/0.67 = 0.49$, we expect the proportion of females in the lithium group who have episodes, denoted by $\hat{p}_{1;\text{fem}}$, to be such that the male and female odds ratios are equal, that is,

$$0.16 = \frac{\hat{p}_{1;\text{fem}}/[1 - \hat{p}_{1;\text{fem}}]}{0.49}.$$

Solving gives us $\hat{p}_{1;\text{fem}} = 0.085$.

Suppose that 8.5% of the females in the lithium group had an episode. We have just shown that for both males and females the sample odds ratio is equal to 0.16. It is easy to show that if we consider the odds of not having an episode instead of the odds of having an episode, then the odds ratios for both the males and females are also equal (they are equal to $1/0.16 = 6.25$). This demonstrates the usefulness of the odds ratio for comparing different populations.

Not only is the odds ratio useful for comparing the association between two dichotomous variables for different populations, it also has a great advantage over the relative risk and the risk difference for a single population when a retrospective sampling scheme is utilized, as shown by the following example. Consider the data for our retrospective study of the association between family history of alcoholism and a particular psychiatric disorder given in Table 3 and summarized in Table 7. From Table 7 we estimated that 40% of the disorder population have a positive family history of alcoholism compared with 8.333% of the control population. Let $p_1^{(f)}$ denote the probability of a subject with the disorder having a positive family history of alcoholism and $p_2^{(f)}$ denote the probability of a subject without the disorder having a positive family history of alcoholism. Because samples were taken from the populations with and without the disorder, the sample estimates $\hat{p}_1 = 0.4$ and $\hat{p}_2 = 0.08333$ estimate $p_1^{(f)}$ and $p_2^{(f)}$, respectively, and thus estimates for the relative difference $p_1^{(f)} - p_2^{(f)}$, the relative risk $p_1^{(f)}/p_2^{(f)}$, and the odds ratio $[p_1^{(f)}/(1 - p_1^{(f)})]/[p_2^{(f)}/(1 - p_2^{(f)})]$ can be estimated by replacing the population probabilities by the sample estimates.

However, since family history of alcoholism is the risk factor, we would like to relate family history of alcoholism to the probability of having the disorder. That is, we are more interested in measures of association that are functions of the risk of having the disorder rather than the risk of having a positive family history of alcoholism. Let $p_1^{(d)}$ denote the probability of a subject with a positive family history of alcoholism having the disorder and $p_2^{(d)}$ denote the probability of a subject without a positive family history of alcoholism having the disorder. Because of the retrospective sampling scheme, these probabilities refer to subjects belonging to either of the two populations (disorder or control) from which the samples were taken. Now, although the relative risk and risk difference based on $p_1^{(d)}$ and $p_2^{(d)}$ are not the same as those based on $p_1^{(f)}$ and $p_2^{(f)}$, it can be shown that the odds ratios are the same; that is,

$$\frac{p_1^{(f)}/(1 - p_1^{(f)})}{p_2^{(f)}/(1 - p_2^{(f)})} = \frac{p_1^{(d)}/(1 - p_1^{(d)})}{p_2^{(d)}/(1 - p_2^{(d)})}$$

Hence, even though $\hat{p}_1 = 0.4$ and $\hat{p}_2 = 0.08333$ are estimates of $p_1^{(f)}$ and $p_2^{(f)}$ and do not estimate $p_1^{(d)}$ and $p_2^{(d)}$, the sample odds ratio $[\hat{p}_1/(1 - \hat{p}_1)]/[\hat{p}_2/(1 - \hat{p}_2)] = [O_{11}/O_{21}]/[O_{12}/O_{22}] = [20/30]/[5/55] = 7.33$ estimates the common odds ratio. Thus we can say that 1) the odds of a subject with a positive family history of alcoholism having the disorder is 7.33 times greater than the odds of a subject without a positive family history of alcoholism having the disorder, or 2) the odds of a subject with the disorder having a family history of alcoholism is 7.33 times greater than the odds of a subject without the disorder having a family history of alcoholism. Clearly the first statement is more meaningful.

In contrast, the risk difference $p_1^{(d)} - p_2^{(d)}$ and relative risk $p_1^{(d)}/p_2^{(d)}$ cannot be estimated by replacing $p_1^{(d)}$ and $p_2^{(d)}$ by $\hat{p}_1$ and $\hat{p}_2$, since these are estimates of $p_1^{(f)}$ and $p_2^{(f)}$. Furthermore, because of the sampling scheme, sample estimates of $p_1^{(d)}$ and $p_2^{(d)}$ are not available. However, if $p_1^{(d)}$ and $p_2^{(d)}$ are small, then it can be shown that the odds ratio provides an approximation to the relative risk $p_1^{(d)}/p_2^{(d)}$, showing yet another advantage of the odds ratio.

INFERENCE FOR THE ODDS RATIO FOR A SINGLE 2 × 2 TABLE

For a retrospective study, the population and sample odds ratios are defined in the same way as for a prospective study, except with the roles of variable 1 and variable 2 reversed. Thus for a prospective study the sample odds are defined by

$$\hat{\psi} = (O_{11}/O_{12})/(O_{12}/O_{22}), \tag{1}$$

and for a restrospective study the sample odds are defined by

$$\hat{\psi} = (O_{11}/O_{21})/(O_{21}/O_{22}), \tag{2}$$

But Eqs. 1 and 2 are both equal to

$$\hat{\psi} = \frac{O_{11}O_{22}}{O_{21}O_{12}}, \tag{3}$$

which estimates the population odds ratio, which is the same regardless of whether we define the risk as the probability of a subject having the variable 1 characteristic or as the probability of a subject having the variable 2 characteristic. For a cross-sectional study the population odds ratio is defined in terms of conditional probabilities, treating one of the variables as fixed (that is, as a risk variable) and the other variable as the response variable. The sample odds ratio for a cross-sectional study is also given by Eq. 3. Thus, inference using the odds ratio does not depend on which sampling design—prospective, retrospective, or cross-sectional—is employed, which is another desirable quality of the odds ratio.

We discuss two methods for obtaining a confidence interval for the odds ratio. Let ψ denote the true odds ratio. A 95% confidence interval for ψ using the method proposed by Miettinen (1976), which is a test-based method, is given by

$$\hat{\psi}^{(1 \pm 1.96/\sqrt{\chi^2})}. \tag{4}$$

More generally, to obtain a $(1 - \alpha)100\%$ confidence interval, replace 1.96 by $z_{\alpha/2}$ in the confidence interval expression. Although this confidence interval method is strictly valid only if the odds ratio is equal to 1, for most practical purposes it is sufficiently accurate. Rosner (1990) cautions that this method should be used only if $0.2 \leq \hat{\psi} \leq 5.0$. This confidence interval procedure has the desirable property of always agreeing with the chi-squared test in the sense that if the chi-squared test statistic is significant at, say, the 0.05 significance level, then the 95% confidence interval for the common odds ratio defined by Eq. 4 will not include 1, while if the chi-squared test is not signficant, then the confidence interval will include 1.

Alternatively, a 95% confidence interval for $\log \hat{\psi}$ is given by

$$\log \hat{\psi} \pm 1.96 z_{\alpha/2} \hat{\sigma}_{\log \hat{\psi}}, \tag{5}$$

where

$$\hat{\sigma}^2_{\log \hat{\psi}} = \frac{1}{O_{11}} + \frac{1}{O_{12}} + \frac{1}{O_{21}} + \frac{1}{O_{22}}.$$

is the estimated variance of $\log \hat{\psi}$. It is assumed that each $O_{ij} > 0$; if not, then 0.5 is added to each cell. A 95% confidence interval for ψ is obtained by taking antilogarithms of the endpoints of the confidence interval for $\log \psi$. This procedure requires a large sample size, as does the previous procedure, but, unlike the previous procedure, it is valid regardless of the value of ψ. More generally, a $(1 - \alpha)100\%$ confidence interval results if 1.96 is replaced by $z_{\alpha/2}$ in the confidence interval expression.

Usually the interpretation of the odds ratio and its confidence interval compares the odds of the variable 2 (or outcome variable) characteristic occurring for each level of variable 1 (the antecedent or risk variable), regardless of which sampling method is used.

Example 2. Again consider the data for the retrospective study of the association between family history of alcoholism and a particular psychiatric disorder given in Table 3. We have

$$\hat{\psi} = \frac{O_{11} O_{22}}{O_{21} O_{12}} = \frac{20(55)}{30(5)} = 7.33,$$

and

$$\hat{\sigma}^2_{\log \hat{\psi}} = \frac{1}{O_{11}} + \frac{1}{O_{12}} + \frac{1}{O_{21}} + \frac{1}{O_{22}} = \frac{1}{20} + \frac{1}{5} + \frac{1}{30} + \frac{1}{55} = 0.3015.$$

Thus $\hat{\sigma}_{\log \hat{\psi}} = \sqrt{0.3015} = 0.549$, and a 95% confidence interval using Eq. 5 for $\log \psi$ is given by

$$\log(7.33) \pm 1.96(0.549) = (0.91594, 3.0680).$$

Taking the antilogs of the endpoints gives the 95% confidence interval for ψ:

$$[\exp(0.91594), \exp(3.0680)] = (2.50, 21.50).$$

Interpretation: We have 95% confidence that the odds of a subject with a positive family history of alcoholism having the disorder are between 2.50 and 21.50 times greater than the odds of a subject without a positive family history of alcoholism having the disorder.

In the SAS output in Table 8 (under "Estimates of the Common Relative Risk" for the case–control study) the test-based confidence interval given by Eq. 4 is labeled "Mantel-Haenszel," while the one based on Eq. 5 is labeled "Logit." Our calculation of the Logit confidence interval agrees (except for a slight rounding error) with the SAS confidence interval of (2.500, 21.513). From the SAS output the 95% confidence interval using the test-based method is (2.714, 19.817). Since the estimated odds ratio ($\hat{\psi} = 7.33$) is greater than 5, the Logit confidence interval is preferable.

ODDS RATIO INFERENCE AND TESTS OF ASSOCIATION FOR SEVERAL 2 × 2 TABLES

Consider the data for the study of the effect of lithium on manic depression in males given in Table 2. In Table 9 are hypothetical data collected for female manic depressives.

If the probability of an episode is related to sex (that is, sex is a confounding variable), then the combined population odds ratio can be quite different from the sex-specific odds ratios, even if the sex-specific odds ratios are equal, and thus we would want to control for the sex variable. This can be done by testing the null hypothesis of no association between treatment and episodes for males and for females using the Mantel-Haenszel test (Mantel and Haenszel, 1959; Mantel, 1963) described below. If there is a significant association, then the degree of association between the treatment and episodes variables can be estimated separately for males and females. If the two odds ratios are similar, then it is also meaningful to estimate a weighted average of the odds ratios to summarize the degree of association.

More generally, in this section we consider the situation where the data have been stratified into K subgroups (or strata) with respect to one or more suspected confounding variables, in order to make the subjects within each stratum more homogeneous. The data

TABLE 9. Data Layout for a Hypothetical Randomized Study of the Effect of Lithium on Manic Depression in Females

		Episodes within 3 months		
		Present	Absent	
Treatment	Lithium	15	105	120
	Placebo	43	57	100
		58	162	220

TABLE 10. Data Layout for a 2 × 2 Contingency Table for the kth Stratum, for $k = 1, \ldots, K$

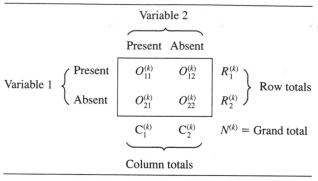

for the kth stratum ($k = 1, \ldots, K$) can be summarized in a 2 × 2 contingency table relating variable 1 to variable 2, as shown in Table 10. The Mantel-Haenszel test, described below, is used to test the null hypothesis of no association between variables 1 and 2 for each of the K strata.

The rationale for the Mantel-Haenszel test is as follows: Under the null hypothesis of no association for each stratum and conditional on the row and margin totals, the expected value of $O_{11}^{(k)}$, the frequency in the first cell of the kth table, is given by

$$E_{11}^{(k)} = R_1^{(k)} C_1^{(k)} / N^{(k)}$$

and the variance of $O_{11}^{(k)}$ is

$$V_{11}^{(k)} = \frac{C_1^{(k)} C_2^{(k)} R_1^{(k)} R_2^{(k)}}{N^{(k)} N^{(k)} [N^{(k)} - 1]}.$$

Let X denote the sum of the frequencies in the first cells of the K tables; that is,

$$X = \sum_{k=1}^{K} O_{11}^{(k)}.$$

It follows that the expected value and variance of X are

$$E(X) = \sum_{k=1}^{K} E_{11}^{(k)} \quad \text{and} \quad V(X) = \sum_{k=1}^{K} V_{11}^{(k)}.$$

The Mantel-Haenszel test statistic is given by

$$\chi_{MH}^2 = \frac{[X - E(X)]^2}{V(X)} = \frac{\left[\sum_{k=11}^{K} O_{11}^{(k)} - \sum_{k=1}^{K} E_{11}^{(k)} \right]^2}{\sum_{k=1}^{K} V_{11}^{(k)}},$$

which has an approximate chi-squared distribution with one degree of freedom under the null hypothesis. Thus, for a significance level equal to α, we reject the null hypothesis of no association if $X^2_{MH} > \chi_{\alpha;1}$. The Mantel-Haenszel test can be used if either the $N^{(k)}$ are large or if K is large (even if the $N^{(k)}$ are small.)

Since we have conditioned on the row and column totals in each table (that is, we have treated them as fixed), then, from knowing the frequency in the first cell of a table the other three cell frequencies can be found. Hence they do not provide any additional information concerning the association, explaining why the Mantel-Haenszel statistic is based only on one of the frequencies in each table.

Note that X^2_{MH} tends to be large if $O^{(k)}_{11}$ is consistently larger or consistently smaller than $E^{(k)}_{11}$, while it can be close to zero if $O^{(k)}_{11}$ is greater than $E^{(k)}_{11}$ for some strata and $O^{(k)}_{11}$ is less than $E^{(k)}_{11}$ for other strata. Thus the Mantel-Haenszel test is designed for the alternative hypothesis of a consistent association between variable 1 and variable 2 across the K strata—that is, most of the strata-specific odds ratios are greater than 1 or most of them are less than 1. The test has little power to detect an association where some of the stratum-specific odds ratios are less than 1 and some are greater than 1.

An estimate of a weighted average of the stratum-specific odds ratios is provided by the Mantel-Haenszel estimator

$$\hat{\psi}_{MH} = \frac{\sum_{k=1}^{K}[O^{(k)}_{11}O^{(k)}_{22}/N^{(k)}]}{\sum_{k=1}^{K}[O^{(k)}_{21}O^{(k)}_{12}/N^{(k)}]}.$$

If the stratum-specific odds ratios are equal, then $\hat{\psi}_{MH}$ estimates the common odds ratio. If the individual odds ratios differ greatly, then usually we would want to estimate them separately rather than estimate an average of them.

We discuss two methods for finding a confidence interval for the common odds ratio (or for a weighted average of the odds ratios if they are not equal) that are similar to those discussed above for a single 2×2 table (see Inference for the Odds Ratio for a Single 2×2 Table). A 95% confidence interval using the test-based method proposed by Miettinen (1976) is given by

$$\hat{\psi}_{MH}^{(1 \pm 1.96/\sqrt{X^2_{MH}})}. \tag{6}$$

More generally, to obtain a $(1 - \alpha)100\%$ confidence interval, replace 1.96 by $z_{\alpha/2}$ in the confidence interval expression. Remarks similar to those made about the test-based confidence interval of Eq. 4 also pertain to this method: the method is strictly valid only if the common odds ratio is equal to 1, Rosner (1990) cautions that this method should be used only if $0.2 \leq X^2_{MH} \leq 5.0$, and this procedure always agrees with the Mantel-Haenszel test.

The second confidence interval method is similar to the confidence interval given by Eq. 5. Let

$$\hat{\psi}^{(k)} = \frac{O^{(k)}_{11}O^{(k)}_{22}}{O^{(k)}_{21}O^{(k)}_{12}}$$

denote the odds ratio estimate for the kth stratum. Define the "pooled estimate" by

$$\log \hat{\psi}_p = \frac{\sum_{k=1}^{K} w^{(k)} \log \hat{\psi}^{(k)}}{\sum_{k=1}^{K} w^{(k)}},$$

where

$$w^{(k)} = [\hat{\sigma}^2_{\log \hat{\psi}(k)}]^{-1} = \left(\frac{1}{O_{11}} + \frac{1}{O_{12}} + \frac{1}{O_{21}} + \frac{1}{O_{22}}\right)^{-1}$$

Thus $\log \hat{\psi}_p$ is a weighted average of the stratum-specific sample log odds ratio estimates, with each $\log \hat{\psi}^{(k)}$ weighted by the inverse of its estimated variance, and it provides an estimate of the corresponding weighted average of the population log odds ratios. A 95% confidence interval is obtained by taking the antilogarithms of the endpoints of the interval

$$\log \hat{\psi}_p \pm 1.96 \hat{\sigma}_{\log \hat{\psi}_p}, \tag{7}$$

where

$$\hat{\sigma}^2_{\log \hat{\psi}_p} = \left[\sum_{k=1}^{K} w^{(k)}\right]^{-1}.$$

Note that the estimate $\hat{\psi}_p$ of the common odds ratio differs from the Mantel-Haenszel estimate $\hat{\psi}_{MH}$.

The Breslow-Day (1980) test can be used to test the null hypothesis of homogeneity of odds ratios, that is, that the strata-specific odds ratios are equal. Although this test is not suited for hand calculation, it is included in the SAS FREQ procedure. This test requires a large sample size within each stratum. However, even if the assumption of homogeneity of odds ratios does not hold, the two confidence interval procedures discussed are still valid procedures for estimating a weighted average of the odds ratios, although it usually will be more useful to examine confidence intervals for individual odds ratios when the odds ratios differ substantially. In addition to performing the Breslow-Day test, it is advisable to compute the stratum-specific odds ratios in order to get some idea of the degree of heterogeneity.

Example 3. For the data for the randomized study of the effect of lithium on manic-depression in males and females given in Tables 2 and 9: 1) estimate the sex-specific odds ratios; 2) test if the sex-specific odds ratios are equal using the Breslow-Day test; 3) test the null hypothesis of no association, controlling for sex, using the Mantel-Haenszel test; 4) estimate a weighted average of the odds ratios using the Mantel-Haenszel estimate and $\hat{\psi}_p$; and 5) give 95% confidence intervals for the weighted average of the odds ratios. In Table 11 is a partial output from a SAS analysis of these data. Pertinent results are indicated by an arrow.

TABLE 11. SAS Statements and Partial SAS Output for Example 3

SAS Statements

```
data data1;
    input sex $ treatmnt episodes count ;
cards;
    male 1 1 8
    male 1 2 22
    male 2 1 28
    male 2 2 12
    female 1 1 15
    female 1 2 105
    female 2 1 43
    female 2 2 57
;
proc freq; weight count;
    table sex*treatmnt*episodes / chisq cmh;
run;
```

Partial SAS output

Summary of Cochran-Mantel-Haenszel Statistics (Based on Table Scores) for Treatment by Episodes Controlling for Sex

	Statistic	Alternative Hypothesis	DF	Value	Prob
→	1	Nonzero correlation	1	38.655	0.000
→	2	Row mean scores differ	1	38.655	0.000
→	3	General association		38.655	0.000

Estimates of the Common Relative Risk (Row1/Row2)

	Type of Study	Method	Value	95% Confidence	Bounds
→	Case–Control	Mantel-Haenszel	0.179	0.104	0.308
→	(Odds ratio)	Logit	0.179	0.102	0.315
	Cohort	Mantel-Haenszel	0.321	0.225	0.460
	(Col1 risk)	Logit	0.325	0.217	0.486
	Cohort	Mantel-Haenszel	1.664	1.417	1.954
	(Col2 risk)	Logit	1.616	1.360	1.921

The confidence bounds for the M-H estimates are test based.

→ Breslow-Day Test for Homogeneity of the Odds Ratios

Chi-squared = 0.093   DF = 1   Prob = 0.760

Total sample size = 290.

Solutions:

1. Letting $\hat{\psi}_1$ and $\hat{\psi}_2$ denote the sample odds ratio for the males and females, respectively, we have $\hat{\psi}_1 = 8(12)/[28(22)] = 0.1558$ and $\hat{\psi}_2 = 15(57)/[43(105)] = 0.1894$. Thus we see that the two odds ratio estimates are quite close. *Interpretation:* We es-

timate that the odds of a male manic-depressive on lithium having an episode within 3 months are 16% of the odds for a male manic-depressive in the control group. For a female manic-depressive on lithium, the estimated odds for the lithium group are 19% of the odds for the control group.

2. Based on the Breslow-Day test results reported in the SAS output in Table 11 there is not sufficient evidence to conclude that the sex-specific odds ratios are different ($p = 0.76$). (Note: we would have rejected the null hypothesis of homogeneity at, say, the 0.05 significance level if the p value was less than 0.05.)

3. Computations for the Mantel-Haenszel test statistic:

$$O_{11}^{(1)} = 8 \qquad O_{11}^{(2)} = 15 \qquad X = 8 + 15 = 23$$

$$E_{11}^{(1)} = 36(30)/70 = 15.4286 \quad E_{11}^{(2)} = 58(120)/220 = 31.6364$$

$$E(X) = 15.4286 + 31.6364 = 47.065$$

$$V_{11}^{(1)} = \frac{36(34)(30)40}{70(70)69} = 4.3443 \qquad V_{11}^{(2)} = \frac{58(162)(120)100}{220(220)219} = 10.6374$$

$$V(X) = 4.3443 + 10.6374 = 14.9817$$

$$\chi_{MH}^2 = \frac{[X - E(X)]^2}{V(X)} = \frac{(23 - 47.065)^2}{14.9817} = 38.655$$

Since $\chi_{MH}^2 = 38.655 > \chi_{0.05;1} = 3.84$, we reject the null hypothesis of no association and conclude that there is an association between treatment and episodes, controlling for sex ($\alpha = 0.05$). In agreement with our calculations, the SAS output also gives the same value for the Mantel-Haenszel statistic and gives a corresponding p value of 0.000.

4.
$$\hat{\psi}_{MH} = \frac{8(12)/70 + 15(57)/220}{28(22)/70 + 43(105)/220} = .179$$

is the Mantel-Haenszel estimate of the weighted average of the odds ratios.
Computations for $\hat{\psi}_p$:

$$w^{(1)} = \left(\frac{1}{8} + \frac{1}{28} + \frac{1}{22} + \frac{1}{12} \right)^{-1} = 3.4542$$

$$w^{(2)} = \left(\frac{1}{15} + \frac{1}{43} + \frac{1}{105} + \frac{1}{57} \right)^{-1} = 8.5477$$

$$\log\hat{\psi}_p = \frac{(3.4542)\log(0.1558) + 8.5477\log(0.1894)}{3.4542 + 8.5477} = -1.720099$$

$$\hat{\psi}_p = \exp(-1.720099) = 0.1790$$

In this example the two estimates $\hat{\psi}_{MH}$ and $\hat{\psi}_p$ are the same. Since the Breslow-Day test is not significant, the sample sizes are large (hence the Breslow-Day test is valid), and the sample odds ratios are close, we consider that these estimates are for a common odds ratio. *Interpretation:* We estimate that the odds of a manic-depressive on lithium having an episode within 3 months is 18% of the odds of a manic-depressive in the control group having an episode, controlling for sex.

5. Computations for a 95% confidence interval using Eq. 7:

$$\hat{\sigma}^2_{\log\hat{\psi}_p} = [w^{(1)} + w^{(2)}]^{-1} = (3.4542 + 8.5477)^{-1} = 0.0833201$$

$$\hat{\sigma}_{\log\hat{\psi}_p} = \sqrt{0.0833201} = 0.2886$$

$$\log\hat{\psi}_p \pm 1.96\,\hat{\sigma}_{\log\hat{\psi}_p} = -1.720099 \pm 1.96(0.2886) = (-2.285755, -1.154443)$$

95% confidence interval for $\hat{\psi}_p$:

$$[\exp(-2.285755), \exp(-1.154443)] = (0.1017, 0.3152).$$

Interpretation: We have 95% confidence that the odds of having an episode within 3 months for a manic-depressive lithium patient is between 10% and 32% of the odds for a manic-depressive control patient, controlling for sex.

This confidence interval can be found in the section "Estimates of the Common Relative Risk" in the SAS output in Table 11 and is called the "Logit" method for the case–control type of study, The first confidence interval (0.104, 0.308) for the case–control type of study, labeled "Mantel-Haenszel," is the 95% confidence interval using the test-based interval given by Eq. 6.

MATCHED-PAIRS ANALYSIS

A matched-pairs analysis is a stratified analysis where each stratum consists of a sample size of two, with one subject at one level of the risk variable (variable 1) and the other subject at the other level of the risk variable. For example, in a randomized prospective study comparing two treatments (drug vs. placebo), subjects are matched according to similarity of suspected confounding variables (such as age and sex), and then one member of each pair is randomly assigned to one of the treatments, with the other member receiving the other treatment. Table 12 shows how matched-pairs data are usually summarized.

TABLE 12. Data Layout for Matched-Pairs Data

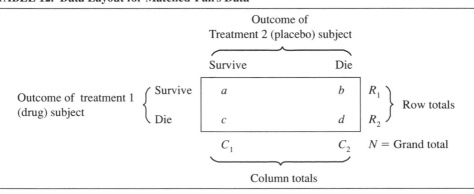

Although Table 12 looks similar to the 2×2 contingency table in Table 1 for un-matched data, it is quite different in that it treats the matched pair as the basic unit rather than the individual subject. For example, in Table 12, a is the number of matched pairs for which both subjects survived, while b is the number of matched pairs for which the subject assigned to treatment 1 survived while the subject assigned to treatment 2 died. Furthermore, there are N pairs, or $2(N)$ subjects.

Using the analysis methods of the previous section, it can be shown the Mantel-Haenszel test statistic for testing the null hypothesis of no association is given by

$$\chi^2_{MH} = \frac{(b - c)^2}{b + c}.$$

The null hypothesis of no association is rejected if $\chi^2_{MH} > \chi^2_{\alpha;1}$. This test is equivalent to McNemar's test. An estimate of the common odds ratio (odds of a treatment 1 subject surviving divided by the odds of a treatment 2 subject surviving) is

$$\hat{\psi}_{MH} = b/c.$$

If homogeneity of the odds ratios is not assumed, then $\hat{\psi}_{MH}$ is an estimate of a weighted average of the odds ratios. A 95% confidence interval for the common odds ratio (or weighted average) is given by

$$(b/c)\exp(\pm 1.96 \sqrt{1/b + 1/c}),$$

where it is assumed that b and c are greater than 0.

Example 4. Consider the following randomized matched prospective study of the effect of lithium on manic-depression in males. Sixty manic-depressive males are matched according to age (within 5 years) and clinical condition (mild, moderate, or severe), resulting in 30 matched pairs. Using random assignment, one member of each pair is assigned to the lithium treatment and the other member to the placebo. The data for this study are summarized in Table 13. We see, for example, that there are two matched pairs where both subjects had seizures within 3 months.

An estimate of the common odds ratio is $\hat{\psi}_{MH} = 6/19 = 0.316$, and a 95% confidence interval for the common odds ratio is given by

TABLE 13. Data Summary for a Randomized Matched-Pairs Prospective Study of the Effect of Lithium on Manic-Depression in Males

		Episodes within 3 months for subject on placebo		
		Present	Absent	
Episodes within 3 months for subject on lithium	Present	2	6	8
	Absent	19	3	22
		21	9	30

$$(6/19)\exp(\pm 1.96 \sqrt{1/6 + 1/19}) = (0.045, 2.24).$$

Interpretation: We have 95% confidence that the odds of having an episode within 3 months for a male manic-depressive lithium patient is between 0.045 and 2.24 times the odds for a male manic-depressive control patient, controlling for age and clinical condition.

LOGISTIC REGRESSION

We conclude this chapter by showing how the ideas discussed thus far can be viewed within the more general logistic regression framework. For our discussion it is assumed that the reader is acquainted with multiple linear regression analysis.

We consider the situation where we are interested in studying the relationship between a dichotomous outcome (or response or dependent) variable and several independent (or explanatory) variables; the independent variables can be either quantitative (continuous or discrete) or qualitative. The two levels of the outcome variable will be coded as 1 and 0, with 1 corresponding to the occurrence of the event of interest. For example, in our randomized prospective study of the effect of lithium on manic-depression, we consider episodes (1 = presence of episodes, 0 = absence of episodes) to be the outcome variable and treatment and sex to be the independent variables. We are interested in how treatment and episodes are related after controlling for sex. Although all of these variables are qualitative, we might also want to consider controlling for quantitative variables, such as age or income. Using the Mantel-Haenszel procedure, we can control for quantitative variables only if we categorize them (for example, age: <30, 30−50, >50).

In least-squares regression, the mean of the outcome variable is modeled as a linear function of the independent variables. For example, in the simple linear regression model, the model is

$$E(Y|x) = \beta_0 + \beta_1 x,$$

where x is a value of the independent variable and $E(Y|x)$ is the mean (or expected value) of Y given x. In this model, each unit increase in x results in an increase equal to β_1 in the expected value of Y.

Now suppose that Y is a dichotomous variable with its levels coded as 1 and 0. Then the expected value of Y is just the probability of the event corresponding to level 1; that is, $p_x = E(Y|x)$ is the probability that $Y = 1$ given x. Thus we might consider a model similar to the one above where we model p_x as a linear function of the independent variable:

$$p_x = \beta_0 + \beta_1 x. \tag{8}$$

However, there are two problems with this model. First of all, p_x is bounded by 0 and 1, but the equation $\beta_0 + \beta_1 x$ is not bounded by 0 and 1; hence this model could produce absurd estimates for p_x. Second, we have already argued that an increase in p_x from, say, 0.01 to 0.10, is intuitively more of an increase than an increase from 0.50 to 0.60. Thus, although each unit increase in x results in an increase equal to β_1 in p_x, the practical effect of the change depends on the base value of p_x and hence on the value of x.

The *logistic regression model* models the log of the odds as a linear function of the independent variables. For one independent variable the model is

$$\log \frac{p_x}{1 - p_x} = \beta_0 + \beta_1 x.$$

The function $\log[p_x/(1 - p_x)]$ is called the *logit function* of p_x. This model overcomes the two problems inherent in Eq. 8. Since the odds can be between 0 and ∞, then the range of the log of the odds is $(-\infty, \infty)$, which is the same as the range of the function $\beta_0 + \beta_1 x$. Furthermore, now a one unit increase in x results in a *proportionate* increase in the odds equal to $\exp(\beta_1)$. For example, if an increase in x from 1 to 2 doubles the odds, similarly an increase in x from 10 to 11 will also double the odds. Hence, the practical effect of a unit increase in x on p_x does not depend on the value of x.

The logistic regression approach has two main advantages over the stratification approach described in the previous sections: 1) Quantitative independent variables do not have to be categorized, and 2) the investigator can much more thoroughly investigate the relationship between the response probability and the independent variables. The advantage of the stratification approach is its conceptual simplicity. In the following example we show how the stratification approach can be viewed within the context of the logistic regression framework, but it is beyond the scope of this chapter to demonstrate the flexibility of analysis provided by the logistic regression model that is not available with the stratification approach (for a more detailed discussion, see Kleinbaum et al., 1982, Chapter 21).

Example 5. For the male manic-depressive data in Table 2 the outcome variable is episodes and the independent variable is treatment. Consider the logistic regression model

$$\log \frac{p_x}{1 - p_x} = \beta_0 + \beta_1 x, \tag{9}$$

where x is the treatment ($x = 1$ if lithium, $x = 0$ if placebo) and p_x is the probability of a subject given treatment x having episodes within 3 months. Thus $p_{x=1}$ is the probability of a subject on lithium having episodes within 3 months, while $p_{x=0}$ is the probability of a subject on placebo having episodes within 3 months. In Eq. 9 the log of the odds of having episodes is modeled as a function of treatment only.

In Table 14 are the SAS statements and output for fitting Eq. 9 and two other models using the method of maximum likelihood estimation. The output for Eq. 9 is titled "Males only." We see that the treatment variable is statistically significant (p value $= 0.0006$) from the "Analysis of Maximum Likelihood Estimates" section of the SAS output, and thus we conclude that there is an association between treatment and episodes. The parameter estimates are $\hat{\beta}_0 = 0.8473$ and $\hat{\beta}_1 = -1.8589$. Since the odds ratio (the odds of a lithium group subject having an episode divided by the odds of a control group subject having an episode) is given by

$$\psi = \frac{\dfrac{p_{x=1}}{1 - p_{x=1}}}{\dfrac{p_{x=0}}{1 - p_{x=0}}},$$

it follows from Eq. 9 that $\psi = \exp(\beta^1)$. Hence the maximum likelihood estimate of ψ is $\hat{\psi} = \exp(\hat{\beta}_1) = \exp(-1.8589) = 0.156$, which is the same as $\hat{\psi} = 8(12)/[28(22)]$, as calculated using Eq. 3.

In the second model we use the male and female manic-depressive data from Tables 2 and 10 and model the log of the odds of having an episode as a function of treatment and sex by fitting the model

$$\log \frac{p_{x_1,x_2}}{1 - p_{x_1,x_2}} = \beta_0 + \beta_1 x_1 + \beta_2 x_2. \tag{10}$$

In this model x_1 is the treatment variable ($1 =$ lithium, $0 =$ placebo), x_2 is the sex variable ($1 =$ male, $0 =$ female), and p_{x_1,x_2} is the probability of an episode for a subject with treatment $= x_1$ and sex $= x_2$. It can be shown that this model assumes a common odds ratio—that is, the odds of a lithium group subject having an episode divided by the odds of a control group subject having an episode is the same for each sex. From the SAS output (titled "Males and females—main effects model") we see that treatment and sex are each significant. Since the p value for treatment is 0.0001, we conclude that there is a significant asociation between treatment and episodes, controlling for sex ($p = 0.0001$). Note that this was the same conclusion reached in Example 3 using the Mantel-Haenszel test (there $p = 0.000$).

We can also compute an estimate for the common odds ratio by noting that, for a given value of x_2, the common odds ratio is given by

$$\psi = \frac{\dfrac{p_{x_1 = 1,x2}}{1 - p_{x_1 = 1,x2}}}{\dfrac{p_{x_1 = 0,x2}}{1 - p_{x_1 = 0,x2}}},$$

and hence it follows from (10) that $\psi = \exp(\beta^1)$. Thus the maximum likelihood estimate of ψ is $\hat{\psi} = \exp(\hat{\beta}_1) = \exp(-1.7211) = 0.1789$, which agrees with $\hat{\psi}_{MH}$ and $\hat{\psi}_p$ computed in Example 3.

A 95% confidence interval for the common odds ratio is given by the interval $\exp(\hat{\beta}_1 \pm 1.96\ \hat{\sigma}_{\hat{\beta}_1})$, where $\hat{\sigma}_{\hat{\beta}_1}$ is the estimated standard deviation for $\hat{\beta}_1$. From the SAS output we have $\hat{\sigma}_{\hat{\beta}_1} = 0.2891$. Thus our 95% confidence interval is $(0.1015, 0.3152)$, which agrees very closely with the intervals given in Example 3.

The third model is

$$\log \frac{p_x}{1 - p_x} = \beta_0 + \beta_1 x_1 + \beta_2 x_2 + \beta_3 x_1 x_2, \tag{11}$$

TABLE 14. SAS Statements and Partial SAS Output for Three Logistic Regression Models Fitted to the Manic-Depressive Data

SAS Statements

```
data data1;
   input treatmnt episodes n;
cards;
   1  8  30
   0  28  40
;
proc logistic data=data1;
   model episodes/n = treatmnt;
   title 'males only'
data data2;
   input sex treatmnt episodes n;
   sex_trmt = sex*treatmnt;
cards
   1  1  8   30
   1  0  28  40
   0  1  15  120
   0  0  43  100
;
proc logistic data=data2;
   model episodes/n = sex treatmnt;
   title 'males and females -- main effects model';
proc logistic data=data2;
   model episodes/n = sex treatmnt sex_trmt;
   title 'males and females -- full model';
```

SAS output

Males only

The LOGISTIC Procedure

Data Set: WORK.DATA1
Response Variable (Events): EPISODES
Response Variable (Trials): N
Number of Observations: 2
Link Function: Logit

Response Profile

Ordered Value	Binary Outcome	Count
1	EVENT	36
2	NO EVENT	34

Analysis of Maximum Likelihood Estimates

Variable	Parameter Estimate	Standard Error	Wald Chi-Square	Pr > Chi-Square	Standardized Estimate
INTERCEPT	0.8473	0.3450	6.0305	0.0141	
TREATMNT	−1.8589	0.5381	11.9360	0.0006	−0.510838

TABLE 14. SAS Statements and Partial SAS Output for Three Logistic Regression Models Fitted to the Manic-Depressive Data *(Continued)*

Males and females—main effects model.

The LOGISTIC Procedure

Data Set: WORK.DATA2
Response Variable (Events): EPISODES
Response Variable (Trials): N
Number of Observations: 4
Link Function: Logit

Response Profile

Ordered Value	Binary Outcome	Count
1	EVENT	96
2	NO EVENT	196

Analysis of Maximum Likelihood Estimates

Variable	Parameter Estimate	Standard Error	Wald Chi-Square	Pr > Chi-Square	Standardized Estimate
INTERCEPT	−0.2622	0.1912	1.8803	0.1703	
SEX	−1.0525	0.3088	11.6149	0.0007	0.248751
TREATMNT	−1.7211	0.2891	35.4318	0.0001	−0.474985

Males and females—full model.

The LOGISTIC Procedure

Data Set: WORK.DATA2
Response Variable (Events): EPISODES
Response Variable (Trials): N
Number of Observations: 4
Link Function: Logit

Response Profile

Ordered Value	Binary Outcome	Count
1	EVENT	94
2	NO EVENT	196

Analysis of Maximum Likelihood Estimates

Variable	Parameter Estimate	Standard Error	Wald Chi-Square	Pr > Chi-Square	Standardized Estimate
INTERCEPT	−0.2819	0.2020	1.9471	0.1629	
SEX	1.1291	0.3998	7.9762	0.0047	0.266854
TREATMNT	−1.6641	0.3420	23.6694	0.0001	−0.459242
SEX_TRMT	−0.1948	0.6376	0.0934	0.7599	−0.032771

with x_1 and x_2 being defined as in Eq. 10. The output for this model is titled "Males and females—full model." In this model we have included the interaction term x_1x_2, which represents the interaction between treatment and sex. It can be shown that this third model does not assume a common odds ratio, unless $\beta_3 = 0$. From the output we see that the p value for the interaction term is 0.7599. Thus there is not sufficient evidence to conclude that $\beta_3 \neq 0$; that is, there is not sufficient evidence to conclude that the odds ratios are not homogeneous. Note that this p value agrees with the Breslow-Day p value of 0.760 in Example 3.

ACKNOWLEDGMENTS

This work was partially supported by The University of Iowa Psychiatric Epidomiology/Biostatistics Training Program, NIMH grant MH15168.

REFERENCES

Breslow N, Day NE (1980). "Statistical Methods in Cancer Research, vol I, The Analysis of Case–Control Studies." Lyon: IARC.

Kleinbaum DG, Kupper LL, Morgenstern H (1982)."Epidemiologic Research: Principles and Quantitative Methods." Belmont, CA: Wadsworth.

Mantel N (1963). Chi-square tests with one degree of freedom: Extensions of the Mantel-Haenszel procedure. J Am Stat Assoc 58:690–700.

Mantel N, Haenszel W (1959). Statistical aspects of the analysis of data from retrospective studies of disease. J Natl Cancer Inst 22:719–748.

Miettinen OS (1985). "Theoretical Epidemiology: Principles of Occurrence, Research in Medicine." New York: Wiley.

Miettinin OS (1976): Estimability and estimation in case-referent studies. Am J Epidemiol 103:226–235.

Rosner B (1990). "Fundamentals of Biostatistics." Boston, MA: PWS-Kent.

CHAPTER 4

Methods in Psychiatric Genetics

STEPHEN V. FARAONE and MING T. TSUANG

Harvard Medical School Department of Psychiatry at the Massachusetts Mental Health Center and Brockton-West Roxbury Veterans Affairs Medical Center, Boston, MA 02401 (S.V.F., M.T.T.); Pediatric Psychopharmacology Unit, Psychiatry Service, Massachusetts General Hospital (S.V.F.); Department of Epidemiology, Harvard School of Public Health, Boston, MA 02115 (M.T.T.)

INTRODUCTION

Psychiatric genetics is a multidisciplinary field with roots in human genetics, psychiatry, molecular biology, statistics, and epidemiology. Thus, students of psychiatric genetics face a difficult challenge: to acquaint themselves with diverse methodologies and specialize in those needed to achieve their scientific goals. In this chapter we introduce these methods and provide references for more advanced studies of particular issues.

Some readers may be surprised to find discussions of genetics in a textbook of psychiatric epidemiology. After all, epidemiologists usually concern themselves with describing the distribution and determinants of disease as a function of exposure to some environmental variable. This leads naturally to the goal of finding *environmental* risk factors that cause illness. In contrast, classic genetics focuses on genetic mechanisms and, in experimental studies, may even seek to strictly control the environment and eliminate environmental variance. Put simply, epidemiologic research often treats genetic determinants as noise and environmental agents as the signal; genetic studies reverse the roles of genes and environment.

Psychiatric genetics favors neither extreme and adopts the position of genetic epidemiology, which has been defined as "a science that deals with the etiology, distribution, and control of disease in groups of relatives and with inherited causes of disease in populations" (Morton, 1982). Genetic epidemiologists examine the distribution of illness within families with the goal of finding genetic *and* environmental causes of illness. Thus, psychiatric genetics considers both environmental and genetic risk factors—and their interaction—to be on an equal footing. In this paradigm the epidemiologists' concept of "exposure" must extend to genes and family relationships.

It is crucial to recognize the importance of environmental factors in psychiatric genetics because genetic epidemiologists have been accused (incorrectly) of ignoring the envi-

Genetic and statistical terms set in bold italics are defined in the Appendix in the back of the book (pages 453–456).

Textbook in Psychiatric Epidemiology, Edited by Tsuang, Tohen, and Zahner
ISBN 0-471-59375-3 © 1995 Wiley-Liss, Inc.

ronment. Of course, much of the literature in psychiatric genetics does sounds purely genetic. Studies seek to demonstrate familiality, find genes, and estimate heritability. However, in many of these studies, the role of environment is always implicit, even when not mentioned directly. Our point is simple. Although psychiatric genetics seeks to clarify how genes lead to psychiatric illness, most researchers agree that the pathway from *genotype* to *phenotype* cannot be understood without reference to environmental agents that trigger illness in susceptible individuals.

Ironically, psychiatric genetics has provided the strongest evidence supporting the idea that nongenetic factors play a causal role in the expression of psychiatric illness. Most notable in this regard are twin studies. These show that both members of a pair of *monozygotic (MZ)* twins will be affected with schizophrenia or mood disorder only between 50% and 70% of the time, depending on the disorder (Faraone and Tsuang, 1985; Tsuang and Faraone, 1990). By revealing that 30%–50% of MZ co-twins are unaffected, despite sharing 100% of their genes in common, the twin method clearly points to the influence of environmental factors in the etiology of these disorders.

THE CHAIN OF PSYCHIATRIC GENETIC RESEARCH

Work in psychiatric genetics tends to follow a series of questions in a logical progression (Table 1). This sequence, which has been called the *chain of genetic epidemiologic research* (Faraone and Santangelo, 1992), is as follows: First, we ask "Is the disorder familial?" In other words, does it run in families? Second, "What is the relative magnitude of genetic and environmental contributions to disease etiology and expression?" Third, "How is the disease transmitted from generation to generation?" Fourth, "If genes mediate this transmission, where are they located?" Fifth, "What are the genetic and environmental mechanisms of disease?"

Is the Disorder Familial?

Since this question is the easiest to answer it frequently is the first to be asked. For example, observations of disorders "running in families" may come from clinicians who often treat patients from the same family. Of course, once familiality is informally established in a clinical setting, it remains to be confirmed with a rigorous research design, known as the *family study method.*

TABLE 1. Chain of Psychiatric Genetic Research

Questions	Methods
Is disorder familial?	Family study
What are the relative contributions of genes and environment?	Twin and adoption studies
What is the mode of transmission?	Segregation analysis
Where is the gene (or genes) located?	Linkage and association studies

Selection of Probands. Ideally, a family study should use the blind case–control paradigm, a staple of epidemiology and behavioral science. The cases and controls used in genetic studies are known as ***probands.*** We usually select probands with the disorder from a source that is "enriched" with the diagnosis of interest. For example, patients in psychiatric clinics are more likely to have bipolar disorder than patients in a family practice clinic. Furthermore, patients in a bipolar specialty clinic are more likely to have bipolar disorder than patients in a general psychiatric clinic.

Selection from clinics instead of the general population is useful for two reasons. First, to achieve an adequate number of cases from the general population we would need to screen many individuals. This is costly and of dubious benefit. Second, multiple stages of ascertainment increase the probabilities of ill probands being "true cases" and of normal probands not having the disorder under study. Individuals who seek treatment and are given a clinical diagnosis are more likely to have experienced the level of distress and disability that the diagnostic nosology requires for psychiatric illness. This combined with the fact that individuals free of illness are rarely referred means that psychiatric clinic populations have a higher base rate of all psychiatric illnesses than does the general population.

The positive predictive power of a diagnosis (the proportion of those with the disorder among all patients receiving the diagnosis) increases with increases in the base rate of the disorder being diagnosed (Meehl and Rosen, 1955). Thus, multiple stage ascertainment increases the positive predictive power by using clinic status to increase the proportion of "true cases" in the sample that is assessed by the research protocol. Unavoidably, this method of increasing the positive predictive power will increase the false-negative rate. In this context, false-negatives reflect those who have a disorder but are 1) not referred to a clinic or 2) referred but do not receive a clinical diagnosis. Thus, the generalizability of results will be limited to the degree that these false negatives differ from the probands enrolled in our study. Treatment is, of course, the most notable factor that will differentiate these groups.

Likewise, multistage screening of controls decreases the probability of misclassifying someone with the disorder as a control. Of course, since screened controls are selected for absence of the disorder of interest, they cannot be considered representative of the general population. However, work in psychiatric epidemiology indicates that screened controls are very effective when the goal of a project is to delineate factors that differentiate controls from cases (Tsuang et al., 1988). Furthermore, unscreened controls frequently have rates of psychopathology and its correlates that are above the population expectation (Gibbons et al., 1990; Kruesi et al., 1990; Shtasel et al., 1991). Thus, unscreened controls are often heavily contaminated with cases, thereby obscuring the effects of the variable of interest.

We emphasize that controls should be screened only for the disorder being studied, not for other psychiatric disorders or conditions. When controls are screened for additional disorders, the results can spuriously indicate a familial relationship between the disorder used to select cases and the disorders that were screened from controls (Kendler, 1990). For example, we know that alcoholism and anxiety disorders both run in families. Consider a family study of alcoholism that screens control, but not alcoholic, probands for anxiety disorders. Since anxiety is familial, the rates of anxiety among relatives of controls will be decreased by the screening process. In contrast, the rates in relatives of alcoholics will not be decreased. Thus, anxiety disorders will be more prevalent among the relatives of alcoholics due to the choice of control group.

The selection of controls should satisfy the comparability principles required for meaningful inferences in case–control epidemiologic studies (Miettinen, 1985; Wacholder et al., 1992a–c). It is usually not possible to establish a primary study base with a geographically defined population. This is so because the clinics from which probands are selected may serve a broad geographic region that is difficult to delineate. This is especially true for specialty clinics at universities. In many cases the reputation of the clinic attracts patients from great distances.

The usual approach is to establish a secondary study base defined by the ascertainment source. The use of secondary study bases limits generalizability and does not produce a representative sample from a geographical population. Nevertheless, it does allow for meaningful case–control comparisons if the controls are individuals who could have been cases had they developed the disorder of interest during the time of investigation (Miettinen, 1985; Wacholder et al., 1992a–c). When sampling from a clinic, this requires that if the control subjects had needed treatment for the disorder, they would have been referred to the clinics that provided the case probands. For example, in a general hospital outpatient setting, it is likely that patients who seek treatment for medical disorders in medical clinics would go to the same hospital's psychiatric clinic for the treatment of a psychiatric disorder.

Of course, instead of establishing a secondary study base, it is possible to match cases and controls on "relevant" variables. One problem here is defining what is and is not a "relevant" variable. Age, sex, and socioeconomic status are usually considered, but others may be appropriate. However, matching should be used cautiously so as to avoid the "matching fallacy" (Meehl, 1970; Resnick, 1992) and "overmatching" (Miettinen, 1985; Greenland and Morgenstern, 1990). As discussed by Meehl (1970), matching on specific variables often unmatches on others. In addition to creating unusual samples, this also leads to reduced statistical efficiency and biased estimates (Wacholder et al., 1992c). These problems are most severe when the matching variable is strongly associated with the disorder under study.

An obvious example of the matching fallacy is as follows. Numerous studies find that attention deficit hyperactivity disorder (ADHD) interferes with school achievement (Faraone et al., 1993; Faraone et al., in press). Thus, matching controls to ADHD subjects on school achievement would create an unusually high functioning ADHD sample or an unusually low functioning control sample. It may be difficult to draw meaningful inferences from such samples. Instead of matching, we use statistical methods to examine and control for the effects of potentially confounding variables.

Following the selection of cases and controls, the study attempts to assess the diagnostic status of as many of the relatives of cases and controls as possible. The aim is to compare rates of illness in relatives of cases to rates in the relatives of controls. To estimate these rates of illness accurately care must be taken to assess as many relatives as possible. However, psychiatric disorders affect emotions, thinking, and interpersonal relationships. Thus, nonparticipation may not be random with respect to illness status: Family members who are ill may be more likely to refuse participation than those who are well. Paranoid schizophrenia provides a good example of this problem. Paranoia leads to distrusts of strangers, friends, and family. This makes it difficult for a paranoid person to agree to answer the many questions required by psychiatric interviews.

If a disorder has a genetic etiology, then relatives of ill probands should carry a greater risk for the illness than relatives of controls. In addition, the risk to relatives of probands should be correlated with their degree of relationship to the proband or with the amount of genes they share in common. First-degree relatives such as parents, siblings, and children share 50% of their genes, on average, with the proband. They should be at greater risk for the disorder than second-degree relatives (grandparents, uncles, aunts, nephews, nieces, and half-siblings) because second-degree relatives share only 25% of their genes with the proband.

A genetic hypothesis predicts that the risk for relatives of ill probands is higher than that for relatives of controls and that the risk for relatives of probands increases as the amount of genes shared increases. In practice, however, it is rare that a family study will have the resources to diagnose second- or third-degree relatives. Most studies assess only first-degree relatives. Table 2 displays the familial pattern of risk found in the families of schizophrenic probands. These risk figures come from many of the earlier European family studies and conform to the expectation that first-degree relatives are at highest risk, followed by second- and then third-degree relatives.

Family Study Versus Family History. In planning a family study of psychiatric illness we must choose between two approaches for the evaluation of family members: the *family history* and *family study* methods. The family history method collects diagnostic information about all family members by interviewing only one or several informants per family. This method uses a specialized instrument such as the interview for Family History Research Diagnostic Criteria (FH-RDC; Andreasen et al., 1977) or the Family Interview for Genetic Studies (FIGS; NIMH Genetics Initiative, 1992b).

TABLE 2. Rates of Schizophrenia Among Relatives of Schizophrenic Patients[a]

Relatives	Percent at Risk
First degree	
Parents	4.4
Children	12.3
Both parents schizophrenic	36.6
Brothers and sisters	8.5
Neither parent schizophrenic	8.2
One parent schizophrenic	13.8
Fraternal twins of opposite sex	5.6
Fraternal twins of same sex	12.0
Identical twins	57.7
Second degree	
Uncles and aunts	2.0
Nephews and nieces	2.2
Grandchildren	2.8
Half brothers/sisters	3.2
Third degree	
First cousins	2.9
General population	0.86

[a]Based on Slater and Cowie (1971), with the exception of twin data from Shields and Slater (1975). Adapted, with permission, from Tsuang and Vandermey (1980).

In contrast, the family study method determines diagnoses by interviewing all family members directly. Several excellent structured psychiatric interviews are available, but only one was designed specifically for genetic studies: the Diagnostic Interview for Genetic Studies (DIGS; NIMH Genetics Initiative, 1992a; Nurnberger et al., 1993).

An obvious advantage of the family history method is its low cost: Interviewing a few family members is less costly then interviewing all family members. However, several researchers have shown that family history data underestimate true rates of many psychiatric disorders. The overall strategy of these studies has been to collect family history data on the same subjects who have also been diagnosed by the family study method. By using the family study method as the "gold standard" they can estimate the accuracy of the family history method.

Mendlewicz et al. (1975) examined the accuracy of the family history method in the context of a family study of mood disorders. The probands were 140 patients with either bipolar disorder or major depressive disorder. When the probands were used as informants for the family history method, the rates of mood disorders in the family were underestimated. The family history method was most accurate when the informant was the child or spouse of the person being diagnosed.

Similar results were reported by Andreasen et al. (1977). They determined the specificity and sensitivity of family history diagnoses using an adaptation of the Research Diagnostic Criteria they termed the Family History Research Diagnostic Criteria. *Specificity* is the probability of correctly classifying a subject as well by the family history method if that subject is assessed as well by the family study method. *Sensitivity* is the probability that the subject is diagnosed ill by family history if they are diagnosed ill by the family study method. In their application to mood disorders, the specificity was high but the sensitivity was low. For example, among family members classified as having a mood disorder by direct interview, only 59% were so classified by the family history method.

It is possible to improve the sensitivity of the family history method by using several informants to provide information about the subject being diagnosed. In the Andreasen et al. study, when only probands were interviewed via the FH-RDC, the lifetime prevalence of mood disorders among relatives was 11%. This rate increased to 17% when other relatives were interviewed along with the proband. However, both rates underestimated the 25% rate obtained by the family study method.

Orvaschel et al. (1982) found that the family history method was better for some types of relatives than for others. For example, in their study, the sensitivity of the family history method was lower when the subject being diagnosed was male. Sensitivity was also higher if the relative being diagnosed was ill at the time of the family history interview. This latter finding makes intuitive sense: We are more likely to know of a relative's problems if, for example, they are in a psychiatric hospital at the time we are asked about their condition.

Other studies have shown that the accuracy of family history assessments varies by diagnosis. Thompson et al. (1982) found that sensitivities for major depression and alcoholism were much higher than for generalized anxiety, drug abuse, phobic disorder, and depressive personality. Moreover, diagnoses based on spouse or offspring reports were more sensitive than those based on parent or sibling reports.

In the family study of mood disorders by Gershon and Guroff (1984), the family history method was most sensitive (96%) when the informant was being asked about a proband. It was halved to 48% when the relative being diagnosed was not a proband. Notably, there was a positive linear relationship between sensitivity and the number of informants. The sensitivity was only 15% with one informant, but increased to 67% when five informants were used. Specificity decreased only a little, from 99% to 92%, when the number of informants was increased from one to five.

In a relatively large study of 609 mood disordered probands and 2,216 first-degree relatives, Andreasen et al. (1986) confirmed the results from previous validity studies of the family history method. Relative to the family study method, rates of illness in relatives were always underestimated by the family history method using the FH-RDC. One key exception was the diagnosis of antisocial personality: The family history rate of this disorder was three times greater than the direct interview estimate. Thus, it may be that the family history method is *more* valid than direct interview when the disorder in question has a pejorative connotation.

In the Andreasen et al. (1986) study the sensitivities and specificities of the family history method were consistent with previous reports. The sensitivities were low. They ranged from 31% for schizophrenia to 69% for "psychotic disorder." As expected, the specificities were higher. These ranged from 84% for probable depressive disorder to 100% for schizophrenia and schizoaffective disorder. The sensitivity of the family history method was best when the informant was a parent of the subject being asked about. For depression the sensitivities were 62% for parent informants, 51% for sibling informants, and 37% for child informants.

Ideally, the diagnoses of subjects should use three sources of information: direct interviews with the subject, family history interviews with informants who are familiar with the subject, and medical records when available. All sources of information about a given individual are then combined into a consensus diagnosis (Leckman et al., 1982; Gershon and Guroff, 1984). As suggested by the research reviewed above, the direct interview and medical record usually provide more useful information than the family history assessment. In fact, two studies find that diagnoses based on direct interviews alone closely approximate best estimate diagnoses (Leckman et al., 1982; Gershon and Guroff, 1984). However, a diagnosis based only on medical records is often a suitable proxy to the best estimate diagnosis (Gershon and Guroff, 1984).

Silverman and colleagues (1986) evaluated the reliability of the family history method for dementing illnesses such as Alzheimer's disease. When rating the same individual, different informants had high levels of agreement on the presence of dementia and its age at onset. The rates of dementia found in this family history study were similar to what had been found in previous family studies using direct methods of assessment. The authors concluded that multiple informants would likely increase the validity of the family history method, but, because they did not directly evaluate relatives, inferences about validity were limited.

Kosten et al. (1992) examined the validity of the family history method for five diagnoses used in a family study of opiate addiction: depression, anxiety, antisocial personality, alcoholism, and drug abuse. For diagnosing family members, the sensitivities were uniformly low, ranging from 6% to 39%. Specificities were greater than 95%, with the exception of depression, which had a specificity of 54%.

The authors also provided data about the type and number of informants. Spouses and children were better informants than parents or siblings. For alcoholism and drug abuse females were better informants than males. Increasing the number of informants improved the accuracy of the family history method for depression, antisocial personality, and alcoholism, but not for anxiety disorders or drug abuse.

Collection of data using the family history method may be influenced by the presence of psychiatric illness in the informant. Kendler and colleagues (1991) asked *discordant* twins about depression, anxiety, and alcoholism in their parents. Twins are discordant if only one has the disease being studied. Compared with the unaffected twin, those with a history of major depression or generalized anxiety were more likely to report the same disorder in their parents. This effect was not observed for alcoholism. However, since direct interview data had not been collected on the parents, it is not certain if the affected twin was over-reporting psychopathology or the unaffected twin was under-reporting it. Nevertheless, this study underscores the need for more methodologic work to clarify the utility of the family history method for specific disorders.

Table 3 outlines the advantages and disadvantages of the family history and family study methods. The choice between the two requires a trade-off between data quality and the expense of data collection. The family history method is the method of choice when there are not sufficient data to justify the expense of a family study. Thus, it is a good choice for initial pilot phases of a genetic investigation. However, after the family history method demonstrates familiality, the family study is the tool of choice for examining the details of familial transmission.

If the question at hand dictates the use of the family history method, the following recommendations should be considered: 1) use the FH-RDC, FIGS, or some other semistructured method for eliciting the family history; 2) because the family history method has low sensitivity, use less stringent diagnostic criteria than for direct interview data; 3) use multiple informants for each person to be diagnosed; 4) seek out informants who have had substantial contact with the person to be diagnosed; 5) remember that the method is most valid when the person to be diagnosed is ill at the time of interviewing the informant. These "rules of thumb" provide a rough guide for planning a family history study. The studies discussed above should be consulted for information about specific disorders.

Caveats. The family study is a practical and robust tool for psychiatric genetics. In many cases, it has provided the initial hint that a disorder might have a genetic component. However, we must be cautious in concluding that a disorder is caused by genes after we observe that it is familial. Disorders can "run in families" for nongenetic reasons such as shared environmental adversity, viral transmission, and social learning. Also, since the culture and environment shared by family members tends to increase as the degree of relationship decreases, the pattern of risk due to environmental factors may mimic the pattern expected for genetic relationships.

Family data on tuberculosis provide a good example of such confounding. Data collected in the 1940s showed that the risk to family members related to probands who had tuberculosis increased with the degree of genetic relationship. That is, first-degree relatives had higher rates of tuberculosis than second-degree relatives (McGue et al., 1985). McGue et al. (1985) pointed out that the distribution of familial risk for schizophrenia and that for tuberculosis both showed that the risk to relatives of ill probands increased

TABLE 3. Family Study Versus Family History Method

Method	Pros	Cons
Family history	Practical, high specificity	Low sensitivity
Family study	High quality data	Expensive

with the amount of genes shared with the proband. However, the patterns differed in a few subtle ways that allowed them to show that the risk for schizophrenia was transmitted genetically whereas tuberculosis was transmitted through the environment.

Our point is straightforward: The finding of familial transmission cannot be unambiguously interpreted. Although family studies are indispensable for establishing the familiality of disorders they cannot, by themselves, establish what type of transmission. All mechanisms that could lead to a familial clustering of disease should be considered.

What Are the Relative Contributions of Genes and Environment?

Genes, environment, and their interaction: These are the ingredients of the pathophysiological brew that engenders psychopathology. Psychiatric genetics seeks to assay these ingredients and determine their relative proportions. The tools for this venture are twin and adoption studies.

Unfortunately, twin and adoption studies are fairly difficult to implement because of the difficulty in finding and collecting large enough samples that are informative for the disorder to be studied. Twin births are rare, and twins with psychopathology are even rarer. Adoption is relatively common, but laws in most countries make it impossible to study the biologic relatives of adopted children.

However, valuable resources for twin and adoption studies do exist, and these have fueled work in this area for many decades. For example, countries like Denmark have extensive adoption and twin registries in addition to psychiatric registries. By recording all twin births, adoptions, and psychiatric contacts in a specified geographic region, these registries have allowed researchers to proceed with genetic studies of gene–environment relationships. Linkage of the psychiatric registries with the twin and adoption registries has created unique opportunities for genetic epidemiologic investigations of some psychiatric disorders.

Twin Studies. The biologic process of twinning creates a natural experiment in psychiatric genetics. Identical or ***monozygotic (MZ)*** twins inherit identical ***chromosomes*** and thereby have 100% of their genes in common. In contrast, the genetic similarity of fraternal or ***dizygotic (DZ)*** twins is no different than that of siblings. On average, DZ twins share 50% of their genes. Thus, MZ and DZ twins are markedly different with regard to their genetic similarity. However, if twin pairs are reared in the same household, then the degree of environmental similarity between MZ twins should be no different than that between DZ twins. The astute reader will note that our comments regarding genetic similarity are *facts* of inheritance, but our comments about the environment are *assumptions*. The correctness of these assumptions is key to the valid use of the twin method.

Since MZ twins are genetic copies of one another, any differences between a pair of MZ twins are assumed to be due primarily to environmental influences. In contrast, differences between DZ twins could be due to either genetic or environmental influences. Thus, comparing the co-occurrence of a psychiatric disorder in the two types of twins provides information about the relative contributions of genetic and environmental factors in the etiology of the disorder. The co-occurrence of a disorder in both twins is called *concordance*; if one twin has the disorder and the other does not, the twins are *discordant* for the disorder.

Twin data for psychiatric disorders are usually expressed as concordance rates. Because we assume the same environmental similarity for both types of twins, a higher concordance rate for MZ than for DZ twins indicates the operation of genetic mechanisms. We can use pairwise or probandwise concordance rates, depending on the method of sampling the twins. The ***pairwise concordance*** rate is defined as the proportion of twin pairs in which both twins are ill. To compute this, count the number of twin pairs ***concordant*** for the disorder and divide the result by the total number of pairs. We use this method of computing concordance when the probability of sampling any specific ill individual is so low that two ill co-twins are never independently sampled as probands.

However, when the sampling probability is higher, the probandwise concordance rate is the method of choice. ***Probandwise concordance*** is the proportion of proband twins who have an ill co-twin. Thus, it is the number of concordant pairs plus the number of concordant pairs in which both the twins are probands, divided by the total number of pairs.

Frequently, twin data are used to estimate the ***heritability*** of a disorder. Heritability measures the degree to which genetic factors influence variability in the manifestation of the disorder (the phenotype). We divide phenotypic variability (V_p) into two components: genetic variability (V_g) and environmental variability (V_e). This partitioning of phenotypic variability assumes that genetic and environmental factors are statistically independent (i.e., $V_p = V_g + V_e$). Heritability in the broad sense (h^2) is the ratio of genetic and phenotypic variances (i.e., $h^2 = V_g/V_p$).

As these formulas show, a heritability of 1 indicates that variability in the phenotype is due to genetic factors alone. In contrast, a heritability of 0 attributes all phenotypic variation to environmental factors. However, a key point here is that a zero heritability does not mean that the etiology of the phenotype can be explained solely by environmental influence. Retardation due to phenylketonuria (PKU) is a classic case for demonstrating this point.

PKU is caused by a ***recessive*** gene. Infants who inherit two copies of this gene (they are ***homozygous***) suffer from a complete deficiency of the enzyme required to metabolize phenylalanine. These children will become retarded only if they ingest phenylalanine. Heritability estimated on a sample of individuals who have the pathogenic genotype will be zero simply because there is no genetic variability in the sample. In this case, any variability in the PKU trait must be due to the environment.

The details of methods for calculating heritability are beyond the scope of this chapter. Smith (1974) and Plomin et al. (1990) provide information about the calculation and interpretation of this measure (see also LaBuda et al., 1993).

Figure 1 gives an example of how twin data can shed light on the etiology of psychiatric illnesses. It presents results from six different twin studies of broadly defined mood disorders or "manic-depressive disorder" (Tsuang and Faraone, 1990). Each bar on the graph represents a single study. The cross-hatched part of each bar indicates what percentage of the disorder could be attributed to genetic factors. The black part of the bar indicates what percentage could be attributed to common or shared environmental factors. The white part of the bar indicates the proportion of variance due to unique environmental factors or events experienced by one twin but not the other. This pattern of results attributes approximately 60% of the variance in mood disorders to genetic factors; it attributes 30%–40% of the variance to common environmental factors. Unique environmental effects appear to have accounted for less than 10% of the variance in these six studies.

This is a relatively simple analysis of twin data. Twin methodology can become math-

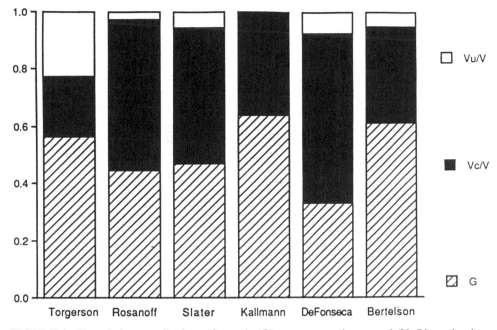

FIGURE 1. The relative contributions of genetic (G), common environmental (Vc/V), and unique environmental (Vu/V) variance to the liability to mood disorders.

ematically sophisticated. If we have data from parents and siblings of twins or indices of the environment, then specialized methods can provide information about gene–environment interaction and gene–environment correlation. An excellent reference for these methods is the book by Neale and Cardon (1992).

Two additional twin study designs deserve special mention. When monozygotic twins are reared apart, we have a unique—but rare—opportunity to study the relative importance of genes and environment. Since MZ twins reared apart do not share a common environment, any phenotypic similarity must be due to genetic factors. We cannot invoke shared environment as a cause of phenotypic concordance. However, MZ twins with psychiatric illness are rare, and cases of such twins reared apart are even rarer. Thus, this design cannot be routinely used.

A second twin study design uses the children of discordant MZ twins. The logic of this design is straightforward. If a disorder is caused by a genotype in combination with environmental factors, then the well member of a discordant MZ twin pair should carry the genotype. Presumably, they did not develop the disorder because they had not been exposed to a relevant environmental cause. If so, then the children of the well twin should have the same risk for the disorder as the children of the ill twin.

A good example of this design is a Danish study by Fischer (1971). She examined 71 offspring of MZ twin pairs who were discordant for schizophrenia. The offspring of the schizophrenic twins had a 9.6% rate of schizophrenia; the rate among offspring of the nonschizophrenic twins was 12.9%. These two rates were not significantly different. Thus, the risk to the children of these MZ twins did not depend on the presence of schizophrenia in the twin. From this we infer that the twins who did not have schizophrenia did have the genetic susceptibility to schizophrenia and passed it on to their children in the same manner as did the ill twins. Since Gottesman and Bertelsen (1989) confirmed these results in an 18 year follow-up study of Fischer's sample, the finding constitutes strong evidence that environmental factors may prevent gene expression in the unaffected twin.

Adoption Studies. Like twinning, adoption creates a useful paradigm for psychiatric genetic studies. Children adopted at an early age have a genetic relationship to their biologic parents and an environmental relationship to their adopted parents. Thus, adoption studies can determine if biologic or adoptive relationships account for the familial transmission of disorders. If genes are important, then the familial transmission of illness should occur in the biologic but not the adoptive family. In contrast, if culture, social learning, or other sources of environmental transmission cause illness, then familial transmission of illness should occur in the adoptive but not the biologic family.

There are three major adoption study designs. The parent-as-proband design compares rates of illness in the adopted offspring of parents with and without the disorder. If genetic factors mediate the disorder then rates of illness should be greater in the adopted children of ill parents compared with the adopted children of well parents.

As its name suggests, the adoptee-as-proband design starts with ill and well adoptees and examines rates of illness in both biologic and adoptive relatives. If the biologic relatives of ill adoptees have higher rates of illness than the adoptive relatives of ill adoptees, then a genetic hypothesis is supported. In contrast, if the adoptive relatives show higher rates of illness, then an environmental hypothesis gains support.

The third design is the cross-fostering design. This approach compares rates of illness for two groups of adoptees: One has well biologic parents and is raised by ill adoptive parents and the other has ill biologic parents and is raised by well adoptive parents. Higher rates of illness in the former group of adoptees than in the latter group would imply a primarily nongenetic mode of illness transmission.

Although they are difficult to execute, adoption studies have provided extensive data for both mood disorders (Mendlewicz and Rainer, 1977; Cadoret, 1978; Cadoret et al., 1985; Wender et al., 1986; Tsuang and Faraone, 1990) and schizophrenia (Heston, 1966; Kety et al., 1968, 1978; Tsuang et al., 1993). Taken as a group, these studies support the hypothesis that the familial transmission of these disorders is due to genetic, not environmental factors.

Despite their power to disentangle genetic and environmental factors, adoption studies must be viewed with some caution due to potential methodologic problems that cloud their unambiguous interpretation. First, adoptees and their families are not representative of the general population. This may limit the generalizability of results. Furthermore, adoptees are at greater risk for psychiatric illness than nonadopted children (Deutsch et al., 1982; Kotsopoulos et al., 1988). Although the reasons for this are not clear, this increased risk for psychiatric disorders requires that we use an adoptee control group. For example, in the adoptee-as-proband design, the relatives of ill adoptees must be compared with the relatives of well adoptees. Some other control group should not be used, even if it is matched to the ill adoptee group on demographic measures.

Another potential problem is that it may be difficult to find a sample of adoptees who were all separated from their parents at birth. If the child has lived with a parent for even a short period of time prior to adoption, the biologic relationship will have been "contaminated" by environmental factors. Some might even argue that the child's contact with the mother immediately after birth creates a residue of environmental influence that affects subsequent psychopathology.

Kety et al. (1968, 1978) presented a compelling design that deals with this problem. Their method requires a sample of biologic paternal half-siblings of ill and well adoptees. Paternal half-siblings share a common father yet have different mothers. Therefore, they do not share prenatal, perinatal, or neonatal environmental exposure to the same mother. Thus, this design rules out confounding by in utero influences, birth traumas, and early mothering experience. In the work of Kety and colleagues, the biologic paternal half-siblings of schizophrenic adoptees were at greater risk for schizophrenia than the biologic paternal half-siblings of control adoptees. Such a finding clearly bolsters the hypothesis that schizophrenia is caused, at least in part, by genetic factors.

Of course, there are some environmental correlates of the biologic parents that cannot be handled by the paternal half-sibling design. For example, children born to fathers of the lowest social class may share toxic environmental factors such as poor pre- and peri-natal care, poor nutrition, and an adverse social environment; these may confound the genetic parent–child relationship.

Despite these potential confounds and the difficulty of ascertaining appropriate cases and controls, the adoption study remains a valuable tool for disentangling genetic and environmental contributions to the familial aggregation of psychiatric disorders. The problems we note serve to underscore a basic tenet of psychiatric genetic research: Any assertion that a disorder is caused by genetic factors must refer not to a single study but to a series of studies using different paradigms.

What Is the Mode of Transmission?

After demonstrating that a disorder is influenced by genetic factors, the next logical task is to determine the mechanism of transmission from parent to child. This information is useful from two perspectives. Showing that the transmission of a disorder corresponds to a known mode of transmission provides clues for subsequent research steps. For example, if the transmission is clearly due to a single gene, the next step might be linkage analysis, which uses family psychiatric data and samples of *DNA* to find mutant genes (see discussion below). In contrast, if environmental factors are implicated, then a search for such factors would be warranted.

Moreover, the mode of transmission has implications for genetic counseling. Genetic counseling is the process whereby clinical professionals inform people about either their probability of developing a genetic disorder or that of any children they are planning to conceive. Ideally, in the absence of genetic linkage data, such counseling should be based on risk figures from a known model of genetic transmission. This model can be applied to an individual's pedigree to determine that individual's risk for a disorder. Morton et al. (1979) demonstrated that the degree of risk predicted depends on the model of transmission. They also found that clinically important errors in risk prediction were made when they used the wrong genetic model to make predictions.

A model of familial transmission translates assumptions about genetic and environmental causes into mathematical equations. These equations are then used to predict the distribution of a disorder that we observe in pedigrees or twin pairs. If the pattern of a disorder predicted by the model is close to what we observe, we say that the model fits the data. This provides evidence in favor of the model being tested. In contrast, if the predicted pattern of disorder differs from what is observed, we reject the model and seek another mechanism of transmission. The term *segregation analysis* is used to describe analyses that assess the mode of disease transmission.

As the reader might suspect, the methods we discuss in this section require a good deal of mathematical and statistical expertise to be understood and correctly implemented. In the short space of this chapter we cannot present these mathematical details, but instead provide an overview of the different classes of methods used to test hypotheses about genetic and environmental transmission (however, a detailed discussion of two segregation analysis algorithms is given in a subsequent section). Several excellent texts, review articles, and computer program documentation provide a detailed guide to these methods (Elston and Stewart, 1971; Morton, 1982; Lalouel et al., 1983; Bailey-Wilson and Elston, 1989).

Mathematical Modeling of Genetic and Environmental Transmission.

A genetic model comprises two major components. First, we must describe how the disorder is transmitted. For example, if we believe the disorder is due to a single dominant gene, our model must include the frequency of the gene in the population. It must also require that the transmission of the gene from parent to child follow the laws of genetic transmission. For example, if a mother carries one pathogenic gene the probability that she transmits this gene to a child must be 50%. Genetic models can specify environmental effects in several ways. Consider some simple examples: In a single gene model we can specify the *penetrance* of each genotype. Penetrance indicates the probability that each genotype causes disease. If we believe that disease occurs when an environmental event (e.g., head injury) occurs in someone carrying the pathogenic gene, then our model should allow some gene carriers to be well. Another possibility is that other causes for the disease exist. If so, then people who do not carry the gene will have some probability of becoming ill. That is, the penetrance is greater than zero for those who do not carry the hypothetical disease gene.

The second component of a genetic model is a procedure for determining whether the predictions made by the model adequately describe the pattern of illness observed in families. One modeling approach attempts to predict rates of illness in various classes of relatives. The pedigree data are reduced to a table of numbers indicating the rate of illness in these classes (e.g., mothers, fathers, brothers, sisters, sons, daughters, and more distant relatives). The mathematical model is then estimated by choosing values for the model parameters (e.g., gene frequency and penetrance) that most accurately reproduce the observed rates. The observed and predicted rates can then be compared with a chi-square test to determine if any deviation between predicted and observed rates is large enough to warrant rejecting the model.

Modeling rates of illness does not capitalize on all the information available in pedigree data. By lumping all families together within one data table, we cannot directly model the transmission of genes from one generation to the next. In contrast, pedigree analysis computes the *likelihood* of the pattern of illness in each family. For this approach the raw data are not summarized into a table. Instead, the analysis uses the status of all persons and their relationship to others in the pedigree who are and are not affected. An algorithm then computes the probability or likelihood that the assumed model is correct given the pedigree data and the value of model parameters. Those parameter values yielding the most likely model are used as final estimates. With this approach we establish the model's *goodness of fit* with a likelihood ratio chi-square test.

For example, when we estimate parameters for a single gene model we assume that a

pair of genes at a single location or *locus* on a chromosome is responsible for the transmission of a disorder. If *b* represents the pathogenic version of the gene (or *allele*) and *B*
represents the normal allele at the same locus, then there are three possible genotypes:
BB, Bb, and *bb*. Under a mendelian genetic model, the probability that a *BB* father transmits the *b* gene to his daughter must be zero. Likewise, the transmission probability that a
parent of each genotype transmits *B* or *b* is fixed by the laws of mendelian inheritance.
This leads to a straightforward statistical test: compute the likelihood of a mendelian
model and compare this with a model that allows the transmission probabilities to deviate
from their mendelian values. A significant difference would indicate that the single gene
model could be rejected.

Types of Transmission Models. Single gene mendelian transmission is only one of
many transmission mechanisms that we use to describe family and twin data. There are
three broad classes of transmission mechanisms: genes, environment, and their interaction. We find it useful to classify the genetic mechanisms into three types of models: single major gene, *oligogenic,* and *multifactorial polygenic.* The word *major* indicates that
one gene can account for most of the genetic transmission of a disorder. Other genes and
environmental conditions may play minor roles in modifying the expression of the disease or determining its age of onset. In contrast, an oligogenic model assumes that the
combined actions of several genes cause illness. These genes may combine in an additive
fashion such that the probability of illness is a function of the number of pathogenic
genes. Alternatively, the mechanism may be interactive. For example, three abnormal alleles at different chromosomal locations may be needed for disease to occur. Of course a
combination of additive and interactive mechanisms can also be considered.

One difficulty in testing oligogenic models is that there are many ways in which several genes might combine to cause a disorder. For example, there are 100 possible two-
locus models that can describe a dichotomous trait. If the trait is trichotomous, there are
2,634 possible models (Elston and Namboodiri, 1977). A plausible argument can be made
for excluding many of these possibilities because they either do not fit hypotheses about
the disorder or they are biologically meaningless. Nevertheless, the number of models
that remain to be tested is daunting.

The multifactorial polygenic (MFP) model proposes that a large, unspecified number
of genes and environmental factors combine in an additive fashion to cause disease. The
difference between oligogenic and polygenic models is one of degree. The former contain
"several" genes (e.g., less than 10), whereas the latter include a "large number" of genes
(e.g., 100). Geneticists originally developed polygenic models to describe quantitative
traits such as height and intelligence. By specifying a "large number" of genes, these
models could explain how discrete genes could cause traits that were continuously distributed in the population.

Since many diseases are qualitative categories — not quantitative dimensions — geneticists developed the concept of *liability* (Falconer, 1965). Liability describes an unobservable trait: the predisposition to onset with disease. As liability increases so does the probability of disease onset. Alternatively, we might assume that disease occurs when one's
liability crosses a specific threshold.

In some ways, the MFP model is easier to handle statistically than oligogenic inheritance, despite the large number of components involved. Although the MFP model posits
that many genes and environmental factors contribute additively to disease causation,
these individual factors are not directly modeled. According to the model, liability is nor-

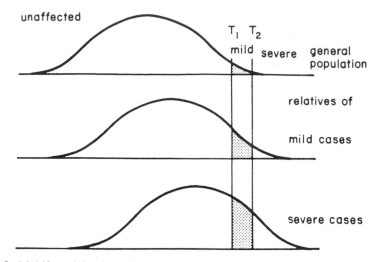

FIGURE 2. Multifactorial polygenic liability threshold model. The two thresholds delimit mild and severe forms of the disorder.

mally distributed. Individuals above a certain threshold on the liability scale manifest the disorder. More than one threshold may be placed along the liability continuum, representing varying degrees of severity, as illustrated in Figure 2. Individuals to the right of the right-hand threshold will develop a severe form of the disorder. Those to the left of the left-hand threshold may have minor problems or be unaffected, while those whose liability falls between the two thresholds would have an intermediate form of the disorder.

For example, some researchers have suggested that bipolar and unipolar disorders might be severe and mild variants of mood disorders. In this case, individuals above the highest threshold develop bipolar disorder, those below the lowest threshold are normal, and those in between have unipolar disorder.

Using the statistical method of path analysis, the MFP model has been generalized to evaluate the relative contributions of genetic and environmental effects. Path analysis models partition the observed covariances or correlations between family members (with regard to a trait or disorder) into several components. Examples of such components are 1) the effect of transmissible environment on phenotype (the cultural heritability); 2) the effect of genotype on phenotype (the genetic heritability); 3) the effect on phenotype of environmental factors unique to twins or siblings; 4) the effect of transmissible parental environment on the transmissible environment of a child raised by the parent; 5) the correlation between transmissible parental environments (i.e., nonrandom mating); 6) interactions between genes and environment; and 7) correlations between genes and environment.

McGue and colleagues (1985) applied a path analytic model to family data on schizophrenia and tuberculosis. Like schizophrenia, tuberculosis aggregates in families. Unlike schizophrenia, the etiology of tuberculosis is known: Originally thought to be a genetic disease, it is now known to be transmitted through a bacterial infection. The parameter estimates obtained from the path analysis of schizophrenia family data indicate a high and significant genetic heritability (0.67) along with a low and nonsignificant cultural heritability (0.19). For tuberculosis these estimates were reversed: Genetic heritability was estimated to be 0.06, while the estimate for cultural heritability was 0.62. The familial aggregation of tuberculosis was correctly attributed to environmentally transmitted factors. This validation of the path analytic MFP model on a disorder with a known mode of transmission further validates the results of the analysis of the schizophrenia data in this study.

The *mixed model* posits that both MFP and single gene components may be involved in disease etiology. Statistical analysis of the mixed model can determine if either component alone can provide an adequate fit to the data or if the null hypothesis of no single gene effect and no MFP effect fits best. For example, one report of a mixed model analysis of data on 79 chronic schizophrenic probands and their families (Risch and Baron, 1984) concluded that although a polygenic model also fit, these family data were consistent with a mixed model in which the major gene was recessive and had a high gene frequency and a very low penetrance.

Unfortunately, segregation analysis techniques have not yet been successful in demonstrating a definitive mode of transmission for most psychiatric disorders. There are many such studies of families with mood disorders (Faraone et al., 1990; Tsuang and Faraone, 1990) and schizophrenia (Faraone and Tsuang, 1985). One exception may be Tourette's syndrome, a neuropsychiatric disorder characterized by multiple vocal and motor tics. Some data show the transmission of this disorder to be autosomal dominant with incomplete and sex-specific penetrance and variable expression (Pauls and Leckman, 1986).

Where Are the Gene(s) Located?

Eventually, psychiatric genetic research leads to questions such as, "Where is the gene located?" and "What are the genetic and environmental mechanisms of disease?" This stage of inquiry requires input from colleagues from molecular genetics, because they can provide the methods for tracking the inheritance of these disorders through families. Linkage analysis is a more powerful method of establishing genetic etiology for the psychiatric disorders than the statistical methods of segregation analysis. Segregation analysis can only show that the pattern of disease is consistent with a specific genetic model. Linkage analysis can actually determine where the gene is located on the human genome.

The search for disease genes faces formidable obstacles. Paramount among these is the number of potential disease genes. Each of us has over 100,000 genes. Moreover, only 10% of our chromosomal material (DNA) contains the coding sequences (i.e., instructions) for these genes. The average gene is made up of 3,000 base pairs (the building blocks of DNA). But the entire set of chromosomes (the *genome*) contains 3 billion base pairs. Thus, searching for disease genes might seem as difficult as looking for a needle in a haystack.

Fortunately, geneticists and statisticians have solved this genetic needle in a haystack problem. Today, there is no question that current molecular genetic and statistical technologies can find the genes that cause genetic disorders (Ott, 1992). In fact, the list of diseases with known disease genes grows each year. Examples include Huntington's disease, Alzheimer's disease, cystic fibrosis, Duchenne's muscular dystrophy, myotonic dystrophy, familial colon cancer, von Recklinghausen neurofibromatosis, and a form of mental

98   FARAONE AND TSUANG

retardation due to the fragile X syndrome. The methodology for finding genes, known as linkage analysis, is now fairly routine.

Background for Linkage Analysis. Linkage analysis is made possible by the "***crossing over***" that takes place between two ***homologous*** chromosomes during ***meiosis***, the process whereby ***gametes*** are created. Genetic transmission occurs because we inherit one member of each pair of chromosomes from our mother and one from our father. However, these inherited chromosomes are not identical to any of the original parental chromosomes. During meiosis, the original chromosomes in a pair cross over each other and exchange portions of their DNA. After multiple crossovers, the resulting two chromosomes each consist of a new and unique combination of genes.

Figure 3 schematically demonstrates the result of a single crossover. The original pair of chromosomes is represented as one dark and one light strand. Three different genes are represented with uppercase and lowercase letters signifying different alleles at the same locus.

Figure 4 represents the new chromosome pair produced by multiple crossovers. When meiosis is complete, each gamete will contain one chromosome from each of the newly formed pairs. As Figure 4 indicates, the probability that two genes on the same chromosome will recombine during meiosis is a function of their physical distance from one another. We say that two loci on the same chromosome are "linked" when they are so close to one another that crossing over rarely or never occurs between them. Closely linked genes usually remain together on the same chromosome after meiosis is complete.

In addition to the physical distance between loci, the number of crossovers that occurs between them will determine whether or not they will recombine. An odd number will result in recombination, whereas an even number will not. If two loci are very far apart, the probability of an odd number of crossovers between them is equal to the probability of an even number. As a result, the probability of recombination is 50%. Therefore, genes on the same chromosome that are very far apart from one another are transmitted independently, as are genes on different chromosomes.

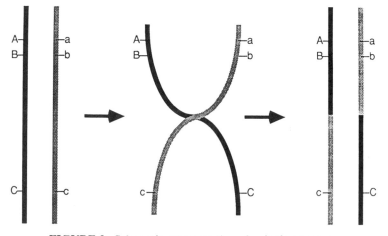

FIGURE 3. Schematic representation of a single crossover.

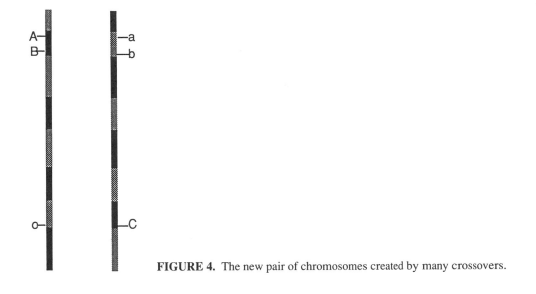

FIGURE 4. The new pair of chromosomes created by many crossovers.

Genetic Markers for Linkage Analysis. Linkage analysis determines if a putative disease gene is closely linked to a known ***genetic marker.*** A genetic marker is a measurable human trait controlled by a single gene with a known chromosomal location. The marker must be ***polymorphic*** (i.e., more than one version of the gene exists with high frequency), and its mode of inheritance must be known. Early linkage studies used genetically controlled traits as genetic markers. Examples include color blindness, blood groups, enzymes, proteins, and systems such as human leukocyte antigen (HLA) that control immune response.

The use of genetically determined traits as genetic markers greatly restricted the use of linkage analysis because, compared with the size of the genome, relatively few markers were available. Because of their rarity, the a priori probability that a trait or disorder might be mapped to a known chromosomal location was low. Moreover, although these markers were polymorphic, they were not remarkably so. As we discuss below, highly polymorphic markers are best because they increase the statistical power of linkage analyses. Fortunately, molecular geneticists developed laboratory methods that directly characterize DNA samples. Because of this, it is now possible to have genetic markers useful for testing linkage to all portions of the genome.

An early example of a DNA marker is the restriction fragment length polymorphism (RFLP) (Botstein et al., 1980). Restriction endonucleases cut DNA into pieces. The locations of the cuts are determined by the sequence of the ***nucleotides*** in the DNA. There are four nucleotides: adenine (A), guanine (G), cytosine (C) and thymine (T). For example, the restriction endonuclease known as AluI cuts DNA between the nucleotides guanine and cytosine wherever the nucleotide sequence AGCT occurs. The size of the resulting fragments is determined by the particular sequence of base pairs in the gene. Since these fragments can be measured in the laboratory, family members can be classified according to the length of the fragment that results from cutting their DNA with AluI.

The discovery of loci in the human genome that contained repeated sequences of DNA was especially useful because the number of base pair repetitions varied a great deal among individuals. That is, the length and number of fragments produced by a restriction endonuclease on the same chromosomal fragment taken from different individuals varied substantially. These are called **VNTR** markers because they result from a variable number of tandem repeats (Nakamura et al., 1987, 1988).

Another class of markers, the **CA repeats**, has provided additional highly polymorphic markers (Weber and May, 1989). These are based on variations in the number of times the nucleotide sequence CA is repeated. These markers appear to be quite frequent in the genome and may provide a more efficient and rapid means for genotyping than the conventional RFLP or VNTR markers. The advantage of this type of marker is its increased level of polymorphism. Moreover the experimental procedures required to examine these markers are simpler than those required for RFLP type markers. To date, thousands of DNA markers have been cataloged and identified along the human genome. In the near future, we expect that most of the human genome will be mapped with closely spaced DNA markers, making it possible to search exhaustively for single major genes responsible for psychiatric disorders.

Statistical Methods for Linkage Analysis. The statistical methods of linkage analysis capitalize on both the occurrence of crossing over and the availability of polymorphic genetic markers. They seek to compute a statistic indicating the probability that the cosegregation of genetic markers and disease within pedigrees exceeds what we would expect from the play of chance alone. Thus, linkage analysis assesses the association of disease and marker *within* families.

Linkage methods must be distinguished from the association method (discussed in a later section). The latter method assesses the association of disease and marker in individuals from different families. As an example, we would say that a population association exists between a gene and schizophrenia if schizophrenics are more likely than suitable controls to have a specific version of the gene. For example, if 80% of unrelated schizophrenics had the A version of the gene compared with only 10% of unrelated controls, we would conclude that the gene is associated with schizophrenia.

In contrast, a linkage study attempts to show that, within pedigrees, schizophrenic family members tend to have the same version of the gene. For example, consider a finding of linkage between schizophrenia and a DNA marker that is expressed as one of two alleles, A or B. This means that in some families the schizophrenic members would be more likely to carry the A allele at the marker locus. If they transmitted the schizophrenia gene to offspring they would also be very likely to transmit the A allele at the marker locus. However, in other schizophrenia families, the schizophrenic patients might be more likely to carry the B version of the marker allele. If they transmitted the schizophrenia gene to offspring they would be very likely to transmit the B allele at the marker locus. The key point is that ill members from the *same* family tend to carry the same marker allele near the disease locus. If this seems confusing it may be helpful to note that the marker gene is *not* the disease gene; it is only physically close to the disease gene. By chance different families will have different versions of the marker gene linked to the disease gene.

The Affected Relative Pair Method. The affected relative pair method of linkage analysis evolved from the affected sib-pair method (Weeks and Lange, 1988; Ward, 1993). The original "identity by descent" affected sib-pair method worked with pairs of ill siblings having parents with four different alleles at the marker locus. That is, the father carried two versions of the gene and the mother carried two versions that differed from the father's. For example, the father might have alleles A and B and the mother might have C and D. Under the null hypothesis of no linkage, the distribution of alleles shared by siblings at the locus is well defined. For example, consider any of the alleles, say A. The probability that the father transmitted it to the first child is 0.50. The probability of transmitting it to the second child is also 0.50. Therefore, the probability that he transmits A to both children is 0.50 times 0.50 or 0.25.

Now assume that the marker locus is close to a disease locus and that the two children have the disease. Because both have the disease gene, both share a segment of DNA that contains the gene and surrounding loci. The size of this segment is not fixed (it depends on where crossovers occurred). However, the probability that the marker locus is on this segment increases with the proximity of the marker to the disease locus. If the marker and disease loci are contiguous, then the children who inherited the disease gene should also have inherited the same allele at the marker locus. We say that the shared marker allele is "identical by descent" to indicate that the alleles observed in the children are copies of the same parental allele. We know this is so only because the sib-pair method requires parents to have four different alleles at the marker locus. For example, suppose the father has alleles A and B and the marker locus and the mother has C and D. If two of their children each have allele C at the marker locus then (ignoring the very small probability of mutation), we know that their C alleles are copies of their mother's C allele. Thus their C alleles are identical by descent.

A statistical test was developed to determine whether the observed distribution of marker alleles differed significantly from what was expected under the hypothesis of no linkage. The method was later generalized to the case in which the parental marker alleles were not all unique. In this situation we can determine if alleles are "identical by state" but not if they are "identical by descent." Identity by state means that the two alleles are the same but we cannot be certain if they are copies of the same parental gene. For example, suppose the father has alleles A and B and the marker locus and the mother has A and C. If two of their children each have allele A at the marker locus, then we cannot determine if both received it from the father, both from the mother, or one from the mother and the other from the father. Identity by state methods are needed when the marker is not polymorphic enough to result in four different alleles in the parents. Unfortunately, the loss of identity by descent information reduces statistical power (Bishop and Williamson, 1990).

The affected relative pair method is a general form of the sib-pair method. It allows all ill relative pairs to be included in the analysis. As is the case with siblings, linkage between a marker and a disorder increases the probability that any pair of ill relatives will share the same version of the DNA marker. The major advantage of the affected relative pair method is that we can use it without knowing the mode of inheritance of the disease. This makes it very appealing for studies of psychiatric disorders: As we discussed above, segregation studies have not been able to confirm specific modes of inheritance for these disorders. Thus, we can detect linkage with no a priori knowledge of the genetic and environmental parameters that mediate familial transmission. However, by eliminated information about the mode of inheritance, the method sacrifices some statistical power.

The Lod Score Method. In contrast to affected relative pair methods, the lod score method requires knowledge of the mode of inheritance. Although it is possible to estimate the mode of inheritance and test for linkage simultaneously, the usual practice is to test for linkage under an assumed genetic model. We do so by estimating the ***recombination fraction:*** the probability that the disease and marker genes will recombine during meiosis (Ott, 1992). The lower the probability, the greater the likelihood of linkage. The most widely used method is to compute a maximum likelihood estimate of the recombination fraction. Then a likelihood ratio test compares the odds of the data occurring given that estimate with the odds of the data if the true recombination fraction is 0.5 (this is our null hypothesis because unlinked loci recombine with a probability of 0.5).

This likelihood ratio is an odds ratio comparing the probability that linkage is present with the probability of no linkage. Since we usually examine the base 10 logarithm of the odds ratio, the test statistic is known as the *lod score* (log of the odds ratio). Lod scores can be summed over pedigrees. Lod scores greater than 3 are considered to be evidence in favor of linkage, while lod scores less than -2 constitute evidence against linkage. Thus, a linkage analysis will support the hypothesis of linkage if the odds favoring linkage are 1,000 to 1 (i.e., $\log[1,000/1] = 3$).

As noted above, the main drawback of the lod score method is that we must specify parameters that describe the mode of genetic transmission. However, there is a way around this problem. Greenberg (1989) showed that if we analyze our data several time under different modes of inheritance, the lod score will be greatest for the model that is closest to the true mode of inheritance. For example, we might choose to examine two dominant models and two recessive models. We might also vary the assumed frequency of the gene in the population.

So far, we have been discussing linkage analyses that involve only two loci: one marker locus and one disease locus. Since a disease gene will be surrounded by many potential marker loci, these "two-point" analyses will not have optimal power to detect linkage and locate the gene. Multipoint analyses use several markers simultaneously during the linkage analysis. Multipoint mapping improves statistical power by using all available marker information in the area of the putative disease locus (Spence, 1987). Lander and Botstein (1986a, b, 1988; Lander, 1988) proposed "interval mapping," which assesses linkage, not to a single marker, but to an interval flanked by a pair of markers. Xu et al. (1992) recently evaluated interval mapping with statistical simulations. Compared with single point analyses, interval mapping was much more powerful, requiring 30% fewer families to detect linkage. Moreover, interval mapping was more robust to misclassification of penetrances, diagnoses, and phenocopies. Although these considerations favor a multipoint approach, the method must be used with caution. Risch and Guiffra (1992) showed that, if the mode of transmission is complex, multipoint analyses can spuriously reject linkage. However, they also show that this problem is mitigated when using high estimates of the disease allele frequency.

The lod score method has been generalized for the detection of linkage heterogeneity. That is, we can test the null hypothesis that all families are linked in favor of an alternative hypothesis that only a proportion are linked. Ott (1983) demonstrated that the Admixture test of linkage heterogeneity had better statistical properties than the Predivided Sample test. Risch (1988) developed a Bayesian procedure (the B-test) and compared it with the Admixture and Predivided Sample tests. He concluded that the Predivided Sample test was the least suitable and that the B-test and Admixture test were similar in power. The Admixture test also has the advantage of providing estimates of 1) the recombination fraction for the linked form and 2) the proportion of linked families in the sample.

In lod score analyses, the statistical test for linkage is the lod score obtained at the maximum likelihood estimate of the recombination fraction. As this lod score increases, the evidence favoring linkage also increases. Traditionally, a lod score of three or more had been considered to be statistically significant evidence of linkage. As Ott (1992) showed, this corresponds, asymptotically, to a type I error rate of 0.0001 with 0.001 as an upper bound. This rather stringent significance level is necessary due to the low prior probability of linkage.

However, the lod score criterion of three (LOD3) may not be appropriate for complex genetic diseases like schizophrenia. A number of concerns that have been raised in the literature are worth noting. First, the LOD3 criterion was originally designed by Morton (1955) for mendelian diseases for which it was reasonable to compute a prior probability of linkage. For nonmendelian diseases the prior probability is unknown (Clerget-Darpoux et al., 1990; Green, 1990). Morton also assumed that the test was carried out sequentially as pedigrees were collected. Thus, LOD3 does not apply to analyses of fixed sample sizes (Clerget-Darpoux et al., 1990).

The LOD3 criterion must also be adjusted for the effects of testing multiple markers. This includes both the assessment of linkage at multiple loci and the use of multiple markers to assess linkage at a single locus (Edwards and Watt, 1989; Clerget-Darpoux et al., 1990; Edwards, 1990). When there is a meaningful prior probability of linkage, Ott (1992) demonstrated that the critical α level should be no greater than 0.001 for as many as 100 markers but should be no greater than $1/[1,000 \times (g - 100)]$ when the number of markers, g, is greater than 100. For the nonmendelian case there is no simple analytical solution because the prior probability of linkage is unknown (Green, 1990).

Another procedure that inflates the type I error rate is the use of multiple disease definitions in sequential linkage analyses (Goldin, 1990). For a mendelian disease assessed with m different phenotype definitions, Green (1990) suggested adding $\log_{10}\{m\}$ to the lod score criterion. Although this is a relatively small effect, the simulation study of Clerget-Darpoux et al. (1990) showed that the error rate at LOD3 may be greater for complex diseases. Moreover, by maximizing the lod score over different modes of inheritance we are also inflating the type I error rate. Both Green (1990) and Ott (1990a) suggested that simulation methodology may be the only means of effectively controlling the type I error rate when studying nonmendelian disorders.

The use of computer simulation methods to determine the appropriate lod score criterion was demonstrated by Weeks et al. (1990 a,b). Briefly, the procedure is as follows. First, the linkage analysis is performed on real data by maximizing the lod score over genetic models and phenotype definitions. After a high lod score is found a second analysis is performed on the same pedigrees. The only difference between the two analyses is that the first analysis uses the real marker data and the second uses simulated marker data. In the second analysis the markers are simulated under the assumption that the disease and marker are not linked. In the simulation, marker genotypes are assigned to subjects whose parents were not studied based on the marker gene frequencies used in the first analysis and the assumption of ***Hardy-Weinberg equilibrium.*** Marker genotypes are assigned to other pedigree members by simulating mendelian laws of transmission on the pedigree. The simulation step is replicated many times and, for each replicate, we record the maximum lod score attained. This provides us with the distribution of maximum lod scores expected under the null hypothesis of no linkage. To set a type I error rate of α, we choose the lod score corresponding to the $1 - \alpha$ point on the cumulative maximum lod score distribution computed by the simulation. To estimate probabilities in the upper tail of the maximum lod score distribution accurately, many replications are necessary.

When the observed maximum lod score from the actual linkage analysis exceeds all of the simulated maximum lod scores, the estimated type I error rate is 0. In this case, to ensure that the true type I error rate is no greater than 0.001 with $100(1 - \phi)\%$ confidence, Weeks at al. showed that the number of simulation replicates should be greater than $\log\{\phi\}/\log\{.999\}$. Thus, for a 95% confidence interval, 2,995 replicates are required. By maintaining a comprehensive and systematic record of all linkage analyses performed, we can generate accurate rules for declaring the statistical significance of lod scores.

Another concern in assessing the statistical significance of a linkage finding is the fact that all individuals in the sample do not contribute equally to the lod score. For example, although several factors led to the reversal of the highly significant linkage finding for bipolar disorder by Egeland et al. (1987), one of these was a change in affection status of several pedigree members (Kelsoe et al., 1989). Clearly, a significant linkage finding will be more compelling if we can demonstrate that it would not lose significance if a follow-up study of the sample were to find a few changes in diagnosis. The computer program VaryPhen determines the degree to which the magnitude of lod scores depends on each individual in the pedigree (Xie and Ott, 1990).

A final caution in the use of linkage methods is the specification of marker allele frequencies. Linkage analysis algorithms require the user to specify the population frequencies of the different alleles at the DNA marker locus. Freimer et al. (1993) provide a discussion of this issue. They point out that, for some markers, it may be difficult to get correct allele frequencies because these can vary dramatically between ethnic subgroups. They note that this problem is relevant when the linkage analysis must reconstruct marker genotypes, a situation that is not unusual. Their simulations show that misspecification of allele frequencies does not affect statistical power, but can lead to both false-negative and false-positive linkage results. Thus, they suggest that linkage analysts determine how sensitive their results are to changes in marker allele frequencies by running several analyses.

Nechiporuk et al. (1991) provided an empirical example of how misspecification of marker allele frequencies can modify results. In a genetic linkage study of Alzheimer's disease they found that "assumptions regarding marker allele frequencies had a major and often unpredictable effect on calculated lod scores."

Statistical Power. In planning and conducting a linkage study, it is important to consider the number of pedigrees (or ill relative pairs) needed to show linkage. Although the detection of heterogeneity is also of interest, it requires a much larger sample size than does the detection of linkage under heterogeneity (Cavalli-Sforza and King, 1986; Ott, 1986; Clerget-Darpoux et al., 1987; Martinez and Goldin, 1989, 1990).

Goldin and Gershon (1988) calculated the number of schizophrenic sib pairs needed to detect linkage. Their autosomal dominant model assumed a population prevalence of 1% and no *phenocopies* (subjects without the pathogenic gene who develop the disease). The probability of a person becoming schizophrenic was 0.5 if they had one or two copies of the disease allele. They also assumed that 1) the identity by descent (IBD) of marker alleles is known exactly, i.e., the marker was highly polymorphic; and 2) 50% of sibships were linked. They examined results for two values of the recombination fraction: 0.01 (which indicates very close linkage) and 0.1 (which indicates linkage, but at a 10-fold greater distance). Under these conditions, 50 pairs achieved 80% power for a recombination fraction of 0.01, while 120 pairs achieved the same level of power for a value of 0.10. Since, given the degree of polymorphism of most DNA markers, the sib-pair method usually needs information from parents, this would require data from 200 and 440 people (two siblings and two parents per family), respectively, for recombination fractions of 0.01 and 0.1.

Bishop and Williamson (1990) investigated the power to detect linkage by using identity-by-state (IBS) methods. For a rare dominant disease, they found that pairs of affected grandparent–grandchild or affected first cousins were more informative for linkage analysis than pairs of affected siblings. Assuming that a marker of four alleles with equal frequency is used and that all affected relative pairs were linked with the marker, they calculated the sample size needed to detect linkage for pairs of affected grandparent–grandchild or affected first cousins. For example, for a dominant disease gene with a frequency of 0.022 and no phenocopies, 50 pairs of first cousins had 80% power to detect linkage if the recombination fraction was 0.05; the power was 20% if it was 0.20. The sample size needed increased when heterogeneity and phenocopies were allowed. Unlike the determination of IBD scores, the determination of the IBS distribution does not require information from other relatives. Thus, although in principle the power to detect linkage per pair is lower for the IBS method than the IBD method, the number of individuals needed for genotyping of the marker may not differ greatly between these two methods.

As pointed out by Goldin and Gershon (1988) and Bishop and Williamson (1990), the power calculations for affected sib pairs or affected relative pairs are usually based on a 0.05 significance level; this is much less stringent than the traditional lod score significance cutoff of 3, which is approximately equal to 0.001. If the 0.001 significance level is used, the number of affected sib pairs needed increases about 1.7-fold (Goldin and Gershon, 1988). Thus 200 sib pairs (400 individuals) rather than 120 pairs (240 individuals) would be needed to achieve 80% power for a recombination fraction of 0.1. To make the affected relative pair significance level comparable with traditional lod score method, Risch (1990c) proposed a maximum lod score criterion of 3 to assess the significance of linkage for relative pairs.

Risch (1990c) parameterized the IBD distribution for various relative pairs in terms of a risk ratio λ_R, which is the risk to type R relatives divided by the population prevalence. He demonstrated that λ_R is the critical parameter in determining the power to detect linkage using affected relative pairs. Based on data of McGue et al. (1983), Risch (1990b) estimated that λ_R is approximately 10 for schizophrenia. Assuming that there is no genetic heterogeneity and that a fully informative and tightly linked marker (recombination fraction = 0.0) is used, approximately 50 affected sib pairs would have 80% power to detect linkage. If the recombination fraction is 0.10, approximately 170 pairs are needed to achieve 80% power. Risch (1990d) also showed that the power of relative pairs is very sensitive to the polymorphism of the marker. For example, although 40 sib pairs have 70% power when the marker is fully informative (i.e., very polymorphic), the power falls to 10% when the informativeness decreases by 30%.

The work of Cavalli-Sforza and King (1986) shows that it is relatively easy to achieve high power to detect linkage by using the lod score method if the disease has a clear mendelian mode of transmission. For a fully penetrant dominant disease without phenocopies, 14 nuclear families each comprising 2 parents and 3 children would achieve a 50% power of detecting linkage for a recombination fraction of 0.1. This assumes that the affected parent is *heterozygous* at the marker locus and that all families are linked. If only

50% or 30% of the families were linked, then the number of families required would be 52 and 138, respectively. These figures are optimistic for psychiatric genetics since psychiatric disorders are unlikely to be fully penetrant, *phenocopies* probably exist, and genetic heterogeneity is likely.

Martinez and Goldin (1989) used a more complex model of disease in their assessment of the sample size needed for the detection of linkage. In their study, the disease prevalence was fixed at 2%. For a dominant disease with a penetrance of 0.9 and a phenocopy rate of 5%, the average number of nuclear families (three siblings with at least one affected) needed to achieve 50% power at a recombination fraction of 0.01 was 28; this assumed that 50% of the families were linked to a fully informative marker (Martinez and Goldin, 1989). If the penetrance decreased to 0.5 then the number of families needed to maintain 50% power increased to 101. When analyses were limited to families having sibships of three with at least two affected, the power increased substantially. Using the same marker and assuming the penetrances of 0.9 and 0.5, the number of families (three siblings with at least two affected) needed to achieve a 50% power were 25 and 53, respectively.

Chen et al. (1992b) assessed the statistical power for linkage studies of schizophrenia by simulating schizophrenia pedigrees. These simulations used the known demographic, epidemiologic, and familial features of the disorder to create pedigrees that one would expect to ascertain in a linkage study of schizophrenia. They then evaluated the power of the pedigrees using simulation methodology. They assumed that penetrance was incomplete (0.189) and age dependent, 16% of cases were phenocopies, and markers were moderately informative. Compared with Martinez and Goldin (1989), they assumed a much lower penetrance (0.189 vs. 0.5), a higher phenocopy rate (16% vs. 5%), and a 30% less informative marker. Nevertheless, for a given level of power, the sample size needed under their assumptions was not much greater than that reported by Martinez and Goldin.

For example, consider the sample size needed to attain 50% power when the recombination fraction is approximately 0.01 and 50% of families are linked with the marker. For a penetrance of 0.5, Martinez and Goldin (1989) showed that any one of the following three types of families were needed: 1) 101 nuclear families of sibship size 3 with at least 1 affected child (202 of 505 individuals affected); 2) 53 nuclear families of sibship size 3 but with at least 2 affected children (146 of 265 individuals affected); or 3) 41 nuclear families of sibship size 4 with at least 2 affected children (117 of 246 individuals affected). In these nuclear families, about one-half of the obligatory gene-carrying parents would also be affected. In the simulations by Chen et al. (1992b), 50 multigeneration pedigrees with at least 3 affected individuals were needed to achieve the same level of power. These pedigrees contained approximately 150 affected individuals and 500 subjects in total. This total is nearly identical to that in No. 1 above, but the proportion affected is lower (30% vs 40%). The total number of subjects is about twice that in Nos. 2 and 3 above, but these latter methods require approximately half the sample to be affected. Although cases 2 and 3 require only half the sample needed, this difference is not that dramatic given that, compared with the findings of Chen et al., the results for 1, 2, and 3 assume a much higher penetrance and a much lower phenocopy rate.

What is perhaps most notable in this comparison is that the number of *affected* individuals required to achieve the same power is very similar. This suggests that the contribution of unaffected individuals to the linkage analysis is limited. Indeed, Goldin and Martinez (1989) demonstrated that ignoring marker and disease loci information of unaffected individuals results in only a small increase in the average sample size needed to detect linkage. This is intuitively reasonable. Because models of psychiatric disorders assume low penetrance, unaffected individuals are ambiguous. They may be gene carriers—who do not express the gene—or they may not carry the gene. This conceptual ambiguity translates into a loss of statistical power for the unaffected cases.

We can refer to the above-referenced papers on power analysis for a general idea of how to plan for a linkage study (see also Levinson, 1993a,b). However, once the diagnostic data are collected, we can use simulation methods to estimate the power for a specific sample. Boehnke (1986) proposed using statistical simulations to evaluate the power of known pedigrees. The method now handles reduced penetrance, phenocopies, and heterogeneity (Ott, 1989a; Ploughman and Boehnke, 1989). Specialized computer programs such as SIMLINK (Ploughman and Boehnke, 1989) accomplish this purpose.

SIMLINK needs only information about phenotype, age, and pedigree structure from generated pedigrees. Genotypes must be simulated in the power analysis. To simulate genotypes, SIMLINK requires the genetic parameters of the disease locus, including the gene frequency, penetrance of each genotype, and the disease's age at onset distribution.

After generating trait genotypes, SIMLINK generates marker genotypes according to a given marker allele frequency, mendelian transmission, and the recombination fraction between trait and marker. To compute the statistical power under genetic heterogeneity, SIMLINK allows us to specify that only a proportion of pedigrees are linked to the marker. After simulating trait and marker genotypes, a maximum likelihood algorithm estimates the recombination fraction and the proportion of pedigrees linked to the marker.

For a user-specified number of replications, SIMLINK simulates the cosegregation of the disease locus with a marker locus under the assumption of a true recombination fraction r. For each replication, SIMLINK computes lod scores for several test recombination fractions (e.g., 0.01, 0.05, 0.10, 0.20, 0.30, 0.40, 0.50). For each replication, SIMLINK determines the maximum lod score for that replication. After the user-specified number of replications, say N, we are left with a distribution of N maximum summed lod scores. For a specified lod score threshold of declaring linkage, the relative frequency that the maximum summed lod score exceeds the threshold is the power of the linkage test.

Alternatives to Linkage Analysis. Linkage analysis has been extremely successful for diseases with well-defined modes of inheritance. However, it has not yet gleaned genes for psychiatric disorders. Because of this, some investigators have turned to association studies and related techniques.

Association Studies. As we discussed above, the process of crossing over during meiosis shuffles the parental genes so that the chromosomes we receive from our fathers and mothers are not identical to any of their original chromosomes. Thus, through the generations, genes are constantly shifting from one chromosome to another. As a result, we should expect no association between alleles of loci on the same chromosome. For example, assume that locus 1 can have allele a or A and locus 2 can have allele b or B. If the two loci are on the same chromosome then the probability that any chromosome contains the pair Ab, P(Ab), should be equal to the probability of A, P(A), times the probability of b, P(b). That is, P(Ab) = P(A) $\times$ P(b). Similarly, P(AB) = P(A) $\times$ P(B) and so on. Put simply, if we know that a chromosome contains allele A at locus 1, this tells us nothing about the probability of locus 2 containing allele B or b.

This random distribution of alleles at different loci on the same chromosome is only partially true. It is an empirical fact that some loci are associated with one another so that

P(*Ab*) ≠ P(*A*) × P(*b*) (Vogel and Motulsky, 1986). For example, it may be that chromosomes with allele *A* at locus 1 are more likely to have allele *b* at locus 2 than we would expect by chance (i.e., than we would expect from the frequency of allele *b* in the population). Now, assume that locus 1 is a disease locus and that *A* is a dominant pathogenic allele. Also assume that locus 2 is a DNA marker locus. If the two loci are associated as indicated above, then people with the disease should be more likely to have marker allele *b* than people without the disease.

This nonrandom association of alleles at different loci is called ***linkage disequilibrium***. Knowledge of its causes is essential if it is to be a tool for finding disease genes. One cause of linkage disequilibrium is the fact that the reshuffling of genes on chromosomes depends on genetic distance. If two genes are very close to one another, then they will rarely be separated by crossing over and will usually be transmitted together. Thus, due to close linkage, the alleles at two loci will tend to be transmitted together. We say "tend to" because eventually crossing over will separate them.

Fortunately, the reshuffling of linked genes can take many thousands of years. This means that, theoretically, we should be able to detect associations between diseases and DNA markers if the marker locus is *very close* to the disease locus. Compared with a linkage study, the design and analysis of an association study is straightforward. We do not require pedigrees with multiple ill members. Samples of unrelated patients and controls will suffice. Instead of a complex linkage analysis, all we need do is compare the rates of marker alleles (or genotypes) in patients and controls with standard statistical tests (Vogel and Motulsky, 1986).

A major disadvantage of association studies is that the DNA marker must be tightly linked to the disease gene. This is in contrast with the linkage method, which can detect linkage over relatively large distances. Thus, with linkage analysis it is possible to "scan the genome," which is a shorthand way of saying that, if we use many markers, we can test for linkage to all chromosomal loci. In contrast, for an association study to succeed we need to know where to look for the gene. But, the reason for doing linkage and association studies is to find the gene. So how do we know where to look?

Since we do not know where to look, we can make some educated guesses. When we make such a guess we are specifying a *candidate gene*. Once we have a candidate gene we find a DNA marker that is very close to that gene and proceed with our association study. Ideally a candidate gene would have a known pathophysiologic significance. For example, Alzheimer's disease leaves a clear pathophysiologic signature on the brain (senile plaques containing β-amyloid). Since the production of β-amyloid requires the amyloid precursor protein (APP), the APP gene was a logical candidate gene for Alzheimer's disease. The examination of APP as a candidate gene was further motivated by symptomatic and pathophysiologic correspondences between Alzheimer's disease and Down's syndrome (Schweber, 1985). The latter syndrome was known to be caused by a trisomy of chromosome 21, and the APP gene had been mapped to chromosome 21 (Korenberg et al., 1988). Thus, APP was clearly a candidate gene for Alzheimer's disease, and, eventually, studies of the APP gene among Alzheimer's disease patients found unequivocal mutations (Chartier-Harlin et al., 1991; Goate et al., 1991; Naruse et al., 1991; van Duijn et al., 1991).

Unlike Alzheimer's disease, most psychiatric disorders do not have a known pathophysiology that points to an obvious candidate gene. For example, although schizophrenia is undoubtedly a disease of the brain, the pathophysiologic details have eluded careful investigation (Tsuang and Faraone, 1994). There are many genes that *might* be relevant to schizophrenia, but none of these are credible candidate genes in the sense that the APP gene was a credible candidate for Alzheimer's disease. For example, neurotransmitter systems are dysregulated in many psychiatric disorders, and the location of relevant genes is now known. Examples include genes for monoamine oxidase (Bach et al., 1988; Hsu et al., 1988a,b), dopamine-β-hydroxylase (Lamouroux et al., 1987; Kobayashi et al., 1989), tyrosine hydroxylase (Grima et al., 1987), and dopamine receptor subtypes (Zander et al., 1981; Bunzow et al., 1988; Grandy et al., 1989; Dearry et al., 1990; Sunahara et al., 1990).

Psychiatric geneticists have tried to capitalize on plausible links between such genes and psychiatric illness (Blum et al., 1990; Gelernter et al., 1991; Nothen et al., 1992; Schwartz and Moises, 1993), but not without controversy (Conneally, 1991; Kidd, 1993; Pato et al., 1993). The failure of association studies to produce consistently reproducible results supports Crowe's (1993, p 76) contention that "candidate genes in psychiatry are lottery tickets." As Crowe discussed, there are approximately 30,000 genes expressed in the human brain. Any of these could be a "candidate" for psychiatric disease, yet none are well justified to the same degree that the APP gene was a credible candidate for Alzheimer's disease. As a result, the a priori probability is low that any one of these is associated with a specific disease.

Crowe computed that the likelihood of a false-positive result is so high that one would have to set a statistical significance level of 0.00001 to achieve a false-positive rate of 5%. If we were to use a significance level of 0.001, 80% of positive findings would be false. The traditional α level of 0.05 would yield 99.5% false-positive results.

The problem of false-positive results is exacerbated by the fact that close linkage is not the only cause of disease–marker associations (Vogel and Motulsky, 1986; Crowe, 1993; Kidd, 1993). The frequencies of DNA marker alleles varies among ethnic groups. Thus, if patient and control groups are not carefully matched for ethnicity, spurious differences in allele frequencies between groups will emerge. Also, closely linked loci can exhibit linkage disequilibrium—but this is not a necessity. Kidd (1993) gave the example of PKU, a single gene disorder of amino acid metabolism. Although the PKU gene is close to several DNA markers, none of these show linkage disequilibrium.

Because of the problems discussed above, association studies must be used and interpreted with caution. Kidd (1993) suggested that consistent replication would be the best evidence for a true association. However, he also cautioned that, to be a true replication, a subsequent study should use methods that are similar if not identical to the methods of the original study. Crowe (1993) also emphasized the importance of standardized research methods and suggested selecting probands from multiplex pedigrees to ensure that we are studying a genetic form of the illness.

Because it may be difficult to find patient and control groups that are suitably matched for ethnicity, several investigators have developed tests of linkage disequilibrium that use the parents of ill individuals as controls (Rubinstein et al., 1981; Falk and Rubinstein, 1987; Ott, 1989b; Knapp et al., 1993; Spielman et al., 1993). For example, the transmission test for linkage disequilibrium (TDT) uses families having at least one affected offspring and one parent who is heterozygous for the DNA marker to be tested (Spielman et al., 1993). The TDT compares the number of times heterozygous parents transmit the associated marker allele to affected offspring with the number of times they transmit the other marker allele. If these probabilities differ from what is expected by chance, then we can conclude that linkage disequilibrium exists. Although the TDT solves the problem of ethnicity matching, it still faces the problem of false positives and must be cautiously interpreted in the absence of a credible candidate gene.

Mutation Screening. Since psychiatry has few (some would say no) good candidate genes, some investigators have suggested that, instead of demonstrating associations with polymorphic DNA markers, we should demonstrate associations with mutations that have pathophysiologic significance. As we discussed above, DNA markers are often selected because many variants exist. These markers are usually in "noncoding" portions of the genome. In other words, they occur in stretches of DNA that have no physiologic significance. This has been referred to as *junk* DNA: It is the DNA that evolution "threw away" because it was not needed to create adaptive organisms.

Linkage studies value the high level of polymorphism of junk DNA because it increases statistical power. The physiologic function of the marker is irrelevant. But, in the absence of a candidate gene, associations with junk DNA can be meaningless because such DNA could not cause the disease being studied. Because of this, several investigators have suggested that we search directly for mutations that have pathophysiologic significance (Sobell et al., 1992; Crowe, 1993). In short, the goal of these methods is to find an association between an allele and a disease not because the two are closely linked but because the allele causes the disease. Several variants of this approach have been proposed.

One approach identifies a candidate gene that is known to have two or more alleles that are of functional significance. For example, the D_4 dopamine receptor gene has several allelic forms that differ in their abilities to bind the neuroleptic drugs that treat schizophrenia (Sommer et al., 1993). Thus, Sommer and colleagues (1993) compared the D_4 dopamine alleles of schizophrenics with those of controls. Although they found no differences, their work illustrates an important point: Group differences in the D_4 dopamine gene would have been more compelling than differences in a DNA marker that is next to the D_4 dopamine gene.

This first approach is useful but lacks a key ingredient: It is possible for a gene to have several different "normal" alleles of no pathophysiologic significance. Thus, investigators have sought methods that identify clear mutations. For example, Crowe (1993) noted that the nature and location of apparent mutations provide information about the probability of their being pathologic. He also discussed how laboratory methods can be used to demonstrate the effects of an apparently mutant gene.

A second approach to finding mutations comprises several methods that have been described as *mutation screening*. Gejman and Gelernter (1993) described the strengths and weaknesses of three types of mutation screening: Single-stranded conformational polymorphisms, denaturing gradient gel electrophoresis, mismatch cleavage, and DNA sequencing. The epidemiologist need not know the details of each method. The key point to remember is that each method searches candidate genes for allelic variants that should have pathophysiologic significance.

Sobell, et al. (1992, 1993) describe an approach to mutation screening they called *VAPSE-based case–control association studies*. A VAPSE is a DNA sequence Variation Affecting Protein Structure or Expression. We find VAPSEs with DNA sequencing, which is the direct examination of the nucleic acid sequence that forms the DNA. Any modified sequence that changes the DNA blueprint is a VAPSE. By definition, VAPSEs occur only in regions of the genome that code for proteins or regulate biologic processes—junk DNA cannot constitute a VAPSE.

Sobell and colleagues (1992) describe five phases of a VAPSE study: 1) Select a candidate gene; 2) use a subset of patients to search for VAPSEs; 3) if you find a VAPSE, use a large case–control association study to see if the disease is associated with the VAPSE; 4) replicate the observed association, and determine if the VAPSE and disease are linked using linkage analyses in families that exhibit the VAPSE; and 5) estimate the population attributable risk of the VAPSE.

Methods of mutation screening represent a major advance in the application of the case–control association study. However, these methods are only a beginning. Replicating the finding and demonstrating linkage will be necessary before any "plausible mutation" can be seriously considered as a cause of disease. Replication may be difficult because, like the traditional association study, these methods are subject to the problem of false positives created by case–control differences in ethnicity and the absence of credible candidate genes.

SAMPLING, DESIGN, AND STATISTICAL ISSUES

This section contains a discussion of some of the methodologic issues facing the genetic epidemiologist working in psychiatry.

Ascertainment

Ascertainment or sampling is critical to an accurate assessment of the mode of inheritance. In epidemiology, sampling bias occurs when the sampling procedure creates a sample that systematically differs from the population it purports to represent. For example, we know that people who volunteer to be part of a "normal" control group have rates of psychopathology and its correlates that exceed the population expectation (Gibbons et al., 1990; Kruesi et al., 1990; Risch et al., 1990; Thaker et al., 1990; Shtasel et al., 1991; Buckley et al., 1992). Another type of bias occurs when we want to generalize our results to all people with a disorder but sample patients from a psychiatric clinic. Clearly, people who seek treatment will differ systematically from those in the community who do not.

There are many ways for a sample to be biased. However, in genetic epidemiology we use the term *ascertainment bias* to refer only to biases that affect the distribution of illness in the family. By *distribution* we mean the number of ill family members and the pattern of illness in the family. For example, if we design a project that recruits families having one ill parent and one ill child, we create a sample that appears to have a dominantly transmitted disorder (because, unlike recessive disorders, these are usually seen in both generations of a nuclear family).

Ascertainment bias occurs when we do not sample families randomly. It is a ubiquitous problem for genetic epidemiology because the low prevalence of most genetic disorders makes it impractical to sample families randomly. For example, in a study of schizophrenia, which has a base rate of about 1% in the population, we would have to screen many hundreds of families before obtaining a sufficient sample size. Since random sampling is not feasible, we must resort to proband sampling.

A proband is a person with the illness under study who brings the family to the attention of the investigator. We say that a family has multiple probands if we independently ascertain more than one family member with the disease from the sampling frame. This will occur, for example, when we are sampling from a clinic if ill family members use the same clinic.

The literature on ascertainment problems and their remediation is complex. We restrict our comments to the "classic" model of ascertainment developed by Weinberg (1925) and Fisher (1934)[1]. There are two types of ascertainment: complete and incomplete. ***Complete ascertainment*** is difficult to attain. It refers to a simple random sampling of families to find those that have one or more members with the disease of interest. With proband sampling we have ***incomplete ascertainment.*** There are three types of incomplete ascertainment. In ***truncate ascertainment,*** the probability of an ill individual's being sampled (represented as π) is high. Therefore, all ill members of a family will be probands, and everyone in the population with the disorder is sampled. From the point of view of statistics, this is the most desirable method of accomplishing incomplete ascertainment since, as Weinberg (1925) and Fisher (1934) demonstrated, it is not necessary to adjust data analyses statistically for this type of sampling. The estimation of genetic parameters under truncate ascertainment produces essentially the same result as under random sampling. This is so because the probability that a family is ascertained is not dependent on family size. Thus, we are not biasing families to have unusually high (or low) rates of illness. Unfortunately, truncate ascertainment is very difficult to carry out. It is only feasible for rare disorders treated in a tertiary care setting, where it is fairly certain that every ill person in a defined population will eventually be seen.

The other extreme of sampling is ***single ascertainment.*** In this case, π, the probability of sampling any one person who is ill, is very low. Because of this there will be only one proband per family. In other words, assume we are sampling bipolar patients from the Boston metropolitan area. Under single ascertainment the likelihood that any specific bipolar patient in Boston will be in our sample will be very low (e.g., 0.01). Because of this, the likelihood of sampling two bipolar patients from the same family is extremely low.

Single ascertainment creates a very specific type of bias: Families with many ill members are more likely to enter a given sample. For instance, if, in a family of 10, there are 6 people with bipolar disorder, whereas only 1 of a family of 3 has the disorder, then the first family has six chances to be ascertained but the second family has only one chance. Thus, under single ascertainment, the probability of sampling a family is proportional to the number of ill members. This means that our estimate of the proportion of ill siblings in any sibship will be too high.

The goal of genetic modeling is to correct for this sampling bias. Fortunately, it is easy to correct our estimate of the proportion of ill siblings: We merely exclude the proband from the analysis. Thus, the proportion of ill siblings of the probands estimates the proportion of ill siblings (among sibships expressing the disorder) that we would have found had we used random sampling.

Sometimes, a proband sampling procedure is neither single nor truncate ascertainment. We call this intermediate case ***multiple ascertainment.*** As its name suggests, under multiple ascertainment more than one family member is independently sampled as a proband, but not all ill family members are probands. Thus, π, the probability of sampling any given person who is ill, is between 0 and 1. In this situation, we correct our estimate of the proportion of ill siblings by weighting multiple proband families by the number of probands in the family.

---

[1]The classic model may not always be appropriate, for a variety of reasons (see Ewens and Shute, 1986; Greenberg, 1986; Shute and Ewens, 1988a,b, for discussions of relevant issues).

As discussed in a prior section, correction for ascertainment is necessary for segregation analysis if we are to estimate correctly the parameters of genetic transmission. Thus, it is of paramount importance, in genetic epidemiologic studies, to specify the ascertainment scheme as precisely as possible before data collection begins. If the ascertainment is uncertain, an investigator cannot accurately estimate genetic parameters. If the ascertainment scheme is misspecified, then inferences drawn from the data may be false. Sometimes, investigators who have collected family data without intending to estimate genetic parameters as one of their original goals will decide later that they are interested in doing just that. Then, when these investigators consult a genetic epidemiologist about carrying out segregation analyses, they are disappointed to learn that their data are unsuitable for such analyses simply because the ascertainment scheme was either not clearly specified or was nonsystematic.

The distinction between sampling procedures that are ill specified and those that are nonsystematic deserves some comment. An ill-specified sampling plan is one that cannot be reproduced because the methods of ascertainment were never recorded. Ascertainment is nonsystematic if we cannot determine which ill family members brought the family to the attention of the study. In other words, we cannot be certain who the probands are. For example, if we use advertisements soliciting families with "two or more cases of schizophrenia" we are often not certain which patients in, say, a family with four schizophrenic siblings "caused" the family to be sampled. Because of this, if we ascertain families nonsystematically they cannot be used for segregation analysis to estimate genetic parameters. A second problem is that we often cannot define the population base from which we nonsystematically sampled families. This hinders our ability to generalize results.

Although these last two points argue against nonsystematic approaches to sampling, other factors must be considered as well. Paramount among these are issues of cost and efficiency. For example, families with more than one case of schizophrenia are rare (McGue and Gottesman, 1989, 1991; Pulver and Bale, 1989); systematic surveys can find such families but only at a very high cost. Since linkage studies do not *require* prior segregation analyses, it is reasonable to argue that the costs of systematic ascertainment cannot be justified. This argument gains more strength by the observation that, in the past, segregation analyses of psychiatric disorders have sometimes led to conflicting results (Faraone and Tsuang, 1985; Faraone et al., 1990; Tsuang and Faraone, 1990).

Before leaving our discussion of ascertainment bias, we must emphasize that although investigators can choose to ascertain systematically or not, they do not have complete control over the type of systematic ascertainment (i.e., single, multiple, truncate, complete). For example, in planning a family study of a common disorder we may decide to sample from a hospital clinic. Although characteristics of the disorder may lead us to expect single ascertainment, it is always possible for us to learn that some of our probands come from the same family. Thus, it is necessary for genetic epidemiologic investigations to keep track of who is and is not a proband so that multiple ascertainment can be detected—and corrected for—should it occur.

Estimating Risk to Relatives

The simplest and perhaps most common means of analyzing genetic epidemiologic data is to compute the rate of illness among relatives of ill probands and compare this with the rate observed among relatives of suitable control probands. As we discussed in the previous section, to be meaningful, these rates must be corrected for ascertainment bias. In this section we discuss two other issues that must be considered: the correlation in risk among relatives and the variable age at onset of most psychiatric disorders.

Lack of Statistical Independence Among Family Members. When comparing a group of relatives of bipolar patients with relatives of normal controls regarding the presence or absence of bipolar disorder, one of the many statistics available for assessing association in a 2×2 contingency table would seem to be suitable. The rows of the table would be formed by the proband's diagnosis (bipolar or not) and the columns by the relative's diagnosis (bipolar or not). This would be fine if we had sampled only one relative from each family.

However, it is usually more cost effective (and genetically interesting) to sample as many relatives from a specified class (e.g., siblings) as possible. In this case, the outcomes of the relatives are not necessarily statistically independent of one another. That is, the probability of one relative being bipolar may vary with the number and pattern of bipolar relatives in the family. Since this would be true under a variety of models of genetic and/or environmental transmission, it is a priori unreasonable to assume statistical independence when analyzing such data (Weissman et al., 1986).

The statistical dependence among relatives is *theoretically* a problem. However, we know of no available statistical research that indicates to what extent this problem invalidates inferences made from statistical tests that ignore it. It seems unlikely that the estimate of rates would be biased, but the p values from statistical tests will probably not be accurate. The degree and direction of this inaccuracy are unknown, but it is reasonable to speculate that the increased similarity of relatives (compared with unrelated subjects) would decrease the variance of estimates and increase the type I error rate.

Fortunately, there are several statistical approaches that can handle this problem. The most straightforward way to compute an accurate significance level is to use the proportion of probands having at least one ill relative as the index of familiality. Thus, the unit of analysis becomes the proband. Since the sampling design can ensure that the probands are statistically independent, we can proceed with traditional statistics (e.g., the chi-squared test, logistic regression). If we are assessing a quantitative outcome (e.g., the intelligence scores among siblings of probands), we can use the mean of all relatives from a class (e.g., compute the mean intelligence score for each sibship). These means can then be analyzed with traditional statistics (if other assumptions are not violated).

Another approach is to use statistical models that do not assume independence of observations. The problem of nonindependence can be handled with the regressive models developed by Bonney (1984, 1986, 1987) and Borecki et al. (1990). These models can use either categorical or continuous traits as dependent variables. They flexibly expand the well-known linear regression and logistic regression models to incorporate situations of nonindependence. The regressive logistic framework is particularly suitable for genetic work because in controlling for nonindependence due to familial correlations it allows for the estimation of parameters of genetic and environmental transmission (see discussion below). The major drawback to this approach is that it sets the data analyst along the path of segregation analysis, which can be very time consuming and may not be in the statistical repertoire of many investigators doing family studies.

Variable Age at Onset. Most psychiatric disorders have a variable age at onset. In some cases the range of age at onset is very wide. For example, although most patients with schizophrenia experience their first symptoms in their 20s or early 30s, some cases can begin in childhood and others after 50. Variable age at onset hinders any interpretation of simple rates of illness because these will depend on the age of the sample. For example, say that the rate of schizophrenia was 10% in a sample of adolescents and 10% in a sample of 50 year olds. We ought to have some means of adjusting these rates to reflect our intuitive sense that the rate among adolescents—who have only just entered the period of risk—indicates a greater risk for schizophrenia than the rate among the 50 year olds—who have lived through most of the period of risk.

We achieve this adjustment by computing the ***morbidity risk:*** the probability that the subjects being studied are susceptible to the illness of interest (Vogel and Motulsky, 1986). An individual who is susceptible may not have onset at the time of examination or may have died due to an unrelated cause. Thus, the morbidity risk is a probability, not a rate. It is the probability that a person will manifest the disorder if he or she lives (or had lived) long enough. For this reason, the morbidity risk is sometimes called the ***lifetime risk.*** Methods to estimate morbidity risk adjust the raw rate of illness in a sample to account for the well subjects who have not lived through the risk period.

If n is the total number of subjects, and m is the total number of affected, then the raw rate of illness is simply $^m/_n$. Since some of the *n* subjects who are well may eventually have onset of the disorder, the raw rate will always underestimate the morbidity risk. Thus, one approach to morbidity risk estimation has been to adjust the denominator downward. The adjusted denominator has traditionally been called the ***Bezugsziffer (BZ).***

The BZ is a sum of weights reflecting each subject's length of exposure to risk up to the age of examination. If w_i is the weight for the ith individual, then the morbidity risk, MR, is estimated by

$$\hat{MR} = \frac{m}{\sum_{i=1}^{n} w_i} .$$

To assign w_i, Weinberg (1925) suggested that we empirically define a risk interval from the lowest to highest possible age at onset. For the ith individual whose age at examination is y_i, we assign $w_i = 0$ if y_i is less than the lowest age at onset, $w_i = 1/2$ if y_i is within the risk period, and $w_i = 1$ if y_i is greater than the oldest age at onset. This method is easy to use, but limited because it assumes that the risk for onset is uniform from the lowest to highest age at onset. Chase and Kramer (1986) demonstrated that these problems could lead to a biased estimation of the true morbidity risk.

Strömgren (1935) proposed a method that assumes we know the age at onset distribution of the disease. He suggested we use the cumulative distribution function of age y at time i (y_i) to create weights (w_i), i.e., $w_i = F(y_i)$. For example, if the 50th percentile of the age at onset distribution was at age 25, then 25 year olds would be given a weight of 0.50 because they have lived through only half the period of risk. If the 90th percentile was at age 60, then 60 year olds would have a weight of 0.90.

With this approach, the estimated morbidity risk is unbiased (Larsson and Sjögren, 1954; Risch, 1983). Strömgren (1938) realized that his original method would estimate the morbidity risk to be greater than 1 under some conditions (e.g., when every subject in the sample is affected). Thus, he modified the formula such that the affected cases contribute one to the denominator and are thereby not weighted by their age at examination. However, several researchers have shown that this modified estimator is biased and have advised against its use (Larsson and Sjögren, 1954; Thompson and Weissman, 1981; Risch, 1983).

For computing confidence intervals or testing hypotheses, we must calculate the variance of the estimated morbidity risk. In a simplified form, the variance of the morbidity risk is a modification of the variance of a proportion, with the sample size replaced by the BZ:

$$\text{Var} (\hat{\text{MR}}) = \frac{\hat{\text{MR}} (1 - \hat{\text{MR}})}{\sum_{i=1}^{n} w_i}.$$

This equation is sufficient for an approximate estimate of the MR such as Weinberg's shorter method. However, for Strömgren's estimator, a more exact form should be used (Larsson and Sjögren, 1954; Risch, 1983):

$$\text{Var} (\hat{\text{MR}}) = \frac{\hat{\text{MR}}}{\sum_{i=1}^{n} w_i} (1 - \frac{\hat{\text{MR}} \sum_{i=1}^{n} w_i^2}{\sum_{i=1}^{n} w_i}).$$

Given that a prior age at onset distribution is available, Risch (1983) derived a maximum likelihood estimate (MLE) of the morbidity risk. The MLE estimate of the morbidity risk has a smaller variance than Strömgren's estimator and, for small samples, is less biased (Risch, 1983). Moreover, the MLE method can estimate the age at onset distribution simultaneously with the morbidity risk (Risch, 1983). This is useful when the age at onset distribution is unknown. Also, other methods assume that the age at onset distribution is known without error. However, it has always been estimated from a sample. By simultaneously estimating the morbidity risk and the age at onset distribution, the MLE method computes a more accurate estimate of the variance of the morbidity risk. However, with simultaneous estimation, other factors, such as missing data and the form of the age at onset distribution, must be considered (for a more detailed discussion, see Cupples et al., 1991; Chen et al., 1992a).

To compute unbiased estimates of risk, Strömgren's method and the maximum likelihood approach must either assume or estimate the correct age at onset distribution. In practice, the required age at onset distribution is usually estimated from the observed ages at onset observed among the proband sample. However, the observed age at onset is biased toward younger ages by the underlying age structure of the susceptible population (Heimbuch et al., 1980; Baron et al., 1983; Chen et al., 1992a, 1993). Using the observed age at onset distribution from prevalent cases can lead to a non-negligible bias in samples of young subjects (Chen et al., 1993). Thus, it is important to obtain an age at onset distribution corrected for the underlying population age structure rather than relying on the observed distribution.

Morbidity risk estimation must address the differential probability of disappearance from observation at any particular age between susceptible and nonsusceptible groups (Sturt, 1985). In practice, one main cause of disappearance is mortality; others include loss to follow up and refusal of participation. Both may be increased in samples of psychiatric patients. Strömgren's method is biased by such effects but Risch's maximum likelihood method (1983) is not.

A second approach to estimating morbidity risk uses concepts from survival analysis (Lee, 1980). Statisticians developed this method to model the time to a specific outcome (e.g., the death of a patient or the failure of a machine). The survival function is the cumulative probability that the outcome does not occur as a function of time. A key feature of survival analysis is that it handles censored data; a censored datum comes from a subject who does not die, but is not observed for the entire study period.

For morbidity risk estimation, the outcome of interest is onset of illness, and the survival function presents the cumulative probability of being free from illness as a function of age. Censored cases are subjects who are unaffected at the time of examination. Thus, to apply this approach we need to know the subjects' age at onset (if they have the disorder) or their age at examination (if they do not).

An early survival analysis approach to morbidity risk estimation was the Weinberg morbidity table (Slater and Cowie, 1971). This was an approximation of the life table approach to survival analysis (Lee, 1980). Both methods have been superseded by the Kaplan-Meier approach (Kaplan and Meier, 1958). This latter method is approximately unbiased in large samples; the other methods are not (e.g., Breslow and Crowley, 1974). Since the information needed to compute the morbidity risk for both the actuarial and Kaplan-Meier methods is the same, the latter is the method of choice.

The Kaplan-Meier method is as follows. Suppose there are n individuals whose survival times, $t_{(i)}$, i = 1 to n, are available. First, we sort the n survival times in increasing order such that $t_{(1)} \leq t_{(2)} \leq t_{(n)}$. If there are tied survival times, uncensored ones are put before censored ones. Then the survival function at time t, S(t), is

$$\hat{S}_{(t)} = \prod_{t_{(r)} \leq t} \left(\frac{n-r}{n-r+1}\right),$$

where r runs through those positive integers for which $t_{(r)} \leq t$ and $t_{(r)}$ is uncensored. The morbidity risk to time t, MR(t), equals $1 - S(t)$. The variance of the Kaplan-Meier estimate of S(t) is given by Greenwood's formula:

$$\text{Var}\,[\hat{S}\,(t)] = [\hat{S}\,(t)]^2 \prod_{t_{(r)} \leq t} \frac{1}{(n-r)\,(n-r+1)}.$$

Survival analysis uses the age at onset of ill relatives to compute the morbidity risk MR(t) up to the largest age in the sample. In contrast, Strömgren's method using the age at onset distribution in probands computes the full lifetime risk. Since the available data dictate the maximum age at which we can compute MR(t), the risk to ages greater than those observed is undefined. This creates some problems in application. First, if the largest observed onset is well below the upper boundary of a known risk interval, then it is difficult to justify the MR(t) as a morbidity risk estimate. Second, comparisons of morbidity risks between groups are meaningful only when the MR(t) in each group is computed at a similar age. Third, since the number of subjects still at risk usually becomes small at large ages, the variance for MR(t) may be large.

In summary, morbidity risk estimation is needed to determine the risk for manifesting disorders having a variable age at onset. Two sets of methods are available. One uses a known age at onset distribution as a weighting system; the other uses methods from survival analysis. Strömgren's estimator or Risch's maximum likelihood estimate is the method of choice among weighting methods; the Kaplan-Meier estimator is preferable when using the survival analysis approach. Further work is needed to choose between weighting and survival analysis methods.

Family Study Designs

The Familial–Sporadic Design. It is likely that many psychiatric disorders are etiologically heterogeneous. That is, there may be different genetic and nongenetic forms of the disease. The familial–sporadic design seeks to develop diagnostic rules that discriminate between genetic and nongenetic forms of an illness. We say that a patient has a familial form of disease if at least one relative also has the disease (or a genetically related disorder). Otherwise, we say that the patient has a sporadic form. Thus, the familial–sporadic strategy attempts to distinguish cases of illness that are more likely to be of the genetic type from those that are more likely to be of the sporadic type. Some day, when we know which mutations cause psychiatric disorders, it may be possible to specify exact diagnostic criteria for genetic and nongenetic subforms. In the meanwhile, we must use the familial–sporadic distinction as a "proxy" for the genetic–nongenetic distinction.

The familial–sporadic method assumes that patients having one or more ill relatives are more likely to have a genetic form of the disorder; these are designated as *familial cases*. Patients having no ill relatives are assumed to be more likely to have an environmental form of the disorder; they are designated as *sporadic cases*. The designations *familial* and *sporadic* are imperfect indicators of the probability of membership in the latent, unobservable categories of "genetic" and "environmental."

As Lewis et al. (1987) pointed out, the classification of cases as familial or sporadic is a research strategy—not an etiologic model. If clinical or neurobiologic measures discriminate these groups, we can learn something about the relative importance of genetic and environmental factors in subgroups defined by these factors. Also, comparisons between familial and sporadic subgroups can help us develop criteria that identify a more homogeneously familial form of the illness. The familial–sporadic strategy cannot determine the mechanism of familial aggregation (e.g., single gene vs. multigene vs. environmental transmission). We must base such inferences on other information (e.g., twin, segregation analysis, and linkage studies).

A powerful version of the familial–sporadic strategy involves the comparison of concordant and discordant MZ twins. Because MZ twins share identical genotypes, an illness having complete genetic determination should be observed in both twins. Thus, it is useful to separate MZ twin pairs that both have the disease (concordant pairs) from pairs where only one has the disease (discordant pairs). Clearly, genetic factors should be more prominent in the concordant than the discordant pairs.

The success of the familial–sporadic strategy relies on its ability to assign correctly "true genetic" cases to the familial category and "true environmental" cases to the sporadic category. We cannot do this without error. Notably, the method is insensitive to differences in the size and age structure of families (Kendler and Hays, 1982; Kendler, 1987). For example, a patient with 10 relatives available for study is more likely to have an ill relative than a patient with only 1 relative. Therefore, the availability of relatives for study will influence the accuracy of classification.

Lyons et al. (1989a) suggested that, under some conditions even a modest relationship between the familial–sporadic and genetic–nongenetic distinctions might be useful. They conducted a power analysis employing a Monte Carlo simulation procedure based on the rates of misclassification determined by Kendler (1987). They concluded that for a sample size of 175, statistical power was moderate to good for effect sizes greater than or equal to one standard deviation unit. Put simply, the utility of the familial–sporadic strategy depends on the size of the samples studied (the larger the better) and the size of the true, unobservable differences between the genetic and nongenetic forms of illness.

The analysis conducted by Lyons et al. (1989a) assumed that the genetic form of the disorder was caused by a single major genetic locus. Eaves et al. (1986) conducted a power analysis of the familial–sporadic distinction assuming a multifactorial polygenic process in which there is a normally distributed liability to illness that is due to numerous genes and environmental factors acting in an additive fashion. They concluded that large sample sizes of probands and relatives are required to detect etiologic heterogeneity with "substantial probability" when using first-degree relatives. However, these authors calculated that use of MZ twins is a much more powerful approach; when MZ twins are used as probands compared with singletons with three first-degree relatives for each proband, there is an 85% reduction in the number of probands required for equal statistical power. For example, to achieve comparable power to a family study using one first-degree relative per proband with 1,026 relatives and probands, a study of MZ twins would require 65 subjects.

Since power analyses show that the familial–sporadic strategy has low statistical power, it is notable that—even with small sample sizes—this method has produced positive results. For example, sporadic cases of schizophrenia are more likely to have had perinatal complications and brain abnormalities by computed tomography. Familial cases are more likely to have attentional deficits (Lyons et al., 1989b). We are far from having diagnostic criteria for "familial" schizophrenia, but the available data suggest that this is a possibility.

The High-Risk Design. The high-risk design has two major goals: 1) to identify risk factors that increase the probability of onset in susceptible individuals and 2) to define manifestations of psychiatric genotypes that are expressed in the absence of frank illness.

To achieve the first goal, the investigator must select a sample of subjects at high risk for the disorder who have not already had onset of symptoms. Ideally, these should be as young as possible so that many risk factors can be studied. This has led to the children-at-risk paradigm in which the investigator finds parents with the disease of interest and studies their children. This design has been successfully employed in studies of schizophrenia (Mednick et al., 1971; Erlenmeyer-Kimling, 1975; Fish et al., 1992) and mood disorders (Orvaschel, 1990; Biederman et al., 1991).

The cited studies (and many others) show that the children-at-risk design yields valuable information about the early signs of illness and risk factors for onset. However, such studies are difficult to perform for two reasons. First, to define *at risk* we must use parental illness. This is reasonable, but we should be aware that not all of our at-risk sample is truly susceptible to the illness. For example, we know from family studies that approximately 10% of the children of schizophrenic patients will eventually experience schizophrenia or some other psychotic disorder (Tsuang et al., 1993). Thus, if we start with a sample of 100 children of schizophrenic patients, only 10 will eventually become psychotic. Clearly, large samples are needed if we are to be able to observe many onsets of illness.

A second burden of the children-at-risk study is the need for longitudinal follow up. In order to predict who does, and does not, become schizophrenic, the children need to be followed for many years into adolescence and adulthood. Since some subjects will be lost to follow up, we need to plan our initial sample size accordingly. We should also plan our assessments so that we can determine if there are meaningful differences between subjects lost versus those not lost to follow up.

The second goal of the high-risk study is to define manifestations of psychiatric genotypes that are expressed in the absence of frank illness. Such phenomena are of interest because they may provide clues to the etiology or pathophysiology of disease. They may also facilitate the discovery of genes by linkage analysis. Since this type of high-risk study does not seek to predict which susceptible people develop disease, it is easier to implement than the children-at-risk design. The basic design is straightforward. We compare the biologic relatives of patients with the biologic relatives of controls using some indicator that we believe to measure the unobservable liability to disease.

Guidelines for validating such indicators have periodically been presented in the literature (Reider and Gershon, 1978; Gershon and Goldin, 1986; Garver, 1987; Keefe et al., 1991; Kremen et al., 1992). These provide some guidance for choosing measures with which to design phenotypes for linkage analysis. A summary of these follows.

Specificity requires that the indicator be more strongly associated with the disease of interest than with other psychiatric conditions. Putative genotype indicators should exhibit *state independence*. The measure should be stable over time and should not be an epiphenomenon of the illness or its treatment. The putative indicator should be *heritable*. An indicator that does not show familial transmission will not be helpful for linkage analyses.

We should be able to demonstrate a *familial association* between the illness and the indicator. Relatives of ill probands should express the indicator to a greater degree than an appropriate control group. The illness and the indicator should also show *cosegregation* within families. The prevalence of illness among relatives who manifest the indicator should be higher than among relatives who do not.

Finally, an indicator should have *biological* and *clinical plausibility*: Even if shoe size met other criteria, it would be suspect as a valid indicator due to its lack of biologic or clinical plausibility. Clinical plausibility might be demonstrated by showing that the indicator resembles the clinical phenomenology of the illness. For example, negative symptoms are a prominent feature of schizophrenia that may be an expression of the genotype among relatives of schizophrenic patients (Tsuang et al., 1991). Neurodiagnostic indicators will have some biologic plausibility if they assess brain regions believed to be impaired by the disorder (Kremen et al., 1994).

Examples of Algorithms for Segregation Analysis

This section provides some detailed information on two popular segregation analysis models, the unified model as implemented in POINTER (Morton et al., 1983) and the regressive logistic model (Bonney, 1984; Bonney, 1986; Bonney, 1987) as implemented in REGTL (Sorant and Elston, 1989a) of the Statistical Analysis for Genetic Epidemiology computer programs (Bailey-Wilson and Elston, 1989). In discussing these methods, we focus on how the algorithms deal with issues that are particularly relevant to the genetic epidemiology of psychiatric disorders.

POINTER was originally based on the mixed model proposed by Morton and MacLean (1974). In this model, a genetic trait is assumed to be due to the influence of a major locus with mendelian transmission, a polygenic component, and random environmental effects. For qualitative traits like psychiatric disorders, the model assumes an underlying "liability" or predisposition to illness, x, that is normally distributed, $N(\mu, V)$. Illness occurs only in those individuals who exceed a threshold on the liability continuum. The liability is composed of three components: 1) a major locus effect, g, with two alleles A and B; 2) a multifactorial transmissible effect, c, with normal distribution $N(0,C)$; and 3) a random, nontransmitted environmental component e, also normally distributed $N(0,E)$, with $x = g + c + e$ and $V = G + C + E$. For qualitative traits such as diagnoses, the mean (μ) and variance (V) of liability are assumed to be 0 and 1, respectively.

At the major locus, the A allele is responsible for the increase of liability, i.e., it is the disease gene. The three genotypes AA, AB, and BB have mean liabilities of μ_{AA}, μ_{AB}, and μ_{BB}, respectively. The frequency of A is q. The displacement between the two homozygotes (AA and BB) on the scale of x is t, and the degree of dominance of the A allele is indexed by $d = (\mu_{AB} - \mu_{AA})/(\mu_{BB} - \mu_{AA})$. For dominant traits, $\mu_{AB} = \mu_{BB}$ and $d = 1$; for recessive traits, $\mu_{AB} = \mu_{AA}$ and $d = 0$.

The unified model extends the mixed model by including parameters to model the probabilities that individuals with the genotypes AA, AB, and BB transmit the B allele to offspring (Elston and Stewart, 1971; Lalouel et al., 1983). We use τ_{AA}, τ_{AB}, and τ_{BB} to denote these probabilities. The multifactorial polygenic component is indexed by the heritability parameter, h. Heritability is the ratio of the variance of the multifactorial effect to the total variance of the trait. It ranges from a low of 0, indicating no multifactorial effect, to a high of 1, indicating that the trait being modeled can be completely accounted for by multifactorial polygenic factors. POINTER can correct for variable age at onset by specifying age-specific liability classes. However, this approach assumes that risk to relatives is associated with the age at onset of the proband. Unfortunately, Iselius and Morton (1991) indicated that genetic transmission probabilities are not correctly implemented in POINTER. As a result, nonmendelian transmission probabilities are not interpretable when families are selected through probands.

In the REGTL logistic regressive model, the likelihood of the data is modeled as function of the following parameters: 1) each person can be one of three types, AA, AB, or BB, with the following respective population frequencies: Ψ_{AA}, Ψ_{AB}, or Ψ_{BB}. For a genetic model, A refers to the gene that predisposes to illness, and AA, AB, and BB are genotypes; 2) each type is associated with a probability that expresses the susceptibility to become ill: γ_{AA}, γ_{AB}, and γ_{BB} (under a genetic model these are termed the *penetrances* of each genotype); 3) for disorders having a variable age at onset, the probability of becoming ill is also a function of two age distribution parameters: β (the baseline effect) and α (the age adjustment coefficient) (these parameters determine the mean and variance of the logistic distribution of age at onset); 4) each type (AA, AB, or BB) is also associated with a probability that an individual of the type will transmit the A factor to a child. These are the transmission probabilities τ_{AA}, τ_{AB}, and τ_{BB}.

POINTER computes the maximum likelihood estimates of parameters using the numerical maximization algorithm GEMENI (Morton et al., 1983). REGTL uses MAXFUN of the Statistical Analysis for Genetic Epidemiology computer programs (Sorant and El-ston, 1989b). The likelihood ratio statistic for a test of two nested models is twice the difference of log likelihoods, $-2[\ln(L_1) - \ln(L_2)]$; L_1 is the likelihood of the restricted model, and L_2 is the likelihood of the general model. The restricted model is defined by placing restrictions on the parameters of the general model. A significant chi-square test statistic indicates that the restricted model provides a significantly poorer fit to the data than does the general model.

For example, under the most general model, all three transmission probabilities are estimated; in contrast, the genetic model restricts these probabilities to follow the laws of mendelian transmission (i.e., $\tau_{AA} = 1$, $\tau_{AB} = 0.5$, and $\tau_{BB} = 0.0$). Comparing this restricted model to the general model, a significant test would indicate that the genetic model could be rejected. The degrees of freedom of the chi-squared test statistic are equal to the difference in the number of estimated parameters between the two models. When a parameter is estimated to equal its minimum or maximum possible value (i.e., the estimate went to a bound), the parameter is usually not counted as an estimated parameter for the purposes of computing degrees of freedom.

The likelihood ratio statistic is only appropriate when the parameters of the restricted model are a proper subset of the parameters of the general model. To test genetic and nongenetic hypotheses, a variety of restricted models can be compared with more general models. Non-nested models can be compared using Akaike's Information Theoretic Criterion (AIC) (Akaike, 1974; Buckley et al., 1992):

$$AIC = -2\ln(\text{likelihood}) + 2(\text{number of estimated parameters}).$$

Although tests of statistical significance are not possible, smaller AICs correspond to better-fitting models.

To be certain that the maximization routines converge at the true maximum, it is a good idea to estimate each model several times using different sets of starting parameter values. For POINTER, a strategy for hypothesis testing is as follows: 1) For the *Mixed model*, estimate the polygenic heritability parameter (h) along with three single gene parameters: the gene frequency (q), the degree of dominance (d), and the displacement (t). The transmission probabilities, τ_{AA}, τ_{AB}, and τ_{BB} should be fixed at mendelian values (i.e., $\tau_{AA} = 1$, $\tau_{AB} = 0.5$, and $\tau_{BB} = 0.0$). 2) for the *Generic Mendelian* model, fix the polygenic heritability parameter to zero. 3) For the *Dominant, Codominant, and Recessive Mendelian* models, restrict the Generic Mendelian model by fixing the dominance parameter, d, to 1.0, 0.5, and 0.0, respectively. 4) For the *Multifactorial Polygenic* model, restrict the mixed model by estimating only the heritability parameter, h.

For REGTL, the strategy for hypothesis testing is as follows: 1) For the *General* model, the type frequencies must sum to one, and each must be greater than or equal to 0 and less than or equal to 1. The transmission probabilities and the susceptibilities should be free to vary between 0 and 1; the susceptibilities can be different for males and females. 2) For the *Hardy-Weinberg* model, restrict the general model by estimating a gene frequency (q_A), and use the genetic principle of Hardy-Weinberg to compute the type frequencies from the gene frequency. 3) For the *Sex-Independent* model, require males and females to have equal susceptibilities for each type (i.e., $\gamma_{ij[\text{female}]} = \gamma_{ij[\text{male}]}$). This tests whether the effect of type varies with gender. 4) For the *Environmental Transmission* model, restrict the three transmission probabilities to be equal to one another (i.e., $\tau_{AA} = \tau_{AB} = \tau_{BB}$). By setting the transmission probabilities equal to one another, this model assumes that the type of the parent does not determine the type of the child. This tests whether the hypothesized pathogenic factor (the *A* factor) is transmitted from parent to offspring. The acceptance of this model would imply that the distribution of illness in families can be accounted for by *nonfamilial* attributes of the environment. 5) For the *Cultural Transmission* model, set the transmission probabilities as $\tau_{AA} = \tau_{AB} = 1$ and $\tau_{BB} = 0$. That is, individuals with the pathogenic *A* factor always transmit the factor, regardless of the presence of a possible second dose of that factor. Those without the pathogenic factor cannot transmit the factor. The acceptance of this model would implicate, as etiologic agents, environmental factors transmitted from ill parents to their children. 6) For the "τ_{AB}-*Free*" model, set the τ_{AB} parameter equal to its mendelian value of 0.5. This is a frequently used test of mendelian transmission (Chartier-Harlin et al., 1991). 7) For the *generic* Mendelian model, set the transmission probabilities to mendelian values (i.e., $\tau_{AA} = 1$, $\tau_{AB} = 0.5$, and $\tau_{BB} = 0.0$). The susceptibilities (i.e., the penetrances for each genotype) should be allowed to vary freely between zero and one. 8) For the *Dominant, Codominant, and Recessive Mendelian* models, set the transmission probabilities to mendelian values. Model dominance by requiring the penetrance of the *AB* genotype to equal that of the *AA* genotype (i.e., $\gamma_{AA} = \gamma_{AB}$). For the recessive model, set the penetrance of the *AB* genotype to be equal to that of the *BB* genotype (i.e., $\gamma_{BB} = \gamma_{AB}$). For codominance, require the penetrance of the *AB* genotype to be midway between the penetrances of the *AA* and *BB* genotypes (i.e., $\gamma_{AB} = 5[\gamma_{AA} + \gamma_{BB}]$).

POINTER and REGTL use different methods to correct for the ascertainment (i.e., sampling) bias caused by the nonrandom sampling of families through probands. POINTER uses the classic approach to ascertainment correction by requiring the specification of π, the probability that an ill individual is ascertained as a proband. It is a good idea to test the robustness of POINTER's results by performing analyses with π equal to 0.1, 0.5, and 0.9. REGTL takes a conditional likelihood approach in which the likelihood one would compute for a random sample is divided by the likelihood of a conditioned subset (in our cases, the probands). In REGTL analyses, all probands from each family should be included in the conditioned subset. The nonparametric approach taken by REGTL frees one from making strong assumptions regarding ascertainment that, if incorrect, could bias parameter estimation.

The population prevalence used for the calculation of likelihoods also differs between the two models. POINTER requires the user to specify the population prevalence based on prior knowledge of the epidemiology of the disease. Genetic parameters may be biased if the prevalence is specified incorrectly. In contrast, REGTL can estimate the gene frequency from the family data used for the segregation analysis. Since the method of ascertainment used by REGTL allows us to use normal control families in the segregation analysis, we can obtain a reasonably precise estimate of population prevalence because the ascertainment method corrects for the fact that the control probands were selected on the basis of not having the disease. Although the control families provide little statistical information about the segregation of illness, they provide much information about the population prevalence. Since this information influences the likelihood function, it influences the final maximum likelihood estimate of prevalence.

The two algorithms take different approaches to modeling gender differences, which are common in psychiatric illness (Cloninger et al., 1978; Pauls, 1979; Berney, 1989; DeLisi et al., 1989; Goldstein et al., 1989; Faraone et al., 1991; Harris et al., 1991). In REGTL, we can test for a significant sex effect by comparing a model with sex-specific penetrances for each genotype to a model in which penetrance is not sex dependent. In

POINTER, we cannot test for a sex effect but must model sex differences by specifying sex-specific prevalences prior to the analysis. To do this we must assume sex-specific liability classes. POINTER models these classes by estimating sex-specific thresholds on the liability continuum. The threshold for expressing the disorder would be higher for the sex that has the lower population prevalence of the disorder.

PSYCHIATRIC GENETICS AND PSYCHIATRIC EPIDEMIOLOGY

As this chapter shows, psychiatric genetics is a multidisciplinary endeavor. In combines the methodologic talents of the epidemiologist, the mathematical proficiency of the statistician, and the laboratory wizardry of the molecular geneticist. It is notable that the great pioneers of psychiatric genetics — Weinberg, Strömgren, Rüdin, Slater, Essen-Möller, and others — used epidemiologic methods to show that major psychiatric disorders were heritable. This set the stage for the biologic revolution in psychiatry.

Although we now look toward molecular genetics and neuroscience to clarify the etiologic and pathophysiologic details of psychiatric illness, these are unlikely to succeed without a continued partnership with epidemiology. Indeed, with the exception of Alzheimer's disease, attempts to find genes for psychiatric illness have been disappointing (Tsuang et al., 1993).

Because of this, there has been a growing methodologic literature pertaining to the linkage analysis of complex diseases such as schizophrenia (Lander, 1988; Merikangas et al., 1989; Ott, 1990a,b; Risch, 1990a–d; Weeks et al., 1990a,b; Spence et al., 1992). In this context "complex" is a shorthand way of saying that the disease is not transmitted in a simple mendelian fashion.

Many complexities plague psychiatric genetics, and many solutions have been proposed in the above referenced articles. We summarize them in 10 key points as follows: 1) use standardized diagnostic criteria; 2) define diagnoses that will be included as affected cases before the data collection; 3) use assessment and diagnostic procedures that minimize false-positive diagnoses; 4) ascertain pedigrees and collect data in a manner that can be reproduced by other investigators; 5) collect detailed clinical and demographic data to allow comparisons with other samples; 6) maintain complete blindness between the psychiatric diagnoses and marker statuses of all subjects; 7) implement procedures to facilitate the follow-up of pedigree members; 8) implement procedures to minimize laboratory errors; 9) use a threshold of statistical significance that takes into account the data analytic issues unique to complex nonmendelian disorders; 10) allow other investigators access to complete pedigree and clinical information relevant to any publications of linkage results.

It is instructive to note that most of these points are directly relevant to the epidemiologic foundation of a linkage study. This suggests to us that advances in psychiatric epidemiology may be needed to expedite work in psychiatric genetics.

ACKNOWLEDGMENTS

Preparation of this chapter was supported in part by National Institute of Mental Health grants 1R01MH41879-01, 5 UO1 MH46318-02, and 1 R37MH43518-01 to M.T.T. and the Veterans Administration's Medical Research, Health Services Research and Development and Cooperative

Studies Programs. We thank Wei J. Chen, M.D., Sc.D., Michael Lyons, Ph.D., and Susan Santangelo, Sc.D., for their collaboration on related manuscripts.

REFERENCES

Akaike H (1974): A new look at statistical model identification. IEEE Tran Auto Con AC-19:716–723.

Andreasen NC (1986): The family history approach to diagnosis: How useful is it? Arch Gen Psychiatry 43:421–429.

Andreasen NC, Endicott J, Spitzer RL, Winokur G (1977): The family history method using diagnostic criteria. Reliability and validity. Arch Gen Psychiatry 34:1229–1235.

Bach AWJ, Lan NC, Johnson DL, Abell CW, Bembenek ME, Kwan S-W, Seeburg PH, Shih JC (1988): cDNA cloning of human liver monoamine oxidase A and B: molecular basis of differences in enzymatic properties. Proc Nat Acad Sci 85:4934–4938.

Bailey-Wilson JE, Elston RC (1989): "Statistical Analysis for Genetic Epidemiology." New Orleans: Department of Biometry and Genetics, LSU Medical Center.

Baron M, Risch N, Mendlewicz J (1983): Age at onset in bipolar-related major affective illness: Clinical genetic implications. J Psychiatry Res 17:5–18.

Berney TP (1989): Fragile X syndrome and disorders of the sex chromosome. Curr Opin Psychiatry 2:593–598.

Biederman J, Rosenbaum JF, Bolduc EA, Faraone SV, Hirshfeld DR (1991): A high risk study of young children of parents with panic disorder and agoraphobia with and without comorbid major depression. Psychiatry Res 37:333–348.

Bishop DT, Williamson JA (1990): The power of identity-by-state methods for linkage analysis. Am J Hum Genet 46:254–265.

Blum K, Noble EP, Sheridan PJ, Montgomery A, Ritchie T, Jagadeeswaran P, Nogami H, Briggs AH, Cohn JB (1990): Allelic association of human dopamine D2 receptor gene in alcoholism. JAMA 263:2055–2060.

Boehnke M (1986): Estimating the power of a proposed linkage study: A practical computer simulation approach. Am J Hum Genet 39:513–527.

Bonney GE (1984): On the statistical determination of major gene mechanisms in continuous human traits: Regressive models. Am J Hum Genet 18:731–749.

Bonney GE (1986): Regressive logistic models for familial disease and other binary traits. Biometrics 42:611–625.

Bonney GE (1987): Logistic regression for dependent binary observations. Biometrics 43:951–973.

Borecki IB, Lathrop GM, Bonney GE, Yaouanq J, Rao DC (1990): Combined segregation and linkage of genetic hemochromatosis using affection status, serum iron, and HLA. Am J Hum Genet 47:542–550.

Botstein D, White RL, Skolnick M, Davis RW (1980): Construction of a genetic linkage map in man using restriction fragment length polymorphisms. Am J Hum Genet 32:314–31.

Breslow N, Crowley J (1974): A large sample study of the life table and product limit estimates under random censorship. Ann Stat 2:437–453.

Buckley P, O'Callaghan E, Larkin C, Waddington JL (1992): Schizophrenia Research: The problem of controls. Biol Psychiatry 32:215–217.

Bunzow JR, Van TH, Grandy DK, Albert P, Salon J, Christie M, Machida CA, Neve KA, Civelli O (1988): Cloning and expression of a rat D2 dopamine receptor cDNA. Nature 336:783–787.

Cadoret RJ (1978): Evidence for genetic inheritance of primary affective disorder in adoptees. Am J Psychiatry 135:463–466.

Cadoret RJ, O'Gorman TW, Heywood E, Troughton E (1985): Genetic and environmental factors in major depression. J Affect Disord 9:155–164.

Cavalli-Sforza LL, King M-C (1986): Detecting linkage for genetically heterogeneous diseases and detecting heterogeneity with linkage data. Am J Hum Genet 38:599–616.

Chartier-Harlin M-C, Crawford F, Houlden H, Warren A, Hughes D, Fidani L, Goate A, Rossor M, Roques P, Hardy J, Mullan M (1991): Early-onset Alzheimer's disease caused by mutations at codon 717 of the b-amyloid precursor protein gene. Nature 353:844–846.

Chase GA, Kramer M (1986): The abridged census method as an estimator of lifetime risk. Psychol Med 16:865–871.

Chen WJ, Faraone SV, Orav EJ, Tsuang MT (1993): Estimating age at onset distributions: The bias from prevalent cases and its impact on risk estimation. Genet Epidemiol 10:43–60.

Chen WJ, Faraone SV, Tsuang MT (1992a): Estimating age at onset distributions: A review of methods and issues. Psychiat Genet 2:219–238.

Chen WJ, Faraone SV, Tsuang MT (1992b): Linkage studies of schizophrenia: A simulation study of statistical power. Genet Epidemiol 9:123–139.

Clerget-Darpoux F, Babron M-C, Banaïti-Pellié C (1987): Power and robustness of the linkage homogeneity test in genetic analysis of common disorders. J Psychiatr Res 21:625–630.

Clerget-Darpoux F, Babron M-C, Banaïti-Pellié C (1990): Assessing the effect of multiple linkage tests in complex diseases. Genet Epidemiol 7:245–253.

Cloninger CR, Christiansen KO, Reich T, Gottesman II (1978): Implications of sex differences in the prevalences of antisocial personality, alcoholism, and criminality for familial transmission. Arch Gen Psychiatry 35:941–951.

Conneally PM (1991): Association between the D_2 dopamine receptor gene and alcoholism. A continuing controversy. Arch Gen Psychiatry 48:757–759.

Crowe RR (1993): Candidate genes in psychiatry: An epidemiological perspective. Am J Med Genet Neuropsychiatry Genet 48:74–77.

Cupples LA, Risch N, Farrer LA, Myers RH (1991): Estimation of morbid risk and age at onset with missing information. Am J Hum Genet 49:76–87.

Dearry A, Gingrich JA, Falardeau P, Fremeau RTJ, Bates MD, Caron MG (1990): Molecular cloning and expression of the gene for a human D1 dopamine receptor. Nature 347:72–76.

DeLisi LE, Dauphinais ID, Hauser P (1989): Gender differences in the brain: Are they relevant to the pathogenesis of schizophrenia? Comp Psychiatry 30:197–208.

Deutsch CK, Swanson JM, Bruell JH, Cantwell DP, Weinberg F, Baren M (1982): Short communication: Overrepresentation of adoptees in children with attention deficit disorder. Behav Genet 12:231–238.

Eaves LJ, Kendler KS, Schulz SC (1986): The familial sporadic classification: Its power for the resolution of genetic and environmental etiological factors. J Psychiatr Res 20:115–130.

Edwards JH (1990): The linkage detection problem. Ann Hum Genet 54:253–275.

Edwards JH, Watt DC (1989): Caution in locating the gene(s) for affective disorder. Psychol Med 19:273–275.

Egeland JA, Gerhard DS, Pauls DL, Sussex JN, Kidd KK, Allen CR, Hostetter AM, Housman DE (1987): Bipolar affective disorders linked to DNA markers on chromosome 11. Nature 325:783–787.

Elston RC, Namboodiri KK (1977): Family studies of schizophrenia. Bull Int Stat Inst 47:683–697.

Elston RC, Stewart J (1971): A general model for the genetic analysis of pedigree data. Hum Hered 21:523–542.

Erlenmeyer-Kimling L (1975): A prospective study of children at risk for schizophrenia: Methodological considerations and some preliminary findings. In Wirt R, Winokur G, Ross M (eds): "Life History Research in Psychopathology." Minneapolis, MN: University of Minnesota Press, pp 22–46.

Falconer DS (1965): The inheritance of liability to certain disease, estimated from the incidence among relatives. Ann Hum Genet 29:51–71.

Falk CT, Rubinstein P (1987): Haplotype relative risks: An easy reliable way to construct a proper control sample for risk calculations. Ann Hum Genet 51:227–233.

Faraone SV, Biederman J, Keenan K, Tsuang MT (1991): A family-genetic study of girls with DSM-III attention deficit disorder. Am J Psychiatry 148:112–117.

Faraone SV, Biederman J, Krifcher B, Keenan K, Moore C, Sprich S, Ugaglia K, Jellinek MS, Spencer T, Norman D, Seidman L, Kolodny R, Benjamin J, Kraus I, Perrin J, Chen W, Tsuang MT (1993): Evidence for independent transmission in families for Attention Deficit Hyperactivity Disorder (ADHD) and learning disability: Results from a family-genetic study of ADHD. Am J Psychiatry 150:891–895.

Faraone SV, Kremen WS, Tsuang MT (1990): Genetic transmission of major affective disorders: Quantitative models and linkage analyses. Psychol Bull 108:109–127.

Faraone SV, Santangelo S (1992): Methods in Genetic Epidemiology. In Fava M, Rosenbaum JF (eds): "Research Designs and Methods in Psychiatry." Amsterdam, the Netherlands: Elsevier, pp 93–118.

Faraone SV, Tsuang MT (1985): Quantitative models of the genetic transmission of schizophrenia. Psychol Bull 98:41–66.

Fischer M (1971): Psychosis in the offspring of schizophrenic monozygotic twins and their normal co-twins. Br J Psychiatry 118:43–52.

Fish B, Marcus J, Hans SL, Auerbach JG, Perdue S (1992): Infants at risk for schizophrenia: Sequelae of a genetic neurointegrative defect. A review and replication analysis of pandysmaturation in the Jerusalem infant development study. Arch Gen Psychiatry 49:221–235.

Fisher, RA (1934): The effect of methods of ascertainment upon the estimation of frequencies. Ann Eugen 6:13–25.

Freimer NB, Sandkuiji LA, Blower SM (1993): Incorrect specification of marker allele frequencies: Effects on linkage analysis. Am J Hum Genet 52:1102–1110.

Garver DL (1987): Methodological issues facing the interpretation of high risk studies. Schiz Bull 13:525–529.

Gejman PV, Gelernter J (1993): Mutational analysis of candidate genes in psychiatric disorders. Am J Med Genet Neuropsychiat Genet 48:184–191.

Gelernter J, O'Malley S, Risch N, Kranzler HR, Krystal J, Merikangas K, Kennedy JL, Kidd KK (1991): No association between an allele at the D_2 dopamine receptor gene (DRD2) and alcoholism. JAMA 266:1801–1807.

Gershon ES, Goldin LR (1986): Clinical methods in psychiatric genetics. Acta Psychiatr Scand 74:113–118.

Gershon ES, Guroff JJ (1984): Information from relatives. Diagnosis of affective disorders. Arch Gen Psychiatry 41:173–180.

Gibbons RD, Davis JM, Hedeker DR (1990): A comment on the selection of "healthy controls" for psychiatric experiments. Arch Gen Psychiatry 47:785–786.

Goate A, Chartier-Harlin M-C, Mullan M, Brown J, Crawford F, Fidani L, Giuffra L, Haynes A, Irving N, James L, Mant R, Newton P, Rooke K, Roques P, Talbot C, Pericak-Vance M, Roses A, Williamson R, Rossor M, Owen M, Hardy J (1991): Segregation of a missense mutation in the amyloid precursor protein gene with familial Alzheimer's disease. Nature 349:704–706.

Goldin LR (1990): The increase in type I error rates in linkage studies when multiple analyses are carried out on the same data: A simulation study (abstract). Am J Hum Genet 47:A180.

Goldin LR, Gershon ES (1988): Power of the affected-sib-pair method for heterogeneous disorders. Genet Epidemiol 5:35–42.

Goldin LR, Martinez MM (1989): The detection of linkage and heterogeneity in nuclear families when unaffected individuals are considered unknown. In Elston RC, Spence MA, Hodge SE, MacCluer JW (eds): "Multipoint Mapping and Linkage Based Upon Affected Pedigree Members." New York: Alan R. Liss, pp 195–200.

Goldstein JM, Tsuang MT, Faraone SV (1989): Gender and schizophrenia: Implications for understanding the heterogeneity of the illness. Psychiatr Res 28:243–253.

Gottesman II, Bertelsen A (1989): Confirming unexpressed genotypes for schizophrenia. Risks in the offspring of Fischer's Danish identical and fraternal discordant twins. Arch Gen Psychiatry 46:867–872.

Grandy DK, Litt M, Allen L, Bunzow JR, Marchionni M, Makam H, Reed L, Magenis RE, Civelli O (1989): The human dopamine D2 receptor gene is located on chromosome 11 at q22–q23 and identifies a TaqI RFLP. Am J Hum Genet 45:778–785.

Green P (1990): Genetic linkage and complex diseases: A comment. Genet Epidemiol 7:25–27.

Greenberg DA (1989): Inferring mode of inheritance by comparison of lod scores. Am J Med Genet 34:480–486.

Greenland S, Morgenstern H (1990): Matching and efficiency in cohort studies. Am J Epidemiol 131:151–159.

Grima B, Lamouroux A, Boni C, Julien J-F, Javoy-Agid F, Mallet J (1987): A single human gene encoding multiple tyrosine hydroxylases with different predicted functional characteristics. Nature 326:707–711.

Harris T, Surtees P, Bancroft J (1991): Is sex necessarily a risk factor to depression? Br J Psychiatry 158:708–712.

Heimbuch RC, Matthysse S, Kidd KK (1980): Estimating age-of-onset distributions for disorders with variable onset. Am J Hum Genet 32:564–574.

Heston LL (1966): Psychiatric disorders in foster home-reared children of schizophrenic mothers. Br J Psychiatry 112:819–825.

Hsu Y-PP, Powell JF, Chen S, Weyler W, Ozelius L, Bruns G, Utterback M, Mallet J, Gusella JF, Breakefield XO (1988a): Molecular genetic studies of MAO genes. In Dalstrom A, Belmaker H, Sandler M (eds): "Progress in Catecholamine Research: Part A. Basic and peripheral Mechanisms." New York: Alan R Liss, pp 89–95.

Hsu Y-PP, Weyler W, Chen S, Sims KB, Rinehart WB, Utterback MC, Powell JF, Breakefield XO (1988b): Structural features of human monoamine oxidase A elucidated from cDNA and peptide sequences. J Neurochem 51:1321–1324.

Iselius L, Morton NE (1991): Transmission probabilities are not correctly implemented in the computer program POINTER. Am J Hum Genet 49:459.

Kaplan EL, Meier P (1958): Nonparametric estimation from incomplete observations. Am Stat Assoc J 53:457–481.

Keefe RSE, Silverman JM, Siever LJ, Cornblatt BA (1991): Refining phenotype characterization in genetic linkage studies of schizophrenia. Soc Biol 38:197–218.

Kelsoe JR, Ginns EI, Egeland JA, Gerhard DS, Goldstein AM, Bale SJ, Pauls DL, Long RT, Kidd KK, Conte G, Housman DE, Paul SM (1989): Re-evaluation of the linkage relationship between chromosome 11p loci and the gene for bipolar affective disorder in the old order Amish. Nature 342:238–243.

Kendler KS (1987): Sporadic vs familial classification given etiologic heterogeneity: II Sensitivity, specificity and positive and negative predictive power. Genet Epidemiol 4:313–330.

Kendler KS (1990): The super-normal control group in psychiatric genetics: Possible artifactual evidence for coaggregation. Psychiat Genet 1:45–53.

Kendler KS, Hays P (1982): Familial and sporadic schizophrenia: A symptomatic, prognostic and EEG comparison. Am J Psychiatry 139:1557–1562.

Kendler KS, Silberg JL, Neale MC, Kessler RC, Heath AC, Eaves LJ (1991): The family history method: Whose psychiatric history is measured? Am J Psychiatry 148:1501–1504.

Kety SS, Rosenthal D, Wender PH, Schulsinger F (1968): The types and prevalence of mental illness in the biological and adoptive families of adopted schizophrenics. J Psychiat Res 1:345–362.

Kety SS, Rosenthal D, Wender PH, Schulsinger F, Jacobsen B (1978): The biologic and adoptive families of adopted individuals who became schizophrenic: Prevalence of mental illness and other characteristics. In Wynne LC, Cromwell RL, Matthysse S (eds): "The Nature of Schizophrenia: New Approaches to Research and Treatment." New York: John Wiley & Sons, pp 25–37.

Kidd KK (1993): Associations of disease with genetic markers: Deja vu all over again. Am J Med Genet Neuropsychiat Genet 48:71–73.

Knapp M, Souchter SA, Baur MP (1993): The haplotype-relative-risk (HRR) method for analysis of association in nuclear families. Am J Hum Genet 52:1085–1093.

Kobayashi K, Kurosawa Y, Fujita K, Nagatsu T (1989): Human dopamine-beta hydroxylase gene: Two mRNA types having different 3'-terminal regions are produced through alternative polyadenylation. Nucleic Acids Res 17:1089–1102.

Korenberg J, West R, Pulst S (1988): The amyloid protein precursor gene maps to chromosome 21 sub-bands q21.15–q21.1. Neurology 38:265.

Kosten TA, Anton SF, Rounsaville BJ (1992): Ascertaining psychiatric diagnoses with the family history method in a substance abuse population. J Psychiatr Res 26:135–147.

Kotsopoulos S, Côte A, Joseph L, Pentland N, Stavrakaki C, Sheahan P, Oke L (1988): Psychiatric disorders in adopted children: A controlled study. Am J Orthopsychiatry 58:608–612.

Kremen WS, Seidman LJ, Pepple JR, Lyons MJ, Tsuang MT, Faraone SV (1994): Neuropsychological risk indicators for schizophrenia: A review of family studies. Schiz Bull 20:103–119.

Kremen WS, Tsuang MT, Faraone SV, Lyons ML (1992): Using vulnerability indicators to compare conceptual models of genetic heterogeneity in schizophrenia. J Nerv Ment Dis 180:141–152.

Kruesi MJP, Lenane MC, Hibbs ED, Major J (1990): Normal controls and biological reference values in child psychiatry: Defining normal. J Am Acad Child Adolesc Psychiatry 29:449–452.

LaBuda MC, Gottesman II, Pauls DL (1993): Usefulness of twin studies for exploring the etiology of childhood and adolescent psychiatric disorders. Am J Med Genet Neuropsychiat Genet 48:47–59.

Lalouel JM, Rao DC, Morton NE, Elston RC (1983): A unified model for complex segregation analysis. Am J Hum Genet 35:816–826.

Lamouroux A, Vigny A, Faucon BN, Darmon MC, Franck R, Henry JP, Mallet J (1987): The primary structure of human dopamine-beta-hydroxylase: insights into the relationship between the soluble and the membrane-bound forms of the enzyme. Eur Mol Biol J 6:3931–3937.

Lander ES (1988): Splitting schizophrenia. Nature 336:105–106.

Larsson T, Sjögren T (1954): A methodological, psychiatric and statistical study of a large Swedish rural population. Acta Psychiatr Neurol Scand (Suppl) 89:40–54.

Leckman JF, Sholomska D, Thompson WD, Belanger A, Weissman MM (1982): Best estimate of lifetime diagnosis: A methodological study. Arch Gen Psychiatry 39:879–883.

Lee EL (1980): "Statistical Methods for Survival Data Analysis." Belmont: Lifetime Learning.

Levinson DF (1993a): Linkage information in small family structures: Comparison of pedigrees with three to five affected members. Psychiatry Genet 3:45–57.

Levinson DF (1993b): Power to detect linkage with heterogeneity in samples of small nuclear families. Am J Med Genet Neuropsychiatry Genet 48:94–102.

Lewis SW, Reveley AM, Reveley MA, Chitkara B, Murray RM (1987): The familial/sporadic distinction as a strategy in schizophrenia research. Br J Psychiatry 151:306–313.

Lyons MJ, Faraone SV, Kremen WS, Tsuang MT (1989a): Familial and sporadic schizophrenia: A simulation study of statistical power. Schiz Res 2:345–353.

Lyons MJ, Kremen WS, Tsuang MT, Faraone SV (1989b): Investigating putative genetic and environmental forms of schizophrenia: Methods and findings. Int Rev Psychiatry 1:259–276.

Martinez MM, Goldin LR (1989): The detection of linkage and heterogeneity in nuclear families for complex disorders: One versus two major loci. Am J Hum Genet 44:552–559.

Martinez MM, Goldin LR (1990): Power of the linkage test for a heterogeneous disorder due two independent inherited causes: A simulation study. Genet Epidemiol 7:219–230.

McGue M, Gottesman II (1989): Genetic linkage in schizophrenia: Perspectives from genetic epidemiology. Schiz Bull 15:453–464.

McGue M, Gottesman II (1991): The genetic epidemiology of schizophrenia and the design of linkage studies. Eur Arch Psychiatr Neurol Sci 240:174–181.

McGue M, Gottesman II, Rao DC (1983): The transmission of schizophrenia under a multifactorial threshold model. Am J Hum Genet 35:1161–1178.

McGue M, Gottesman II, Rao DC (1985): Resolving genetic models for the transmission of schizophrenia. Genet Epidemiol 2:99–110.

Mednick SA, Mura E, Schulsinger F, Mednick B (1971): Perinatal conditions and infant development in children with schizophrenic parents. Soc Biol (Suppl) 18:103.

Meehl P, Rosen A (1955): Antecedent probability and the efficiency of psychometric signs, patterns, or cutting scores. Psychol Bull 52:194–216.

Meehl PE (1970): Nuisance variables and the ex post facto design. In Radner M, Winokur S (eds): "Minnesota Studies in the Philosophy of Science." Minneapolis, MN: University of Minnesota Press, pp 373–402.

Mendlewicz J, Fleiss JL, Cataldo M, Rainer JD (1975): Accuracy of the family history method in affective illness. Arch Gen Psychiatry 32:309–314.

Mendlewicz J, Rainer JD (1977): Adoption study supporting genetic transmission in manic-depressive illness. Nature 268:327–329.

Merikangas KR, Spence A, Kupfer DJ (1989): Linkage studies of bipolar disorder: Methodologic and analytic issues. Report of MacArthur foundation workshop on linkage and clinical features in affective disorders. Arch Gen Psychiatry 46:1137–1141.

Miettinen OS (1985): "Theoretical Epidemiology." New York: John Wiley.

Morton LA, Kidd KK, Matthysse SW, Richards RL (1979): Recurrence risks in schizophrenia: Are they model dependent? Behav Genet 9:389–406.

Morton NE (1955): Sequential tests for the detection of linkage. Am J Hum Genet 7:277–318.

Morton NE (1982): "Outline of Genetic Epidemiology." Basel: Karger.

Morton NE, MacLean CJ (1974): Analysis of family resemblance. III. Complex segregation analysis of quantitative traits. Am J Hum Genet 26:489–503.

Morton NE, Rao DC, Lalouel J-M (1983): "Methods in Genetic Epidemiology." New York: Karger.

Nakamura Y, Carlson M, Krapcho D, Kanamori M, White R (1988): New approach for isolation of VNTR markers. Am J Hum Genet 43:854–859.

Nakamura Y, Leppert M, O'Connell P, et al. (1987): Variable number of tandem repeat (VNTR) markers for human gene mapping. Science 235:1616–1622.

Naruse S, Igarashi S, Kobayashi H, Aoki K, Inuzuka T, Kaneko K, Shimizu T, Iihara K, Kojima T, Miyatake T, Tsuji S (1991): Mis-sense mutation Val-Ile in exon 17 of amyloid precursor protein gene in Japanese familial Alzheimer's disease. Lancet 337:978–979.

Neale MC, Cardon LR (1992): "Methodology for Genetic Studies of Twins and Families." the Netherlands: Kluwer Academic Publishers.

Nechiporuk A, Fain P, Kort E, Nee LE, Frommelt E, Polinsky RJ, Pulst SM (1991): Linkage of familial Alzheimer disease to chromosome 14 in two large early onset pedigrees: Effects of marker allele frequencies on lod scores. Am J Med Genet Neuropsychiatry Genet 48:63–66.

NIMH Genetics Initiative (1992a): "Diagnostic Interview for Genetic Studies." Rockville, MD: National Institute of Mental Health.

NIMH Genetics Initiative (1992b): "Family Interview for Genetic Studies." Rockville, MD: National Institute of Mental Health.

Nothen MM, Erdmann J, Korner J, Lanczik M, Fritzer J, Fimmers R, Grandy DK, O'Dowd B, Propping P (1992): Lack of association between dopamine D_1 and D_2 receptor genes and bipolar affective disorder. Am J Psychiatry 149:199–201.

Nurnberger JI, Blehar MC, Kaufmann CA, York-Cooler C, Simpson SG, Harkavy-Friedman J, Severe JB, Malaspina D, Reich T (1994): Diagnostic interview for genetic studies: Rationale, Unique Features, and Training. Arch Gen Psychiatry 51:849–859.

Orvaschel H (1990): Early onset psychiatric disorder in high risk children and increased familial morbidity. J Am Acad Child Adolesc Psychiatry 29:184–188.

Orvaschel H, Thompson WD, Belanger A, Prusoff BA, Kidd KK (1982): Comparison of the family history method to direct interview: Factors affecting the diagnosis of depression. J Affect Disord 4:49–59.

Ott J (1983): Linkage analysis and family classification under heterogeneity. Ann Hum Genet 47:311–320.

Ott J (1986): The number of families required to detect or exclude linkage heterogeneity. Am J Hum Genet 39:159–165.

Ott J (1989a): Computer-simulation methods in human linkage analysis. Proc Natl Acad Sci USA 86:4175–4178.

Ott J (1989b): Statistical properties of the haplotype relative risk. Genet Epidemiol 6:127–130.

Ott J (1990a): Genetic linkage and complex diseases: A comment. Genet Epidemiol 7:35–36.

Ott J (1990b): Invited editorial: Cutting a Gordian knot in the linkage analysis of complex human traits. Am J Hum Genet 46:219–221.

Ott J (1992): "Analysis of Human Genetic Linkage." Baltimore: The Johns Hopkins University Press.

Pato CN, Lander ES, Schulz SC (1989): Prospects for the genetic analysis of schizophrenia. Schiz Bull 15:365–372.

Pato CN, Macciardi F, Pato MT, Verga M, Kennedy JL (1993): Review of the putative association of dopamine D2 receptor and alcoholism: A meta-analysis. Am J Med Genet Neuropsychiatry Genet 48:78–82.

Pauls DL (1979): Sex effect on the risk of mental retardation. Behav Genet 9:289–295.

Pauls DL, Leckman JF (1986): The inheritance of Gilles de la Tourette's syndrome and associated behaviors. Evidence for autosomal dominant transmission. N Engl J Med 315:993–997.

Plomin R, Defries JC, McLearn GE (1990): "Behavioral Genetics. A Primer." New York: Freeman.

Ploughman LM, Boehnke M (1989): Estimating the power of a proposed linkage study for a complex genetic trait. Am J Hum Genet 44:543–551.

Pulver AE, Bale SJ (1989): Availability of schizophrenic patients and their families for genetic linkage studies: Findings from the Maryland epidemiology sample. Genet Epidemiol 6:671–680.

Reider RO, Gershon ES (1978): Genetic strategies in biological psychiatry. Arch Gen Psychiatry 35:866–873.

Resnick SM (1992): Matching for education in studies of schizophrenia. Arch Gen Psychiatry 49:246.

Risch N (1983): Estimating morbidity risks with variable age of onset: Review of methods and a maximum likelihood approach. Biometrics 39:929–939.

Risch N (1988): A new statistical test for linkage heterogeneity. Am J Hum Genet 42:353–364.

Risch N (1990a): Genetic linkage and complex diseases, with special reference to psychiatric disorders. Genet Epidemiol 7:3–7.

Risch N (1990b): Linkage strategies for genetically complex traits. I. Multilocus models. Am J Hum Genet 46:222–228.

Risch N (1990c): Linkage strategies for genetically complex traits. II. The power of affected relative pairs. Am J Hum Genet 46:229–241.

Risch N (1990d): Linkage strategies for genetically complex traits. III. The effect of marker polymorphism on analysis of affected relative pairs. Am J Hum Genet 46:242–253.

Risch N, Baron M (1984): Segregation analysis of schizophrenia and related disorders. Am J Hum Genet 36:1039–1059.

Risch N, Giuffra L (1992): Model misspecification and multipoint linkage analysis. Hum Hered 42:77–92.

Risch SC, Lewine RJ, Jewart RD, Eccard MB, McDaniel JS, Risby ED (1990): Ensuring the normalcy of "normal" volunteers. Am J Psychiatry 147:682–683.

Rubinstein P, Walker M, Carpenter C, Carrier C, Krassner J, Falk C, Ginsberg F (1981): Genetics of HLA disease associations: The use of the haplotype relative risk (HRR) and the "haplo-delta" (Dh) estimates in juvenile diabetes from three racial groups. Hum Immunol 3:384.

Schwartz XL, Moises HW (1993): No association between schizophrenia and homozygosity at the D_3 dopamine receptor gene. Am J Med Genet Neuropsychiatry Genet 48:83–86.

Schweber MA (1985): A possible unitary genetic hypothesis for Alzheimer's disease and Down's syndrome. Ann NY Acad Sci 450:223–238.

Shields J, Slater E (1975): Genetic aspects of schizophrenia. Br J Psychiatry (Spec Pub) 9:32–40.

Shtasel DL, Gur RE, Mozley D, Richards J, Taleff MM, Heimberg C, Gallacher F, Gur RC (1991): Volunteers for biomedical research. Recruitment and screening of normal controls. Arch Gen Psychiatry 48:1022–1025.

Silverman JM, Breitner JCS, Mohs RC, Davis KL (1986): Reliability of the family history method in genetic studies of Alzheimer's disease and related dementias. Am J Psychiatry 143:1279–1282.

Slater E, Cowie V (1971): "The Genetics of Mental Disorder." London: Oxford University Press.

Smith C (1974): Concordance in twins: Methods and interpretation. Am J Hum Genet 26:454–466.

Sobell JL, Heston LL, Sommer SS (1992): Delineation of genetic predisposition to multifactorial disease: A general approach on the threshold of feasibility. Genomics 12:1–6.

Sobell JL, Heston LL, Sommer SS (1993): Novel association approach for determining the genetic predisposition to schizophrenia: Case–control resource and testing of a candidate gene. Am J Med Genet Neuropsychiatry Genet 48:28–35.

Sommer SS, Lind TJ, Heston LJ, Sobell JL (1993): Dopamine D_4 receptor variants in unrelated schizophrenic cases and controls. Am J Med Genet Neuropsychiatry Genet 48:90–93.

Sorant AJM, Elston RC (1989a): Segregation analysis of a truncated (censored) trait with logistic P.D.F. (REGTL version 1.0). In Bailey-Wilson JE, Elston RC (eds): "Statistical Analysis for Genetic Epidemiology." New Orleans: Department of Biometry and Genetics, LSU Medical Center.

Sorant AJM, Elston RC (1989b): A subroutine package for function maximization (A users guide to MAXFUN version 5.0). In Statistical Analysis for Genetic Epidemiology. Bailey-Wilson JE, Elston RC (eds): New Orleans: Department of Biometry and Genetics, LSU Medical Center.

Spence MA (1987): Genetic linkage: Sampling issues and multipoint mapping. J Psychiatr Res 21:631–637.

Spence MA, Bishop DT, Boehnke M, Elston RC, Falk C, Hodge SE, Ott J, Rice J, Merikangas K, Kupfer D (1992): Methodological issues in linkage analyses for psychiatric disorders: Secular trends, assortative mating, bilineal pedigrees. Report of the MacArthur Foundation Network I Task Force on Methodological Issues. Hum Hered (in press).

Spielman RS, McGinnis RE, Ewens WJ (1993): Transmission test for linkage disequilibrium: The insulin gene region and insulin-dependent diabetes mellitus (IDDM). Am J Hum Genet 52:506–516.

Strömgren E (1935): Zum ersatz des Weinbergschen "abgekurzten verfahrens" zugleich ein beitrag zur Frage von der Erblichkeit des Erkrankungsalters bei der Schizophrenie. Z Ges Neurol Psychiatrie 153:784–797.

Strömgren E (1938): Beitrage zur psychiatrischen erblehre auf grund von Untersuchungen an einer Inselbevolkerung. Acta Psychiatr Neurol Scand (Suppl) 19:1–257.

Sturt E (1985): Estimating morbidity risks with variable age of onset (correspondence). Biometrics 41:311–313.

Sunahara RK, Niznik HB, Weiner DM, Stormann TM, Brann MR, Kennedy JL, Gelernter JE, Rozmahel R, Yang Y, Israel Y, Seeman P, O'Dowd BF (1990): Human dopamine D1 receptor encoded by an intronless gene on chromosome 5. Nature 347:80–83.

Thaker GK, Moran M, Lahti A, Adami H, Tamminga C (1990): Psychiatric morbidity in research volunteers. Arch Gen Psychiatry 47:980.

Thompson WD, Orvaschel H, Prusoff BA, Kidd KK (1982): An evaluation of the family history method for ascertaining psychiatric disorders. Arch Gen Psychiatry 39:53–58.

Thompson WD, Weissman MM (1981): Quantifying lifetime risk of psychiatric disorder. J Psychiatr Res 16:113–126.

Tsuang MT, Faraone SV (1990): "The Genetics of Mood Disorders." Baltimore: Johns Hopkins.

Tsuang MT, Faraone SV (1994): Schizophrenia. In Winokur G, Clayton P (eds): "Medical Basis of Psychiatry." Philadelphia, PA: Harcourt Brace Jovanovich (in press).

Tsuang MT, Faraone SV, Lyons MJ (1993): Advances in psychiatric genetics. In Costa e Silva JA, Nadelson CC, Andreasen NC, Sato M (eds): "International Review of Psychiatry," vol I. Washington, DC: American Psychiatric Press.

Tsuang MT, Fleming JA, Kendler KS, Gruenberg AM (1988): Selection of controls for family studies: Biases and implications. Arch Gen Psychiatry 45:1006–1008.

Tsuang MT, Gilbertson MW, Faraone SV (1991): Genetic transmission of negative and positive symptoms in the biological relatives of schizophrenics. In Marneros A, Tsuang MT, Andreasen N (eds): "Positive vs. Negative Schizophrenia." New York: Springer-Verlag, pp 265–291.

Tsuang MT, Vandermey R (1980): "Genes and the Mind: Inheritance of Mental Illness." London: Oxford University Press.

van Duijn CM, Hendriks L, Cruts M, Hardy JA, Hofman A, Van Broeckhoven C (1991): Amyloid precursor protein gene mutation in early-onset Alzheimer's disease. Lancet 337:978.

Vogel F, Motulsky AG (1986): "Human Genetics: Problems and Approaches." Berlin: Springer-Verlag.

Wacholder S, McLaughlin JK, Silverman DT, Mandel JS (1992a): Selection of controls in case–control studies. I. Principles. Am J Epidemiol 135:1019–1028.

Wacholder S, Silverman DT, McLaughlin JK, Mandel JS (1992b): Selection of controls in case–control studies. II. Types of controls. Am J Epidemiol 135:1029–1041.

Wacholder S, Silverman DT, McLaughlin JK, Mandel JS (1992c): Selection of controls in case–control studies. III. Design options. Am J Epidemiol 135:1042–1050.

Ward PJ (1993): Some developments on the affected-pedigree-member method of linkage analysis. Am J Hum Genet 52:1200–1215.

Weber JL, May PE (1989): Abundant class of human DNA polymorphisms which can be typed using the polymerase chain reaction. Am J Hum Genet 44:388–396.

Weeks DE, Brzustowicz L, Squires-Wheeler E, Cornblatt B, Lehner T, Stefanovich M, Bassett A, Gilliam TC, Ott J, Erlenmeyer-Kimling L (1990a): Report of a workshop on genetic linkage studies in schizophrenia. Schiz Bull 16:673–686.

Weeks DE, Lange K (1988): The affected-pedigree-member method of linkage analysis. Am J Hum Genet 42:315–326.

Weeks DE, Lehner T, Squires-Wheeler E, Kaufmann C, Ott J (1990b): Measuring the inflation of the lod score due to its maximization over model parameter values in human linkage analysis. Genet Epidemiol 7:237–243.

Weinberg W (1925): Methoden und Technik der Statistik mit besonderer Berücksichtigun der Sozialbiologie. In: Gottstein A, Schlossmann A, Teleky L (eds): "Handbuch der sozialen Hygiene und Gesundheitsfürsorge 1. Grundlagen und methoden." Berlin: Verlag von Julius Springer, pp 71–148.

Weissman MM, Merikangas KR, John K, Wickramaratne P, Prusoff BA, Kidd KK (1986): Family-genetic studies of psychiatric disorders. Developing technologies. Arch Gen Psychiatry 43:1104–1116.

Wender PH, Kety SS, Rosenthal D, Schulsinger F, Ortmann J, Lunde I (1986): Psychiatric disorders in the biological and adoptive families of adopted individuals with affective disorders. Arch Gen Psychiatry 43:923–929.

Xie X, Ott J (1990): Determining the effect of a change in affection status on the lod score. (abstract). Am J Hum Genet 47:A205.

Xu JF, Taylor EW, Meyers DA (1992): Interval mapping in the genetic linkage study of complex disorders: A simulation study (abstract). Am J Hum Genet 53.

Zander KJ, Fischer B, Zimmer R, Ackenheil M (1981): Long-term neuroleptic treatment of chronic schizophrenic patients: Clinical and biochemical effects of withdrawal. Psychopharmacology 73:43–47.

CHAPTER 5

The Epidemiologic Catchment Area (ECA) Program: Studying the Prevalence and Incidence of Psychopathology

DARREL A. REGIER and CHARLES T. KAELBER

Division of Epidemiology and Services Research, National Institute of Mental Health, National Institutes of Health, Rockville, MD 20857

BACKGROUND AND PURPOSES OF THE ECA PROGRAM

The Epidemiologic Catchment Area (ECA) program was a targeted collaborative research effort, launched by the National Institute of Mental Health (NIMH) in the 1980s, to fill a significant void in documenting the frequency of specific mental disorders and the utilization of health services associated with mental and behavioral disorders in the United States. Propelled by needs identified in the 1978 President's Commission on Mental Health, the ECA program built on significant developments in the field of psychiatric diagnoses and community field trial methodology that occurred during the years preceding its implementation. From an epidemiologic design perspective, the ECA includes components of both a cross-sectional (prevalence) and a prospective (incidence) study.

One of the most important of these developments in the epidemiologic study of mental disorders was the publication in the *Diagnostic and Statistical Manual* (DSM-III) of specific criteria for the diagnosis of mental disorders to promote more reliable and more specific assessment than had been the case previously (American Psychiatric Association, 1980). With the improvement in case definitions promulgated by the publication of DSM-III, the incidence and prevalence of the major psychiatric disorders could be more accurately determined. In addition, by surveying community samples (rather than clinical samples), more accurate estimates of the number of both treated and untreated persons with mental disorders could be derived to help plan for the delivery of mental health services.

While the 1978 President's Commission expressed interest in evaluating the effect that establishing community mental health centers had on reducing the frequency of institutionalization for persons with mental disorders, changes in diagnostic criteria and case

The opinions expressed in this chapter are those of the authors only and do not necessarily reflect those of the National Institute of Mental Health.

Textbook in Psychiatric Epidemiology, Edited by Tsuang, Tohen, and Zahner
ISBN 0-471-59375-3   © 1995 Wiley-Liss, Inc.

definition limited possibilities for providing information of high scientific quality to enumerate persons with major mental disorders and their use of services.

Furthermore, a complete clinical picture of the spectrum of mental disorders in the general population could not be provided. Being able to identify persons with mild or even subclinical states offers promise for effective prevention or early intervention to avert progression and more severe disability. Knowledge about the full spectrum of clinical presentations may also contribute to the identification of new syndromes or subtypes that may have differing etiologies or differing responses to treatment. Conducting the ECA study in large community-based samples made it possible to close some of these gaps in information in the evaluation of both patients and nonpatients. Incorporating the DSM-III diagnostic criteria into the ECA interview schedule elevated the assessment and enumeration process to a level of scientific objectivity and precision not previously attained in surveys of mental illness in community population groups. Beyond determining the prevalence of mental disorders in the general population, the ECA study also sought to identify persons at both increased and decreased risk of developing specified disorders. Establishing variations in risk status may provide clues to possible causes and identify groups for targeted intervention to prevent or moderate the course of illness. By surveying contacts with specialty mental health, general medical, and other human services settings, the ECA study also attempted to determine how well needs of the mentally ill for mental health services were being met. Epidemiologic and mental health services research data are closely linked in the ECA, and service utilization experience of both diagnostic and community groups can be enumerated.

Events that occurred during World War II heightened concern about the prevalence of mental illness in the general population. Not only were many potential recruits evaluated as being unfit for military service because of some mental health impairment, but the war itself produced a large number of psychiatric casualties, associated with the stress of battlefield and other wartime conditions. The presumed role of stress in the causal pathway of mental disorders, especially under wartime conditions, popularized the notion that stress was an important, if not critical, determinant in the development of some mental disorders even in peacetime (Regier and Robins, 1991).

The post-World War II concerns about mental illnesses led to the creation of NIMH by the U.S. Congress and to its support of several large community surveys to help evaluate the role of stress in the etiology and development of mental disorders (Leighton et al., 1963; Srole et al., 1962; Commission on Chronic Illness, 1957). While these community surveys used relatively advanced sampling methods, carefully trained interviewers, and structured interview schedules to collect information on the prevalence of symptoms, syndromes, and impairment levels, they produced estimates of mental illness that were considered widely disparate. The apparent explanation for these differences focused more on interstudy differences in case definition and assessment procedures rather than presumed differences in prevalence between surveyed communities (Kramer, 1969). When more uniform case definitions and a standardized assessment instrument were employed, disparate rates of psychiatric disorders tended to be reduced (Cooper et al., 1972). These findings led to increased interest in improving the objectivity of diagnostic criteria and emphasizing the importance of diagnostic reliability (Feighner et al., 1972; Spitzer et al., 1978; Endicott and Spitzer, 1978).

In conducting large-scale epidemiologic research, case identification may require that nonclinicians conduct interviews in homes or other locations in the community. For these sampling techniques to work well, a highly structured interview instrument is required to minimize or avoid any need for nonclinicians to interpret the clinical significance of responses to open-ended questions. Community-based studies prior to the ECA documented that lay or nonclinical interviewers can obtain reliable information on psychiatric symptoms that could generate specific diagnoses according to defined criteria. However, when the ECA was being planned, no interview schedule existed that incorporated the newly developed DSM-III diagnostic criteria and was also appropriate for large community sampling.

In a series of consultation meetings involving a broadly based group of national and international consultants, a decision was made to develop a new instrument for use in the ECA program, based on the Renard Diagnostic Interview (Helzer et al., 1981). The resulting revised instrument, the NIMH Diagnostic Interview Schedule (DIS), incorporated coverage of DSM-III diagnostic criteria for selected mental and behavioral disorders (Robins et al., 1981a,b).

The ECA was anticipated to represent an authoritative national effort that merited involving the highest possible level of scientific and research skill to develop assessment instruments, to deal with complex sampling problems involved in combining both community and institutional populations, and to develop and conduct the necessary data collection and analysis efforts. A major early NIMH decision to help fulfill these research aspirations led to selecting investigators at multiple collaborating sites. This approach permitted selection from among competitive applications from the interested research community and also utilized the interests and community variations with access to special population groups (e.g., African-Americans, Hispanics, the elderly, and urban and rural populations). Furthermore, each site represented a replication of efforts at other sites to help enhance overall credibility by guarding against chance single-center variations in findings (Regier and Robins, 1991).

A primary intent was to estimate the prevalence of mental disorders in both treated and untreated community "catchment areas" of at least 200,000 persons at each site. This approach permitted the generation of estimates to include both severe mental disorders, most likely to be represented in institutional populations, and less severe forms of mental disorder, mostly likely to be under-represented or absent from institutional populations, but occurring in the general community.

Sample size estimation took into account the objective of estimating mental disorders and their associated risk factor levels in both community and institutional population groups. About 3,000 interviews at each site were judged to be needed to generate estimates of risk factors for schizophrenia, which afflicts about 1% of the general population. Based on information about the relation of the number of beds in long-term institutions, institutions were sampled at a rate about 10 times the rate of households. Accordingly, about 3,000 households and about 500 institutional residents were targeted for interview at each site to estimate prevalence rates of specific disorders and to assess the occurrence of risk factors among both institutional and household residents. These estimates projected an overall sample size substantially larger than any previously conducted survey of mental disorders.

Five sites were selected through a peer-review process from among all applications received in response to the NIMH solicitation. These five institutions were Yale University, The Johns Hopkins University, Washington University, Duke University, and the University of California in Los Angeles that respectively surveyed communities and institutions in New Haven, Baltimore, St. Louis, Durham, and Los Angeles. Carefully sampled communities were surveyed to permit estimation of results in other defined population groups, as well as to project estimates for the entire United States. While each site coordinated its own local survey and data collection activities, all interviewer trainers received their instruction in a common program at Washington University to promote the comparability of interviews conducted at all sites (Regier and Robins, 1991).

THE DIAGNOSTIC INTERVIEW SCHEDULE

The DIS is a highly structured interview schedule that can be administered by trained lay interviewers to identify persons in the community who meet criteria for specific psychiatric disorders. The interview elicits information on diagnostic criteria to assess the occurrence of selected mental or behavioral disorders and the utilization of both general medical and mental health services. The DIS was specifically developed to collect information that would permit assessment using DSM-III diagnostic criteria from information obtained by lay interviewers.

Evaluation of the diagnostic reliability and concordance of results with clinical interviews were carried out in various ways. At one site, clinician interviews using the Schedule for Affective Disorders and Schizophrenia, Lifetime Version (SADS-L) were compared with lay interviews using the DIS (Orvaschel et al., 1985). The SADS-L had been previously shown to increase diagnostic reliability by reducing information variance (Endicott and Spitzer, 1978), and reviewing the lifetime prevalence would permit comparison with past episodes of a disorder obtained by lay interviewers using the DIS. At another site, clinical reappraisal, using a standardized psychiatric examination, was conducted to compare with results from the DIS (Folstein et al., 1985). A psychiatrist or clinical psychologist re-examined a sample of persons who had been interviewed within the prior 3 weeks using the DIS. At another site specially trained physicians participated in several comparison evaluations involving lay-administered DIS with physician assessments using the DIS, a checklist, or neither (Helzer et al., 1985a,b). These studies helped to ensure that the information collected by trained lay interviewers would correspond closely with information gathered in a clinical setting by fully trained professional clinicians (Anthony et al., 1985; Helzer et al., 1985a,b; Robins et al., 1985).

Conducting interviews of this type presented formidable challenges. For example, since the interviewers were not required to have clinical training, the questions had to be simple enough to take into account limited educational levels, meaningful enough to recall significant experiences and symptoms, and sensitive enough to cause neither embarrassment nor offense. Extensive pilot testing and pretesting helped to ensure that these issues were dealt with satisfactorily. Overall, less than 1% of those who agreed to participate did not complete the interview. While the accuracy with which respondents answered the questions cannot be assured, a number of measures were evaluated both before and during the data collection to help ensure that reliable and accurate information was obtained (Burke, 1986; Dohrenwend, 1989; Robins et al., 1982; Robins, 1985).

In administering the DIS the interviewer follows explicit instructions by reading each specified question and follows up responses with additional specified questions. The interview is highly structured and does not rely on the interviewer to assess the presence of any diagnosis. The questions are structured and sequenced to determine whether a symptom has occurred, and, if so, whether it has sufficient clinical significance to lead to consultation with a health professional, whether medication has been taken because of the symptom, or whether the symptom has interfered in a significant way with social or occupational activities.

After systematically exploring the nature and quality of these symptoms, additional inquiry is made to determine whether the symptom had only occurred in association with a medical illness, an injury, some other physical condition (e.g., pregnancy) or in association with alcohol or other drug use. Careful exclusion of these physical causes of symptoms is required before the possibility of a psychiatric condition is considered. In addition to the quality and severity of the symptoms, information on duration and frequency of appearance of symptoms and the age of onset of symptoms is also obtained. All interviewees are asked all symptom questions, and the resulting data base allows evaluation of subthreshold symptom patterns as well.

While the DSM-III encompasses over 120 diagnoses for adults, the DIS included only a portion of these disorders, focusing on those of greatest frequency and for which the diagnostic criteria were explicit enough to be evaluated from a single interview. Table 1 lists the disorders covered in the DIS, as used at all sites in the ECA (Leaf et al., 1991).

Prevalence estimates of psychiatric disorders from the DIS can be generated for different time periods, including lifetime prevalence. If criteria for a disorder have been met at

TABLE 1. Psychiatric Disorders Assessed by the Diagnostic Interview Schedule (DIS)[a]

Affective disorders
    Major depressive disorder
    Dysthymia
    Bipolar
    Atypical bipolar
Schizophrenia and schizophreniform
Substance use disorders
    Alcohol abuse or dependence
    Sedative, hypnotic abuse or dependence
    Opioid abuse or dependence
    Amphetamine abuse or dependence
    Cocaine abuse
    Hallucinogen abuse
Cannabis abuse or dependence
Anxiety disorders
    Obsessive-compulsive
    Agoraphobia
    Social phobia
    Simple phobia
    Panic
    Post-traumatic stress disorder
Anorexia nervosa
Somatization
Antisocial personality
Cognitive impairment[b]
    Severe
    Mild

[a]In the ECA study some but not all sites assessed other disorders as well, e.g., generalized anxiety, tobacco use disorder, pathological gambling. Adapted from Leaf et al; 1991.)
[b]Not a DSM-III diagnosis

any time in the person's life, that person is included in the count of lifetime prevalence. One of the research interests in the ECA was to evaluate risk factors for various major disorders. All other things being equal, disorders that last a long time are more likely to be active than those lasting only a brief period. Thus, the association of active disorders with possible predictors of occurrence (i.e., risk factors) is confounded with their association with possible predictors of duration of illness. These two factors cannot be separated in cross-sectional studies. However, lifetime prevalence estimates are not confounded by the duration of disorder and are to be preferred when attempting to evaluate risk factor relationships in cross-sectional studies.

Even so, cross-sectional studies like the ECA may have other complicating interpretative features. For example, since the ECA surveyed persons aged 18 years and older, persons within the sample varied considerably in the length of time at risk of developing a disorder. That is, some young people who did not have the disorder at the time of the survey might develop it as they age, and the association they have with the risk factor would be missed at the time of the survey.

In addition, only living persons are surveyed in cross-sectional studies, and missing from the study sample are persons who have died. Youthful deaths have been shown to be increased in younger persons with psychiatric disorders, and these persons will be absent from the study sample (Tsuang and Woolson, 1978). Still another limitation in the interpretation of results from cross-sectional studies is the capacity to assess whether an association with a lifetime disorder is a potential cause of the disorder or its consequence. For example, depressive symptoms are often associated with alcohol abuse/dependence, but it is not clear whether depressive symptoms predispose to excess alcohol intake or whether heavy alcohol consumption causes depression. Cross-sectional studies have only a limited capacity to clarify these issues.

ECA SAMPLE SELECTION

An important objective of the ECA was to measure the prevalence of specific psychiatric disorders in selected samples of residents, whether they lived in the community or in institutional facilities serving the designated "catchment areas." Institutionalized persons were anticipated to account for a substantial number of persons with psychiatric disorders. Prisons were expected to include many persons with antisocial personality and substance abuse disorders, many persons with dementia would reside in nursing homes, and the more severely afflicted persons with mental disorders would be found in psychiatric facilities. As noted above, a sampling fraction for institutions about 10 times that for households was selected to take into account that only a small proportion of the total population is institutionalized and even a large study like the ECA would survey too few institutionalized cases unless specific oversampling procedures were used.

NIMH required that each site obtain a representative sample of its selected mental health catchment area (Holzer et al., 1985). In addition, some sites oversampled selected subgroups to be able to derive estimates for these subgroups as well. For example, a predominately Hispanic area was selected by the site in Los Angeles, and in St. Louis African-Americans were oversampled by using a stratified block design based on estimated ethnic mix. Elderly persons were oversampled in New Haven, Baltimore, and Durham.

Results of the ECA have been projected to provide national estimates, weighted to take into account the age, gender, and ethnicity of the entire United States, based on the 1980 national population census. Even so, none of the study sites included many Asian-American or Native American persons. Hispanic persons are represented primarily through the site in Los Angeles, which is largely of Mexican background, so that Hispanics of Cuban and Puerto Rican background are not well represented.

The ECA program combined five independent surveys to generate estimates of the frequency of mental disorders at the national level. While the accuracy of interview responses cannot be ensured, the fact that the results across all study sites are fairly consistent lend additional credibility to them. Details of sampling procedures at each site have been described elsewhere (Holzer et al., 1985; Leaf et al., 1985, 1991).

SELECTED ECA FINDINGS

The ECA program provides estimates of the current and lifetime prevalences of common psychiatric disorders; the ages of onset for specific disorders; their duration, age, gender, and ethnic variations in development of and recovery from these disorders; and which population groups are most likely to need care. This information can be critical for planners who have responsibility for developing prevention and intervention programs.

Overall Prevalence Estimates

As with any large-scale survey, estimates from the ECA data are subject to some methodologic limitations. These limitations include the facts that not all psychiatric disorders were considered by the DIS, persons interviewed varied in their willingness and ability to answer questions accurately, there were nonrandom refusals to be interviewed, and the five collaborating sites did not represent random samples of the U.S. population (Robins et al., 1991).

Even with these limitations, the ECA represents a major step forward in the epidemiologic study of psychiatric disorders. The ECA is the first large survey to provide estimates based on specific diagnostic criteria of the DSM-III and in which respondents reported symptoms for well-specified time periods. The questions of the DIS were carefully worded to elicit information dealing with each criteria for the covered disorders. Interviews were standardized by the use of this highly structured interview schedule, reliably administered across all study sites. Interviewer comparability was promoted by using fully elaborated questions and by having common training programs and thorough supervision during the conduct of the survey. Independent editing of interviews and a standard data cleaning procedure helped to reduce interviewer error. Response rates that exceeded 75% overall were sufficiently high to make it probable that the study samples were representative of the surveyed catchment areas. National estimates were derived by adjusting the demographic profiles of each sampled area to those for the 1980 census of the entire country.

Data from the ECA program yield estimates that from a single interview about 32% of adults in the United States report symptoms meeting criteria for one or more psychiatric disorders during their lifetimes. About 20% had an active disorder, that is, one for which criteria had been met at some time during the past with at least one symptom (or episode) occurring in the year before the interview (Table 2) (Robins et al., 1991). Among men 36% met criteria for a mental or addictive disorder at some point in their

TABLE 2. Prevalence of Any Psychiatric Disorder in Particular Groups

	No.	Lifetime Prevalence	Active Cases in Last Year	Remission[b]
		Prevalence of Any Disorder[a] in Percent (SE)		
Total	19,640	32 (0.48)	20 (0.41)	38
Gender				
Men	8,419	36 (0.72)	20 (0.59)	44
Women	11,221	30 (0.65)***	20 (0.57)	33
Age				
<30	4,872	37 (0.90)	25 (0.80)	32
30–44	4,650	39 (0.97)	23 (0.84)	41
45–64	4,194	27 (0.88)***	15 (0.69)	44
65+	5,912	21 (1.10)***	13 (0.90)	38
Ethnicity				
White	13,091	32 (0.53)	19 (0.44)	41
Black	4,697	38 (1.56)***	26 (1.40)***	32
Hispanic	1,606	33 (2.10)	20 (1.78)**	39
Education				
Not complete high school	8,818	36 (0.86)	23 (0.76)	36
High school or more	10,565	30 (0.58)***	18 (0.48)***	40
Financial dependence				
Yes	2,767	47 (1.67)	31 (1.55)	34
No	16,318	31 (0.50)***	18 (0.42)***	42
Occupational status of men 30–64				
Total	3,452	35 (0.81)	17 (0.77)	51
Unemployed	774	48 (2.46)	29 (2.24)	40
Unskilled	599	40 (2.48)*	19 (2.00)*	53
Skilled or higher	2,061	30 (1.15)***	14 (0.86)*	53
Site[c]				
Baltimore	3,586	41 (0.98)	27 (0.89)	34
Durham	4,123	35 (1.00)***	23 (0.88)	34
Los Angeles	3,503	33 (0.94)	18 (0.78)***	45
St. Louis	3,327	31 (1.12)	18 (0.92)	42
New Haven	5,101	28 (0.85)*	18 (0.37)	36
Rural–urban[c]				
Urban	4,694	34 (0.89)	21 (0.77)	38
Rural	2,107	32 (1.37)	20 (1.18)	38
Marital history				
Married and never div/sep	9,216	24 (0.63)	13 (0.50)	46
Single and never cohabited for 1 year	3,424	33 (1.07)***	22 (0.95)***	33
Ever divorced/separated	5,906	44 (0.99)***	27 (0.88)***	39
Unmarried and cohabited	986	52 (2.77)**	36 (2.66)**	31

[a]Negative cases, patients who failed to answer questions in person about one-third or more of the specific diagnoses, are considered uninformative and are not included in these analyses. Significantly different from group just above: *p <0.05, **p<.0.01, ***p<0.001.

[b]Lifetime minus active (1 year) divided by lifetime (Lt − 1 Yr)/Lt.

[c]Weighted to local populations rather than the nation. The two sites for which rural–urban comaprisons were made were Durham and St. Louis.

SOURCE: Robins et al. (1991).

lives, while 30% of women met criteria for a disorder. Men and women had similar rates of active disorder—20% of each had symptoms in the last year. These results differ from some previous studies that reported that mental disorders in women are higher than those for men (Leighton et al., 1963; Srole et al., 1962). One explanation of this difference is that gender variation occurs for specific disorders, and the overall prevalence will be determined by the coverage of disorders included in the survey (Robins et al., 1991).

If one assumes that the incidence of psychiatric disorders were stable over time and did not affect survival, increasing rates of lifetime disorder should be found as each birth cohort progresses through the life cycle. The ECA data indicate that age cohorts 18–29 years (i.e., under 30) and 30–44 years have the highest lifetime rates of disorder (Table 2). Curiously, for those aged 65 years and older, only 21% met criteria for any lifetime disorder, the lowest prevalence among the various age cohorts. Lower rates of active cases among older persons is also at variance from some previous studies (Leighton et al., 1963; Srole et al., 1962), but these studies did not exclude persons whose symptoms might have been attributed to physical rather than psychiatric disorders. This is an important consideration, since older persons are much more likely than younger persons to have physical illnesses. Possible explanations for lower symptom reporting among the elderly include 1) attributing symptoms to physical rather than psychiatric causes, 2) regarding symptoms as being "trivial," and 3) forgetting (Robins et al., 1991).

The finding of lower lifetime prevalence rates was largely but not entirely limited to white elderly. In addition the lower lifetime prevalence rates among the elderly have not been replicated in surveys of other non-U.S. cultures, suggesting that the instrument itself is not producing artifactual findings (Canino et al., 1987; Lee et al., 1987; Yeh et al., 1984). One possible interpretation for a lower lifetime rate among elderly persons than younger cohorts is that those with psychiatric disorders might have reduced life spans due to premature deaths. Evidence for this increased death rate among the psychiatrically impaired has been reported (Tsuang and Woolson, 1978). Another explanation is that psychiatric disorders have increased over time, producing higher rates in younger birth cohorts. Suggestive evidence for this interpretation is supported by temporal increases in alcohol consumption, drug use, criminal offenses, and suicide rates (Robins and Kulbok, 1986).

Higher rates occurred for African-Americans for both lifetime (38%) and active (26%) disorders than for whites or Hispanics (Table 2). However, this difference in rates is confounded by socioeconomic status (SES). When SES is controlled, rates for African-Americans are no higher than for whites. In the ECA, assessment of SES was based on each person's own educational level, current income, and current occupation. Because of the cross-sectional nature of the data, assignment of cause–effect relationships is not possible, since observed associations may be explained either as a risk factor for psychiatric disorder or as a consequence of a disorder.

Persons who did not complete high school had an increased risk of any disorder compared with those who were high school graduates (36% vs. 30%) (Table 2). Nearly half (47%) of those persons receiving public support had a lifetime disorder, and 31% had active symptoms. In relation to occupation, 35% of men aged 30–64 years had a lifetime disorder, nearly the same as all men in the study, but only 17% had active disorder. While the highest rates of lifetime and active disorder occurred among men who were not working full time, men employed in unskilled jobs also had higher rates than men in more skilled positions. Only small urban–rural differences were noted at the two sites (St. Louis and Durham) that included rural areas (Robins et al., 1991).

In relation to marital status, 44% of those who had been separated or divorced and 52% of those who had cohabited without ever marrying had experienced a disorder over the lifespan. Rates for active disorder were also high for these groups (27% and 36%, respectively). The rates for those who married and were never divorced or separated had the lowest rates (24% lifetime and 13% active)—rates that were lower than those for single persons who had never cohabited for more than a year (Robins et al., 1991).

Prevalence Estimates for Specific Disorders

Phobias and alcohol abuse are the most prevalent disorders in the United States (Table 3) (Robins et al., 1991). Over 14% of persons reported a phobia during their lifetime, and nearly 9% during the past year. For alcohol abuse and dependence nearly 14% met criteria for their lifetime, and over 6% during the past year. Other frequently occurring disorders include generalized anxiety disorder, major depressive episode, and drug abuse/dependence. Cognitive impairment, assessed only for active disorder, occurred in about 5%. Somatization disorder occurred in about 1 per 1,000 persons (Robins et al., 1991).

Unemployed men aged 30–64 had at least a twofold rate of every disorder except drug abuse compared with employed men (Robins et al., 1991). Prevalence rates of more than four times those for the employed were found among the unemployed for mania, schizophrenia, and panic disorder. These same disorders were also more common among men holding unskilled jobs. These disorders may both keep men from working and also, if working, may interfere with their possibilities for promotion (Robins et al., 1991).

In relation to marital status, drug abuse is the only disorder in which a majority of those affected (61%) had never married (Table 4) (Robins et al., 1991). Other disorders with more than a third of affected persons being single include schizophrenia (36%),

TABLE 3. Prevalence of Specific Disorders (Percent)

	Lifetime	Active (One Year)
Phobia	14.3	8.8
Alcohol abuse/dependence	13.8	6.3
Generalized anxiety	8.5	3.8
Major depressive episode	6.4	3.7
Drug abuse/dependence	6.2	2.5
Cognitive impairment mild or severe	—[a]	5.0
Dysthymia	3.3	—[a]
Antisocial personality	2.6	1.2
Obsessive compulsive	2.6	1.7
Panic	1.6	0.9
Schizophrenia or schizophreniform	1.5	1.0
Manic episode	0.8	0.6
Cognitive impairment: severe	—[a]	0.9
Somatization	0.1	0.1

[a]Not ascertained.
SOURCE: Robins et al. (1991).

TABLE 4. Marital Status of Those With Active Mental Disorders

	No. With Active Disorder	Divorced/ Separated (%)	Single (%)	Widowed (%)	Married (%)	Divorced/ Separated of Those Ever Married (%)
Schizophrenia	229	26	36	5	33	41
Depressive episode	812	22	26	8	44	30
Panic	196	22	22	6	51	28
Somatization	64	21	25	26	28	28
Generalized anxiety	359	20	25	5	49	27
Manic episode	112	20	37	5	39	31
Alcohol abuse/ dependence	1,018	18	39	3	40	30
Antisocial personality	295	18	35	2	44	28
Phobia	2,118	16	22	7	55	21
Obsessive compulsive	385	16	25	7	52	21
Drub abuse/dependence	602	14	61	1	24	26
Cognitive impairment:						
Mild or severe	2,039	12	16	27	45	14
Severe	421	12	23	37	28	16
None of the diagnoses	5,777	8	23	8	61	10

SOURCE: Robins et al. (1991).

manic episode (37%), alcohol abuse (39%), and antisocial personality (35%). More striking than the associations of disorders with not marrying are associations of disorders with marital difficulties. Rates of being currently separated or divorced are at least twice as high for those with almost any active disorder as for those without the disorder. The apparent nonassociation with drug abuse relates primarily to the fact that many of these individuals were single. The highest proportion of being currently divorced or separated is found among persons with schizophrenia (26%). The high rates of divorce and/or separation among those ever married shows that marriages tend to be more unstable and remarriage more difficult for persons with this disorder (Robins et al., 1991).

Age of Onset and Duration of Disorders

Adult psychiatric disorders often begin at early ages. For example, the median age of onset for the first symptom of those affected with some disorder was 16 years. The first symptom for any disorder occurred by age 24 years for over 75%, and 90% had their first symptom by age 38 years. Since the average age of the U.S. population is about 40 years, younger people may have many years of continued risk to develop one or more psychiatric disorders. Those over age 40 added few late-life onset cases except for cognitive impairment, which increases in frequency after age 70 (Robins et al., 1991).

Since about 20% have an active disorder (one within the past year) and 32% had a disorder at some time in life, about 37% of those with a lifetime diagnosis of a disorder (32%–20%/32%) had recovered at the time of the first or Wave 1 survey. The median age of persons with no active disorder but who had a past disorder was 19 years, suggesting that persons who have a later onset of disorder are more likely to recover. The last symptom of a disorder from which recovery occurred seemed to be about 30 years, with a mean interval of 10.4 years between the first and last symptom (Robins et al., 1991).

In DSM-III a maximum age of onset was included in the criteria for only three disorders: 1) age 15 years for antisocial personality, 2) 30 years for somatization disorder, and 3) 45 years for schizophrenia. In the ECA survey the maximum age limitation is about twice the age at which each of these disorders usually becomes manifest (about age 8 years for antisocial personality, age 15 for somatization disorder, and age 19 for schizophrenia) (Robins et al., 1991).

The age of onset for most of the major psychiatric disorders is usually in the teenage or young adult years of life. In addition to antisocial personality, somatization disorder, and schizophrenia, other disorders with typical ages of onset in the teenage years include phobias, drug abuse/dependence, and manic episodes.

The average duration of illness for those who recover can be estimated by subtracting the age of onset of the first symptom or episode from the age at which the last symptom appeared. The disorder with the longest average duration was antisocial personality, with an average duration of 19.7 years among those who recovered. Other disorders with long average durations include phobia (15.4 years) and alcohol abuse/dependence (8.7 years) (Robins et al., 1991).

Prevalence Estimates Among Institutionalized Persons

Not unexpectedly, rates of psychiatric disorder among those institutionalized were much higher than those not in institutions (Table 5) (Robins et al., 1991). About 65% of persons institutionalized in psychiatric hospitals, prisons, or residential alcohol/drug centers and nursing homes or hospitals for the chronically ill had a psychiatric disorder at some time in their life, and the disorder was active for 51%. Persons in psychiatric facilities who did not report any psychiatric disorders may be accounted for by the occurrence of disorders not covered by the DIS, persons whose insight into their own conditions was too poor to report symptoms accurately, and those hospitalized even though criteria for a disorder were not meet (e.g., hospitalization for a suicide attempt) (Robins et al., 1991).

The distribution of disorders present in institutionalized persons is also quite different from those present in persons not institutionalized. For example, 51% of the institutionalized population have current cognitive impairment, a rate more than 10 times the rate in households (Robins et al., 1991). Twenty-four percent had severe cognitive impairment

TABLE 5. Psychiatric Disorder and Institutionalization

	No.	Lifetime Prevalence (%)	Active (One Year) (%)	Proportion of Affected in Remission (%)
No institutionalized	18,059	32	19	41
Any institution	1,581	65	51	22
Psychiatric hospital	174	78	73	6
Prison or residential alcohol/drug center	709	83	57	31
Nursing home or chronic hospital	698	57	46	19

SOURCE: Robins et al. (1991).

(24 times the household rates); and another 27% had mild cognitive impairment (about 7 times the household rate). Other disorders with three or more times the rate in households are drug abuse (9% of the institutionalized sample), antisocial personality (5% of the institutionalized sample), schizophrenia (3% of the institutionalized sample), and somatization disorder (2%) (Robins et al., 1991).

Not unexpectedly, different types of institutions have different distributions of disorders. For example, 92% of those with cognitive impairment, mild or severe, were in nursing homes and similar settings, while 78% of those institutionalized with alcohol or drug substance abuse/dependence were in prisons or residential substance abuse programs (Robins et al., 1991). Persons with schizophrenia or manic episodes were widely distributed in all three types of institutions—prisons, mental hospitals, and chronic care settings. The de-institutionalization of persons with chronic severe mental disorders has contributed to their more widespread distribution in other types of institutions (Redick, 1974).

Risk Factors for Prevalence of Specific Disorders

Overall, the ECA data indicate that over their lifetimes more men meet criteria for having any disorder than do women, that younger persons have more disorders than older persons, African-Americans more than whites, and less educated more than well educated. Furthermore, active disorders are more likely to be reported among those who are financially dependent, unemployed, and or have low job status even if employed. Persons who are divorced, separated, or cohabiting also have more active disorders. While men have more lifetime disorders than women, only two disorders—alcohol abuse and antisocial personality—have a sizable male excess. On the other hand, lifetime rates for women exceeded those for men for somatization disorder, obsessive-compulsive disorder, and major depressive episodes (Robins et al., 1991).

Overall, younger adults had more psychiatric disorders than older adults. The higher lifetime rates among younger adults are largely related to antisocial personality, drug disorders, and manic episodes. An increase in prevalence was noted for each of these disorders in successively younger cohorts, suggesting that the incidence of these disorders may be increasing over time. Alternatively, these disorders may lead to premature death, with the risk of excess mortality continuing over the lifetime (Robins et al., 1991).

The prevalence of schizophrenia was highest among those aged 30–44 years, with those 45–64 having a lower prevalence and those over 65 still lower. Since the risk of onset continues through at least age 35 years, a lower prevalence in these younger cohorts may reflect that some persons have not yet developed their first schizophrenic episode. Major depression and panic disorders have low rates in the elderly. Somatization, generalized anxiety, phobia, and panic showed no excess among younger persons (Robins et al., 1991). Severe cognitive impairment was more common with each successively older cohort, with a more than doubling of the prevalence rates (George et al., 1991).

Comorbid Disorders

Data from the ECA can also be used to describe the co-occurrence of disorders in persons. Knowledge about comorbid conditions has important evaluation and treatment implications and raises questions about possible common etiologic or risk factors for each disorder. From a nosologic perspective, co-occurring conditions stimulate inquiry about the appropriate grouping of shared clinical features. Since DSM-III is based on shared clinical features without making assumptions about etiology or pathophysiology, co-occurrence might be expected for disorders that share clinical features. Some exclusion rules and criteria built into DSM-III result in pre-emptive diagnoses for some disorders. When these exclusion rules are disregarded, about 18% of the total population or about 60% of those with at least one disorder had at least two lifetime psychiatric disorders. Somatization, antisocial personality, panic, and schizophrenia had rates of comorbidity that exceeded 90% (Robins et al., 1991).

Disorders that co-occur within the last year provide some indication that some persons experience multiple disorders simultaneously. Odds ratios for estimating the co-occurrence of two disorders were computed as the ratio of the frequency of the two disorders being simultaneously present or absent compared with the frequency of each one appearing alone. Overall, the occurrence of any one disorder doubled the chances of having any second disorder. Among the 15.7% who had a disorder in a 1 month period, 23% had some other co-occurring disorder. For the 6 month prevalence period in which 19.5% had a disorder, 25% had one or more comorbid disorder during the same 6 month period. Over the lifespan 35% had one or more comorbid conditions (Bourdon et al., 1992).

The co-occurrence of mental disorders with alcohol abuse/dependence and drug abuse/dependence seems especially noteworthy. The lifetime prevalence rates were estimated to be 22.5% for any nonsubstance abuse mental disorder, 13.5% for alcohol dependence/abuse, and 6.1% for other drug dependence/abuse (Regier et al., 1990). Among persons with any mental disorder, the odds ratio for having an addictive disorder was 2.7, and the lifetime prevalence rate was about 29%. This group includes an overlap of 22% with an alcohol disorder and 15% with another drug disorder. Persons with either an alcohol or other drug disorder had a sevenfold greater increase compared with the general population for having the other addictive disorder. Thirty-seven percent of persons with an alcohol disorder also had a co-morbid mental disorder. The greatest mental-addictive disorder association occurred for those with a drug (other than alcohol) disorder and a mental disorder, with 53% occurrence and an odds ratio of 4.5. Persons treated in specialty mental health and addictive disorder clinics had substantially higher odds of having a comorbid disorder. The prison population had the highest comorbidity rates of addictive and severe mental disorders among those in institutions. The most frequently occurring mental disorders were antisocial personality, schizophrenia, and bipolar disorder (Regier et al., 1990).

Follow-Up for Incidence and Prospective Prevalence Rates

While the ECA program surveyed community populations cross-sectionally, the program also conducted follow-up surveys after 6 and 12 months to gather additional information on the incidence of specific disorders and the utilization of mental health services. The original or Wave 1 survey included 20,291 directly interviewed persons (i.e., without a proxy), and at the 12 month follow up or Wave 2 interview, all but 4,442 (21.9%) were reinterviewed (Regier et al., 1993). While these sample sizes at both Waves 1 and 2 are quite large, even the most common psychiatric disorders have low annual incidence rates, and few new cases occur over the course of a single year. Even so, estimates of annual incidence can be derived (Eaton et al., 1989).

More recently the ECA data have been used to generate a prospective 1 year prevalence estimate of 28.1%, composed of a 1 month prevalence of 15.7% and a 1 year inci-

TABLE 6. Prevalence per 100 Persons 18 Years and Older: Five ECA Sites Combined Community and Institutionalized Population[a]

Disorders	1 Month at Wave 1	1 Year New at Wave 2	1 Year Prevalence	No. of Persons[b]
Any DIS ADM disorder	15.7±0.4	12.3±0.4	28.1±0.5	44,679,000
Any DIS disorder except alcohol or drug	13.0±0.4	9.0±70.3	22.1±0.4	35,139,000
Any mental disorder with comorbid substance use	1.0±0.1	2.3±0.1	3.3±0.2	5,283,000
Any substance use disorder	3.8±0.2	5.6±0.3	9.5±0.3	15,054,000
Any alcohol disorder	2.8±0.2	4.6±0.2	7.4±0.3	11,766,000
Any drug disorder	1.3±0.1	1.8±0.1	3.1±0.2	4,929,000
Schizophrenic/schizophreniform	0.7±0.1	0.3±0.1	1.1±0.1	1,749,000
Affective	5.2±0.2	4.3±0.2	9.5±0.3	15,143,000
Any bipolar	0.6±0.1	0.5±0.1	1.2±0.1	1,908,000
Unipolar major depression	1.8±0.1	3.2±0.2	5.0±0.2	7,950,000
Dysthymia	3.3±0.2	2.1±0.1	5.4±0.2	8,586,000
Anxiety	7.3±0.3	5.3±0.2	12.6±0.3	20,034,000
Phobia	6.3±0.2	4.7±0.2	10.9±0.3	17,331,000
Panic	0.5±0.1	0.7±0.1	1.3±0.1	2,067,000
Obsessive-compulsive disorder	1.3±0.1	0.8±0.1	2.1±0.1	3,339,000
Somatization	0.1±0.0	0.1±0.0	0.2±0.2	365,000
Antisocial personality	0.5±0.1	1.0±0.1	1.5±0.1	2,385,000
Cognitive impairment (severe)	1.7±0.1	1.0±0.1	2.7±0.1	4,293,000

[a]ADM, alcohol, drug, and mental. Rates are standardized to the age, sex, and race distribution of the 1980 institutionalized and noninstitutionalized population of the United States aged 18 years and older. Data are mean 6 SE.
[b]The combined community and institutional, civilian adult population was 159 million in 1980, 167 million in 1983, and 184 million in 1990. A 16.5% increase from 1980 to 1990 is an adjustment factor that may be applied to these data to estimate the number of persons with disorders or service use in 1990. For example, the 44,679,000 with any mental or addictive disorder in 1980 would be increased to 52,051,000 in 1990.
SOURCE: Regier et al. (1993).

dence of new or recurrent disorders of 12.3% (Table 6) (Regier et al., 1993). About 6.6% of the sample developed one or more new disorders after being evaluated as having no previous lifetime diagnosis at the time of the initial Wave 1 survey. To these new episodes were added another 5.7% with an identified disorder at the first survey who either relapsed or experienced a new disorder at the 1 year follow-up survey.

Using additional information available to estimate 1 year prevalence prospectively (Waves 1 and 2 data together) identifies about one-third more cases (a 20% 1 year prevalence from Wave 1 data only [Table 2] compared with a 28% 1 year prevalence from Waves 1 and 2 [Table 6]). This higher estimate of 1 year prevalence based on prospectively collected data is observed for most specific disorders, although the increase in estimate varies by disorder. Table 6 also provides population estimates of the number of persons with mental and addictive disorders based on the 1980 U.S. population. The U.S. population increased about 16.5% from 1980 to 1990 (Regier et al., 1993).

In addition to data on the prevalence of any DIS ADM (alcohol, drug, mental) disorder, Table 6 also displays incidence and prevalence rates for specific DIS disorders. Nine and a half percent had any substance use disorder in the prospectively determined 1 year prevalence. Corresponding rates for any alcohol disorder and any drug disorder were 7.4% and 3.1%, respectively. In comparing the 1 year prevalence rates with 1 month prevalences and 1 year new cases at Wave 2, the episodic character of addictive disorders is shown by the relatively low point-prevalence/incidence ratio. That is, more new cases occurred during the year than there were current cases at the beginning of the year. A stable point-prevalence rate indicates that a significant rate of recovery has occurred during the year (Regier et al., 1993).

The relative chronicity of other disorders can be assessed in this way as well. For example, unipolar depressive disorder has the highest annual incidence rate among the group of affective disorders, but it appears to be more episodic than bipolar disorder or dysthymia. Dysthymia, by definition, requires at least 2 years of depressive symptoms. The value for the 1 month prevalence includes persons with a lifetime diagnosis. The 1 year incidence includes persons who did not meet lifetime criteria at Wave 1 but did meet criteria at Wave 2 for the first time. The 1 month and 1 year new rates for bipolar disorder are quite close (0.6% and 0.5%, respectively), suggesting that the average duration of a bipolar episode is slightly longer than 1 year (Regier et al., 1993).

Somatization disorder is a chronic disorder by definition, and, while it has a low prevalence, these persons tend to be high users of both general medical services and mental health services. Antisocial personality disorder, also a chronic condition by definition, has a 1 year prevalence of 1.5% and a 1 year incidence of 1.0%. In the ECA the diagnosis of severe cognitive impairment was based on a current mental status examination. Incidence cases include only those persons who were not evaluated as severely impaired at Wave 1. Among the 1.7% 1 month prevalence at Wave 1, about half (0.9%) had the same level of severe impairment at Wave 2. The other portion (0.8%) appeared to function at a higher level at the Wave 2 evaluation (Regier et al., 1993).

Services Utilization Associated With Mental and Addictive Disorders

Nearly 15% (14.7%) reported use of service in one or more sectors of the mental and addictive service system. While some overlap of utilization occurred, 5.9% received treatment from specialists in mental and addictive disorders, 6.4% obtained treatment from general medical physicians, 3.0% sought services from other human service professionals, and 4.1% turned to the voluntary support sector for care (Regier et al., 1993).

Only a little more than a quarter (28.5%) of persons with any disorder sought mental health or addictive services. This proportion varied by disorder—over 60% for somatization, schizophrenia, and bipolar disorder to less than 25% for addictive disorders and severe cognitive impairment. Persons with somatization disorder have the highest rates of use of any mental/addictive disorder, reaching nearly 70% in a 1 year period. They also have the highest use of general medical services (49.4%), the highest overall health subsystem use (63.4%), the highest use of other human services (15.3%), the highest use of services involving any professional (67.2), and the second highest use (second to unipolar major depression) of the voluntary support network. While the total number of persons with somatization disorder is relatively small, their use of services in the general medical and mental health systems is substantial (Regier et al., 1993).

These data on incidence of disorder and utilization of services can contribute to discussions about national health policy issues. The data quantify the burden of mental disorders in the population and the utilization of health services and identify the gaps in utilization of mental health services, which have been shown to have efficacy in the treatment of mental disorders.

The characteristics of persons successfully followed after 1 year have also been evaluated (Eaton et al., 1992). Attrition from the Wave 2 reinterview was considered in two ways: 1) persons who were not located after 1 year and 2) persons who were located but refused to participate. Being male, Hispanic, young, and unmarried were associated with not being found 1 year later, while those who were found but refused to participate tended to be older, married, and have lower educational attainment than those who did participate. Persons with panic and depression were less likely to be found at the Wave 2 reinterview.

CONCLUDING REMARKS

The goals of the ECA included gathering information to increase knowledge about the frequency of psychiatric disorders in the community, especially the frequency of major specific disorders (both active and lifetime), and the utilization of mental health services in the general population. While not specifically identified as goals, the ECA has also provided important information about the age of onset and average duration of disorders, the frequency of remission or relapse, and comorbidity.

Knowledge about the natural history of disorders helps to evaluate the impact of various interventions aimed at reducing the prevalence and cost of mental disorders. A reduced prevalence might occur through reductions in incidence, reductions in relapse, and reductions in the average duration of episodes. Targeted programs like the NIMH D/ART to promote early recognition and early intervention for depression can be evaluated to assess progress over time (Regier et al., 1988). Efforts directed toward preventing the occurrence of mental disorders can focus on identified risk factors and reductions in symptoms before diagnostic threshold levels are reached. The high levels of comorbidity noted in the ECA data can encourage caregivers to make thorough assessments to be certain that the full range of morbidity is identified and direct intervention efforts toward each disorder.

An additional important finding from the ECA data is that only a small fraction of persons with psychiatric disability seek professional assistance, in spite of evidence that significant levels of impairment exist in their capacity for work, for self-support, and for satisfactory interpersonal relationships. To improve this situation will require more efforts to promote the early recognition of these disorders and increase knowledge that treatment can be accessible and effective (Robins et al., 1991).

The ECA data also show that many persons with substantial psychopathology reside in community institutions, including those not specifically for the treatment of the mentally disabled. Examples of this include the large number of persons with schizophrenia who are in prisons and nursing homes, where recognition and treatment for their disorder may not be available (Robins et al., 1991).

The ECA data have also helped to highlight that psychiatric disorders in men are as common as in women, although the frequency of specific disorders differ by gender. Women suffer more frequently from depression and anxiety disorders, while men suffer more from substance dependence/abuse disorders and antisocial personality. The data also document that many disorders may have their onset in early adult life but that recovery is not uncommon.

An additional unanticipated contribution of the ECA survey was to reveal some difficulties in dealing with the co-occurrence of multiple disorders and the exclusion criteria for some disorders within the DSM-III classification system. Analyses of the ECA data contributed to revisions in the DSM classification system (Boyd et al., 1984; American Psychiatric Association, 1987).

The importance of reliable diagnostic assessment has been recognized internationally, in no small part due to the wide acceptance of DSM-III and DSM-III-R. When the section of the Tenth Revision of the International Classification of Diseases (ICD-10), dealing with mental and behavioral disorders, was being prepared, an important effort was made to develop clinical descriptions and diagnostic guidelines that encouraged more objective assessment (Sartorius et al., 1993). In addition, a version of the ICD-10 was also developed for research that identified explicit diagnostic criteria to improve diagnostic reliability still further. Concurrently, a new assessment instrument, the Composite International Diagnostic Interview (CIDI), is being developed for use in community surveys of adults (Robins, et al., 1989; Wittchen et al., 1991). The CIDI directly evolved from the DIS and incorporates revised diagnostic criteria for the ICD-10 and DSM classification systems.

As a cross-sectional or prevalence survey, the ECA design was not conducted primarily to explore causal relationships, which are difficult to do in cross-sectional surveys as noted above. However, associations of disorders with demographic and other correlates can still provide clues for more specific explorations of causal associations. Since many adult disorders have their roots in childhood, the need to learn more about early childhood experiences and symptom patterns is evident. A limitation of the ECA is that it had to depend on personal retrospective reporting of symptoms by those interviewed. Personal reporting bias that may occur can be reduced or eliminated by prospectively gathered information. Such prospectively conducted studies, starting in early childhood, should seek to encompass a full range of child and adolescent disorders, as well as adult disorders, in due order. Validation of interview data should come from parents, schools, medical records, and other available sources. It is hoped that such a prospective study might be undertaken in the near future.

REFERENCES

American Psychiatric Association (1980): "Diagnostic and Statistical Manual of Mental Disorders," 3rd ed. Washington, DC: American Psychiatric Association.

American Psychiatric Association (1987): "Diagnostic and Statistical Manual of Mental Disorders," 3rd ed, revised. Washington, DC: American Psychiatric Association.

Anthony JC, Folstein M, Romanoski AJ, Korff MR, Nestadt G, Chahal R, Merchant A, Brown C, Shapiro S, Kramer M, Gruenberg E (1985): Comparison of lay Diagnostic Interview Schedule and a standardized psychiatric diagnosis. Arch Gen Psychiatry 42:667–676.

Bourdon KH, Rae DS, Locke BZ, Narrow WE, Regier DA (1992): Estimating the prevalence of mental disorders in US adults from the epidemiologic catchment area survey. Public Health Rep 107:663–668.

Boyd JH, Burke JD, Gruenberg EM, et al. (1984): Exclusion criteria of DSM-III: A study of cooccurrence of hierarchy-free syndromes. Arch Gen Psychiatry 41:983–989.

Burke JD (1986): Diagnostic categorization by the Diagnostic Interview Schedule (DIS): A comparison with other methods of assessment. In Barrett JH, Rose RM (eds): "Mental Disorders in the Community." New York: Guilford Press, pp 255–285.

Canino GJ, Bird H, Shrout P, Rubio-Stipec M, Geil KP, Bravo M (1987): The prevalence of alcohol abuse and/or dependence in Puerto Rico. In Gaviria M, Arana J (eds): "Health and Behavior: Research Agenda for Hispanics." Chicago, IL: Public-Services of the University of Illinois at Chicago, Research Monograph Series No. 1, pp 127–144.

Commission on Chronic Illness (1957): "Chronic Illness in a Large City," vol 4. Cambridge, MA: Harvard University Press.

Cooper JE, Kendell RE, Gurland BJ, Sharpe L, Copeland JRM, Simon R (1972): "Psychiatric Diagnosis in New York and London." London: Oxford University Press.

Dohrenwend BP (1989): The problem of validity in field studies of psychological disorders revisited. In Robins L, Barrett J (eds): "The Validity of Psychiatric Diagnoses." New York: Raven Press, pp 35–55.

Eaton WW, Anthony JC, Tepper S, Dryman A (1992): Psychopathology and attrition in the epidemiologic catchment area surveys. Am J Epidemiol 135:1051–1059.

Eaton WW, Kramer M, Anthony JC, Dryman A, Shapiro S, Locke BZ (1989): The incidence of specific DIS/DSM-III mental disorders: Data from the NIMH Epidemiologic Catchment Area Program. Acta Psychiatr Scand 79:163–178.

Endicott J, Spitzer RL (1978): A diagnostic interview: The Schedule for Affective Disorders and Schizophrenia. Arch Gen Psychiatry 35:837–844.

Feighner PJ, Robins E, Guze SB, Woodruff RA, Winokur G, Munoz R (1972): Diagnostic criteria for use in psychiatric research. Arch Gen Psychiatry 26:57–63.

Folstein M, Romanoski A, Chahal R, Anthony J, VonKorff M, Nestadt G, Merchant A, Gruenberg E, Kramer M (1985): Eastern Baltimore Mental Health Survey Clinical Reappraisal. In Eaton WW, Kessler LG (eds): "Epidemiologic Field Methods in Psychiatry: The NIMH Epidemiologic Catchment Area Program." Orlando, FL: Academic Press, pp 253–284.

George L, Landerson R, Blazer D, Anthony J (1991): Cognitive impairment. In Robins LN, Regier DA (eds): "Psychiatric Disorders in America." New York: Free Press, pp 291–327.

Helzer JE, Robins LN, Croughan JL, Welner A (1981): Renard diagnostic interview: Its reliability and procedural validity with physicians and lay interviewers. Arch Gen Psychiatry 38:393–398.

Helzer J, Robins L, McEvoy L, Spitznagel E (1985a): A comparison of clinical and diagnostic interview schedule diagnoses. Arch Gen Psychiatry 42:657–666.

Helzer JE, Stolzman R, Farmer A, Brochington IF, Plesons D, Singerman B, Works J (1985b): Comparing the DIS with a DIS/DSMIII based physician reevaluation. In Eaton WW, Kessler LG (eds): "Epidemiologic Field Methods in Psychiatry: The NIMH Epidemiologic Catchment Area Program." Orlando, FL: Academic Press, pp 285–308.

Holzer CE, Spitznagel E, Jordan KBV, Timbers DM, Kessler L, Anthony JC (1985): Sampling the household population. In Eaton WW, Kessler LG (eds): "Epidemiologic Field Methods in Psychiatry: The NIMH Epidemiologic Catchment Area Program." Orlando FL: Academic Press, pp 23–48.

Joint Commission on Mental Illness and Health (1961): "Action for Mental Health." New York: Basic Books.

Kramer M (1969): Cross national study of diagnosis of the mental disorders: Origins of the problem. Am J Psychiatry 125(Suppl I–II).

Leaf PJ, German P, Spitznagel E, George L, Landsverk J, Windle C (1985): The institutional population. In Eaton WW, Kessler LG (eds): "Epidemiologic Field Methods in Psychiatry: The NIMH Epidemiologic Catchment Area Program." Orlando, FL: Academic Press, pp 49–66.

Leaf PJ, Myers JK, McEvoy LT (1991): Procedures used in the epidemiologic catchment area study. In Robins LN, Regier DA (eds): "Psychiatric Disorders in America." New York: Free Press.

Lee CK, Kwak YS, Rhee H, Kim YS, Han JH, Choi JO, Lee YH (1987): The national epidemiological study of mental disorders in Korea. J Korean Med Sci 2:1:19–34.

Leighton DC, Harding JSD, Macklin DB, MacMillan AM, Leighton AH (1963): "The Character of Danger: Psychiatric Symptoms in Selected Communities." New York: Basic Books.

Orvaschel H, Leaf P, Weissman M, Holzer C, Tischler G, Myers J (1985): The Yale–ECA Concordance Study: A Comparison of the DIS and the SADS-L. In Eaton WW, Kessler LG (eds): "Epidemiologic Field Methods in Psychiatry: The NIMH Epidemiologic Catchment Area Program." Orlando, FL: Academic Press, pp 235–252.

President's Commission on Mental Health (1978): "Report to the President From the President's Commission on Mental Health," Stock No. 040-000-00390-8, vol 1. Washington, DC: U.S. Government Printing Office.

Redick RW (1974): "Patterns in Use of Nursing Homes by the Aged Mentally Ill," Statistical Note 107. Rockville, MD: Division of Biometry and Epidemiology, National Institute of Mental Health.

Regier DA, Farmer ME, Rae DS, Locke BZ, Keith SJ, Judd LL, Goodwin FK (1990): Comorbidity of mental disorders with alcohol and other drug abuse. J Am Med Assoc 264:2511–2518.

Regier DA, Hirschfeld RMA, Goodwin F, Burke JD, Lazar JB, Judd LL (1988): The NIMH Depression Awareness, Recognition and Treatment (D/ART) program: structure, aims and scientific basis. Am J Psychiatry 145:1351–1357.

Regier DA, Narrow WE, Rae DS, Manderscheid RW, Locke BZ, Goodwin FK (1993): The de facto U.S. mental and addictive disorders service system. Arch Gen Psychiatry 50:85–94.

Regier DA, Robins LN (1991): Introduction. In Robins LN, Regier DA (eds): "Psychiatric Disorders in America." New York: Free Press, pp 1–10.

Robins LN (1985): Epidemiology: Reflections on testing the validity of psychiatric interviews. Arch Gen Psychiatry 42:918–924.

Robins LN, Helzer JE, Croughan J, Ratcliff K (1981a): National Institute of Mental Health Diagnostic Interview Schedule: It history, characteristics and validity. Arch Gen Psychiatry 38:381–389.

Robins LN, Helzer JE, Croughan J, Williams JBW, Spitzer RL (1981b): "NIMH Diagnostic Interview Schedule," Version III, May 1981. Rockville, MD: National Institute of Mental Health.

Robins LN, Helzer JE, Ratcliff K, Seyfried W (1982): Validity of the Diagnostic Interview Schedule: Version II: DSM-III diagnoses. Psychol Med 12:855–870.

Robins LN, Kulbok PA (1986): Methodological strategies in suicide. In Mann J, Stanley M (eds): "Psychology of Suicidal Behavior." Ann NY Acad Sci 487:1–15.

Robins LN, Locke BZ, Regier DA (1991): An overview of psychiatric disorders in America. In Robins LN, Regier DA (eds): "Psychiatric Disorders in America." New York: Free Press, pp 328–366.

Robins LN, Orvaschel H, Anthony J, Blazer D, Burnam A, Burke J (1985): The Diagnostic Interview Schedule. In Eaton WW, Kessler LG (eds): "Epidemiologic Field Methods in Psychiatry: The NIMH Epidemiologic Catchment Area Program." Orlando, FL: Academic Press, pp 285–308.

Robins LN, Wing J, Wittchen HU, Helzer JE, Babor TF, Burke J, Farmer A, Jablensky A, Pickens R, Regier DA, Sartorius N, Towle LH (1989): The Composite International Diagnostic Interview: An epidemiologic instrument suitable for use in conjunction with different diagnostic systems and in different cultures. Arch Gen Psychiatry 45:1069–1077.

Sartorius N, Kaelber C, Cooper JE, Roper M, Rae D, Gulbinat W, Ustun B, Regier DA (1993): Progress toward achieving a common language in psychiatry. Arch Gen Psychiatry 50:115–124.

Srole L, Langer TS, Michael ST, Opler M, Rennie T (1962): "Mental Health in the Metropolis: The Midtown Manhattan Study." New York: McGraw Hill.

Spitzer RL, Endicott J, Robins E (1978): Research diagnostic criteria: Rationale and reliability. Arch Gen Psychiatry 35:773–782.

Tsuang MT, Woolson RF (1978): Excess mortality in schizophrenia and affective disorders. Arch Gen Psychiatry 35:1181–1185.

Wittchen HU, Robins LN, Cottler LB, et al. (1991): Cross cultural feasibility, reliability and sources of variance of the CIDI. Br J Psychiatry 159:645–653.

Yeh E, Hwu HG, Chang LY (1984): Prevalence of mental disorders in Taipei City by Chinese modified Diagnostic Interview Schedule: A preliminary report. Bull Chin Soc Neurol Psychiatry 10:88–103.

CHAPTER 6

Studying the Natural History of Psychopathology

WILLIAM W. EATON

Department of Mental Hygiene, Johns Hopkins University, Baltimore, MD 21205

INTRODUCTION

The purpose of this chapter is to provide a conceptual framework for conducting studies of the natural history of psychopathology in the general population and to illustrate details of the framework with examples from research in the field of psychiatric epidemiology. The three major aspects of the natural history of psychopathology are onset, course, and outcome. Preventive actions directed at onset, course, and outcome are traditionally defined as *primary*, *secondary*, and *tertiary* prevention, respectively. This introductory section is followed by one section on each topic and a conclusion.

This chapter is not intended as a review of studies on natural history of psychopathology. A comprehensive review would be cumbersome and uninformative, because there is so much variation in methodologic quality of studies of natural course. If methodologic standards are set high for such a review (for example, by including only population-based studies with diagnostic information on an adequate number of subjects), there are very few studies that could be included. On the other hand, if methodologic standards are set low for such a review (for example, by including small studies of clinic samples and studies without diagnostic information), there would be a confusing morass of numerous studies with results so mixed and contradictory that the review would be of dubious value. This situation shows the state of the art in this area, indicating that we are still at the beginning stages of learning about the natural history of psychopathology.

The *natural history of psychopathology* is a description, at the level of the population, of the ebbing and flowing of psychopathology from its earliest appearance to its final outcome. It includes signs and symptoms that occur before onset; the fluctuations in signs and symptoms that occur after onset; and consequences of the psychopathology, even those that may occur after remission. It does not include the study of risk factors except as they influence the course. The definition leads to focus in this chapter on descriptive population-based cohort studies. There is relatively little emphasis on cohort studies oriented toward specific risk factors, such as those comparing populations defined as "ex-

Textbook in Psychiatric Epidemiology, Edited by Tsuang, Tohen, and Zahner
ISBN 0-471-59375-3 © 1995 Wiley-Liss, Inc.

posed" and "not exposed" to some risk factor. There is relatively little emphasis on cohort studies that include an intervention trial in an attempt to evaluate risk and protective factors, since the intervention trials are often not based in general populations and since the intervention itself may disrupt the natural history. The primary focus is on population-based studies, since many persons with mental disorder never seek treatment for it.

ONSET

In defining onset, it helps to distinguish the etiologic process from the pathologic process. Pathology occurs when the biologic dynamics have become abnormal—a distinct change in the relationship among variables, the new influence of variables that were not important beforehand, or a new metabolism of some sort. The etiologic process is broader conceptually and includes the period of time when the probability of disorder is heightened, even though the process is still normal. Causes may be present well before the pathologic process has begun. Onset occurs when the pathologic process begins.

The absence of firm data on the validity of the classification system enjoins us to be careful about operationally defining disease onset. It is particularly difficult to establish the validity of a threshold for the presence versus the absence of disorder, because signs and symptoms of psychiatric disorders are widespread in the population, not always reflecting the presence of a psychiatric disorder. From the clinical standpoint, subtle differences in approach to treatment may suggest quite varied thresholds; from the epidemiologic standpoint, subtle differences in threshold may produce widely varying prevalences. A simple definition is that onset occurs when the individual first enters treatment. A related definition is that onset occurs when the symptom is noticeable by a clinician. Another definition is the point when the symptom is first noticed by the individual. With the operational criteria of the Diagnostic and Statistical Manual, it is possible to conceive of onset as the time when full criteria are met for the first time in the life. This definition has been used in studies of incidence (e.g., Eaton et al, 1989,a,b). But it omits that part of the pathologic process that takes place prior to meeting full criteria for disorder. Since the etiologic process may be extended in time, and the operation of etiologic factors distant from when full criteria for disorder are met, this may lead to missing important risk factors.

The definitions above are easy to operationalize but lack a theoretical relationship to the pathologic process. Theoretically, onset is that point in time when the etiologic process becomes irretrievably pathologic; that is, the point when it is certain that the full criteria for disorder will eventually be met. This point of irreversibility is, unfortunately, very difficult to observe.

Prodromes and Precursors

The *prodrome* is the period prior to meeting full-blown criteria of disorder, when some signs or symptoms are nevertheless present. The *speed of onset* is the length of the prodromal period and can be measured in simple units of time (e.g., months or years). The presence of signs or symptoms below the criterion level may help to identify individuals at heightened risk for developing the full-blown disorder, who might be considered targets of prevention. Given the widespread prevalence of individual signs and symptoms of mental disorders in the general population, it is likely that many individuals with signs and symptoms of disorder will not go on to develop the full-blown criteria. In this situation the signs and symptoms are not quite prodromal, in the strict sense of the word, but it seems awkward to refer to them as *risk factors*. Signs and symptoms from a diagnostic cluster that precede disorder, but do not predict the onset of disorder with certainty, are referred to here as *precursor signs and symptoms*. At the present state of our knowledge of the onset of mental disorders, there are few or no signs and symptoms that predict onset with certainty, but precursor signs and symptoms may be helpful in identifying groups at higher risk for onset than the general population. Converting what is known about precursors into true prodromes is an important topic of research for epidemiologists interested in longitudinal research and in prevention.

An illustration of these issues is presented in Figure 1 and Table 1. Figure 1 shows two cumulative distributions for panic disorder. The distribution on the right focuses on the age at which the individual first meets full criteria for DSM-III Panic Disorder. For this distribution, onset must occur during the 1-year follow-up period of the ECA Program, i.e., a true prospective design. The population at risk includes those who had never met criteria for the diagnosis at the beginning of the follow-up period. Thus, the at-risk group includes those with no symptoms, as well as those with some symptoms of disorder, but not meeting full DSM-III criteria. The distribution on the left focuses on the age at which panic first occurred, as reported by the new cases. The dotted line marks the 20th and 50th percentiles, and age values for these are recorded. The figure between the two curves gives a rough outline of the prodromal period.

Panic disorder has onset in young adulthood (Fig. 1). Twenty percent of cases meet criteria for diagnosis for the first time before the age of 27 years and 50% before they are

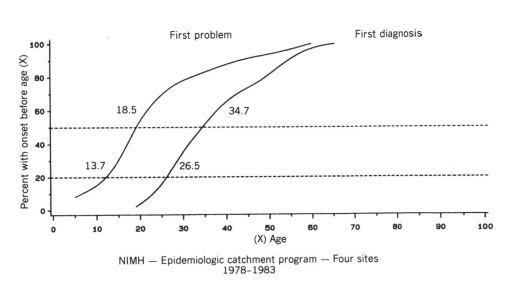

FIGURE 1. Prodromal period for panic disorder. (Adapted from Eaton et al., 1995.)

TABLE 1. Relative and Attributable Risk for Panic Disorder Due to Precursors Epidemiologic Catchment Area Program

Precursor	Precursor Relative Risk	Precursor Prevalence (%)	Precursor Attributable Risk (%)
Nervous person	8.2	24.3	64
Panic attack	24.9	3.8	48
Attack with breathing difficulty	32.9	1.2	28
Attack with heart pounding	30.9	2.7	45
Attack with dizziness	25.1	1.0	19
Attack with fingers tingling	23.4	0.7	14
Attack with pain in chest	24.0	1.0	19
Attack with choking sensation	28.5	0.9	19
Attack with fainting sensation	25.7	1.0	20
Attack with sweating	24.6	2.0	32
Attack with shaking	23.4	2.2	33
Attack with derealization	27.7	1.4	27
Attack with fear of dying	30.4	1.6	32
Attack with hot/cold flashes	27.7	1.8	32

SOURCE: Adapted from Eaton et al., 1995.

35. Twenty percent have their first panic attack before the age of 14 and 50% before the age of 19. The prodromal is about 13 years long for hose with early onset and about 16 years for those with later onset.

Symptoms associated with onset of panic disorder, defined above as *precursors*, are associated with accelerated onset of the disorder. Table 1 shows the prevalence of the precursor, its relative risk in predicting onset of panic disorder during the 1 year of follow-up in the ECA Program, and the attributable risk that can be estimated with the prevalence and the relative risk. The standard formula for attributable risk can be applied here (e.g., Kleinbaum et al., 1982) and is useful because it might prioritize precursors for screening or other prevention programs; but this use of the term is conceptually different from other uses because of the limited duration of the follow up. Therefore, the duration of the follow up is used to qualify the attributable risk. A panic attack with breathing difficulty displays the highest relative risk (32.9), but, due to rarity in the population (prevalence of 1.2% in the population), the attributable risk is only 28%. The occurrence of a simple panic attack is a strong precursor of panic disorder because the relative risk is high (24.9) and the prevalence is not too low (3.8%). A positive response to the question "Are you a nervous person?" is also a strong precursor of panic disorder.

This strategy of searching for precursors is applicable for most disorders. It has been applied to depression previously (Dryman and Eaton, 1991; Horvath et al., 1992).

Population Measures of Onset

Incidence is the rate at which new cases develop in the population. It is essential to distinguish *first incidence* from *total incidence*. The distinction itself is commonly assumed by epidemiologists, but there does not appear to be consensus on the terminology. Most definitions of the incidence numerator include a concept such as "new cases" (Lilienfeld and

Lilienfeld, 1980:138), "illness commencing" (Expert Committee, 1959:6), cases that "come into being" (MacMahon et al., 1960:54), or persons who "develop a disease" (Mausner and Kramer, 1985:44) or "have onset" (National Center for Health Statistics 1977:129). Sartwell and Last (1980) imply total incidence when they state the necessity of allowing "for an individual being counted more than once, if the condition is one for which this is possible (e.g., accidents, colds)." Lilienfeld and Lilienfeld (1980:170) also occasionally equate "incidence" with "attack rate." Kleinbaum et al. (1982) hint at the distinction between first and total incidence, but are not explicit on the issue. Morris (1975) defines incidence as equivalent to our "first incidence" and "attack rate" as equivalent to our "total incidence." Except for the latter text, in none of these definitions is it explicit whether or not an individual who is healthy now, but has had episodes of the disorder over the life course, qualifies for a "new" onset. First incidence corresponds to the most common use of the term *incidence*, but since the usage is by no means universal, the prefix is recommended.

The numerator of *first incidence* for a specified time period is composed of those individuals who have had an occurrence of the disorder for the first time in their lives; the denominator excludes all persons who start the period with any prior history of the disorder. The numerator for *total incidence* includes all individuals who have a new occurrence of the disorder during the time period under investigation whether or not it is the initial episode of their lives or a recurrent episode. The denominator for total incidence excludes only persons who are active cases at the beginning of the follow-up period.

The preference for first or total incidence in etiologic studies depends on hypotheses and assumptions about the way causes and outcomes important to the disease ebb and flow. If the disease is recurrent and the causal factors vary in strength over time, then it might be important to study risk factors not only for first but also for subsequent episodes (total incidence). For example, one might consider the effects of changing levels of stress on the occurrence of episodes of neurotic illness (Tyrer, 1985) or of schizophrenia (Brown and Birley, 1968). For a disease with a presumed fixed progression from some fixed starting point, such as dementia, the first occurrence might be the most important episode to focus on, and first incidence is the appropriate rate. In the field of psychiatric epidemiology, there are a range of disorders with both types of causal structures operating, which leads to discussion of the two distinct types of incidence.

The two types of incidence are functionally related to different measures of prevalence. Kramer et al. (1981) have shown that *lifetime prevalence* (i.e., the proportion of the population who have ever had an attack of a disorder) is a function of first incidence and mortality in affected and unaffected populations. *Point prevalence* (i.e., the proportion of persons in a defined population at a given time who manifest the disorder) is linked to total incidence by the queuing formula $P = I*D$ (Kramer, 1957; Kleinbaum et al., 1982): that is, point prevalence is a function of the total number of cases occurring, and the average duration of their episodes.

Incidence data on specific psychiatric disorders are expensive to gather. A minority of individuals, not necessarily representative of those with disorder, receive treatment, and therefore a field survey is required. Many of the disorders are rare, and many well individuals have to be evaluated, at two distinct points in time, to estimate the incidence rate. The number of prospective studies with sufficiently large samples to estimate rates of incidence is small. If 5,000 person-years of observation is set as the minimum requirement, there are only a handful of studies that cover a range of disorders. These include the ECA study in the United States (Eaton et al., 1989a,b), the Stirling County study in Canada

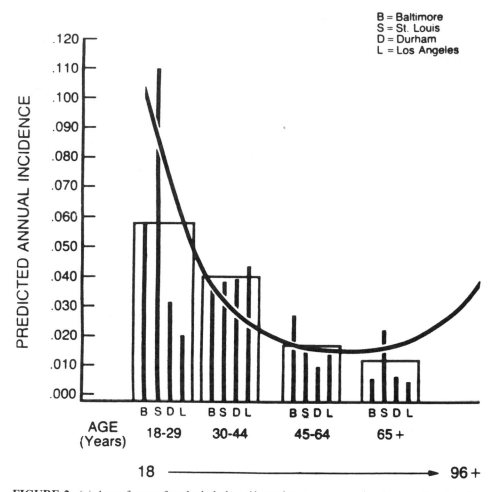

FIGURE 2. (*a*) Age of onset for alcohol abuse/dependence among males. Prospective data from four sites of the Epidemiologic Catchment Area Program. (Adapted from Eaton et al., 1989a. ©1989 Munksgaard International Publishers Ltd., Copenhagen, Denmark.)

(Murphy et al., 1987), the Lundby Study in Sweden (Hagnell et al., 1990), and the Traunstein study in Germany (Fichter et al., 1987).

Comparison of results between these studies is important because the numerators are so small that the findings from any one study are statistically volatile. Figure 2 shows a comparison of results on the incidence of alcoholism in Lundby, Sweden, with the incidence of alcohol abuse or dependence in the ECA cohort. Both studies show sharply declining incidence after young adulthood and a slight rise at the beginning of the seventh decade. The rise shown in the ECA data is caused by five individuals who had incidence in that age range; the rise shown in the Lundby data is caused by only three individuals who had incidence in that age range. These results suggest etiologic clues and have impli-

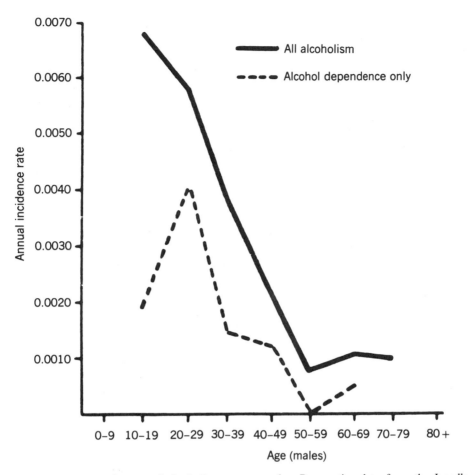

FIGURE 2. (*b*) Age of onset of alcoholism among males. Prospective data from the Lundby study. (Adapted from Ojesjo et al., 1982. Reprinted with permission from *Journal of Studies on Alcohol*, vol. 43, pp. 1190–98, 1943. Copyright by Alcohol Research Documentation, Inc., Rutgers Center of Alcohol Studies, Piscataway, NJ 08855.)

cations for prevention efforts. The results of each study might not be convincing, but the replication of the identical pattern is credible.

Focus on population indicators for the force of morbidity leads to explicit consideration of the idea of a continuous line of development toward manifestation of disease with an as-yet-unknown point of irreversibility. At present we can only hypothesize where the disease begins, so that even the use of a word *symptom* is problematic in the strict medical sense, since we cannot ascribe the complaint or behavior to the disease with perfect accuracy.

There are at least two ways of thinking about the development toward disease. The first way is the increase in severity or intensity of symptoms. An individual could have all the symptoms required for diagnosis but not of them in sufficient intensity or severity as to meet the threshold for disease. The underlying logic of this conception is the relatively high frequency of the symptoms, at a mild level of intensity, in the general population, making it difficult to distinguish normal and subcriterial complaints from manifestations of disease. For many chronic disease, it may be inappropriate to regard the symptom as ever having been "absent" (for example, deviant personality traits on axis II of the *Diagnostic and Statistical Manual*). This type of progression toward disorder is termed *intensification* and leads the researcher to consider whether a crucial level of intensity exists at which the rate of development toward disorder accelerates or becomes irreversible.

A second conceptual approach toward the issue of disease development is the occurrence of new groups of symptoms where none existed. This involves the gradual acquisition of symptoms so that clusters are formed that increasingly approach the constellation required to meet specified definitions for diagnosis. *Present* can be defined as occurrence either at the nonsevere or at the severe level: thus, decisions made about the process of symptom intensification complicate the idea of symptom acquisition. This leads the researcher to consider the order in which symptoms occur over the natural history of the disease and, in particular, whether one symptom is more important than others in accelerating the process.

Figure 3 is an adaptation of a diagram used by Lilienfeld and Lilienfeld (1980; Fig. 6.3) to visualize the concept of incidence as a time-oriented rate. Here the adaptation gives examples of the several distinct forms that onset can take when the disorder is defined by constellations of symptoms varying in intensity, as is the case with mental disorders. The topmost subject ("A") is what might be considered the null hypothesis, and it corresponds to simple onset as portrayed in the original. Figure 3 shows how intensity, represented by the vertical width of the bars, might vary. The threshold of disease is set at

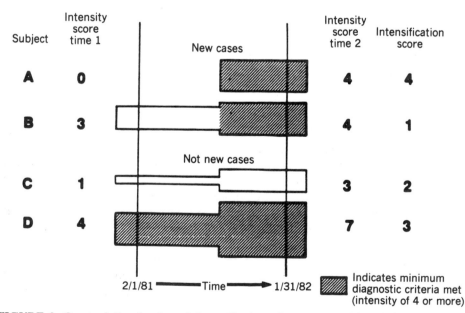

FIGURE 3. Onset of disorder through intensification of symptoms. (Adapted from Eaton et al., 1989b.)

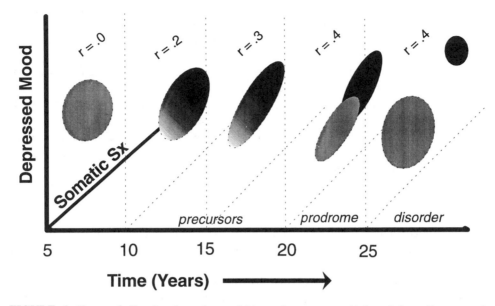

FIGURE 4. Onset of disorder through acquisition of symptoms. (Adapted from Eaton et al., 1989b.)

four units of width, and in the null hypothesis subject A progresses from zero intensity to four units, becoming a case during the observation period. Subject B changes from nearly meeting the criteria (width of three units) to meeting it (four units) during the follow up. Both subjects A and B are new cases, even though the onset was more sudden in subject A than in subject B. Subjects C and D are not new cases, even though their symptoms intensify during the follow up more than do those of the incident case, subject B.

Conceptualizing the force of morbidity as time to a single dichotomous event (i.e., traditional concepts of incidence) is not flexible enough to deal with dimensional constructs, as shown in Figure 3. It is also not flexible enough to deal with changes through time in the convariation of indicators, which can be an important aspect of the force of morbidity. *Emergence* is defined to be the evolution of the relationship of a group of symptoms to each other. Figure 4 shows a simplified view of this developmental phenomenon for the example of the depression syndrome. The vertical axis represents the intensity of mood disturbance, and the diagonal axis, slanting backwards from left to right, the intensity of somatic disturbance. Time is represented by the horizontal axis, passing from left to right. At some early stage of development, the correlation of mood to somatic disturbance is pictured as being 0.0 (round circle representing cross-sectional scatterplot with correlation equal to 0.0). Gradually the mood comes to be associated with the somatic disturbance, shown by the evolution of the circle into an ellipse. At this point, the normal and the abnormal have not split, and the disorder is not inevitable. At this stage both mood and somatic disturbance predict imperfectly to later onset of MDD, and they are precursors. Later, a group begins to emerge for whom mood and somatic disturbance are highly correlated. At this stage, mood and somatic disturbances are prodromal for many. Finally, there emerges a group with very high covariation of mood and somatic disturbance, and a second "normal" group with little covariation remains. An increase in covariation can occur *without* an increase in mean levels of either mood or somatic disturbance. But presumably there is a sharp increase in impairment associated with some threshold of covariation. At some stage in the development of the covariation and impairment, a threshold for disorder might be set.

These concepts allow the study of the progression of disease independently of case definition. The speed of onset can be measured with reference to a threshold of caseness by using growth curve models and slopes (e.g., McArdle and Hamagami, 1992). The development of covariation can be studied with generalized estimating equations (Zeger and Liang, 1986). Risk factors at different stages of the disease may be differentially related to disease progression only above or below the threshold set by the diagnosis. In this situation, the diagnostic threshold might be reconsidered.

Problems in Estimation

Measuring onset in the context of a population requires a prospective approach. It is possible to approximate measures of incidence using data gathered at one point in time, but this requires assumptions that are not generally tenable. Age of onset can be determined in a cross-sectional sample, for example, by asking each respondent who meets lifetime criteria for disorder when the symptoms began. But the distribution of onsets determined in this way are inherently biassed due to truncation and censoring. The truncation occurs because individuals who have onsets and die before the data collection are omitted—they will have had *earlier* onsets than those in the sample. The censoring occurs because individuals will have onsets after the data collection is complete—they will have had *later* onsets than those in the sample. The cross-sectional approach is further compromised because it relies on the respondent's autobiographical memory to recall the time of the onset, which may be quite distant from the time of the data collection. It is likely that those with more recent onsets are less likely to forget the occurrence of the disorder, which biases the onset distribution toward *later* onset. But it is also likely that those with severe cases of disorder are less likely to forget the occurrence of disorder; if severity is associated with earlier onset, this bias would be toward *earlier* onset. Thus, retrospective data from a cross-sectional approach include a mixture of biases that are sometimes undecipherable.

Prospective designs address the issues of truncation and censoring, but they nevertheless rely on an individual's autobiographical memory for estimation of incidence. The minimum design requirement is two waves of data collection. At Wave 1, the lifetime history of psychopathology is determined in order to exclude individuals who have already met the criteria for caseness. At Wave 2, those who have become new cases form the numerator of the incidence rate, and those who were never cases at wave 1 form the risk set, or denominator. The same mistakes in recall can occur in the cross-sectional or prospective design. In the prospective design, the mistakes made by an individual are likely to be smaller than in the cross-sectional design, because the time of data collection is closer to the present for the individual, especially at the second wave where new onsets are determined. But the effects of error are much more complex in the prospective design, because the biases can concatenate in so many different ways. For example, in the East Baltimore ECA panel cohort, there were 2,622 individuals who had never in their lifetimes met criteria for diagnosis of panic disorder by the time of the interview at Wave 1; 20 of these met criteria at Wave 2, giving a cumulative annual incidence rate of about 7 per 1,000 per year (Eaton et al., 1989b). There were 40 individuals at Wave 1 who met criteria for past or present diagnosis; of these, 20 reported never having experienced a panic attack at Wave 2. These 20 might be labeled *reverse incidence*. They represent half (20/40) of those meeting criteria for diagnosis at Wave 1; they match exactly the number (20) of incident cases. This phenomenon is not unique to the ECA surveys (e.g., Newman, personal communication). The existence of "reverse incidence" is due to forgetting and, while disquieting, does not negate the existence of the 20 cases in the numerator of the incidence rate. It does suggest that forgetting of episodes occurs, a tendency that would bias prevalence rates downward and incidence rates upward. The upward bias in incidence would occur because cases that belong in the attack rate would be mixed in with the first incidence rate.

Random error has counterintuitive pernicious effects in prospective research on the natural history of disorder. Indeed, in the context of estimating incidence in field surveys, the concept of *random* error is not very useful. If by random error is meant an equiprobable response, then it is straightforward to show that, for a sample, the bias resulting is moderately upward for prevalence and strongly upward for incidence. The rates of false-positive and false-negative answers to a given question will depend on the question and will not be equiprobable, in general; but many other types of errors in the survey process—mistakes in data entry, for example—will have an equiprobable character to them. Thus, the tendency is for seemingly "random" errors to bias the incidence rates upward.

This discussion leads to the conclusion that incidence rates are likely to be biased upward due to both systematic and random error. There is a need for improvement in measurement of the history of psychopathology (Lyketsos et al., 1994).

COURSE

Remission

Careful definition of terms is essential for studying the natural history of psychopathology (Frank et al., 1991). Conceptualizing and measuring the ebb and flow of psychopathology after onset necessitates focus on duration, measured by units of time, and on recurrence, which is measured in the manner of a risk. *Remission* is a point in time after onset when signs and symptoms diminish sharply. After the first onset has occurred, it is useful to have a measure of level of symptomatology that defines remission unambiguously. Only after setting a threshold for remission can the duration of the episode be studied (Philipp and Fickinger, 1993). The definition of remission has all the complexities of the definition of onset. But as well as a threshold for the presence and absence of signs and symptoms, defined by both intensity and breadth, the definition of remission requires that a threshold of a minimum time period be set below which a remission does not occur. For example, a *remission* may be defined as a continuous period of 3 months or more during which the individual is not meeting full criteria for disorder.

The measure of remission will be most useful if it uses the diagnostic criteria as a comparison or standard value, because the within-diagnostic standard will allow meaningful comparison of qualities of remission between disorders. Therefore, a measure of *completeness of remission* is proposed, to describe that point between episodes that is most free of signs and symptoms. It requires that thresholds be established for the intensity of signs and symptoms, as in, for example, the SCAN (rating scale one value of "1" versus "2" or "3"; Wing et al., 1990). The measure of completeness of remission can be used even if the threshold levels are set differently in different research studies. The measure below takes advantage of the SCAN definitions to set thresholds of symptom intensity and sets 3 months as the minimum time period during which the individual must fail to meet complete diagnostic criteria in order for a remission to be defined and measurable. The proposed levels of completeness of remission are:

Level 1: No signs and symptoms present

Level 2: At least one sign or symptom present, but none above the threshold of intensity

Level 3: One and only one sign or symptom present above the threshold of intensity; other signs and symptoms may or may not be present below the threshold of intensity

Level 4: More than one sign or symptom present above the threshold

Level 5: Full criteria for disorder are present continuously (i.e., remission does not occur). *Continuously* is defined as having no gaps greater than 3 months.

The *speed of remission* is defined similarly to the speed of onset and the prodromal period. It is the time taken from the point at which the disorder is at its symptom peak to the beginning of the remission. The symptom peak is best defined similarly to the concept of acquisition, discussed above: the point in time where highest number of signs and symptoms are above the threshold of intensity. The speed of remission can be measured in standard units of time (e.g., weeks and months).

Recurrence

A *relapse* occurs if the individual meets criteria for disorder after a remission. Relapse requires careful work on terminology and operational definition, as with remission (Falloon et al., 1983). The *speed of relapse* is the time required to move from the state of remission to the symptom peak. As with other duration measures, the metric for speed of relapse is standard units of time.

Recurrence is the risk for relapse and is analogous to incidence in expressing a dynamic or time-oriented risk for onset, as discussed above regarding "attack rate." The rate of recurrence can be estimated similarly to incidence, with the risk set for recurrence being comprised of all those not currently meeting criteria for disorder.

Problems in Estimation

Censoring is the effect produced by the situation that follow up almost always precedes eventual outcome. Data are censored when outcome is known only as of a certain time. Censoring produces important problem in the measurement of durations. For example, a mean duration based on censored data would be downward biassed. Since the mean is highly influenced by observations on the tail of the distribution, the bias in the mean can be quite strong. A body of statistics called *survival analysis* has grown up around this and other related problems (e.g., Lawless, 1982).

Survival analysis has been applied to problems of duration and recurrence of episodes of schizophrenia. Duration and recurrence are two sides of the same coin: Study of the duration of the hospital stay for schizophrenia was most interesting in the days prior to the era of deinstitutionalization, when a large proportion of the life might be spent in a hospital (e.g., Eaton and Whitmore, 1977); duration of tenure in the community after release from hospital became more important as hospital stays shortened to a few weeks, and there was little variation in the population as to length of hospitalization (Mortensen and Eaton, 1994). With better longitudinal survey data, these methods of survival analysis will be increasingly applied to lengths of episodes and remissions for the range of psychiatric disorders.

Attrition is the loss of subjects in longitudinal research usually due to one of three causes: individual mobility outside the study area or to an unknown residence; death; and refusal to participate after some threshold of response burden is reached. In field surveys such as the ECA, attrition after even so short a period of 1 year can be large enough to threaten the credibility of results. The ECA attrition was mostly due to refusal (about 15%) and partly to failure to locate individuals (about 5%). Since the time period was short, there was relatively little attrition due to mortality (less than 1%). With longer time periods between requests for interviews, the components of attrition might be expected to change, with more respondents dying and/or moving away and less refusing.

In population-based psychiatric case registers, attrition is likely to have different causes and a different structure. Refusal is less likely to be important if the level of psychopathology is such as to need or even require treatment, such as might be argued is the case for psychosis. For disorders such as depression, where treatment is often not sought, register data will be severely biassed by attrition.

For registers of limited geographic spread, mobility will be important; for case registers that cover an entire country, such as in Denmark or Israel, mobility will be much less important. The upshot of these comparisons is that population-based psychiatric case registers are a useful source of information on the natural history of severe mental disorders such as psychosis.

Attrition can bias results. In the ECA, older white women and younger black males had about twice the rate of attrition than other respondents, and these differences in attrition were larger than baseline differences related to psychopathology (Eaton et al., 1992a). But the attrition that took place forestalls studying the effect of psychopathology during the interval between baseline and follow up: For example, there may be a tendency for those with new episodes of disorder to move to another location (e.g., a young person might move to another city to live with parents during recovery). In this situation the attrition would bias the rate of incidence downward.

The problems of attrition and censoring are illustrated in Figure 5 with data from the Danish Psychiatric Case Register on hospital admissions during the period 1973 to 1988. Each admission was the first in the individual's lifetime wherein the diagnosis of schizophrenia was given. The figure shows survival curves for the first, fifth, tenth, and fifteenth episodes. Each curve shows the percentage of individuals who remain outside the hospital (vertical axis) according to time since discharge (horizontal axis). Relapse from the first episode tends to occur in the first few years after discharge; by the fifth year, over three-fourths of the cohort have had a second episode of hospitalization. The manner of presentation is immune from the censoring bias, since it correctly portrays the lack of information for the individuals who have not suffered a relapse by the end of the follow up in 1988. Later curves reveal the effects of attrition, however, since they are only computed for individuals suffering 4 or more, 9 or more, and 14 or more relapses, respectively. Survival in the community is less likely for these cohorts because they represent an increasingly severe subsample of the first admission cohort. These data show, in con-

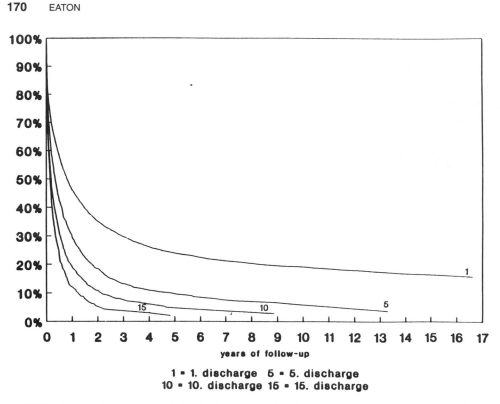

FIGURE 5. Probability of remaining in the community for schizophrenics after discharge from hospital in first, fifth, tenth, and fifteenth episodes. (Adapted from Mortensen and Eaton, 1994.)

trast to ECA data discussed above, that attrition can bias toward portraying more severe psychopathology.

OUTCOME

Outcome refers to the consequences of the psychopathology. These consequences can be immediate, such as impairment and disability resulting from the disorder. The focus here is on important and pernicious consequences of disorder that occur afterward and that are not included in the defining phenomena of the disorder, i.e., future psychopathology of other types and physical illness (comorbidity); overall functioning; and death.

Comorbidity

There has been increasing interest in narrowly defined disorders since the introduction of the DSM-III. Since psychopathology does not always fit into the DSM-III categories and is highly overlapping, the increased "splitting" of disorders has led to increasing interest in *comorbidity*: the occurrence of two or more disorders in the same individual. The disorders can occur simultaneously in the same individual, or they can occur at different points in time—so-called lifetime comorbidity. Comorbidity over the lifetime presumably expresses a genetic diathesis, an early and enduring risk factor, or a long-standing environmental cause. Patterns of differential comorbidity will contribute, eventually, to improved nosology.

Cross-sectional study of comorbidity can focus on the increase in lifetime prevalence for one disorder, given the presence of another. Studies of natural history focus on risk, either through retrospective recall of the timing of one disorder versus the other, or through a true prospective design. For example, in the ECA data, the risk for onset of DSM-III major depressive disorder is 3.4 times higher if the individual has had a panic attack than if they have not suffered a panic attack (Andrade et al., 1993).

Another focus of study in the area of natural history and comorbidity is whether the phenomenology of a given disorder is equivalent when a second disorder has occurred, is present, or will occur in the future. Symptom profiles for panic and major depressive disorders differ in overall level, but not in their pattern, for comorbid cases as compared with those suffering either disorder alone (Fig. 6). These data suggest a common diathesis to panic and depression. Prospective study would contribute valuable information about the overlap between anxiety and depression.

Physical illness is another type of comorbidity and a possible consequence of psychopathology. Study of the relationship of psychopathology to physical illness requires strong shifts in method over the time period of the follow up. For example, psychiatric data can be obtained in field surveys without physical examination or laboratory tests; but evaluation as regards physical illness does require these different modalities of measurement. The shift in modality and intensity of measurement suggests that one of at least two special strategies might be useful. One strategy might be to define cases of psychopathology early in the follow up, with controls from the same population, and to follow up the

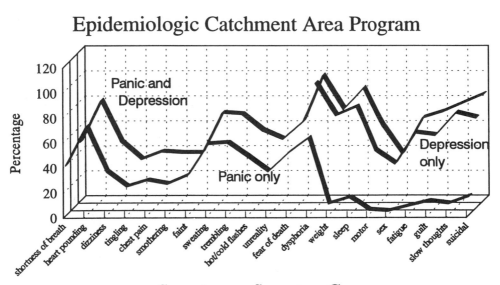

FIGURE 6. Symptom profiles for those with panic only, panic with depression, and depression only (no panic symptoms recorded for depression-only group). Four sites of the Epidemiologic Catchment Area Program.

cases and controls with more regular and more intensive measures than given to the general population. A second strategy would involve a multiple stage screening operation during the follow up to search for possible cases of physical illness for further (expensive) examinations and tests.

In follow ups based on psychiatric case registers, the systems of registration are usually based on the structure of the treatment systems, which tend to separate psychiatry from other areas of medicine. Thus, only highly specialized registration systems, such as the Oxford Record Linkage Study (Acheson, 1967), or the use of two or more illness based registers, such as the Danish Psychiatric and Cancer registration systems (Mortensen and Juel, 1993), is effective.

Functioning

Functioning is the ability to deal with the normal demands of everyday life. Persons with psychopathology are sometime less able to function effectively than the general population. The term as used here includes the WHO definition of disability (WHO, 1980). Impairment and disability resulting from a given disorder such as schizophrenia is widely variable (Jablenski et al., 1980; Eaton, 1991), and most of the costs associated with psychiatric problems come from the reduced functioning, not from the signs and symptoms themselves. The conversion of psychopathology to impairment and disability is thus an important area of study.

Mortality

Mortality, or the rate of death in the population, is usually higher in individuals with psychopathology than in the general population. Increased mortality is associated with schizophrenia (e.g., Babigian and Odoroff, 1969), mood disorders (e.g., Murphy et al., 1987; Black et al., 1985), anxiety disorders (Weissman et al., 1989), and the substance use disorders (Kouzis et al., 1995). For some disorders the increased mortality is associated with the signs and symptoms of the disorder itself, as is the situation for suicide with depression. But the risk for suicide is also high for disorders where the connection is less obvious, as in the controversy over panic and suicide (Weissman et al., 1989; Anthony and Petronis, 1991) and suicide in schizophrenia (Herrman et al., 1987). The rate of accidental death is also sometimes higher among persons with psychopathology. Other causes of death related to psychopathology are more subtle still. For example, it may be the case that individuals with psychopathology are less likely to engage in illness prevention and health promotion behaviors, such as curtailment of smoking or lowering of cholesterol intake, due to preoccupation with psychopathology or less effective functioning generally. Psychopathology involves potent physiologic changes, and there may be important and as-yet-undiscovered biologic connections between psychopathology and risk for major fatal disease such as heart disease, cancer, and diabetes.

Problems in Estimation

Lack of blind measurement is an important problem in estimation as regards outcome. The dependence of outcome on initial state is a central focus of research on natural history, but it is difficult to measure outcome independently of initial state. If the respondent, or the interviewer remembers the initial measurement session, the results of that session are likely to bias measurement of outcome. For example, an interviewer may probe more persistently for the occurrence of panic attacks if it is known that they have occurred in the recent, or even distant, past. Impairment and disability are likely to be rated downward if it is known that the individual once met the criteria for diagnosis of schizophrenia, even if no signs and symptoms are present at the time of the followup. Thus, bias due to lack of blindness is likely to overestimate the relationship of early indicators of psychopathology to later outcomes.

Another problem in estimation of outcome is the *lack of continuity of measurement*, which is a design feature of most follow up studies. The problem is that outcomes such as comorbid disorders and physical illnesses may have occurred after the baseline measurement but before the follow up, and they may be forgotten by the respondent and difficult to observe by the examiner. This situation leads to underestimation of the relationship of baseline psychopathology to outcomes.

Some systems of data collection that cut across different types of illness, such as the Oxford Record Linkage Study, or the use of two or more disease-based registers, as mentioned above, are able to obtain measurements continuous in time; but these suffer from the longitudinal equivalent of Berkson's bias—that is, the tendency for treated persons to show a stronger comorbidity than exists in the untreated population (Berkson, 1946). In this case the bias includes more than just comorbidity of psychopathologies; it includes physical illness, lowered functioning, and mortality as well.

Incomplete ascertainment is a major problem for study of mortality as an outcome of psychopathology. Geographic mobility may be more frequent for those with some types of psychopathology. Deaths of persons who are more mobile will be less likely to enter the local, state, or even national death reporting system. It is also possible that the identification of the dead is less sure for people who have had psychopathology either because they change their names or because they die in uncertain circumstances, with fewer social networks present for identification. Incomplete ascertainment is likely to bias the relationship of psychopathology to mortality in a downward direction.

THE CAREER OF PSYCHOPATHOLOGY

Many of the concepts discussed above present a simplistic point of view by not taking the long-term course into account. For example, incidence, remission, and relapse are all dichotomous outcomes that can be measured with only two waves of observations. One wave defines the sample at risk, which comprises the denominator, and the second wave estimates the numerator. Logistic and proportional hazard regression are appropriate analytic techniques for these measures.

Attempts have been made to categorize or quantify the entire course of psychopathology for a given disorder—what might be termed the *career of psychopathology*. For example, Ciompi (1980) has proposed eight categories for the course of schizophrenia that combine the three dichotomies of onset (acute vs. insidious), course (stable vs. episodic), and outcome (good vs. bad). A visual description of these categories, adapted from Ciompi, is shown in Figure 7. These figures stimulate many interesting questions as to the nature of the course. For example, what is the ultimate outcome? Is the course steadily, progressively deteriorative or progressively ameliorative (Eaton et al., 1992b)? Is the rate of remission related to the speed of onset? Is the risk for recurrence related to the duration of the episode or to the speed of onset? Answers to these questions would be important for clinical treatment, but not much is known because of the difficulties of conducting research on the natural history of psychopathology.

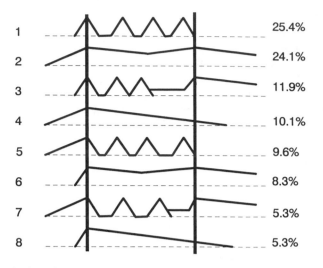

FIGURE 7. Typologies of course of schizophrenia, according to dichotomous criteria for onset, course, and outcome. (Redrawn from Ciompi, 1980.)

Estimation of the percentages for Ciompi's typologies in a prospective study would require a minimum of three waves of observation—one each for the determination of types of onset, course, and outcome, respectively. Psychometricians have known for many years that three waves is the minimum to separate the effect of reliability of measurement from the stability and instability of the construct being measured (Bohrnstedt, 1983). In the case of psychopathology, there appears to be a strong reactivity to the initial wave of measurement (Eaton et al., 1989a,b) so that individuals appear to become healthier between the first and second wave. This reactivity may be due to the stigma associated with mental disorders. It introduces the need for an additional baseline measurement. Therefore, for anything more than very simplistic analyses, the minimum number of waves of measurement required in prospective longitudinal research is four.

Statistical techniques suitable for four or more waves of analysis are currently being developed and will be very useful in future studies. With dichotomous measures of psychopathology and outcome, the appropriate statistical techniques are event history (Allison, 1984) and multiple binary time series analysis (Liang and Zeger, 1989). For continuous measures of psychopathology and outcome, the appropriate statistical techniques are structural equation models (Bollen, 1989) and growth curve/random effects models (McArdle and Hamagami, 1992).

CONCLUSION

Studying the natural history of psychopathology in the general population requires large resources of effort and expense because of the combination of population-based sampling, long-term commitment, and intensity of measurement. Perhaps for these reasons the field is in its infancy. Most data on natural history are based on clinical samples, which are not representative of the population of persons with mental disorders. There are no benchmark estimates for the incidence of most major mental disorders that have been replicated and for which there is a consensus among investigators. The estimates for the long-term courses of disorders are widely varying. Thus, there is plenty of progress to be made!

ACKNOWLEDGMENTS

This work was supported by NIMH grants MH47447 and MH44653. The author is grateful to Beth Melton and Mohamed Badawi for statistical assistance.

REFERENCES

Acheson ED (1967): "Medical Record Linkage." London. Oxford University Press.

Allison P (1984): "Event History Analysis: Regression for Longitudinal Data." Beverly Hills; Sage.

Andrade L, Eaton WW, Chilcoat H (1993): Lifetime comorbidity of panic attacks and major depression in population-based study: Age of onset. Manuscript in preparation.

Andrade L, Eaton WW, Chilcoat H (1995): Lifetime comorbidity of panic attacks and major depression in a population based study: Symptom profiles. Br J Psychiatry (in press).

Anthony JC, Petronis KR (1991): Panic Attacks and Suicide Attempts. Arch Gen Psychiatry 48:1114.

Babigian HM, Odoroff CL (1969): The mortality experience of a population with psychiatric illness. Am J Psychiatry 126:470–480.

Berkson J (1946): Limitations of the application of fourfold table analysis to hospital data. Biom Bull 2:47–53.

Birley JLT, Brown GW. Crises and life changes preceding the onset of relapse of acute schizophrenia: Clinical aspects. Br J Psychiatry 116:327–333.

Black DW, Warrack G, Winokur G (1985): The Iowa record linkage study. I. Studies and accidental deaths among psychiatric patients. Arch Gen Psychiatry 42:71–75.

Bohrnstedt GW (1983): Measurement. In Rossi PH, Wright JD, Anderson AB (eds): "Handbook of Survey Research Research." Orlando: Academic Press, pp 69–121.

Bollen KA (1989): "Structural Equations With Latent Variables." New York: Wiley.

Brown GW, Birley JLT (1968): Crises and life changes and the onset of schizophrenia. J Health Social Behav 9:203–214.

Ciompi L (1980): Catamnestic long-term study on the course of life and aging of schizophrenics. Schiz Bull 6:606–618.

Dryman A, Eaton WW (1991): Affective symptoms associated with the onset of major depression in the community: Findings from the U.S. NIMH Epidemiologic Catchment Area Program. Acta Psychiatr Scand 84:1–5.

Eaton WW (1991): Update on the epidemiology of schizophrenia. Epidemiol Rev, 13:320–328.

Eaton WW, Anthony JC, Tepper S, Dryman A (1992a): Psychopathology and attrition in the epidemiologic Catchment Area Surveys. Am J Epidemiol 134:1041–1059.

Eaton WW, Badawi M, Milton B (1995): Prodromes and precursors. Epidemiologic data for primary prevention of disorders with slow onset. Am J Psychiatry (in press).

Eaton WW, Bilker W, Haro JM, Herrman H, Mortensen PB, Freeman H, Burgess P (1992b): The long-term course of hospitalization for schizophrenia: Change in rate of hospitalization with passage of time. Schiz Bull 18:185–207.

Eaton WW, Kramer M, Anthony JC, Dryman A, Shapiro S, Locke BZ (1989a): The incidence of specific DIS/DSM-III mental disorders: Data from the NIMH Epidemiologic Catchment Area Program. Acta Psychiatr Scand 79:163–178.

Eaton WW, Kramer M, Anthony JC, Chee EML, Shapiro S (1989b): Conceptual and methodological problems in estimation of the incidence of mental disorders from field survey data. In Cooper B, Helgason T (eds): "Epidemiology and the Prevention of Mental Disorders." London: Routledge, pp 108–127.

Eaton WW, Whitmore GA (1977): Length of stay as a stochastic process: A general approach and application to hospitalization for schizophrenia. J Math Sociol 5:273–292.

Expert Committee on Health Statistics (1959): "Sixth Report." Geneva: WHO.

Falloon RH, Grant N, Marshall JLB, et al. (1983): Relapse in schizophrenia: A review of the concept and its definitions (editorial). Psycho Med 13:469–477.

Fichter MM, Koch HJ, Rehm J, Weyerer S (1987): Adversity and the risk of mental illness: preliminary results of the Upper Bavarian Restudy. In Angermeyer MC (ed); "From Social Class to Social Stress." Berlin; Springer-Verlag.

Frank E, Prien RF, Jarrett RB, et al. (1991): Conceptualization and Rationale for consensus definitions of terms in major depressive disorder. Arch Gen Psychiatry 48:851–855.

Hagnell O, Essen-Moller, E, Lanke J, et al. (1990): "The Incidence of Mental Illness Over a Quarter of a Century." Stockholm: Almqvist and Wiksell International.

Herrman HE (1987): Re-evaluation of the evidence on the prognostic importance of schizophrenic and affective symptoms. Aust NZ J Psychiatry 1987 21:424–427.

Horvath E, Johnson J, Klerman GL, Weissman MM (1992): Depressive symptoms as relative and attributable risk factors for first-onset major depression. Arch Gen Psychiatry 49:817–823.

Jablenski A, Schwarz R, Tomov T 91980): WHO collaborative study on impairments and disabilities associated with shizophrenic disorders. Acta Psychiatr Scand Suppl 285 62:152–163.

Kleinbaum DG, Kupper LL, Morgenstern H (1982): "Epidemiologic Research: Principles and Quantitative Methods." Belmost, CA: Lifetime Learning Publications.

Kouzis AC, Eaton WW, Leaf PJ (1995): Psychopathology and mortality in the general population. Soc Psychiatry Psychiatr Epidemiol (in press).

Kramer M (1957): Discussion of the concepts of prevalence and incidence as related to epidemiologic studies of mental disorders. Am J Public Health 47:826–840.

Kramer M, Von Korff M, Kessler L (1981): The lifetime prevalence of mental disorders: Estimation, uses and limitations. Psychol Med 10:429–436.

Lawless JF (1982): "Statistical Models and Methods for Lifetime Data." New York: John Wiley & Sons.

Liang KY, Zeger SL (1989): A class of logistic regression models for multiple binary time series. J Am Stat Assoc 84:447–451.

Lilienfeld AM, Lilienfeld DE (1980): "Foundations of Epidemiology," 2nd ed. New York: Oxford University Press.

Lyketsos CG, Nestadt G, Cwi J, Heithoff K, Eaton WW (1994): The Life Chart Interview: A standardized method to describe the course of psychopathology. Int J Methods Psychiatr Res 4:143–155.

MacMahon B, Pugh TF, Ipsen J. (1960): "Epidemiologic Methods." Boston, MA: Little, Brown and Company

Mausner JS, Kramer S (1985): "Epidemiology: An Introductory Text." Eastbourne, England: WB Saunders.

McArdle JJ, Hamagami F (1992): Modeling incomplete longitudinal and cross-sectional data using latent growth structural models. Exp Aging Res 18:145–166.

Morris JN (1975): "Uses of Epidemiology," 3rd ed. Edinburgh: Churchill Livingstone.

Mortensen PB, Eaton WW (1994): Predictors for readmission risk in schizophrenia. Psychol Med 24:223–232.

Mortensen PB, Juel K (1993): Mortality and causes of death in first-admitted schizophrenic patients. Br J Psychiatry 163:183–189.

Murphy J, Monson RR, Olivier DC, Sobol AM, Leighton AH (1987): Affective disorders and mortality: A general population study. Arch Gen Psychiatry 44:473–480.

National Center for Health Statistics (1977): "Health Interview Survey Procedures (1957–1974): Vital and Health Statistics," Series 1, No. 11. Washington, DC: U.S. Government Printing Office.

Ojesjo L, Hagnell O, Lanke J (1982): Incidence of alcoholism among men in the Lundby Community Cohort, Sweden, 1957–1972.

J Stud Alcohol 43:1190–1198.

Philipp M, Fickinger, MP (1993): The definition of remission and its impact on the length of a depressive episode. Arch Gen Psychiatry 50:407–408.

Sartwell PE, Last JM (1980): Epidemiology. In Last JM (ed): "Maxcy-Rosenau Public Health and Preventive Medicine," 11th ed. New York: Appleton-Century-Crofts, pp 9–85.

Tyrer P (1985): Neurosis divisible? Lancet 8430:685–688.

Weissman MM, Klerman GL, Markowitz JS, Ouelette R, Phil M (1989): Suicidal ideation and suicide attempts in panic disorder and attacks. N Engl J Med 321:1209–1214.

World Health Organization (1980): "International Classification of Impairments, Disabilities, and Handicaps." Geneva: World Health Organization.

Wing JK, Babor T, Brugha T, Burke J, Cooper JE, Giel R, Jablenski A, Regier D, Sartorius N (1990): SCAN: Schedules for clinical assessment in neuropsychiatry. Arch Gen Psychiatry 47:589–593.

CHAPTER 7

Epidemiology of Psychiatric Comorbidity

RONALD C. KESSLER

Institute for Social Research and Department of Sociology, The University of Michigan, Ann Arbor, MI 48106

INTRODUCTION

Studies of diagnostic patterns in both clinical samples (Ross et al., 1988; Rounsaville et al., 1991; Wolf et al., 1988) and general population samples (Boyd et al., 1984; Helzer and Pryzbeck, 1988; Regier et al., 1990a; Kessler et al., 1994c) show that comorbidity among psychiatric disorders is highly prevalent. Over one-half of patients in psychiatric treatment typically receive more than one diagnosis (Wolf et al., 1988), and three out of four patients in treatment for substance abuse or dependence also have a diagnosis of some mental disorder (Ross et al., 1988; Rounsaville et al., 1991). As many as one-half of all lifetime psychiatric disorders in the general population occur to people with a prior history of some other psychiatric disorder (Robins et al., 1991; Kessler et al., 1994c).

Comorbidity presents substantial treatment problems, as standard therapies are either excluded or are complicated when patients have multiple disorders. Many types of comorbidity, moreover, are associated with severe illness course. Unfortunately, most research in psychiatric epidemiology continues to focus on individual diagnostic categories, a bias that must be corrected. This chapter reviews what is currently known about comorbidity and offers directions for future research. The literature on basic patterns of psychiatric comorbidity is reviewed in the following section. The literature on the consequences of comorbidity is then reviewed, followed by a review of the literature on the causes of comorbidity. Future research directions are then discussed.

BASIC PATTERNS OF COMORBIDITY

The Importance of General Population Samples

Most of the published research on psychiatric comorbidity describes treatment samples. Such work attempts to identify patterns of comorbidity and determine whether they respond differentially to treatment. There is encouraging evidence concerning the effective-

Textbook in Psychiatric Epidemiology, Edited by Tsuang, Tohen, and Zahner
ISBN 0-471-59375-3 © 1995 Wiley-Liss, Inc.

ness of this sort of "patient-program matching." For example, Weiss et al. (1988) documented that cocaine abusers who use drugs as a form of self-medication respond differently to treatment depending on the nature of the primary psychiatric disorder that led to their cocaine abuse.

Treatment samples are less well suited, though, to more basic descriptive and analytic epidemiologic research because the patterns of comorbidity found in treatment settings do not reflect the patterns in the community as a whole. This is so because comorbidity is associated with professional help-seeking (Helzer and Pryzbeck, 1988; Regier et al., 1990b; Rounsaville et al., 1987; Woodruff et al., 1973). Because of this problem, it is necessary to turn to community samples for accurate information about the distribution of comorbidity. Such studies are rare. Only two major studies have considered psychiatric comorbidity in the United States. The first is the Epidemiologic Catchment Area (ECA) Study (Robins et al., 1991), a landmark survey of over 20,000 respondents carried out in the early 1980s in five U.S. communities. The ECA generated an enormous amount of information that has fundamentally shaped psychiatric epidemiology, comorbidity included. The second is the National Comorbidity Survey (NCS) (Kessler et al., 1994c), a nationally representative survey of over 8,000 respondents carried out in the early 1990s with the explicit aim of studying psychiatric comorbidity. Results from these two surveys are reviewed below.

Lifetime Comorbidity

The ECA investigators were the first to document that comorbidity is widespread among both patient samples and the general population. Over 54% of ECA respondents with a lifetime history of at least one DSM-III psychiatric disorder were found to have a second diagnosis as well. Fifty-two percent of lifetime alcohol abusers received a second diagnosis, and 75% of lifetime drug abusers had a second diagnosis (Robins et al., 1991). Respondents with a lifetime history of at least one mental disorder compared with respondents with no mental disorder had a relative odds of 2.3 of having a lifetime history of alcohol abuse or dependence and a relative odds of 4.5 of having some other drug use disorder (Regier et al., 1990a).

Similar results were found in the NCS. Fifty-six percent of the respondents with a lifetime history of at least one DSM-III-R disorder also had one or more other disorders (Kessler et al., 1994c). Fifty-two percent of respondents with lifetime alcohol abuse or dependence also had a lifetime mental disorder, while 36% had a lifetime illicit drug use disorder. Fifty-nine percent of the respondents with a lifetime history of illicit drug abuse or dependence also had a lifetime mental disorder, and 71% had a lifetime alcohol use disorder.

Data concerning lifetime comorbidity of specific pairs of disorders in the ECA and NCS are presented in Table 1. Results are shown in the form of odds ratios (ORs). Diagnostic hierarchy rules were not used in constructing this table in order to avoid artificially deflating estimates of comorbidity. The calculations in the ECA, furthermore, were carried out in the subsample of respondents younger than 55 years of age in order to equate results from the NCS, where the sample is in the age range of 15–54 years.

The most striking result in Table 1 is that virtually all of the ORs are greater than 1.0. This means that there is a positive association between the lifetime occurrences of almost every pair of disorders. This is true in both surveys, demonstrating that comorbidity of psychiatric disorders is truly pervasive in the general population.

TABLE 1. Lifetime Comorbidity of ECA (DSM-III) and NCS (DSM-III-R) Disorders[a]

Disorder		1	2	3	4	5	6	7	8	9	10	11	12
A. Affective disorders													
1. Depression		—											
2. Dysthymia	E	14.3											
	N	12.8											
3. Mania	E	31.8	4.1										
	N	16.9	7.3										
B. Anxiety disorders													
4. OCD	E	6.4	4.5	8.7									
	N	—	—	—									
5. Phobia	E	3.5	3.1	3.2	5.2								
	N	4.1	3.0	7.9	—								
6. Panic	E	12.7	8.0	11.6	11.6	4.9							
	N	6.6	4.8	10.4	—	10.8							
7. GAD	E	—	—	—	—	—	—						
	N	9.4	12.5	9.6	—	4.9	11.6						
8. PTSD	E	—	—	—	—	—	—	—					
	N	5.2	4.9	6.2	—	3.3	3.8	3.8					
C. Substance use disorders													
9. Alcohol	E	1.9	2.0	4.6	2.1	1.4	2.6	—	—				
	N	1.9	2.1	4.9	—	1.7	1.6	2.0	1.7				
10. Drug	E	3.5	3.2	7.4	3.3	1.8	3.1	—	—	5.8			
	N	2.4	2.3	4.9	—	2.2	3.0	2.9	3.2	13.7			
D. Other disorders													
11. ASPD	E	2.6	2.7	7.9	3.9	1.6	3.3	—	—	14.6	8.9		
	N	2.0	3.0	5.0	—	2.2	1.7	3.1	3.3	11.3	11.5		
12. NAP	E	8.8	0.1	20.1	13.0	6.1	14.7	—	—	2.9	4.2	5.0	
	N	8.8	8.1	15.9	—	4.7	20.1	15.0	9.4	2.2	2.7	6.6	—

[a]Coefficients in the table are zero-order odds ratios. E, ECA results; N, NCS results. ECA results were computed from the five-site combined ECA public use data tape, using standard ECA post-stratification weights. NCS results were computed from a data tape that included adjustments for systematic nonresponse in addition to post-stratification weights. All disorders are defined without DSM diagnostic hierarchy rules. OCD, obsessive-compulsive disorder; GAD, generalized anxiety disorder; PTSD, post-traumatic stress disorder; Alcohol, alcohol abuse or dependence; Drug, illicit substance abuse or dependence; ASPD, antisocial personality disorder; NAP, schizophrenia or schizophreniform disorder in the ECA and these same disorders plus delusional disorder, schizoaffective disorder, and atypical psychosis in the NCS.

There is considerable variation in the sizes of the ORs. This variation is systematic across the two surveys. For example, the results in the first column show that in both surveys major depression is most strongly comorbid with dysthymia and mania and least strongly comorbid with substance use disorders and antisocial personality disorder. The rank-order correlation between the ORs in the two surveys across the 36 common pairs of disorders is 0.79.

Several patterns related to the variation in ORs are worthy of note. First, one would expect that the relative sizes of the ORs would show that disorders of a single type are more strongly related to each other than to disorders of another type. The results in Table 1 show that this is generally true. However, the strength of pairwise associations within the affective disorders is generally greater than within the anxiety disorders, with an average OR of 14.5 for affective disorders and 6.7 for anxiety disorders.

Second, affective disorders and anxiety disorders are strongly comorbid. In fact, pairwise associations between an affective disorder and an anxiety disorder are generally stronger than between two anxiety disorders (an average OR of 7.0 for affective–anxiety pairs. 6.7 for anxiety–anxiety pairs).

Third, despite a substantial clinical literature pointing to the importance of comorbidity between affective disorders and substance use disorders (Keeler et al., 1979; Allen and Frances, 1986; Demilio, 1989; Hasin et al., 1988; Hesselbrock et al., 1985; Penick et al., 1988; Ross et al., 1988) and between anxiety disorders and substance use disorders (Chambless et al., 1987; Mullaney and Trippett, 1979; Roy et al., 1991a, b; Weiss and Rosenberg, 1985; Hasin et al., 1988; Hesselbrock et al., 1985; Penick et al., 1988), these are among the weakest comorbidities in Table 1 (average ORs of 3.9 for affective–substance pairs and 2.7 for anxiety–substance pairs).

One of the main purposes of investigating comorbid disorders is to help refine definitions of syndromes and diagnoses. With this in mind, it is important to recognize that some of the strongest ORs in Table 1 are associated with clusters that are generally recognized as disorders in their own right. For example, the largest ECA OR and second largest NCS OR describe comorbidity between major depression and mania. This conjunction reflects the fact that people with bipolar disorder usually experience not only mania but also one or more major depressive episodes (Wolf et al., 1988; Andreasen et al., 1988). Another example is the strong comorbidity between mania and nonaffective psychosis, a conjunction that is part of the definition of schizoaffective disorder (American Psychiatric Association, 1987).

There are also a number of strong ORs in Table 1 that are associated with comorbidities that have been discussed in the clinical literature as possibly indicating the existence of a heretofore unrecognized disorder. For example, the suggestion has been made that comorbidity between major depression and panic is due to a phasic "panic–depressive illness" characterized by panic, depressive, and mixed anxious–depressive phases (Akiskal, 1990). This possibility is consistent with the finding in Table 1 of a pronounced association between panic and depression.

Episode Comorbidity

The evidence reviewed thus far has concerned the lifetime comorbidity of multiple disorders. Of even greater clinical interest is the joint occurrence of multiple disorders in the same person at a point in time. Data on this sort of episode comorbidity are reported in Table 2. The format is the same as in Table 1, except that the ORs now refer to 6 month prevalence rather than to lifetime prevalence.

Three broad patterns are worth noting in Table 2. First, the ECA and NCS results concerning the relative magnitudes of the ORs are quite consistent. The rank-order correlation of pairs of ORs across the two surveys is 0.71. Second, there is a very strong consistency in the relative sizes of the ORs in Table 2 compared with Table 1. The rank-order correlation between the ORs for lifetime and 6 month comorbidity is 0.95 in the ECA data and 0.88 in the NCS data. Third, nearly 80% of the ORs in Table 2 are larger than those in Table 1. On average, the Table 2 ORs are approximately 50% greater than the Table 1 ORs.

It is interesting to note that the tendency for the ORs to be larger in Table 2 than Table

TABLE 2. Six-Month Comorbidity of ECA (DSM-III) and NCS (DSM-III-R) Disorders[a]

Disorder		1	2	3	4	5	6	7	8	9	10	11
A. Affective disorders												
1. Depression												
2. Dysthymia	E	10.3										
	N	30.3										
3. Mania	E	45.4	2.2									
	N	30.0	20.0									
B. Anxiety disorders												
4. OCD	E	9.3	3.3	11.1								
	N	—	—	—								
5. Phobia	E	5.6	2.4	4.4	7.6							
	N	6.4	4.4	13.4	—							
6. Panic	E	21.3	5.3	11.7	19.7	8.3						
	N	14.4	12.2	15.8	—	18.1						
7. GAD	E	—	—	—	—	—	—					
	N	17.8	21.5	10.4	—	6.6	17.6					
8. PTSD	E	—	—	—	—	—	—	—				
	N	7.1	7.4	9.4	—	4.1	8.0	7.5				
C. Substance use												
9. Alcohol	E	2.7	1.7	3.8	3.4	1.7	4.6	—	—			
	N	2.6	1.8	5.6	—	2.3	1.4	2.7	2.2			
10. Drug	E	3.4	2.0	3.2	3.4	1.7	1.0	—	—	7.8		
	N	3.0	4.3	5.7	—	3.9	3.9	5.0	2.9	20.6		
D. Other												
11. NAP	E	10.9	0.1	28.2	16.0	8.6	21.0	—	—	4.6	4.7	
	N	—	—	—	—	—	—	—	—	—	—	—

[a]Coefficients in the table are zero-order odds ratios. E, ECA results; N, NCS results. See Table 1 for a description of the samples and diagnoses. Results concerning ASPD are omitted because no recent data are available for this diagnosis. Results for NAP in the NCS are omitted because the number of respondents with recent NAP is too small for stable estimation of odds ratios.

1 is least apparent for the relationships of affective and anxiety disorders with substance use disorders (ORs averaging 3.4 and 2.4, respectively in Table 1 compared with 2.7 and 2.9 in Table 2). This finding is consistent with evidence from the treatment literature that alcohol and drugs are often used to self-medicate depression and anxiety and that this can be effective over short periods of time (thus the comparatively low ratio of 6 month to lifetime ORs) even though prolonged self-medication of this sort leads to an exacerbation of the affective and anxiety disorders (Khantzian et al., 1984).

A good illustration of these opponent processes is found in the work of Stockwell et al. (1982), who studied problem drinkers also suffering from agoraphobia and/or social phobia. It was found that the majority of respondents reported using alcohol as a means of reducing their fears. The same people, however, were also aware of the fact that prolonged drinking had the opposite effect of increasing their anxiety and described how they took care to monitor their alcohol use in order to avoid this negative effect. In a later study it was confirmed that periods of heavy drinking and dependence on alcohol were associated with an exacerbation of agoraphobia and social phobias, while subsequent periods of abstinence were associated with substantial improvements in these phobic anxiety states (Stockwell et al. 1984)

THE CONSEQUENCES OF COMORBIDITY

As noted at the beginning of the chapter, clinical interest in comorbidity is based largely on the realization that episode comorbidity can complicate treatment and that lifetime comorbidity can lead to more severe illness course. Furthermore, recent epidemiologic research has documented that comorbidity can have broader societal costs as well. Evidence concerning these consequences is reviewed in this section of the chapter.

The Impact of Comorbidity on Treatment Effectiveness

Some types of comorbidity are known not to complicate treatment. For example, substance use disorders can cause symptoms of depression and anxiety that are likely to be particularly pronounced at the time of contact with the treatment system, but these symptoms disappear within a few days or weeks of abstinence as the pharmacologic alterations and withdrawal symptoms subside (Schuckit, 1986). In cases of this sort, the clinical course of the primary disorder usually progresses in very much the same way as for patients with pure disorders (Goodwin and Guze, 1984; Merikangas et al., 1985).

In comparison, other types of comorbidity are known to create serious treatment complications. For example, comorbidity of a primary mental disorder with a substance use disorder can create problems for treatment of the mental disorder due to the fact that continued use of substances interfere with therapy for the mental disorder (Marks, 1990) and limits the repertoire of pharmacologic agents available to the clinician to treat the mental disorder (Kranzler and Liebowitz, 1988). Treatment compliance is also likely to be lower and functional impairment higher among patients with a comorbid substance use disorder, and both of these factors are associated with a poorer prognosis (Bukstein et al., 1989).

The Impact of Comorbidity on Course of Illness

There is considerable evidence from both treatment studies (Hirschfeld et al., 1990) and longitudinal community studies (Hagnell and Grasbeck, 1990; Murphy, 1990) that comorbid psychiatric disorders are more chronic than pure psychiatric disorders. Evidence on this issue from the National Comorbidity Survey is reported in Table 3. The coefficients in Table 3 are ORs comparing pure (only one lifetime NCS psychiatric disorder) and comorbid (one or more other disorders) cases of various NCS disorders on three different measures of severity: 1) use of professional services for the focal disorder, 2) use of medications to treat the focal disorder, and 3) current prevalence of the focal disorder. All ORs are adjusted for variation in age of first onset and time since first onset of the focal disorder.

The results in the first two columns show that comorbidity is associated with help-seeking and use of medications, outcomes that can be interpreted as indicators of illness severity. The results in the third column show that comorbidity is also associated with

TABLE 3. The Relationships (Odds Ratios) of Comorbidity With Severity and Chronicity for Selected NCS Disorders[a]

	Help-Seeking	Medications	Recency
Affective disorders			
Depression	2.33	2.77	2.32
Dysthymia	1.70	2.32	1.93
Anxiety disorders			
GAD	2.64	3.78	1.09
Agoraphobia	2.46	7.92	4.76
Simple phobia	1.17	1.97	1.48
Social phobia	2.27	7.84	2.01
Panic	1.18	3.19	3.70
Substance use disorders			
Alc Ab/Dep	3.13	4.95	1.25
Drug	1.82	3.32	3.16

[a]Coefficients are adjusted odds ratios obtained from logistic regression equations that regressed dichotomous measures of the outcomes (help-seeking, lifetime use of professional treatment for the focal disorder; medications, lifetime use of medications to treat the focal disorder; recency, 30-day prevalence of the focal disorder) on dichotomous measures of comorbidity (1, at least one other lifetime disorder; 0, no other lifetime disorder) in subsamples of respondents with a lifetime history of specific DSM-III-R disorders, controlling for age of onset and years since onset. Separate equations were estimated for each of the nine disorders, each equation based on a different sample.

chronicity. More detailed analyses of the NCS data shows that high comorbidity—defined as a lifetime history of three or more disorders—is particularly important in this regard. Fifty-eight percent of all current NCS disorders and 88% of severe current disorders are found among the 13% of the population with a lifetime history of high comorbidity (Kessler et al., 1994c).

Interestingly, similar effects of comorbidity on illness course have been documented when the comorbid condition is a medical illness rather than another mental illness (Keitner et al., 1991). This raises the question whether it is comorbidity that affects illness course or whether comorbidity is merely indicative of a more serious condition (Marlatt and Gordon, 1980; Merikangas et al., 1988; Kovacs, 1990). No systematic research has been done to explore this issue, although several large long-term prospective datasets are available to do so (Angst et al., 1990; Hagnell and Grasbeck, 1990; Murphy, 1990). Such work might show that severity of the focal disorder leads to comorbidity rather than the other way around.

One important result that is inconsistent with the notion that severity of the focal disorder explains the putative affects of comorbidity on illness course is that some types of comorbidity are more important than others in predicting the course of a focal disorder. For example, there is evidence that the course of antisocial personality disorder is much more serious among persons with a comorbid substance use disorder than other forms of comorbidity. This seems to be true, at least in part, because of the disinhibiting effects of substance use (Tardiff et al., 1981; Menuck, 1983). Consistent with this interpretation, epidemiologic evidence documents that the spontaneous remission commonly found among people with antisocial behavior patterns in the age range 30–40 (Robins, 1966;

Guze, 1975) is less likely to occur among those with dependence on alcohol or other drugs (Goodwin et al., 1971). This kind of adverse impact of chronic substance abuse on the course of antisocial personality disorder is not confined to secondary ASPD, but has also been documented in cases where early childhood behavior problems originally led to substance abuse problems (Vaillant, 1980).

An added complication is that the effects of two comorbid conditions may be recipro-cal. The ASPD–substance abuse association again provides a relevant example, as there is evidence that not only does substance abuse adversely affect the course of antisocial personality disorder but that ASPD adversely affects the course of substance abuse disor-der. The later effect occurs, at least in part, because persons with ASPD typically have an earlier age of onset of substance use (Cadoret et al., 1984; Penick et al., 1984) and a more rapid progression to substance abuse and dependence (Hesselbrock et al., 1984, 1985). Furthermore, ASPD is associated with greater problems in everyday living due to sub-stance abuse (Rimmer et al., 1972; Cadoret et al., 1984), with higher rates of substance abuse relapse after treatment (Goodwin et al., 1971), and with a greater likelihood of hav-ing problems with both alcohol and other drugs (Cadoret et al., 1984).

The Social Costs of Psychiatric Disorders

The consequences of comorbidity are not confined to increased treatment complexity and more severe illness course. In addition, and perhaps as a result of these other effects, co-morbid disorders are associated with more social consequences than pure disorders. The NCS shows that persons with a lifetime history of psychiatric comorbidity are signifi-cantly more likely than those with a history of only one psychiatric disorder to experience impairments in a wide range of social roles. These include both social role impairments and work role impairments. Among the social role impairments significantly associated with comorbidity are marital separation and divorce, social isolation, and exposure to conflictual social relationships (Forthofer et al., 1994). Among the work role impairments significantly associated with comorbidity are low educational attainment, unemployment, and chronic financial difficulties (Kessler et al., 1994a).

The NCS data also show that episode comorbidity has important effects on fulfillment of role obligations. NCS respondents with two or more active psychiatric disorders at the time of interview reported an average of over four times as many recent work loss days and three times as many recent work cutback days as respondents with only one active disorder, equivalent to an annualized national projection of over 100 million work loss days and 300 million work cutback days due specifically to active psychiatric comorbid-ity (Kessler et al., 1994d).

THE CAUSES OF COMORBIDITY

Why is it that such a large number of people have multiple disorders? Although this is a question of immense importance, it has not received the empirical attention it deserves, as most research on psychiatric comorbidity has been carried out in treatment samples. Here, the existence of comorbidity is a starting point for investigations of illness course. Nonetheless, a good deal of indirect evidence has accumulated about a number of poten-tially important causal processes that are reviewed in this section of the chapter.

Direct Effects of One Disorder on Another

One possibility is that a primary psychiatric disorder directly influences the onset of other disorders. An example is agoraphobia secondary to panic disorder, which develops when panic leads to a disabling fear of attacks in situations where help is unavailable and escape is impossible (Klein et al., 1987). Another example is chronic mixed anxiety–depression, which can occur when unremitting chronic anxiety leads to feelings of hopelessness and helplessness (Akiskal, 1990).

There is also evidence of direct effects of some primary substance use disorders on later mental disorders. An increasingly important example is cocaine-induced panic (Aronson and Craig, 1986; Liebowitz et al., 1984), which is thought to occur when prolonged cocaine use increases limbic–neuronal excitability (Charney et al., 1987). This pharmacologic "kindling" of the brain can create a permanent change in brain function that decreases the threshold for seizure activity (Goddard et al., 1969). As a result, once the panic attacks begin they become independent of further cocaine use and persist despite discontinuation of the drug. There is evidence that similar long-term patterns of panic disorder can be created by kindling processes linked to the use of psychostimulants (Abraham, 1986). Patients with this sort of disorder seldom have family histories of panic disorder, which is quite different from the case of patients with primary panic disorder (Crowe, 1985). They also respond poorly to first-line medications, although good response has been found to medications with limbic anticonvulsant properties (Louie et al., 1989). Long-term follow ups of patients with this disorder have not yet been reported, so it is uncertain whether prognosis over many years is worse than among primary anxiety patients.

Indirect Effects of One Disorder on Another

A second possibility is that some psychiatric disorders may occur as indirect consequences of others. There are many examples of this in the literature. One of the most important was mentioned earlier in this chapter, that substance abuse can occur as an unintended consequence of self-medicating a mental disorder. Another important example is that secondary substance abuse can occur as a result of participating in deviant peer groups due to primary conduct disorder (Meyer, 1986). In general, the causal processes in these cases involve primary disorders leading to a broad range of experiences that, in turn, predispose to secondary disorders.

Common Causes

A third possibility is that common causes of different psychiatric disorders, such as community context, stress, and lack of social support, lead to comorbidity (National Institute of Mental Health, 1993). An interesting example concerns post-traumatic stress disorder (PTSD), a disorder known to be characterized by extremely high comorbidity (Kilpatrick and Resnick, 1992; Mellman, et al., 1992). Analysis of the National Comorbidity Survey shows that much of this comorbidity is due to the fact that the traumatic experiences that lead to PTSD also cause other stress-related disorders (Kessler et al., 1994e).

Research on juvenile delinquency has been especially influenced by common cause explanations. Researchers working in this area have long been aware that there is a clustering of many different problems among delinquent youth, including various forms of risk taking (e.g., unsafe sex, drunken driving, violent behavior), acting out (e.g., property crimes, substance abuse), and psychological distress (Dryfoos, 1990). Jessor and Jessor (1977) were the first investigators to study this clustering systematically. They concluded that it represents the influence of an underlying "lack of commitment to conventionality." Research on youthful problem behaviors over the past decade has used this idea as an organizing principle and has documented substantial evidence for a clustering of problem behaviors among youth consistent with the ideas of the Jessors (e.g., Barnes and Welte, 1986; Osgood et al., 1988). It is important to note that the measures of psychological distress used in these studies have usually been screening scales of depressed or anxious mood rather than measures of clinically significant psychiatric disorders. Nonetheless, this research offers a provocative hypothesis concerning the common causes of many adolescent problem behaviors that could have important implications for adult comorbidity of psychiatric disorders.

Another important class of common cause explanations concerns biologic causes. Recent twin research by Kendler et al. (1992), for example, has shown that there are common genetic determinants of generalized anxiety disorder and major depression. The distinction between disorders is confused in situations of this sort. Indeed, one might dispute the claim that there are multiple disorders in cases of this sort and argue, instead, that misdiagnosis has merely created the appearance of their being multiple disorders. It must also be recognized, though, that the existence of common genetic causes does not in all cases ensure the eventual onset of the second disorder (or second phase of the single disorder) after the first one has occurred, as genetic influences often have modifiable psychosocial mediators.

FUTURE DIRECTIONS FOR EPIDEMIOLOGIC RESEARCH

Based on the results reviewed above, at least two future directions for epidemiologic research on psychiatric comorbidity seem promising. One is to contribute to the clinical research agenda. The other is to pursue an epidemiologic agenda that would document modifiable risk factors and attempt to prevent comorbidity. In pursuing either of these lines of investigation, it is important that future research avoid the methodologic problems that have plagued previous psychiatric comorbidity research and take advantage of several methodologic opportunities.

Future Directions in Research on the Clinical Agenda

Clinical research on comorbidity is based on the premise that the identification of homogeneous patient groups by means of detailed investigation of complex symptom profiles will both advance our understanding of the pathophysiology of psychiatric disorder and improve our ability to offer effective treatments. The first phase of research is to determine whether patients with particular combinations of disorders are distinct from those with pure disorders in terms of family history, risk factors, and clinical course. If so, the second phase is to carry out laboratory studies, detailed investigations of longitudinal clinical course, and studies that demonstrate a distinct response to treatment.

This clinical research has, up to now, been largely based on treatment samples. There is good reason to believe that the validity of this work is compromised by selection bias. This is especially true for first-phase research. For example, clinical research on generalized anxiety disorder (GAD) has documented such high comorbidity (Brown and Barlow, 1992; Lepine et al., 1994) that questions have been raised concerning whether GAD should be considered an independent disorder (Francis et al., 1990; Cooper, 1990). Yet recent research reporting the first general population data on DSM-III-R GAD shows that a substantial proportion of people with GAD are either pure or primary cases that never come to clinical attention (Wittchen et al., 1994).

Results such as this illustrate clearly the importance of general population psychiatric epidemiologic research for advancing the clinical research agenda. In their absence, clinicians can easily draw incorrect conclusions concerning the prevalence of comorbidity and the implications of comorbidity for illness severity. To avoid these errors, clinical research must rely most heavily on general population studies. This is especially true in first-phase research on family history and risk factors, but also true in second-phase research on clinical course.

Future Directions in Research on the Epidemiologic Agenda

The results reported at the beginning of this chapter suggest that the prevention of comorbidity would reduce a substantial proportion of all lifetime psychiatric disorders and an even greater proportion of ongoing disorders. Yet despite such evidence, comorbidity has been largely ignored in risk factor research, in theorizing about the causes of psychopathology, and in the design of targeted preventive interventions. Interventions aimed specifically at the primary prevention of comorbidity are long overdue. Epidemiologic research is needed to move this agenda forward by pinpointing modifiable risk factors on which such interventions might be based.

Although there are probably some types of comorbidity that would be exceedingly difficult to prevent, the above review has touched on others for which successful prevention is a plausible possibility. Substance use disorders that occur secondary to primary phobias are a good case in point. Comorbidity between phobias and substance use disorders has been found in a number of clinical studies (Chambless et al., 1987; Roy et al., 1991a), with phobias almost always preceding substance abuse in age of onset by as much as a decade (Hesselbrock et al., 1985; Christie et al., 1988). Substance abuse secondary to phobia is particularly common among women, with close to one-third of all female alcoholics reporting an earlier phobia (Helzer and Pryzbeck, 1988). This comorbidity is traditionally attributed to anxiety promoting the use of alcohol and drugs as a form of self-medication (Klein, 1980), an interpretation supported by reports that the vast majority of patients with phobias self-consciously use alcohol or drugs to manage their fears (Bibb and Chambless, 1986). Based on this thinking, interventions might be aimed either at curing the phobia before secondary substance abuse begins or at teaching treatment-resistant phobics alternative strategies for managing their fears. There is good reason to believe that these strategies could be quite effective. They would reduce a substantial percent of lifetime substance use disorders and an even greater percent of current disorders. This is because alcoholics and substance abusers with primary phobias are more chronic than primary alcoholics and substance abusers, presumably because continued fears precipitate further drinking (Marlatt and Gordon, 1980).

The challenge for psychiatric epidemiologists concerned with intervention opportunities such as this is to enhance their understanding of the causal processes that create psychiatric comorbidity enough to select intervention targets. There are formidable methodologic problems involved in doing this, but there are also a number of compensating practical advantages of conducting preventive trials in populations at risk for comorbid disorders (Kessler and Price, 1994). First, the ease of identifying persons at risk for a secondary disorder is greater when they already meet criteria for a primary disorder. Second, already diagnosed groups are at high risk of secondary disorders, increasing the efficiency and power of preventive trials. Third, primary prevention of secondary disorders may allow experimental epidemiologists to use already developed treatment technologies as part of the available technology of preventive intervention strategies. Fourth, conducting preventive trials with diagnosed clinical populations at risk for the development of secondary disorders may increase the social warrant for preventive intervention. Fifth, the prevention of secondary disorders would eliminate the exacerbation of primary disorders, which is known to accompany the onset of secondary disorders. In this way, such interventions would lead to secondary prevention of primary disorders in addition to primary prevention of secondary disorders.

Future Directions in Methodology

In pursuing these new research initiatives it is important to be aware of methodologic problems that have plagued previous research on comorbidity. These include improperly defining the sampling frame, improperly distinguishing between primary and secondary disorders, and failing to consider subgroup differences. It is also important to take advantage of methodologic innovations that can advance our understanding of comorbidity. These problems and innovations are discussed in detail elsewhere (Kessler et al., 1994b; Kessler and Price, 1994). Only a brief overview is presented here.

Sampling was discussed earlier in this chapter, where it was noted that estimates of the prevalence of comorbidity may be biased in treatment samples due to selection into treatment on the basis of comorbidity (Berkson, 1946). Studies of risk factors for comorbidity might be similarly biased when samples are confined to patients. It is, therefore, imperative, that general population surveys assume a more prominent role in future research on patterns and predictors of psychiatric comorbidity than they have in the past.

Once representative data are available, more thoughtful analysis is needed to distinguish primary and secondary disorders. This has been done most commonly in previous research by using retrospective information about which disorder began first to define one as causally "primary" (i.e., typically having an earlier age of onset) and the others in the cluster as causally "secondary." This approach confuses temporal priority with causal priority, though, and can lead to serious errors of inference (Kessler and Price, 1994). These errors can be avoided by using survival models in which first onset of each disorder is treated as a time-varying covariate to predict first onset of subsequent disorders. These models can be elaborated to include risk factors for comorbidity. An illustration of this method applied to the primary–secondary distinction in comorbidity between PTSD and other disorders is presented by Kessler et al. (1994e). A more general discussion of this method is presented by Kessler and Price (1994).

It is important to appreciate in working with these complex models that there may be differences in the effects of risk factors depending on the sex and age of respondents. These specifications have largely been ignored in previous studies of comorbidity. This is a serious limitation, as patterns of comorbidity differ dramatically by these specifiers. For example, comorbid alcoholism is much more often found to be primary and associated with ASPD among men and secondary and associated with affective disorders and anxiety disorders among women (Roy et al., 1991b; Hesselbrock et al., 1986). Furthermore, strong and consistent evidence has been found that depressed patients with an early onset have a stronger family history of both depression and alcoholism than those with a late onset (e.g., Mendlewicz and Baron, 1981).

Social context can also have a powerful effect on comorbidity. The most dramatic illustration of this fact concerns recent changes in patterns of substance use, which affect the base rates on which to evaluate the sensitivity of substance use disorders as predictors of mental disorders. This is illustrated in the work of Weiss et al. (1988), who studied a sample of hospitalized cocaine abusers in 1980–1982 and found very high rates of primary affective disorder. In a replication between 1982 and 1988, however, much weaker evidence of primary affective disorder was found. The authors concluded that this change reflects the fact that cocaine use is more widespread and, at least in some segments of society, becoming normative.

Secular changes of this sort can complicate analysis of the impact of mental disorders on substance use and vice versa. However, they also present special opportunities. For example, Weiss and his colleagues found that the impact of cocaine abuse on course of primary depression decreased as the prevalence of cocaine use increased in the population. This finding suggests that the strong initial effect of cocaine in the early 1980s was due more to the social meanings of cocaine use during that time and to early adopters having higher rates of prior depression than late adopters rather than to any direct effects of the substance itself. Analyses of comorbidity that use short-term historic changes of this sort in creative ways could provide important insights that have been overlooked in prior investigations. The fact that patterns of drug use in America have been changing rapidly in recent years suggests that this strategy could be feasible for many applications.

Other innovative research designs need to be considered in future investigations of comorbidity. For example, while most of the evidence currently available on psychiatric comorbidity is based on retrospective data, a much more persuasive case could be made by using results of retrospective studies to target samples for true prospective analysis. In the latter, persons with a history of a primary disorder who are at risk for the onset of secondary disorders would be followed over time. Young women who contact their primary care physicians about depression, for example, might be targeted as a high-risk group for the subsequent development of prescription drug abuse and studied prospectively to evaluate the importance of a wide variety of potential risk factors. Other innovative research designs include family aggregation designs (Smith, 1976), which can sometimes provide information about causal priorities among comorbid conditions as well as about the contribution of common causes to comorbidity even when the researcher has no specific hypotheses about what the common causes might be (Merikangas et al., 1994). Family-genetic designs (Cadoret and Winokur, 1974; Kendler et al., 1992) can provide information concerning whether common causes are environmental or genetic.

It is also important that future research on comorbidity make more use of experiments than in the past. One unique opportunity to do this involves randomized clinical trials. This would involve modifying the outcomes assessed to include possible secondary disorders and to follow up patients over a longer time interval to see if the experimental intervention reduced risk of first onset of secondary disorders that are known to cluster with the primary disorder. A more ambitious experimental design would embed an experimental intervention in a longitudinal study of risk factors for comorbidity in a sample of people who have already had a first disorder and are in the age range of risk for secondary disorders. In the ideal case, this would be a genetically informative sample. For example, a quasi-cross-fostering design might be embedded in a longitudinal risk factor survey–intervention to prevent alcohol abuse secondary to depression by basing the study on an oversample of depressed children from broken homes who have not had contact with their biologic fathers. This design would require the researchers to know whether these fathers have a history of alcoholism (documented by either maternal report or direct interview with the father). The paternal history of alcoholism could then be used as an indirect indicator of genetic risk for alcoholism as in an adoption design (e.g., Bohman et al., 1981; Cadoret and Gath, 1978; Cloninger et al., 1981), with appropriate controls for confounding covariates (e.g., evaluating the effect of parental divorce and controlling for the possibility of maternal depression). If the intervention is successful in preventing onset of alcoholism, nonexperimental analysis of intervening processes could be used to help interpret the causal pathways involved in this effect in an effort to provide insights concerning future modifications of the intervention.

OVERVIEW

Comorbidity of psychiatric disorders is highly prevalent. In fact, the majority of people who suffer from any one psychiatric disorder also have one or more others. Only 22% of respondents with a lifetime history of major depression in the NCS, for example, were pure depressives, and only 19% of the simple phobics pure phobics. The others had some other lifetime disorder.

Comorbid disorders are, in general, more severe than pure disorders. The NCS results suggest, in fact, that the major societal burden of psychiatric disorder falls on people with comorbidity. Nearly 90% of the people with severe psychiatric impairments in the NCS had a history of three or more comorbid psychiatric disorders.

These results show that comorbidity should be a central focus of both clinical and epidemiologic research on psychiatric disorders. Yet, as noted earlier in the chapter, comorbidity has been largely ignored, until recently, in both theorizing and risk factor research. This situation is now changing.

Psychiatric epidemiology has an important role to play in this new research on comorbidity. We have much to learn about even the most basic questions concerning the distribution of comorbidity in the population, the temporal sequence of onsets among multiple disorders, and the family histories of people with comorbidity compared with those with pure disorders. In addition, general population psychiatric epidemiology is uniquely positioned to investigate risk factors for comorbidity. It is also important to pursue the epidemiologic agenda of searching for modifiable risk factors that can be targeted for preventive interventions. This has been a neglected area of research in comorbidity to date, but one that should be pursued vigorously in the future.

ACKNOWLEDGMENTS

I thank Mike Hughes, Kate McGonagle, and Chris Nelson for carrying out the analyses of the National Comorbidity Survey reported here and Evelyn Bromet, Mike Hughes, and Uli Wittchen for comments on an earlier draft of the chapter.

REFERENCES

Abraham HD (1986): Do psychostimulants kindle panic disorder? [Letter to the editor]. Am J Psychiatry 143:1627.

Akiskal HS (1990): Toward a clinical understanding of the relationship of anxiety and depressive disorders. In JD Maser JD, Cloninger CR (eds): "Comorbidity of Mood and Anxiety Disorders." Washington, DC: American Psychiatric Press, pp 597–610.

Allen MH, Frances RJ (1986): Varieties of psychopathology found in patients with addictive disorders: A review. In Meyer RE (ed): "Psychopathology and Addictive Disorders." New York: Guilford Press, pp 17–38.

American Psychiatric Association (1987): "Diagnostic and Statistical Manual of Mental Disorders," 3rd ed, revised. Washington DC: American Psychiatric Association.

Andreasen NC, Grove WM, Coryell WH, Endicott J, Clayton PJ (1988): Bipolar versus unipolar and primary versus secondary affective disorder: Which diagnosis takes precedence? J Affect Disord 15:69–80.

Angst J, Vollrath M, Merikangas KR, Ernst C (1990): Comorbidity of anxiety and depression in the Zurich Cohort Study of Young Adults. In Maser JD, Cloninger CR (eds): "Comorbidity of Mood and Anxiety Disorders." Washington, DC: American Psychiatric Press, pp 123–138.

Aronson TA, Craig TJ (1986): Cocaine precipitation of panic disorder. Am J of Psychiatry 143:643–645.

Barnes GM, Welte JW (1986): Adolescent alcohol abuse: Subgroup differences and relationships to other problem behaviors. J Adolesc Res 1:79–94.

Berkson J (1946): Limitations of the application of the 4-fold table analyses to hospital data. Biometrics 2:47–53.

Bibb JL, Chambless DL (1986): Alcohol use and abuse among diagnosed agoraphobics. Behav Res Ther 24:49–58.

Bohman M, Cloninger R, Sigvardsson S, von Knorring AL (1981): The genetics of alcoholism and related disorders. J Psychiatric Res 21:447–452.

Boyd JH, Burke JD Jr, Gruenberg E, Holzer CE, Rae DS, George LK, Karno M, Stoltzman R, McEvoy L, Nestadt G (1984): Exclusion criteria of DSM-III: A study of co-occurrence of hierarchy-free syndromes. Arch Gen Psychiatry 41:983–989.

Brown TA, Barlow DH (1992): Comorbidity among anxiety disorders: Implications for treatment and DSM-IV. J Consult Clin Psychol 60:835–844.

Bukstein OG, Brent DA, Kaminer Y (1989): Comorbidity of substance abuse and other psychiatric disorders in adolescents. Am J Psychiatry 146:1131–1141.

Cadoret R, Gath A (1978): Inheritance of alcoholism in adoptees raised apart from alcoholic biological relatives. Br J Psychiatry 13:252–258.

Cadoret R, Troughton E, Widmer R (1984): Clinical differences between antisocial and primary alcoholics. Comp Psychiatry 25:1–8.

Cadoret R, Winokur G (1974): Depression in alcoholism. Ann NY Acad Sci 233:34–36.

Chambless DL, Cherney J, Caputo GD, Rheinstein BJ (1987): Anxiety disorders and alcoholism. J Anxiety Disord 1:24–40.

Charney DS, Woods SW, Goodman WK, Heninger GR (1987): Neurobiological mechanisms of panic anxiety: Biochemical and behavioral correlates of yohimbine-induced panic attacks. Am J Psychiatry 144:1030–1036.

Christie KA, Burke JD Jr, Regier DA, Rae DS, Boyd JH, Locke BZ (1988): Epidemiologic evidence for early onset of mental disorders and higher risk of drug-abuse in young adults. Am J Psychiatry 145:971–975.

Cloninger R, Bohman M, Sigvardsson S (1981): Inheritance of alcohol abuse: Cross-fostering analysis of adopted men. Arch Gen Psychiatry 38:861–867.

Cooper JE (1990): The classification of anxiety states in the International Classification of Diseases. In Sartorius N, Andreoli V, Cassano G, Eisenberg L, Kielholz P, Pancheri P, Racagni G (eds): "Anxiety—Psychobiological and Clinical Perspectives." New York: Hemisphere Publishing Co.

Crowe RR (1985): The genetics of panic disorder and agoraphobia. Psychiatr Dev 2:171–186.

Demilio L (1989): Psychiatric syndromes in adolescent substance abusers. Am J Psychiatry 146:1212–1214.

Dryfoos JG (1990): "Adolescents at Risk: Prevalence and Preventions." New York: Oxford.

Forthofer MS, Kessler RC, Story AL, Gotlieb IH (1994): Selection into and out of first marriage: The effects of mental illness on marital status. Manuscript in preparation.

Francis A, Pincus H, Manning D, Widiger T (1990): Classification of anxiety states in DSM-III and perspectives for its classification in DSM-IV. In Sartorius N, Andreoli V, Cassano G, Eisenberg L, Kielholz P, Pancheri P, Racagni G (eds): "Anxiety—Psychobiological and Clinical Perspectives." New York: Hemisphere Publishing Co.

Goccard GV, McIntyre DC, Leech CK (1969): A permanent change in brain function resulting from daily electrical stimulation. Exp Neurol 25:295–330.

Goodwin DW, Crane JB, Guze SB (1971): Felons who drink—An eight-year follow-up. Q J Stud Alcohol 32:136–147.

Goodwin DW, Guze SB (1984): "Psychiatric Diagnosis," 3rd ed. New York: Oxford University Press.

Guze SB (1975): The validity and significance of the clinical diagnosis of hysteria (Briquet's syndrome). Am J Psychiatry 32:138–141.

Hagnell O, Grasbeck A (1990): Comorbidity of anxiety and depression in the Lundby 25-year prospective study: The pattern of subsequent episodes. In Maser JD, Cloninger CR (eds): "Comorbidity of Mood and Anxiety Disorders." Washington, DC: American Psychiatric Press, pp 139–152.

Hasin D, Grant B, Endicott J (1988): Treated and untreated suicide attempts in substance abuse patients. J Nerv Ment Disord 176:289–294.

Helzer JE, Pryzbeck TR (1988): The co-occurrence of alcoholism with other psychiatric disorders in the general population and its impact on treatment. J Stud Alcohol 49:219–224.

Hesselbrock MN, Hesselbrock VM, Babor F, Stabenau JR, Meyer RE, Weidenman M (1984): Antisocial behavior psychopathology and problem drinking in the natural history of alcoholism. In Goodwin D, Van Dusen K, Mednick S (eds): "Longitudinal Research in Alcoholism." Boston: Nijhoff, pp 197–214.

Hesselbrock VM, Hesselbrock MN, Workman-Daniels KL (1986): Effect of major depression and antisocial personality on alcoholism: Course and motivational patterns. J Stud Alcohol 47:207–212.

Hesselbrock MN, Meyer RE, Keener JJ (1985): Psychopathology in hospitalized alcoholics. Arch Gen Psychiatry 42:1050–1055.

Hirschfeld RMA, Hasin D, Keller MB, Endicott J, Wunder J (1990): Depression and alcoholism: Comorbidity in a longitudinal study. In Maser JD, Cloninger CR (eds): "Comorbidity of Mood and Anxiety Disorders." Washington, DC: American Psychiatric Press, pp 293–304.

Jessor R, Jessor SL (eds) (1977): "Problem Behavior and Psychosocial Development: A Longitudinal Study of Youth." New York: Academic Press.

Keeler MH, Taylor CI, Miller WC (1979): Are all recently detoxified alcoholics depressed? Am J Psychiatry 136:586–588.

Keitner GI, Ryan CE, Miller IW, Kohn R, Epstein NB (1991): 12-Month outcome of patients with major depression and comorbid psychiatric or medical illness (compound depression). Am J Psychiatry 148:345–350.

Kendler KS, Neale MC, Kessler RC, Heath AC, Eaves LJ (1992): Major depression and generalized anxiety disorder. Same genes, (partly) different environments? Arch Gen Psychiatry 49:716–722.

Kessler RC, Foster C, Saunders W, Stagg P (1994a): The social consequences of psychiatric disorders. I. The effects of educational attainment. Manuscript in preparation.

Kessler RC, McGonagle KA, Carnelley KB, Nelson CB, Farmer ME, Regier DA (1994b): Comorbidity of mental disorders and substance use disorders: A review and agenda for future research. In Leaf P (ed): "Research in Community and Mental Health." Greenwich, CT: JAI Press (in press).

Kessler RC, McGonagle KA, Zhao S, Nelson CB, Hughes M, Eshleman S, Wittchen H-U, Kendler KS (1994c): Lifetime and 12-month prevalence of DSM-III-R psychiatric disorders among persons aged 15–54 in the United States: Results from the National Comorbidity Survey. Arch Gen Psychiatry 51:8–19.

Kessler RC, McGonagle KA, Zhao S, Nelson CB, Hughes M, Eshleman S, Wittchen H-U, Kendler KS (1994d): Comorbidity of psychiatric disorders: Prevalence and social consequences. Manuscript in preparation.

Kessler RC, Price RH (1993): Primary prevention of secondary disorders: A proposal and agenda. Am J Community Psychol 21:607–633.

Kessler RC, Sonnega A, Bromet E, Nelson CB (1994e): Posttraumatic stress disorder in the National Comorbidity Survey. Manuscript in preparation.

Khantzian EJ, Gawin FH, Kleber HD, Riordan CE (1984): Methylphenidate treatment of cocaine dependence: A preliminary report. J Subst Abuse Iss 1:107–112.

Kilpatrick DG, Resnick HS (1992): Posttraumatic stress disorder associated with exposure to criminal victimization in clinical and community populations. In Davidson JRT, Foa EB (eds): "Posttraumatic Stress Disorder: DSM-IV and Beyond." Washington, DC: American Psychiatric Press.

Klein D (1980): Anxiety reconceptualized. Comp Psychiatry 21:411–427.

Klein DF, Ross DC, Cohen P (1987): Panic and avoidance in agoraphobia. Arch Gen Psychiatry 44:377–385.

Kovacs M (1990): Comorbid anxiety disorders in childhood-onset depression. In Maser JD, Cloninger CR (eds): "Comorbidity of Mood and Anxiety Disorders." Washington, DC: American Psychiatric Press, pp 271–282.

Kranzler HR, Liebowitz NR (1988): Anxiety and depression in substance abuse: Clinical implications. Med Clin North Am 72:867–885.

Lepine JP, Wittchen H-U, Essau CA (1993): Lifetime and current comorbidity of anxiety and depressive disorders: Results from the International WHO/ADAMHA CIDI Field Trials. Int J Methods Psychiatr Res 3:67–77.

Liebowitz MR, Fyer MR, Gorman J, Dillon D, Appleby IL, Levy G, Anderson S, Levitt M, Palij M, Davies SO (1984): Lactate provocation of panic attacks: I. Clinical and behavioral findings. Arch Gen Psychiatry 41:764–770.

Louie AK, Lannon RA, Ketter TA (1989): Treatment of cocaine-induced panic disorder. Am J Psychiatry 146:40–44.

Marks IM (1990): Mental health care delivery: Innovations, impediments, and implementation. Cambridge: Cambridge University Press.

Marlatt GA, Gordon JR (1980): Determinants of relapse: Implications for the maintenance of behavioral change: In Davidson P, Davidson S (eds): "Behavioral Medicine, Changing Health and Lifestyles." New York: Brunner-Manzel.

Mellman TA, Randolph CA, Brawan-Mintzer O, Flores LP, Milanes FJ (1992): Phenomenology and course of psychiatric disorders associated with combat-related posttraumatic stress disorder. Am J Psychiatry 149:1568–1574.

Mendlewicz J, Baron M (1981): Morbitity risks in subtypes of unipolar depressive illness: Differences between early and late onset forms. Br J Psychiatry 139:463–466.

Menuck M (1983): Clinical aspects of dangerous behavior. J Psychiatry Law 11:227–304.

Merikangas KR, Prusoff BA, Weissman MM (1988): Parental concordance for affective disorders: Psychopathology in offspring. J Affect Disord 15:279–290.

Merikangas KR, Risch NJ, Weissman MM (1994): Comorbidity and co-transmission of alcoholism, anxiety and depression. Psychol Med 24:69–80.

Merikangas KR, Weissman MM, Prusoff BA, Pauls DL, Leckman JF (1985): Depressives with secondary alcoholism: Psychiatric disorders in offspring. J Stud Alcohol 46:199–204.

Meyer RE (1986): "Psychopathological and Addictive Disorder." New York: Guilford.

Mullaney JA, Trippett CJ (1979): Alcohol dependence and phobias: Clinical description and relevance. Br J Psychiatry 135:565–573.

Murphy JM (1990): Diagnostic comorbidity and symptom co-occurrence: The Stirling County study. In Maser JD, Cloninger CR (eds): "Comorbidity of Mood and Anxiety Disorders." Washington DC: American Psychiatric Press, pp 153–176.

National Institute of Mental Health (1993): "The Prevention of Mental Disorders: A National Research Agenda." Unpublished report.

Osgood DW, Johnston LD, O'Malley PM, Bachman JG (1988): The generality of deviance in late adolescence and early adulthood. Am Sociol Rev 53:81–93.

Penick EC, Powell BJ, Liskow BI, Jackson JO, Liskow BI (1988): The stability of coexisting psychiatric syndromes in alcoholic men after one year. J Stud Alcohol 49:395–405.

Penick EC, Powell BJ, Othmer E, Bingham SF, Rice AS, Liese BS (1984): Subtyping alcoholics by co-existing psychiatric syndromes: Course, family history, outcome. In Goodwin DW, VanDusen RT, Mednick SA (eds): "Longitudinal Research in Alcoholism." Hingham MA: Klutter-Nyhoff Publishing Co., pp 167–169.

Regier DA, Burke JD Jr, Burke KC (1990a): Comorbidity of affective and anxiety disorders in the NIMH Epidemiologic Catchment Area Program. In Maser JD, Cloninger CR (eds): "Comorbidity of Mood and Anxiety Disorders." Washington, DC: American Psychiatric Press, pp 113–122.

Regier DA, Farmer ME, Rae DS, Locke BZ, Keith BJ, Judd LL, Goodwin FK (1990b): Comorbidity of mental health disorders with alcohol and other drug abuse. JAMA 264:2511–2518.

Rimmer J, Reich T, Winokur G (1972): Alcoholism. V. Diagnosis and clinical variation among alcoholics. Q J Stud Alcohol 33:658–666.

Robins LN (1966): "Deviant Children Grown Up: A Social and Psychiatric Study of Sociopathic Personality." Baltimore: Williams and Wilkins.

Robins LN, Locke BZ, Regier DA (1991): Overview: Psychiatric disorders in America. In Robins LN, Regier DA (eds): "Psychiatric Disorders in America." New York: Free Press, pp 328–366.

Ross HE, Glaser FB, Germanson T (1988): The prevalence of psychiatric disorders in patients with alcohol and other drug problems. Arch Gen Psychiatry 45:1023–1031.

Rounsaville BJ, Anton SF, Carroll K, Budde D, Prusoff BA, Gawin F (1991): Psychiatric diagnosis of treatment-seeking cocaine abusers. Arch Gen Psychiatry 48:43–51.

Roy A, DeJong J, Lamparski D, Adinoff B, George T, Moore V, Garnett D, Kerich M, Linnoila M (1991a): Mental disorders among alcoholics: Relationship to age of onset and cerebrospinal fluid neuropeptides. Arch Gen Psychiatry 48:423–427.

Roy A, DeJong J, Lamparski D, George T, Linnoila M (1991b): Depression among alcoholics: Relationship to clinical and cerebrospinal fluid variables. Arch Gen Psychiatry 48:428–432.

Schuckit MA (1986): Genetic and clinical implications of alcoholism and affective disorder. Am J Psychiatry 143:140–147.

Smith C (1976): Statistical resolution of genetic heterogeneity in familial disease. Ann Hum Genet 39:281–290.

Stockwell T, Hodgson R, Rankin H (1982): Tension reduction and effects of prolonged alcohol consumption. Br J Addict 77:65–73.

Stockwell T, Smail P, Hodgson R, Canter S (1984): Alcohol dependence and phobic anxiety states: II. A retrospective study. Br J Psychiatry 144:58–63.

Tardiff K, Gross E, Messner S (1981): A study of homicide in Manhattan. Am J Public Health 76:139–143.

Vaillant GE (1980): Natural history of male psychological health VIII. Antecedents of alcoholism and "orality." Am J Psychiatry 137:181–186.

Weiss KJ, Rosenberg DJ (1985): Prevalence of anxiety disorder among alcoholics. J Clin Psychiatry 46:3–5.

Weiss RD, Mirin SM, Griffin ML, Michael JL (1988): Psychopathology in cocaine abusers: Changing trends. J Nerv Ment Disord 176:719–725.

Wittchen H-U, Zhao S, Kessler RC, Eaton WW (1994): DSM-III-R generalized anxiety disorder in the National Comorbidity Survey. Arch Gen Psychiatry 51:355–364.

Wolf AW, Schubert DSP, Patterson MB, Marion B, Grande TP (1988): Associations among major psychiatric diagnoses. J Consult Clin Psychol 56:292–294.

Woodruff RA Jr, Guze SB, Clayton PJ, Carr D (1973): Alcoholism and depression. Arch Gen Psychiatry 28:97–100.

CHAPTER 8

Mental Health Services Research

JACK D. BURKE, JR.

Department of Psychiatry and Behavioral Science, Texas A&M University Health Science Center and Scott & White Clinic and Hospital, Temple, TX 76508

INTRODUCTION

One aim of epidemiology is to understand the functioning of health services (Morris, 1957). Research on mental health services is undertaken on several levels of investigation, including the clinical, program, and systems levels (National Advisory Mental Health Council [NAMHC] 1991). Major questions about the delivery of health services can be summarized with four terms (Teh-wei Hu and Charles E. Windle, personal communication, November 11, 1988):

Equity: Access to health services for the general population can be influenced by socioeconomic, geographic, and cultural factors. In the United States, emphasis is often given to disadvantaged groups, such as the working poor who have no health insurance, residents of sparsely populated rural areas, or minority groups who are alienated from established health care institutions. In addition to access, another problem identified has been the influence of these factors on provision of care, through the diagnostic process as well as choice of treatment.

Efficiency: Providing the right mix of services and delivering the highest level of care possible with a given level of resources have become increasingly important questions as health care expenditures have risen as a proportion of the gross domestic product.

Economy: To some extent, in the United States questions about health economics have been reduced to simple policy questions of how to pay for health care. But more important questions, such as the influence that any particular payment or reimbursement scheme has on the delivery of health care services, and the influence of payment systems on provider behavior, have become increasingly important questions.

Effectiveness: Ensuring the highest quality of care, and presumably through that care ensuring the highest level of health for the population, have become increasingly urgent questions. While a great deal of research has been supported to study the

Textbook in Psychiatric Epidemiology, Edited by Tsuang, Tohen, and Zahner.
ISBN 0-471-59375-3 © 1995 Wiley-Liss, Inc.

fundamental mechanisms of nature and to translate the findings into efficacious therapies, little is known about the way that treatment is provided in everyday clinical practice or how well commonly accepted therapeutic practices promote health of individual patients or the populations from which they come.

Since all four of these questions deal with assessment within populations, with attention to variation across groups, and usually have an integral relationship to questions of type of disease and level of impairment, they are intrinsically based on epidemiologic findings and methods. While health services research is a multidisciplinary field, epidemiology provides the basis for assessing health needs of a population, and its research methods provide a tool to test ways to improve the level of health (Baasher et al., 1982).

In mental health research, the rapid developments in epidemiologic methods have made it possible to begin addressing some of the key questions about delivery of mental health services. In particular, as the distribution of mental illnesses in the population, and the resulting impairment from them, have been clarified through recent epidemiologic studies, and as clinical research has shown the benefit of treatment, mental health services have become a legitimate focus of both research and policy interest. This progress in related fields has helped to overcome the tendency researchers and policy makers have had in the past to dismiss mental health service delivery as an unwieldy or unapproachable subject.

DESCRIPTIVE STUDIES OF MENTAL HEALTH SERVICES

Two of the most important issues from a public health perspective are to determine the need for mental health care in a population and to assess the extent of "unmet need." This issue raises consideration of *equity*, *efficiency*, and *economy* in delivering mental health services. But uncertainty about *effectiveness* of treatment, at the clinical, program, and systems levels, has led to controversy about how to determine when mental health services are needed (Klerman et al., 1992). This controversy leads some policymakers to discuss "demand" for services, to emphasize the consumer's role rather than "need," which might emphasize the provider's view.

To address these issues, studies of services actually provided help to describe the service delivery system and level of care available. These studies provide information about the nature of services provided and the characteristics of patients who use them. Recent studies of the population allow a more direct comparison of an individual's diagnostic status and use of mental health services.

Surveys of Institutions

Until the late 1970s, when epidemiologic methods in psychiatry became more powerful, information on the distribution of mental disorders from most populations in the world came from surveys of the patients in mental institutions. In the United States, these surveys have been sponsored by the U.S. Public Health Service. In the past they have focused on state and county hospitals; with the evolving service delivery system, the periodic census of patients has expanded to include private hospitals, free-standing units (like community mental health centers), general hospitals, and federal hospitals, including veterans' medical centers.

For the last day of 1969, the National Reporting Program of NIMH found that 471,451 patients were in psychiatric inpatient units; by 1981, the number fell to 214,065. The principal location of that care changed as well, with 78.4% in state and county hospitals in 1969 and 58.5% in state and county hospitals by 1981. Another striking finding was the growth in outpatient services, as the estimate of people receiving outpatient services rose from 1.1 million in 1969 to 2.6 million in 1979 (Taube and Barrett, 1985). However, one shortcoming of these data is the lack of comparable information on office visits to individual practitioners, such as psychiatrists, psychologists, and social workers.

Minority Groups. One of the most difficult issues facing services researchers is to determine the relative over-representation of patients who are black or Native American. While the admission rate might be partly explained by socioeconomic factors, the predominance of diagnoses of schizophrenia rather than bipolar disorder among blacks has raised questions about possible bias in the diagnostic practices for different groups (Snowden and Cheung, 1990).

Jails. Studies of special institutions have also been conducted. One of the most important sites to explore has been penal institutions. A study of male detainees in Cook County (Chicago) jails showed that the prevalence of mental disorders among a random sample of 728 males charged with misdemeanors or felonies was two to three times higher than among individuals from the same demographic groups in the general population (Teplin 1990). Results such as these have suggested that the largest mental institution in the United States is apparently the Los Angeles County jail (Torrey et al., 1990).

Surveys of Populations

While data from the NIMH Epidemiologic Catchment Area (ECA) program have been useful in estimating prevalence of mental disorders in the general population (Robins et al., 1984; Myers et al., 1984; Regier et al., 1988a,b), they also provide a basis for estimating use of services by the population. Each respondent in the five-site sample reported on use of mental health services on an inpatient and outpatient basis, with extensive information on the type of provider used.

Initial reports from the ECA demonstrated that about 6%–7% of the adult population reported an ambulatory visit for mental health reasons to a health provider in the 6 month period before the first interview. Of these respondents reporting visits, about half saw a general medical provider only, and half saw a mental health specialist at least once. For all 9,543 respondents in the first three sites, about 16%–25% of all ambulatory health care visits in a 6 month period were reportedly made for mental health problems (Shapiro et al., 1984).

From 14% to 18% of the respondents reported at least one admission for general medical conditions during the year prior to the first ECA interview. For mental health reasons, from 2% to 6% of respondents reported an inpatient admission. This figure was variable across sites, as the community with the highest rate of admissions had the largest number of psychiatric beds available. A similar association was shown for rates of ambulatory mental health visits. Whether these associations of availability of services with higher use of those services depend on reducing unmet need, providing better geographic, financial, or other means to access services, or inducing demand through increased supply is not clear (Shapiro et al., 1984).

More recent analyses of these data have projected estimates of services use to the 1980 adult U.S. population for a 1 year period by combining data from the first ECA interview with the follow-up interview conducted approximately 1 year later. These new estimates suggested that the 1 year prevalence of DSM-III disorders covered by the Diagnostic Interview Schedule (DIS) was 28.1%, or about 44.7 million people aged 18 years or over. About 1% of the population had an inpatient stay for mental health reasons, and about 10.7% had an outpatient visit in this same 1 year period. For outpatient visits, about 5.6% of the population was seen in the mental health specialty sector and about 6.4% in the general medical sector, with some individuals being seen in both. Overall, only about 21.9% of the 44.7 million adults with a currently diagnosable mental disorder received any mental health treatment services from specialty or general medical providers during the 1 year period of study. For patients with schizophrenia, the proportion receiving any mental health service was higher, at 64% of all patients with an active diagnosis, and for major depression it was 54% (Regier et al., 1993).

Minority Groups. National estimates are helpful in determining services use overall and demonstrate that the majority of individuals with mental disorders do not receive mental health treatment. Concerns about *equity* in access and *efficiency* in providing services make it important to examine variations in services use. Another study examining services use in the ECA data demonstrated that individual characteristics associated with using mental health services included being white, female, and aged 25 to 65 years. This study carefully controlled for diagnostic status, so it provides important confirmation that being young or old, nonwhite, and male make people with mental disorders less likely to receive treatment for their disorders (Leaf et al., 1988; Klerman et al., 1992).

Primary Care Populations. Epidemiologic data from studies of general populations suggest that many people with mental disorders are seen primarily or exclusively in general medical settings. Studies assessing the presence of these disorders in patients seen in primary care settings in this country and abroad have verified a high prevalence of serious mental disorders in patient populations. From 15% to 28% of patients have a current mental disorder in a range of studies. The prevalence figure is even higher when more inclusive, but less precise instruments (such as self-report questionnaires rather than research diagnostic interviews) are used as case identification measures (Shepherd et al., 1981; Regier et al., 1988a,b; Katon and Shulberg, 1992). At least one study using a research interview and measures of duration and disability showed that a significant proportion of these conditions are serious and chronic in nature (Regier et al., 1985).

These findings of the importance of primary care in the de facto mental health services system (Regier et al., 1978, 1993) become even more significant when the *effectiveness* of care is examined. A range of studies comparing the primary care clinician's recognition of mental disorders in patients whose interview indicates presence of one show that only 10%–50% of patients are detected as having a diagnosable disorder (Regier et al., 1988a,b; Kessler et al., 1985).

Overview of Services Use. Efforts to compare services use estimates based on surveys of institutional providers with estimates based on surveys of the population have shown reasonable agreement, especially for inpatient care. For example, the ECA estimate for patients receiving care in a state or county mental hospital was 338,000 adults, and the NIMH National Reporting Program estimate was 351,000. For general hospitals, the estimates were 606,000 and 609,000, respectively. However, the ECA estimates for some forms of treatment, such as number of persons with visits to mental health center outpatient clinics, was much lower than reported to the National Reporting Program (Manderscheid et al., 1993). Discrepancies could be accounted for by the fact that the ECA was not designed to provide a nationally representative sample (Regier et al., 1988a). Also, self-reported data on ambulatory health care visits, as used in the ECA, often suffer from inaccuracies in number of visits, time frame, or place of service (Shapiro et al., 1984; Manderscheid et al., 1993).

ANALYTIC STUDIES OF MENTAL HEALTH SERVICES

Epidemiologic data show that the burden of mental disorders in the population is a large one. Even with only about one in five individuals with a diagnosable disorder using services in any 1 year period, the cost of providing treatment is large as well. Mental health services research has been increasingly concerned with *economic* issues, including the cost associated with these disorders, as well as the effect of different payment systems on the way that care is delivered. Data showing that access is uneven, that the general medical system is important in providing care, and that some nonmedical institutions like jails have populations with need for service have also made it increasingly important to examine the interactions between parts of the health care and human service system to see if *efficiency* and *economy* can be improved.

Costs of Mental Disorders

With the data on prevalence in the population and use of mental health services, it has been possible to estimate the costs of providing care to people with mental disorder for the year 1985. The direct costs, in terms of payment for treatment and related services, is estimated at $51.4 billion. More important than this figure for direct costs of treatment is the cost to society resulting from impairment in the individuals with mental disorders through absence from work, unemployment, and need for social services. This core component of indirect costs has been estimated at $116.6 billion. Additional costs of $47.5 billion reflected society's costs in terms of dealing with related accidents, crime, and other problems related to mental disorders. Overall, mental disorders cost $218.1 billion in 1985. With inflation and increases in the population since that time, the figure today is even higher. Corrected just to 1988, for example, the total costs to society were $273.3 billion (Rice et al., 1991).

Paying for Mental Health Services

About 14% of the U.S. population has no health insurance. For people with mental disorders, the figure is even higher, estimated at 18% (NAMHC, 1993). Even for those people with health insurance, from a private source or a government program, the coverage for mental health services is less than for general medical services. Typically insurance plans require the covered individual to assume a higher copayment for each mental health service or a higher deductible than for general medical services. This type of cost-sharing is termed a *demand-side* limit since it serves to reduce the patient's demand for services (Frank et al., 1992). One reason for this discrepancy in copayment and deductibles is that insurers suspect that some services, such as psychotherapy, may have less clearly defined indications or less certain effectiveness than other types of medical services. The higher demand-side limits on mental health services provide a disincentive for use in case covered patients would over-use them without this disincentive.

Evidence exists to show that use of some psychiatric services, notably psychotherapy, may be more sensitive to price than other medical services (Sharfstein et al., 1993). In a large, randomized trial conducted in the 1970s, health insurance benefits with different levels of coverage were provided to residents of six communities across the country. At one extreme, some participants received care that required no copayment, i.e., was "free"; at the other extreme, participants paid 95% of the costs of care. Participants with free care were about twice as likely as those with 95% cost-sharing to use any psychotherapy services. However, the use of services was low even for those in the free care plan, as the total amount was only about $32 per enrollee (in 1984 dollars) (Manning et al., 1986). As health care expenditures have risen over the past 15 years, insurers have sometimes used any measure to reduce their direct costs. In this study, outcome was not measured, so the findings could be interpreted simply as an endorsement of limiting mental health benefits (Borus, 1986).

Another method of controlling health care use, and the corresponding costs of care, has also been developed. It involves the relationship between the insurer and the provider of care rather than the consumer. These limits can be called *supply-side* measures, since they introduce a disincentive to the provider to offer services. The simplest of these methods is to pay the provider a set amount for each covered individual at the beginning of the policy year; under this kind of capitated system, the provider must manage treatment resources to avoid losing money (Frank et al., 1992). Prepaid health plans represent an example of this payment system, which is intended to encourage cost-effective care and avoid overuse of services. For example, use of partial hospitalization programs may reduce the need for admission to a full-time inpatient unit.

In general medical practice, the type of payment system may not influence a clinician's decision making beyond efforts to reduce hospitalization (Greenfield et al., 1992). However, some evidence suggests that general medical clinicians in a health maintenance organization (HMO) are less likely to diagnose depression in their patients than corresponding clinicians in a fee-for-service arrangement (Wells et al., 1988). Evidence from one of the communities studied in the ECA program demonstrates that, for a given severity of illness, patients seen in an HMO received less intensive care than patients in fee-for-service settings (Norquist and Wells, 1991). Psychiatrists have begun to consider what represents a legitimate constriction on services offered to patients in a prepaid health plan, where the provider shares the risks of "overuse" of services compared with the "optimal" treatment that would be offered in a more traditional fee-for-service arrangement (Sabin, 1991). Without more guidance from studies of effectiveness and patient outcomes, these issues will likely be decided simply on the basis of cost containment rather than improving the public mental health (Sharfstein et al., 1993).

Interactions Between Sectors of the Health Care System

Little is known about the pathways taken by patients through the various components of the mental health system. While the components have been identified and services use has been measured, patients have not yet been tracked over time to determine the relative importance of specialty mental health care, general medical care, or other human services and voluntary care (Regier et al., 1993). Jails have been identified as an important institutional residence of individuals with mental disorders, but little is known of how services are provided in penal institutions or how these services supplement or replace other types of mental health services (NAMHC, 1991).

One interaction that has been studied is the relationship of the general medical sector with the specialty mental health sector. For some time, research has shown that people with identified mental disorders have a higher rate of using general medical services than people without a diagnosed mental disorder (Hankin and Oktay, 1979). This finding from a variety of medical settings has been generally confirmed by results from the population-based ECA study (Shapiro et al., 1984; Narrow et al., 1993) and the RAND Health Insurance Experiment (Manning and Wells, 1992).

Of most interest, however, is the finding from a variety of studies that for people with mental disorders who have higher rates of medical services use, there is a reduction of this use once some mental health treatment has been obtained. This "offset effect" for services also results at times in a reduction of overall health care expenditures (Jones and Vischi, 1979; Borus et al., 1985; Mumford et al., 1984; Mumford and Schlesingers, 1987).

At present, the offset effect is still poorly understood. Without a randomized trial, which would be very hard to conduct in most treatment settings, the methodologic limits of retrospective studies may make it difficult for policy makers to bank on any cost-offset effect. The growing focus on measuring outcome and assessing effectiveness of care is likely to receive more research attention in the immediate future.

EXPERIMENTAL STUDIES OF MENTAL HEALTH SERVICES

Finding ways to improve the quality of care offered to people with mental disorders is one of the fundamental goals of an applied research area like mental health services research. Studying "what works, for whom, under what circumstances" is a goal set by the National Institute of Mental Health and its Advisory Council (NAMHC, 1991). Once more is known about ways to maximize the *effectiveness* of mental health services, some of the controversial issues about delivery of services can be addressed. For example, it would be useful to know what impact the limited mental health benefits of most insurance programs have on patient outcome or how to provide the best mix of services to the whole population for a given level of mental health care expenditures.

Formal experimental studies to determine effectiveness of alternative treatment approaches and programs are difficult to undertake. They must be introduced into ongoing systems of care and require extraordinary efforts at maintaining the intervention, reducing attrition, and assessing outcome in both individual and system terms. Unlike studies of new pharmacologic agents, they must enroll a wide range of patients and follow them for long periods of time, much longer than the 6 or 8 weeks that might satisfy studies of new medications. Outcome measures must include assessment of quality of life and not just symptom reduction (NAMHC, 1991). For all of these reasons, studies of mental health treatment effectiveness in day-to-day clinical practice have been difficult to start. But their absence is being felt in current discussions of policy options (NAMHC, 1991, 1993; Ginzberg, 1991; Goldman et al., 1993; Sharfstein et al., 1993).

Effectiveness Studies in Primary Care Settings

One of the first efforts to improve quality of care was to introduce self-report question-naires for mental disorders into primary care settings. If primary care clinicians could be alerted to the presence of a disorder, the diagnosis and subsequent management could presumably be improved. While early pilot studies were encouraging, a formal clinical trial using random assignment into control and experimental groups failed to find a sig-nificant improvement in overall detection of illness. Improved recognition was noted for patients who were elderly, black, or male, but, overall, clinicians tended to ignore the re-sults of the questionnaire, apparently because of the pressure of conducting routine as-sessment of general medical problems (Shapiro et al., 1987).

More recently, efforts of major public health and professional groups has been to em-phasize improved classification systems for mental disorders to be used in primary care. Both the American Psychiatric Association, which publishes the Diagnostic and Statisti-cal Manual, fourth edition, and the World Health Organization's Division of Mental Health, are developing streamlined systems of classification for use by primary care clini-cians.

Under mandate from the U.S. Congress, the Public Health Service is also promoting the use of treatment guidelines for common problems in primary care. The first set of guidelines included Treatment of Depression in Primary Care (Agency for Health Care Policy and Research, 1992), and a new set on anxiety disorders is under preparation. Whether the new classification systems or the treatment guidelines for specific disorders will result in improved patient outcome will need to be assessed by formal studies.

Effectiveness Studies in Mental Health Settings

One of the most pressing issues in delivery of care is to find ways to help patients with severe mental disorders improve their lives in the community. One program that has shown tremendous promise is the Program for Assertive Community Treatment (PACT), which uses multidisciplinary teams, active outreach, and a variety of other measures like job assistance. Initial studies on its effectiveness have shown reduced hospitalization and improved stabilization in the community (Stein, 1992). One problem in having the pro-gram more widely adopted is that replication studies have been somewhat difficult to un-dertake. Without additional studies, it will not be possible to identify the types of settings where it works well or not so well or to disaggregate any key factors that must be present to make the program succeed. (Lalley et al., 1992).

Another important test of program effectiveness is being undertaken as a quasiexperi-mental study of the Robert Wood Johnson demonstration program for services to people with severe mental disorders in nine cities (Goldman et al., 1992). The evaluation is a model in terms of assessing both the individual patients and the impact on the overall sys-tem of care in the cities participating in this long-term project.

To fill the huge gaps in knowledge about improving effectiveness of mental health ser-vices and to promote many more studies like the ones on PACT and the nine city demon-stration program, the Advisory Council of NIMH has recommended a comprehensive re-search effort to find ways to improve care for people with severe mental disorders. In the course of preparing that review, the expert consultants identified a key weakness in out-come studies—the lack of accepted concepts, and corresponding measures, to assess out-come of individual patients. The report suggested that a full assessment of outcome must include not just a measure of clinical signs and symptoms. It must also assess rehabilitative goals, in terms of social and vocational functioning; humanistic goals, in terms of quality of life and personal fulfillment; and public welfare goals, in terms of meeting the family's and society's needs for productivity and safety (NAMHC, 1991; Lalley et al., 1992).

CONCLUSION

At times, mental health services research has seemed close to fulfilling its promise of finding ways to improve the equity, efficiency, economy, and effectiveness of mental health services (Wing and Hailey, 1972; Taube et al., 1988a,b). At other times, it has seemed to fail (Leighton, 1982).

At the verge of the twenty-first century, the task of finding ways to deal with the problems that mental disorders cause for patients seems at least as acute as ever. With the base provided by new epidemiologic methods, with new emphasis on the need for careful research on cost-effective care (Burke and Leshner, 1989; Sharfstein et al., 1993), and with the delineation of specific research agendas (NAMHC, 1991; Lalley et al., 1992), mental health services research now has its best opportunity to improve care for people with mental disorders.

REFERENCES

Agency for Health Care Policy and Research (1992): "Depression in Primary Care: Clinical Practice Guidelines." Washington, DC: Government Printing Office.

Baasher TA, Cooper JE, Davidian H, Jablensky A, Sartorius N, Stromgren E (eds) (1982): "Epidemiology and Mental Health Services: Principles and Applications in Developing Countries." Acta Psychiatrica Scandinavica [Suppl 296] 651.

Borus JF (1986): Coverage, care, cost, and outcome. JAMA 256:1939.

Borus JF, Olendzki MC, Kessler L, Burns BJ, Brandt UC, Broverman CA, Henderson PR (1985): The "offset effect" of mental health treatment on ambulatory medical care utilization and charges. Arch Gen Psychiatry 42:573–580.

Burke JD, Leshner AI (1989): New support for mental health services research. Focus Mental Health Services Res 3:1.

Frank RG, Goldman HH, McGuire TG (1992): A model mental health benefit in private insurance. Health Affairs 11:98–117.

Ginzberg E (ed) (1991): "Health Services Research: Key to Health Policy." Cambridge, MA: Harvard University Press.

Goldman HH, Adler DA, Berlant J, Docherty J, Dorwart R, Ellison JM, Pajer K, Slris S, Kapur S (1993): The case for a services-based approach to payment for mental illness under national health care reform. Hosp Commun Psychiatry 44:542–544.

Goldman HH, Morrissey JP, Ridgely MS, Frank RG, Newman SJ, Kennedy C (1992): Lessons from the program on chronic mental illness. Health Affairs 11:51–68.

Greenfield S, Nelson EC, Zubkoff M, Manning W, Rogers W, Kravitz RL, Keller A, Tarlov AR, Ware JE (1992): Variations in resource utilization among medical specialties and systems of care: Results from the medical outcomes study. JAMA 267:1624–1630.

Hankin JR, Oktay JS (1979): "Mental Disorders and Primary Medical Care: An Analytic Review of the Literature." Washington, DC: Government Printing Office.

Jones K, Vischi T (1979): Impact of alcohol, drug abuse, and mental health treatment on medical care utilization. A review of the research literature. Medical Care 17(Suppl):ii–82.

Katon W, Schulberg H (1992): Epidemiology of depression in primary care. Gen Hosp Psychiatry 14:237–247.

Kessler LG, Cleary PD, Burke JD (1985): Psychiatric disorders in primary care. Arch Gen Psychiatry 42:583–587.

Klerman GL, Olfson M, Leon AC, Weissman MM (1992): Measuring the need for mental health care. Health Affairs 11:23–33.

Lalley TL, Hohmann AA, Windle CD, Norquist GS, Keith SJ, Burke JD (eds) (1992): A national plan to improve care for severe mental disorders. Schiz Bull 18:559–668.

Leaf PJ, Bruce ML, Tischler GL, Freeman DH, Weissman MM, Myers JK (1988): Factors affecting the utilization of specialty and general medical mental health services. Medical Care 26:9–26.

Leighton AH (1982): "Caring for Mentally Ill People: Psychological and Social Barriers in Historical Context." Cambridge, Cambridge University Press.

Manderscheid RW, Rae DS, Narrow WE, Locke BZ, Regier DA (1993): Congruence of Service Utilization Estimates from the Epidemiologic Catchment Area project and other sources. Arch Gen Psychiatry 50:108–114.

Manning WG, Wells KB (1992): The effects of psychological distress and psychological well-being on use of medical services. Med Care 30:541–553.

Manning WG, Wells KB, Duan N, Newhouse JP, Ware JE (1986): How cost sharing affects the use of ambulatory mental health services. JAMA 256:1930–1934.

Morris JN: "Uses of Epidemiology." Edinburgh; Livingstone, 1957.

Mumford E, Schlesinger HJ (1987): Assessing consumer benefit: cost offset as an incidental effect of psychotherapy. Gen Hosp Psychiatry 9:360–363.

Mumford E, Schlesinger HJ, Glass GV, Patrick C, Cuerdon T (1984): A new look at evidence about reduced cost of medical utilization following mental health treatment. Am J Psychiatry 141:1145–1158.

Myers JK, Weissman MM, Tischler GL, Holzer CE, Leaf PJ, Orvaschel H, Anthony JC, Boyd JH, Burke JD, Kramer M, Stoltzman R (1984): Six-month prevalence of psychiatric disorders in three communities: 1980–1982. Arch Gen Psychiatry 41:959–967.

Narrow WE, Regier DA, Rae DS, Manderscheid RS, Locke BZ (1993): Use of services by persons with mental and addictive disorders: Findings from the National Institute of Mental Health Epidemiologic Catchment Area Program. Arch Gen Psychiatry 50:95–107.

National Advisory Mental Health Council (1991): Caring for people with severe mental disorders: A national plan of research to improve services. Washington, DC: Government Printing Office.

National Advisory Mental Health Council (1993): Health care reform for Americans with severe mental illnesses. Am J Psychiatry 150:1447–1465.

Norquist GS, Wells KB (1991): How do HMOs reduce outpatient mental health care costs? Am J Psychiatry 148:96–101.

Regier DA, Boyd JH, Burke JD, Rae DS, Myers JK, Kramer M, Robins LN, George LK, Karno M, Locke BZ (1988a): One-month prevalence of mental disorders in the United States: Based on five Epidemiologic Catchment Area sites. Arch Gen Psychiatry 45:977–986.

Regier DA, Burke JD, Manderscheid RW, Burns BJ (1985): The chronically mentally ill in primary care. Psychol Med 15:265–273.

Regier DA, Goldberg ID, Taube CA (1978): The defacto US mental health services system: A public health perspective. Arch Gen Psychiatry 35:685–693.

Regier DA, Hirschfeld RMA, Goodwin FK, Burke JD, Lazar JB, Judd LL (1988b): The NIMH Depression Awareness, Recognition, and Treatment Program: Structure, aims, and scientific basis. Am J Psychiatry 145:1351–1357

Regier DA, Narrow WE, Rae DS, Manderscheid RW, Locke BZ, Goodwin FK (1993): The de facto U.S. Mental and Addictive Disorders Service System: Epidemiologic Catchment Area Prospective 1-year prevalence rates of disorders and services. Arch Gen Psychiatry 50:85–94.

Rice DP, Kelman S, Miller LS (1991): Estimates of economic costs of alcohol and drug abuse and mental illness, 1985 and 1988. Public Health Rep 106:280–292.

Robins LN, Helzer JE, Weissman MM, Orvaschel H, Gruenberg E, Burke JD, Regier DA (1984): Lifetime prevalence of specific psychiatric disorders in three sites. Arch Gen Psychiatry 41:949–958.

Sabin J (1991): Clinical skills for the 1990s: Six lessons from HMO Practice. Hosp Community Psychiatry 42:605–608.

Shapiro S, German PS, Skinner EA, VonKorff M, Turner RW, Klein LE, Teitelbaum ML, Kramer M, Burke JD, Burns BJ (1987): An experiment to change detection and management of mental morbidity in primary care. Med Care 25:327–339.

Shapiro S, Skinner EA, Kessler LG, VonKorff M, German PS, Tischler GL, Leaf PJ, Benham L, Cottler L, Regier DA (1984): Utilization of health and mental health services: Three epidemiologic catchment area sites. Arch Gen Psychiatry 41:971–978.

Sharfstein SS, Stoline AM, Goldman HH (1993): Psychiatric care and health insurance reform. Am J Psychiatry 150:7–18.

Shepherd M, Cooper B, Brown AC, Kalton G, Clare A (1981): "Psychiatric Illness in General Practice," 2nd ed. Oxford; Oxford University Press.

Snowden LR, Cheung FK (1990): Use of inpatient mental health services by members of ethnic minority groups. Am Psychologist 45:347–355.

Stein LI (1992): On the abolishment of the case manager. Health Affairs 11:172–177.

Taube CA, Barrett SA (eds) (1985): "Mental Health, U.S. 1985." Washington, DC; U.S. Government Printing Office.

Taube CA, Goldman HH, Lee ES (1988a): Use of specialty psychiatric settings in constructing DRGs. Arch Gen Psychiatry 45:1037–1040.

Taube CA, Lave JR, Rupp A, Goldman HH, Frank RG (1988b): Psychiatry under prospective payment: Experience in the first year. Am J Psychiatry 145:210–213.

Teplin LA (1990): The prevalence of severe mental disorder among male urban jail detainees: Comparison with the Epidemiologic Catchment Area Program. Am J Public Health 1990;663–669.

Torrey EF, Erdman K, Wolfe SM, Flynn LM (1990): "Care of the seriously mentally ill: A rating of state programs." Washington, DC: Public Citizen Health Research Group and National Alliance for the Mentally Ill.

Wells KB, Golding JM, Hough RL, Burnam A, Karno M (1988): Factors affecting the probability of use of general and medical health and social/community services for Mexican Americans and non-hispanic whites. Med Care 26:441–452.

Wells KB, Hays RD, Burnam A, Rogers W, Greenfield S, Ware JE (1989): Detection of depressive disorder for patients receiving prepaid or fee-for-service care: Results from the Medical Outcomes Study. JAMA 262:3298–3302.

Wing JK, Hailey AM (1972): "Evaluating a Community Psychiatric Service: The Camberwell Register 1964–1971." London: Oxford University Press.

PART III

ASSESSMENT

CHAPTER 9

Reliability

PATRICK E. SHROUT

Department of Psychology, New York University, New York, NY 10003

INTRODUCTION

Quality of measurement in psychiatry and epidemiology is typically characterized in terms of reliability and validity. *Reliability* is the degree to which a measurement produces systematic or reproducible variation. *Validity* is the degree to which the measurement is useful. Although validity is the ultimate criterion by which to judge a measure, we know that a measure will not be useful if it is contaminated by random variation. In other words, reliability is a necessary condition for validity, but it is not sufficient to guarantee validity.

Even though reliability is only an intermediate step toward quality measurement, it is often methodologically interesting because it is a problem that can usually be fixed. Reliability can be improved by structuring and standardizing the assessment procedure, by improving the training of both the subjects and those carrying out the assessment, and by averaging replicate measurements. If problems of unreliability are not addressed, then subsequent problems of validity are intractable. This is why reliability was given so much attention in developing the Versions III and IV of the *Diagnostic and Statistical Manual* of the American Psychiatric Association (see American Psychiatric Association, 1980).

Epidemiologists must attend both to the reliability of diagnostic measures and of risk measures. Two features of psychiatric epidemiology make reliability more of an enduring problem in this field than in others. One feature is the frequent dependence on self-report information provided by respondents. Self-reports present many opportunities for noise to enter the recorded data: the understanding of the question, the recall and reporting of the answer, and the coding and entry of the data. The other feature is the epidemiologists' search for new populations and risk groups that might provide clues to the etiology of mental disorders. New populations require new assessments of reliability, since populations vary in language, literacy, and cultural expression of disorders. As we will see, the variability of the trait under study in the new population also affects its reliability.

In this chapter I examine methods for evaluating reliability of measures used in psychiatric epidemiology. I first review the classic psychometric theory of reliability. I then

Textbook in Psychiatric Epidemiology, Edited by Tsuang, Tohen, and Zahner
ISBN 0-471-59375-3 © 1995 Wiley-Liss, Inc.

survey the methods used to study reliability, for measures of both psychopathology and epidemiologic risk. In this survey I distinguish quantitative measures and those that classify respondents into categories. I incorporate a set of numerical examples that illustrate the most important measures.

THE RELIABILITY COEFFICIENT

Consider a single measurement procedure. Respondents are sampled from a specific population, measured in some way, and assigned a numerical value that I represent by the variable X. If the characteristic being measured is categorical, then the variable X might be binary, i.e., $X = 1$ if the respondent is in the category, and $X = 0$ otherwise. If the characteristic is quantitative, then X takes some well-defined numerical score.

The variance of X, σ_X^2, is a population parameter that describes how much the measurements differ from person to person in the population being studied. In some populations σ_X^2 might be relatively small, while in other populations the variance might be large. Small variance implies that the measurement distinction is subtle, while large variation implies the opposite. In populations with small overall variation in X, any measurement error may be quite serious.

According to classic reliability theory, it is useful to decompose σ_X^2 into at least two components, $\sigma_X^2 = \sigma_E^2 + \sigma_T^2$, where σ_E^2 is variance due to nonsystematic processes and σ_T^2 is variance due to systematic differences between persons being measured. The idea behind this decomposition is that random errors in measurement appear to increase the total measurement variation. If errors can be eliminated, then the error variance, σ_E^2, goes to zero. If errors dominate the measurement, then the majority of σ_X^2 may be attributable to σ_E^2.

The reliability coefficient, R_X, is a ratio of the population parameters σ_T^2 and σ_X^2:

$$R_x = \frac{\sigma_T^2}{\sigma_X^2} = \frac{\sigma_T^2}{[\sigma_T^2 + \sigma_B^2]} \, . \tag{1}$$

R_X varies from zero (X is due entirely to unsystematic stochastic processes) to unity (X is due entirely to systematic individual differences). It can be thought of as the proportion of σ_X^2 that represents genuine, replicable differences in subjects. It turns out to be a useful quantity in statistical analyses as well. For example, it can be shown that the correlation between X and another variable Y will get smaller as the reliability coefficient of either variable gets smaller. Generally we aim to have measures that have reliability above 0.90, we are happy to find reliability results greater than 0.70, and we may be content to use measures with reliabilities as low as 0.50. If we know that a measure truly has a reliability of 0.50, then we know that only half its variance is systematic.[1] For a complete development of R_X and its implications, see Lord and Novick (1968) or Shrout and Skodol (in press).

---

[1]Landis and Koch (1977) suggested that reliability values as low as 0.41 be considered "fair," but they acknowledged that the designation is completely arbitrary. Fleiss (1981) reported the Landis and Koch labels as one set of conventions. Insofar as these labels encourage researchers to be complaisant with reliabilities known to be as low as 0.41, I find them to be too lenient. In setting standards for reliability, however, we must be aware that *estimates of reliability* may be smaller than the *actual reliability* because of systematic bias, which is discussed later.

DESIGNS FOR ESTIMATING RELIABILITY

To estimate R_X we need to define what is meant by systematic variation of X. Classical psychometric theory defines this hypothetically. Suppose that a subject is selected and is measured once to produce the score X_1. Now suppose that it is possible to make the measurement over and over again without affecting the subject and without recall of the previous X_j values (where j indexes each replicate measure). Classical measurement theory defines the systematic part of X to be the average of all of these hypothetically infinite measurements of the selected subject. This systematic component of the measurement is written as $T = E(X)$, which is interpreted roughly as the expected average of the many replications of X. Note that if the measurement was height or weight, then it would actually be possible to take many repeated measurements of this sort.

In psychiatry and related fields, reliability is estimated by approaching the hypothetical ideal with approximately replicate measurements. If there is virtually no variation across replications of X, then we infer that σ_E^2 is small in magnitude and that reliability is very good. If variation across replications is observed, then the magnitude of the within-subject variation is compared with that of the between-subject variation using the definition of R_X in Eq. (1) above.

The most common replication design calls for making the X measurement at two points in time (the *test–retest design*). Variation in the X values across replications and across respondents is used to estimate σ_E^2, σ_T^2, and σ_X^2, and these can be used to estimate R_X. The formal equations for these estimates are presented in a later section.

Although theoretically and intuitively appealing, the test–retest design falls short of the hypothetical ideal in several ways. On the one hand, the second measurement is often affected by systematic biologic, psychological, and social changes in the respondent. These systematic changes are included with the random variations that make σ_E^2 appear larger. When legitimate change is included with error, the actual reliability of the first assessment is underestimated. By this I mean that the estimate will be too small. On the other hand, if the respondents remember their original responses and then try to be "good" by reporting the same thing, then the reliability estimate may be too large. Methodologists who address these opposing biases recommend that the second assessments be carried out after a long enough period to reduce memory artifacts but promptly enough to reduce the probability of systematic changes. Recommendations of how long the period should be are products more of opinion than science.

Test–retest designs can be used with the whole range of measures made in psychiatric epidemiology. Interviews, questionnaires, ratings, and physical measurements can all be repeated after an appropriate time. It is not always necessary, however, to wait to obtain a replicate measurement. When the measurement is a judgment, such as the Global Assessment Scale (Endicott et al., 1976), it is possible to have two independent ratings made at the same time. Moreover, time can be frozen by videorecording the structured interview so that ratings can be obtained from those viewing the recording. Although these alternatives to traditional test–retest designs overcome the confounding of unreliability with genuine growth or development, they bring with them their own problems. These have been discussed by several authors, including Spitzer (1983). Insofar as the respondent's idiosyncratic responses contribute to unreliability, estimates based on a single interview may underestimate the actual level of random variation in the actual ratings obtained in the field. For this reason, inter-rater reliability studies using recorded interviews are expected to overestimate true reliability.

When the measurement procedure under study is a questionnaire that includes several items pertaining to a single underlying psychological trait or symptom dimension, it is also possible to obtain some information about reliability from a single assessment time. The items that relate to the same underlying concept are considered to be replications of each other. The degree to which the patterns of responses suggest that they are empirically related is used as evidence of reliability. This inference is made on the basis of the *internal consistency* of the questionnaire responses.

Internal consistency measures of reliability are affected by some biases that make them underestimate actual reliability and others that make them overestimate reliability. They will underestimate reliability if the items within the set are not close replications of each other. For example, a scale of depression symptoms may contain some items on mood, others on psychophysiological complaints, and yet others on cognitive beliefs. Although these are all expected to be related to depression, they are not exact replications of each other. To the degree that the correlations among the items are due to the different item content rather than error, the overall reliability estimate will be smaller than it should be.

Reliability may be overestimated by the internal consistency design if the whole interview is affected by irrelevant global response patterns, such as mood or response biases. For instance, some respondents may perceive that acknowledging symptoms is socially undesirable and may systematically under report more bizarre problems. Others may fall into a pattern of denying everything. These so-called *response biases* inflate internal consistency reliability estimates. They are often addressed by mixing the items across many conceptual domains, editing the items so that half are keyed as a symptom when the respondent says "no" and half are keyed the opposite way. Scales of Yea-saying and Need-for-approval are also sometimes constructed to identify those respondents who are susceptible to response biases. The validity of these scales, however, is a subject of open discussion.

Given the possibility of opposing biases, how should we evaluate internal consistency results? If the results appear to indicate high reliability, look for response artifacts that might have inflated the estimate. If provisions have been taken to address response biases, then the high level of reliability might be real. If the results indicate that there is low reliability, then look to see if the items included within the internal consistency analysis are heterogeneous in content. It is possible that a set of items that are heterogeneous might have adequate test–retest reliability even though the internal consistency estimate is low.

Because various reliability designs have different strengths and weaknesses, it is always helpful to incorporate multiple designs into a reliability program. By systematically studying the kinds of replication, one can gain an insight into sources of measurement variation. This is what is recommended by Cronbach and his colleagues (1972) in their comprehensive extension of classical test theory known as *generalizability theory*. This theory encompasses both reliability and validity by asking about the extent to which a measurement procedure works in different populations, at different times, with different raters, who may have different training. This broad perspective easily included designs such as those on the Diagnostic Interview Schedule (DIS) (Anthony et al., 1985; Helzer et al., 1985) that compared results from interviews done by "lay" interviewers to those done by mental health professionals. To the extent that the trained lay interviewers performed like the professionals, the results might be interpreted as test–retest reliability of the DIS. If the level of training actually made a difference, then the results might be interpreted as the validity of using lay interviewers (assuming that the professionals are the ideal interviewers for this structured measure). From the generalizability perspective, it is neither a reliability nor a validity study, but rather a study of the generalizability of DIS results across time and interviewer type. For more information about generalizability theory at an accessible level, see the text by Shavelson (1991).

THE EFFECT OF POPULATION VARIANCE ON RELIABILITY

In all of the reliability designs reviewed above it is assumed that respondents were sampled from the population that is to be studied. By randomly sampling from the population, we can obtain an unbiased estimate of σ_X^2. Note that any bias that is introduced in estimating σ_X^2 can have serious effects on the estimate of R_X. Epidemiologists should be especially sensitive to the fact that samples of patients should not be used in a reliability study if the ultimate survey is to be carried out in the general population. Relative to the variance in community surveys, the variance of most psychiatric measures will be too large in treated samples. The bias is usually concentrated in the σ_T^2 term of $\sigma_X^2 = \sigma_T^2 + \sigma_E^2$, and thus the reliability often appears to be better in the treated population than in a community population. When the reliability study sample has been constructed using stratified samples of cases and noncases, then it is often possible to undo the bias through weighting (e.g., Jannarone et al., 1987).

STATISTICAL REMEDIES FOR LOW RELIABILITY

If an investigator discovers that a quantitative measure is not sufficiently reproducible, there are several remedies that have been mentioned briefly before. The measure itself can be changed, the training of those administering it can be improved, or perhaps some special instructions can be developed for the respondents that improves the purity of the measurement outcome. These are examples of procedural remedies that are often effective. There is also a statistical remedy: Obtain several independent replicate measurements and average their results. The idea is simple: Averages of replicate measures are by definition more systematic than the individual measures themselves, so the reliability of the sum or average of items or ratings will be consistently higher than that of the components. The degree to which reliability is expected to improve in the composites is described mathematically by Spearman (1910) and Brown (1910). Let the sum of k ratings or items $(X_1, X_2, X_3, \ldots X_k)$ be called $W(k)$. Then the expected reliability of $W(k)$ can be written as a function of k and the reliability of the typical measurement, R_X, according to the Spearman-Brown formula:

$$R_{W(k)} = \frac{kR_X}{1 + (k - 1)R_X}. \tag{2}$$

Equation 2 is based on assumptions about the comparability of the measurements that are averaged or summed into $W(k)$, not on the form or distribution of the individual measurements. Because the result is not limited by the distribution of the X measures, the formula is even useful in calculating the expected reliability of a scale composed of k binary (0, 1) items as well as scales composed of quantitative ratings or items. Note that averaging measures only is a remedy for low reliability if there is some evidence of replicability. It is clear that R_W will be zero if R_X is zero, regardless of the magnitude of k.

The Spearman-Brown formula is especially useful for internal consistency studies. Although the items in the scale are the replications in internal consistency design, the scale scores (sums of items) are usually what we want to know the reliability of. This goal can be achieved by calculating the average item reliability and then using that result in Eq. 2 to calculate the expected scale reliability. These steps are combined when one uses certain estimation formulas, such as the classic *coefficient* α of Cronbach (1951).

The relationship described in the Spearman-Brown formula can also be used in studies of inter-rater reliability to determine how many independent ratings need to be averaged to obtain an ideal level of reliability, say C_R. If the obtained level of reliability for a single rater is R_X, then the number of raters that are needed to produce an averaged-rater reliability of C_R is

$$k = \frac{C_R(1 - R_X)}{R_X(1 - C_R)}. \tag{3}$$

For example, if each rater only has a reliability of $R_X = 0.40$ and one wants a reliability of $C_R = 0.75$, then Eq. 3 gives $k = 4.5$. This means that averages of four raters would be expected to have less than 0.75 reliability, while averages of five raters would exceed the target reliability of 0.75.

RELIABILITY THEORY AND BINARY JUDGMENTS

The reliability theory just reviewed does not make strong assumptions about the kind of measurement embodicd in X, and indeed many of the results hold for binary variables such as ones that might represent specific psychiatric diagnoses (e.g., $X = 1$ when the respondent is thought to have current major depression; $X = 0$ otherwise). Kraemer (1979) has shown explicitly how the results work with binary judgments. From her mathematical analysis of the problem it can be seen that the systematic component of X that I have called $T = E(X)$ will end up as a proportion falling between the extremes of 0 and 1. It represents the expected proportion of diagnosticians who would give the diagnosis to the respondent being evaluated. If T is close to 1, then most diagnosticians would say that the respondent is a case, and if T is close to zero, then most would say that the respondent is not a case. Note that while X itself is binary, T is quantitative in the range $(0, 1)$.

Because averages are quantitative (at least for large n), the psychometric results from the Spearman-Brown formula are applicable only when the composite of interest is quantitative. This is often the case when X represents binary items in a symptom scale. Of interest is the count of symptoms, which is closely related to the average of symptom items. However, if we really want a binary variable as the outcome, then the Spearman-Brown result does not apply. For example, diagnoses of several independent judges are sometimes combined into a "consensus diagnosis" that is itself binary. If the consensus rule is one that requires that all judges make the diagnosis before the diagnosis is applied, the result might be less reliable than some of the individual diagnosticians! (see Fleiss and Shrout, 1989). This total consensus rule is as weak as the least reliable diagnostician.

Many of the classic psychometric results depend on the assumed symmetry of errors. Because T is defined as an average, by definition about half the errors go in one direction and half in the other. For diagnoses, however, the errors that attract attention are those that seem to cause clinically relevant discrepancies. For example, if we know that a certain set of presentation facts are viewed by 90% of trained clinicians as indicating schizophrenia, then the clinically relevant discrepancies are those diagnosticians who argue that the diagnosis of schizophrenia is inappropriate. Persons who insist that schizophrenia should be diagnosed with more than 90% certainty are not usually considered in practical terms to be outliers.

The interest in the asymmetry of errors in diagnoses prompts some researchers to decompose inter-rater discrepancies into ones that are consistent with problems of sensitivity and specificity. From this perspective it can be shown that the reliability coefficient of Eq. 1 is a function of both kinds of errors. If we focus on one kind of error only, such as sensitivity, the classic relation between reliability and validity no longer holds necessarily. There are some examples in which different levels of reliability are consistent with the same level of sensitivity. (One usually finds that the assumed specificity or prevalence varies with the reliability in examples such as this [see Carey and Gottesman, 1978].) When asymmetric errors are of central interest, the results reviewed in this chapter may not be totally applicable.

The role of asymmetric errors in binary ratings is only one special aspect of such data. Another is the relation of the expected mean of a binary variable and the expected variance of that variable. For variables that are normally distributed the mean contains no information about the variance of the variable, but, for variables that are binomial (such as binary variables), the variance is necessarily small for variables with means near 0 or 1. This fact has implications in the interpretation of Eq. 1, the definition of the reliability coefficient. If the prevalence of a diagnosis is low in a population, then σ_T^2 will be small. If the level of error variance is held constant, but σ_T^2 is made smaller, then R_X will be smaller. One way to interpret this result is that the level of error must be reduced to study disorders that have smaller base rates in the population. Any randomly false-positive diagnosis makes the diagnostic system seem unreliable for rare disorders. In this case the diagnostic system is unreliable because the precious few true positives are swamped by the random false positives. Nevertheless, the fact that reliability is empirically related to prevalence has caused some commentators to question the utility of reliability measures in binary variables (Grove et al., 1981; Spitznagel and Helzer, 1985). My colleagues and I have argued that this line of questioning is misguided (Shrout et al., 1987).

In the next section I present a survey of reliability statistics that can be used to evaluate data from reliability studies. One of these is Cohen's κ. It is especially designed for categorical outcomes, but it shares with the quantitative statistics its interpretation as estimators of the reliability coefficient in Eq. 1. Although the special features of binary data require a careful consideration of the effects of errors in epidemiologic analyses, the general concerns for the concept of reliability as reviewed in the preceding sections are usually relevant for multivariate analyses that treat binary distinctions as dummy variables.

RELIABILITY STATISTICS: GENERAL

As we have seen, the reliability coefficient of Eq. 1 is defined in terms of variances: variances of systematic person characteristics σ_T^2 and variances of measurements across replications for a single person σ_E^2. There are several ways to estimate the variance ratio shown in Eq. 1 (Dunn, 1989), but one direct method is simply to estimate the separate variance components and then combine them in the form of Eq. 1. Estimates of this sort are called *intraclass correlations*.

Intraclass correlation is not a single statistic, but rather a family of statistics that can be used for estimating reliability. In this section I review several versions that can be used with a wide variety of variables. I focus here on the easiest part of reliability analysis, "point estimation" of the statistic that summarizes the reliability results. Although it is important, there is not space enough to present the methods that must be used to estimate 95% confidence intervals for the study results. The form of the interval estimators depends on the nature and distribution of the data (for information about confidence intervals, see Dunn, 1989; Fleiss, 1981; Shrout and Fleiss, 1979; Shrout and Skodol, in press).

The intraclass correlation estimates are derived from information summarized in the Analysis of Variance (ANOVA) of the data from the reliability study. The ANOVA treats each subject as a level of the SUBJECTS factor. Usually subjects are considered to be a *random factor*, because they are selected to be representative of a population of interest.

If the replicate measurements of the subjects are systematically obtained using a set of k raters or measuring devices, then the ANOVA might involve a two-way SUBJECTS by MEASURES design. If, on the other hand, the replicate measurements of each subject are obtained by randomly sampling k measures, then the analysis would use a one-way ANOVA.

One-Way ANOVA Analyses

Table 1 illustrates data that might be collected in reliability study of ratings made by informants, who in the example are relatives of the study subjects (probands). Each of $N = 10$ probands is rated by $k = 3$ distinct relatives. Between-subject variation can be estimated using all k ratings, and within-subject variation is used to estimate the magnitude of the error variation. When the relationships of the relatives varies from proband to proband, these data do not have a data analytic structure for informant (if there had been such a structure, we might have considered a proband-by-relationship two-way ANOVA). In our analysis we assume that the informants are essentially a random sample of possible informants for a given respondent.

Table 2 shows the layout of the one-way ANOVA, along with the numerical estimates obtained from the data in Table 1. The actual computation of the ANOVA results can be carried out by hand following textbooks such as Hays (1988) or can be obtained from standard computer software, such as SPSS RELIABILITY (e.g., Norusis, 1990). The numerical example illustrates a pattern in which the between-subjects' (probands') mean squares are substantially larger than the within-subjects' mean squares. Consistent with an informal examination of the hypothetical data in Table 1, this pattern suggests that the differences between subjects' mean ratings are larger than the disagreements among relatives regarding the subjects' scores.

The reliability estimate for the one-way ANOVA is calculated using the first formula in Part A of Table 3. This form of the intraclass correlation was called ICR(1, 1) by Shrout and Fleiss (1979), and I retain that designation. To illustrate the calculation with the numerical example from Table 1, we find that

$$\text{ICR}(1, 1) = (251.0 - 22.2)/(251.0 + 2*22.2) = 0.77.$$

This result describes the reliability of a single randomly selected informant. About 77% of the variance of a single informant's ratings is attributable to systematic differences between subjects. Although the stability of the result might be questioned because of the

**TABLE 1. Hypothetical Data on Functioning of 10
Probands by Three of Their Relatives**

Proband	Relatives		
	1	2	3
1	29	32	17
2	23	33	28
3	19	17	18
4	6	10	5
5	13	20	20
6	0	0	2
7	10	11	15
8	5	1	15
9	31	26	19
10	15	17	18

limited sample size, the result is encouraging that *this rating*, in *this population* appears to be made fairly reliably by a single informant.

Suppose that it is possible to obtain three informant ratings for each subject in the survey. How much more reliable would the average of the three ratings be than an individual informant? The answer can be calculated using the Spearman-Brown formula (Eq. 2), with $k = 3$ and $R_X = 0.77$. Alternatively, one can use the formula for ICR(1, k) shown in part B of Table 3. This formula is obtained by algebraically combining the expression for ICR(1, 1) with the Spearman-Brown formula. In this case the answer is ICR(1, k) = 0.91. About 91% of the variance of the average of three randomly chosen informants is attributable to systematic differences between subjects.

Two-Way ANOVA Analyses

Table 4 illustrates data that might be collected in a reliability study of two professional raters or interviewers. As a result of the interview by interviewer 1 we have both a binary diagnosis (disorder present [$X = 1$] vs. disorder absent [$X = 0$]) and a quantitative score such as a total functioning score (called Z in Table 4). Replicate scores and diagnoses are obtained by a second interviewer, interviewer 2. The hypothetical data on $X1$, $X2$, $Z1$, and $Z2$ are shown for 17 respondents. The layout of the two-way ANOVA is shown in Table 5, along with numerical results from the Table 4 examples.

Only two interviewers were used in the reliability study illustrated in Table 4, but we might consider the two to be a random sample from all possible interviewers from the

**TABLE 2. Analysis of Variance When Replications Are Nested Within Subjects:
One-way ANOVA**

Source of Variation	df	Sums of Squares	Mean Squares (MS)	Table 1 Example: MS on *df*
Between subjects	$n - 1$	BSS	BMS = BSS/($n - 1$)	BMS = 251.0 on 9 df
Within subjects	$n(k - 1)$	WSS	WMS = WSS/($n(k - 1)$)	WMS = 22.2 on 20 df

TABLE 3. Versions of Intraclass Correlation Statistics Useful for Various Reliability Designs

Type of Reliability	Raters Fixed or Random?	Version of Intraclass Correlation[a]
Part A: Reliability of single rater		
Nested: n subjects rated by k different raters	Random	$\text{ICR}(1,1) = \dfrac{\text{BMS} - \text{WMS}}{\text{BMS} + (k-1)\text{WMS}}.$
Subject by rater crossed design	Random	$\text{ICR}(2,1) = \dfrac{\text{TMS} - \text{EMS}}{\text{TMS} + (k-1)\text{EMS} + k(\text{JMS} - \text{EMS})/n}.$
Subject by rater crossed design	Fixed	$\text{ICR}(3,1) = \dfrac{\text{TMS} - \text{EMS}}{\text{TMS} + (k-1)\,\text{EMS}}.$
Part B: Reliability of the average of k ratings		
Nested: n subjects rated by k different raters	Random	$\text{ICR}(1,k) = \dfrac{\text{BMS} - \text{WMS}}{\text{BMS}}.$
Subject by rater crossed design	Random	$\text{ICR}(2,k) = \dfrac{\text{TMS} - \text{EMS}}{\text{TMS} + (\text{JMS} - \text{EMS})/n}.$
Subject by rater crossed design	Fixed	$\text{ICR}(3,k) = \dfrac{\text{TMS} - \text{EMS}}{\text{TMS}}.$

[a]BMS and WMS refer to between-subject and within-subject mean squares from a one-way ANOVA. TMS, JMS, and EMS refer to between-subjects (targets), between measures (judges), and error mean squares from two-way ANOVA based on n target-subjects and k raters.

study. If so, then they must *not* be selected on the basis of their special skills as interviewers, but rather should be selected to be representative. When interviewers who are employed in the reliability study represent the population of potential interviewers, we say that they are *random* effects.

In some cases we are interested in the ratings of specific interviewers rather than a population of interviewers. Suppose interviewer 1 is a doctoral candidate who carried out her own data collection and that interviewer 2 is a colleague who is hired to document that the ratings are systematic. In this case we simply wish to describe the quality of data collected by the doctoral candidate, and we say that the interviewers are *fixed* effects.

Depending on whether the raters are considered to be random or fixed, we use different versions of the intraclass correlation to estimate reliability. When we wish to estimate the reliability of a randomly sampled interviewer, we use the expression for ICR(2, 1) shown in Part A of Table 3. This intraclass correlation is not only a function of the between-subjects mean squares and the error mean squares, but also the between-measure (judge) mean squares. If different raters are more or less liberal in assigning high scores, then the final variability of the ratings will be affected. ICR(2, 1) takes this extra variation into account in estimating reliability.

TABLE 4. Hypothetical Data on Assessment of Depression and Functioning[a]

Respondent	X1	X2	Z3	Z2
1	0	1	17	11
2	1	1	17	15
3	0	0	26	25
4	0	0	24	22
5	0	0	19	14
6	0	0	22	16
7	0	0	17	18
8	0	0	23	19
9	1	0	19	16
10	0	1	18	12
11	0	0	21	18
12	1	1	13	11
13	0	0	21	23
14	0	0	22	17
15	0	0	15	12
16	0	0	20	18
17	0	0	21	20

[a]$X1$ and $X2$ represent test–retest diagnoses of major depression ($X = 1$, present; $X = 0$, not present), and $Z1$ and $Z2$ represent ratings of adaptive functioning.

In the two examples of Table 4, one reveals a large between-measure effect and the other does not. From the numbers in Table 4 it can be seen that the $Z2$ ratings are usually smaller than the $Z1$ ratings. Rater 2 seems to believe that most subjects are functioning somewhat worse than perceived by rater 1. Even with this rater difference, the reliability of Z is higher than the reliability of X, according to the data in Table 4. The ICR(2, 1) for Z is calculated as

$$(25.7 - 2.67)/(25.7 + [1]*2.67 + 2*[67.8 - 2.67]/17) = 0.64.$$

The ICR(2, 1) for X is calculated as

$$(0.254 - 0.092)/(0.254 + [1]*0.092 + 2*[0.029 - 0.092]/17) = 0.48.$$

For the rating of adaptive functioning we could consider averaging both individual Z ratings to obtain a more reliable score. We can use either the Spearman-Brown formula, or the expression ICR(2, k) to calculate the reliability of the mean of two such ratings. In this case, the result is 0.78 rather than 0.64.

Although the reliability of the binary X variable is worse than that of the quantitative Z variable, it would not usually be meaningful to rely on an average diagnosis instead of a truly binary rating. For this reason for ICR(2, k) form of the intraclass correlation would not be applied to X in Table 4.

The calculations carried out thus far have assumed that the two sets of ratings in Table 4 are representative of a host of possible interviewers. Now we turn our attention to the

TABLE 5. Analysis of Variance When Replications Have Structure: Two-way ANOVA

Source of Variation	df	Sums of Squares	Mean Squares (MS)	Table 4 Example: MS on df
Between subjects (targets)	$n-1$	TSS	$TMS = TSS/(n-1)$	Variable X: 0.254 on 16 df Variable Z: 25.7 on 16 df
Between measures (judges)	$(k-1)$	JSS	$JMS = JSS/(k-1)$	Variable X: 0.29 on 1 df Variable Z: 67.8 on 1 df
Residual (error)	$(n-1)(k-1)$	ESS	$EMS = \dfrac{ESS}{(n-1)(k-1)}$	Variable X: 0.092 on 16 df Variable Z: 2.67 on 16 df

situation in which the two raters can be considered to be fixed. In this case we can either ignore systematic rater differences in mean ratings or we can adjust for them.

The expression for ICR(3, 1) in part A of Table 3 is appropriate when we wish to describe the reliability of a single fixed rater. Unlike ICR(2, 1), this version of the intraclass correlation is not affected by the between-rater mean squares. On the average, ICR(3, 1) will be larger in magnitude than ICR(2, 1). By fixing the raters to certain persons, the extraneous variation due to sampling of raters is eliminated and the resulting reliability is usually higher.

This effect is especially obvious for Z, which had a large between-rater effect. The ICR(3, 1) for Z is calculated as

$$(25.7 - 2.67)/(25.7 + [1]*2.67) = 0.81.$$

ICR(3, 1) for X is not much different than ICR(2, 1), as the rater effects were small:

$$(0.254 - 0.092)/(0.254 + [1]*0.092) = 0.47.$$

The Reliability of the Average of k Fixed Measures: Cronbach's α

Just as ICR(1, 1) and ICR(2, 1) can be used in the Spearman-Brown formula to determine how much reliability improves by using an average score, so can ICR(3, 1) be used when an average measurement is of interest. In this case the reliability of the averaged measurement can be computed directly using ICR(3, k) from Table 3. For the quantitative Z variable, the reliability of the average is expected to be 0.90.

One common application of ICR(3, k) is to internal consistency analyses of psychometric scales. Items in self-report questionnaires are usually fixed in that the same items are used with all respondents. Suppose that n subjects are administered k scale items, and the results are analyzed using the two-way ANOVA layout of Table 5. The estimate of the reliability of the sum or average of the k fixed items can be computed using ICR(3, k). The result is identical to the internal consistency estimate known as Cronbach's α (Cronbach,

1951). α is computed directly by computer programs such as SPSS RELIABILITY (Norusis, 1990).

OTHER RELIABILITY STATISTICS

Cohen's κ

When binary data such as those for variable X in Table 4 are collected, reliability can be estimated directly using Cohen's κ (Cohen, 1960). Fleiss and Cohen (1973) showed that κ is conceptually equivalent to ICR(2, 1) in Table 3. It can be calculated simply using the entries of a 2×2 table showing the diagnostic agreement. In general, this agreement table might be laid out as follows:

	Rater 1:		Total
Rater 2	$+$	$-$	
$+$	a	b	$a + b$
$-$	c	d	$c + d$
Total	$a + c$	$b + d$	n

Cohen (1960) pointed out that while cells a and d represent agreement, it is not sufficient to evaluate reliability by reporting the overall proportion of agreement, $P_O = (a + d)/n$. This statistic may be large even if raters assigned diagnoses by flipping coins or rolling dice. The κ statistic adjusts for simple chance mechanisms:

$$\kappa = \frac{P_o - P_c}{1 - P_c},$$

where P_O is the observed agreement due to chance:

$$P_c = [(a + c)(a + b) + (b + d)(c + d)]/n^2.$$

When computing κ by hand, it is sometimes more convenient to use the following equivalent expression:

$$\kappa = \frac{ad - bc}{ad - bc + n\,(b + c)/2}.$$

When the X data in Table 4 are tabulated into a 2×2 table like that shown above, we get $a = 2$, $b = 2$, $c = 1$, and $d = 12$. The observed agreement, $P_O = 0.82$, but the expected agreement by chance is $P_C = 0.67$. Using either of the expressions for κ, we find the reliability to be 0.46. As expected, this is quite close to the value of 0.48 obtained using ICR(2, 1).

One advantage of calculating the reliability of binary judgments using κ instead of intraclass correlation methods is that the expressions for κ's standard error and confidence bounds are explicitly suited to binary data (Hale and Fleiss, 1993). κ can also be generalized to describe the overall reliability of a classification into multiple categories. Fleiss (1981) provides an overview of many forms of κ.

Product Moment Correlation

If the reliability study yields two measurements, and if the raters are considered to be fixed (rather than representative of a pool of raters), then reliability can be estimated by computing the product moment correlation between the two measures. This is the usual correlation statistic built into most computer programs and calculators. When the ratings are quantitative, the correlation is known as the *Pearson correlation*, and when the ratings are binary it is known as the *phi coefficient*. Regardless of what they are called, they are comparable to the ICR(3, 1) version of the intraclass correlation described above. For the Z variables the Pearson correlation is $r_p = 0.83$, and for the X variables in Table 4 the phi coefficient is $r_p = 0.47$. These are very close to the ICR(3, 1) values of 0.81 and 0.47 obtained on the same data.

SUMMARY AND CONCLUSIONS

Unreliability is a measurement problem that can often be rectified by improving interview procedures or by using statistical sums or averages of replicate measures. Determining the extent to which unreliability is a problem, however, can be challenging. There are various designs for estimating reliability, but virtually all have some biases and shortcomings. Moreover, different reliability statistics are needed to analyze the reliability data, and the choice of the statistic depends both on the design of the study and on whether the measures are considered to be fixed or representative of a population.

I recommend that reliability studies be considered critically with an eye for ways that measurement quality can be improved. Specifically, if the reliability of a measure appears to be very good, ask whether there are biases in the reliability design that might bias the results optimistically. Were the respondents sampled in the same way in the reliability study that they will be in the field study? Was the respondent given the chance to be inconsistent, or did the replication make use of archived information? If serious biases are not found, then one can put the issue of reliability to rest, at least for the study at hand.

If the reliability of a measure appears to be poor, one should also look for biases in the reliability design. How similar were the replications? Could the poor reliability results be an artifact of legitimate changes over time, heterogeneous items within a scale, or artificially different measurement conditions? Was the sample size large enough to be sure that reliability is in fact bad? One should be especially suspicious if there is evidence of validity of a measure that is purported to be unreliable. Rather than dismissing a measure with apparently poor reliability, ask whether it can be improved to eliminate noise.

REFERENCES

American Psychiatric Association (1980): "Diagnostic and Statistical Manual of Mental Disorders," 3rd ed. Washington, DC: American Psychiatric Association.

Anthony JC, Folstein M, Romanoski AJ, Von Korff MR, Newstadt GR, Chahal R, Merchant A, Brown CH, Shapiro S, Kramer M, Gruenberg EM (1985): Comparison of the lay Diagnostic Interview Schedule and a standardized psychiatric diagnosis. Arch Gen Psychiatry 42:667–675.

Brown W (1910): Some experimental results in the correlation of mental abilities. Br J Psychol 3:296–322.

Carey G, Gottesman II (1978): Reliability and validity in binary ratings: Areas of common misunderstanding in diagnosis and symptom ratings. Arch Gen Psychiatry 35:1454–1459.

Cohen J (1960): A coefficient of agreement for nominal scales. Educ Psychol Measurement 20:37–46.

Cronbach LJ (1951): Coefficient alpha and the internal structure of tests. Psychometrika 16:297–334.

Cronbach LJ, Gleser GC, Nanda H, Rajaratnam N (1972): "The Dependability of Behavioral Measurements: Theory of Generalizability for Scores and Profiles." New York: Wiley.

Dunn G (1989): "Design and Analysis of Reliability Studies." New York: Oxford University Press.

Endicott J, Spitzer RL, Fleiss JL, et al. (1976): The Global Assessment Scale: A procedure for measuring overall severity of psychiatric disturbance. Arch Gen Psychiatry 33:766–771.

Fleiss JL (1981): "Statistical Methods for Rates and Proportions," 2nd ed. New York: Wiley.

Fleiss JL, Cohen J (1973): The equivalence of weighted kappa and the intraclass correlation coefficient as measures of reliability. Educ Psychol Measurement 33:613–619.

Fleiss JL, Shrout PE (1989): Reliability considerations in planning diagnostic validity studies. In Robbins L (ed): "The Validity of Psychiatric Diagnoses." New York: Guilford Press, pp 279–329.

Grove WM, Andreason NC, McDonald-Scott P, Keller MB, Shapiro RW (1981): Reliability studies of psychiatric diagnosis: Theory and practice. Arch Gen Psychiatry 38:408–413.

Hale CA, Fleiss JL (1993): Interval estimation under two study designs for kappa with binary classifications. Biometrics 49:523–534.

Hays WL (1988): "Statistics," 4th ed. Fort Worth, TX: Holt, Rinehart & Winston.

Helzer JE, Robins LN, McEvoy LT, Spitznagel EL, Stoltzman RK, Farmer A, Brockington IF (1985): A comparison of clinical and Diagnostic Interview Schedule diagnoses: Physician reexamination of lay-interviewed cases in the general population. Arch Gen Psychiatry 42:657–666.

Jannarone RJ, Macera CA, Garrison CZ (1987): Evaluating interrater agreement through "case–control" sampling. Biometrics 43:433–437.

Kraemer HC (1979): Ramifications of a population model for kappa as a coefficient of reliability. Psychometrika 44:461–472.

Landis JR, Koch GG (1977): The measurement of observer agreement for categorical data. Biometrics 33: 159–174.

Lord FM, Novick MR (1968): "Statistical Theories of Mental Test Scores." Reading, MA: Addison-Wesley.

Norusis MJ (1990): "SPSS/PC+ Statistics 4.0." Chicago: SPSS Inc.

Shavelson RJ, Webb NM (1991): "Generalizability Theory: A Primer." Newbury Park, CA: Sage.

Shrout PE, Fleiss JL (1979): Intraclass correlations: Uses in assessing rater reliability. Psychol Bull 86:420–428.

Shrout PE, Skodol AE (1994): "Measuring Psychopathology." New York: Oxford University Press.

Shrout PE, Spitzer RL, Fleiss JL (1987): Quantification of agreement in psychiatric diagnosis revisited. Arch Gen Psychiatry 44:172–177.

Spearman C (1910): Correlation calculated from faulty data. Br J Psychol 3:271–295.

Spitzer RL (1983): Psychiatric diagnosis: Are clinicians still necessary? Comprehensive Psychiatry 24:399–411.

Spitznagel EL, Helzer JE (1985): A proposed solution to the base rate problem in the kappa statistic. Arch Gen Psychiatry 42:725–728.

CHAPTER 10

Validity: Definitions and Applications to Psychiatric Research

JILL M. GOLDSTEIN and JOHN C. SIMPSON

Harvard Medical School Department of Psychiatry, Institute of Psychiatric Epidemiology and Genetics, Massachusetts Mental Health Center, Brockton/West Roxbury VA Medical Center, Psychiatry Service, Brockton, MA 02401

INTRODUCTION

Measurement is a process of linking unobservable theoretical concepts to empirical indicators (Carmines and Zeller, 1979). There are two basic properties of measurement that ensure the strength of this linkage: reliability and validity. In this chapter, we discuss the concept and usage of validity. Reliability was discussed fully in a previous chapter, but, for convenience, we define it here simply as the reproducibility of an empirical measure (e.g., internal consistency of the items in a scale, reproducibility of a measurement on different occasions, or agreement between raters). For an empirical indicator to be valid it must first be reliable, but indicators can be reliable without also being valid.

There are a number of ways to assess validity, not all of which are used for every measure of interest. In fact, validity has a number of meanings in different contexts and is perhaps one of the most overused words in the scientific literature. In this chapter, we discuss validity as it applies to the measurement of a construct, i.e., the process of "construct validity." We also discuss validity as it applies to relationships between constructs, i.e., to the "internal validity" and "external validity" of a presumed causal relationship. We provide examples of how validity is applied and statistically evaluated in psychiatric research.

VALIDITY OF A CONSTRUCT

An essential feature of scientific research is often the measurement of abstract concepts and relationships between abstract concepts. *Validity* can be defined as the extent to which an empirical indicator of a concept actually represents the concept of interest (Cronbach and Meehl, 1955; Anastasi, 1976; Nunnally, 1978). For example, if one used a

Textbook in Psychiatric Epidemiology, Edited by Tsuang, Tohen, and Zahner
ISBN 0-471-59375-3 © 1995 Wiley-Liss, Inc.

particular symptom checklist to measure "major depressive disorder," validity asks the question, how accurate is this empirical indicator for diagnosing major depressive disorder? Thus, validity refers to the questions "for what purpose is the indicator being used?" (e.g., to diagnose major depressive disorder) and "how accurate is it for that purpose?" In fact, an indicator (e.g., an instrument such as a test, a rating, or an interview) can be valid for one purpose, but not for another (Carmines and Zeller, 1979; Cronbach, 1971). Thus, one validates the instrument *in relation to its intended purpose* (Cronbach, 1971; Nunnally, 1978; Carmines and Zeller, 1979). If an instrument is to be scientifically useful, it must be both reliable (i.e., result in consistent findings over repeated measurements) and valid (i.e., represent the concept it is intended to represent).

Unlike reliability, validity is an unending process (Nunnally, 1978) in which one attempts to capture the essence of the concept of interest as accurately as possible. It therefore involves a theoretical understanding of the concept of interest in order to measure it accurately. It also involves an assessment of the empirical relationships between an instrument and criteria chosen to evaluate whether the instrument assesses what it is intended to assess. There are three basic ways in which validity is assessed: content validity, criterion validity, and construct validity.

Content Validity

For every abstract concept, there is a universe of items that one might sample in order to measure the concept operationally. *Content validity* involves the adequacy with which one samples the domain of items (Nunnally, 1978). Content validity is ensured by the procedures used to construct items for a test (Nunnally, 1978). One must first specify the universe of items that one hypothesizes will accurately measure the concept of interest. Second, items are then sampled from this domain. If certain kinds of items are central to understanding the concept, one may decide to oversample these types. Finally, selected items are put into a testable form (Carmines and Zeller, 1979).

For example, if one were interested in measuring (diagnosing) "schizophrenia," one would choose, among other things, items such as bizarre delusions or other types of delusions, various kinds of hallucinations, formal thought disorder, and flat affect. An instrument would then be constructed in order to assess these items. Different types of diagnostic instruments have been constructed that are based on certain assumptions about how to acquire accurate assessments of the items.

For example, the Diagnostic Interview Schedule (DIS) (Robins et al., 1981) was designed to allow lay interviewers to assess symptom items in a dichotomous form, i.e., as present or absent, and was wholly dependent on the patient's response to each item. That is, there was an assumption that clinical judgement was unnecessary to assess symptomatology. In contrast, the Schedule for Affective Disorders and Schizophrenia (SADS) (Endicott and Spitzer, 1978) was designed to allow for clinical questioning to assess symptom items. Clinical/diagnostic knowledge was required in order to use the SADS instrument. In addition, ratings of SADS items consisted of a severity scale rather than present versus absent, as in the DIS. As one can see, these two instruments are based on different assumptions regarding how to assess a similar domain of symptom items. One can then assess the content validity of these two approaches, even though the evaluation of content validity alone would provide an incomplete assessment of the validity of these instruments.

There are two standards by which content validity is assessed: the representativeness of the collection of items chosen and the type of test construction used to measure the concept. There are, however, no statistical means of assessing content validity. Essentially, content validity is dependent on appeals to reason regarding the accuracy of the content sampled, or a consensus among experts, and the adequacy with which the items are put into a testable form (Nunnally, 1978; Cronbach and Meehl, 1955).

Examples of Assessment of Content Validity

Streiner (1993) recommended the use of a "content validity matrix" as a means of ensuring that items in a scale are appropriately tapping the intended domains. In such a matrix, each column represents a distinct domain within the general domain of interest, and each row represents a single item. As a means of improving reliability, each domain is represented by several items (i.e., in terms of the content validity matrix, each column should have check marks in several rows). On the other hand, to minimize ambiguity of interpretation, each item should tap only one domain (i.e., each row should have only a single check mark).

As an example of the relevance of domains and items to content validity, we can make use of a study by Schwartz et al. (1975), who devised the Social Adjustment Interview Schedule to investigate outcome in schizophrenia. Within this general domain, the authors conceptually identified eight role areas (i.e., domains) and devised multiple questions (i.e., items) within each role area to address performance and subjective feelings. The different domains included work role (18 items), household role (15 items), marital role (nine items), and social and leisure roles (54 items). Typical items within the work domain included the questions "Are you employed now?" and "Are you confident about your ability to do the job?" Within the marital domain, typical items included "In general, how do you and your spouse get along?" and "Have you been able to talk about feelings and problems with your spouse recently?" There would probably be little disagreement about content validity in this example. In other words, most would agree that these four questions comprise two sets of items, that the first two items are related to work roles, whereas the latter two concern marital roles, and furthermore that there is little if any overlap between the content of these specific items.

Not all applications of content validity will be as straightforward, particularly if the concepts being measured are abstract, i.e., not directly observable. For example, Cloninger (1987) devised an 80 item self-report inventory called the Tridimensional Personality Questionnaire (TPQ) to investigate three hypothesized dimensions of personality: harm avoidance, novelty seeking, and reward dependence. Cloninger's approach to content validity is apparent in his description of how the items were devised (p 580): "To quantify behavioral variation on each dimension separately, questions were specified that were theoretically expected to involve minimal interaction among the dimensions. In practice, this meant that questions were chosen to evaluate the behaviors that were thought to be characteristic of individuals deviant on one dimension and average on the others." As evidence that this standard was achieved, Cloninger reported that the intercorrelations among the three major TPQ scales (calculated using the Pearson product-moment correlation coefficient) were "negligible or weak" and low relative to the reported index of internal consistency (Cronbach's α coefficient; see Chapter 9 for a discussion in the context of reliability). However, the interpretation of these results is complicated because weak intercorrelations were expected in some cases for theoretical reasons (e.g., a weak negative correlation between novelty seeking and harm avoidance).

A somewhat different perspective was presented by Takeuchi et al. (1993), who translated the TPQ into Japanese and replicated Cloninger's study (1987) using a large sample of Japanese university students. Like Cloninger (1987), Takeuchi et al. (1993) reported negligible or weak intercorrelations between the three major scales. However, they also reported results from a factor analysis that were not completely consistent with the theoretical model. (Factor analysis is a multivariate statistical procedure that is used to explain covariation among a set of observed variables in terms of a reduced number of unobserved, latent variables; e.g., see Kim and Mueller, 1978, for an introductory explanation). Within the framework of Streiner's content validity matrix (1993), for example, if each derived factor was considered to define a separate domain (i.e., column) in the matrix, then the harm avoidance, novelty seeking, and reward dependence items should have loaded on different factors. While this was by and large the result for harm avoidance and reward dependence, "the novelty seeking scale showed a scattering factor structure, with several equivocal items loaded on two or more factors; reduction or reorganization of items might be required here" (Takeuchi et al., 1993, p. 277). On the other hand, all reported items had factor loadings above the cutoff of 0.4 on only one of the six factors, and this was consistent with Streiner's ideal (1993) of only one check mark per item in the content validity matrix.

Criterion Validity

The second type of validity is referred to as *criterion validity* (or *predictive validity*). It is concerned with measuring something that is *external* to the measurement of the concept itself, called the *criterion* (Cronbach and Meehl, 1955; Nunnally, 1978). For example, one dimension of predictive criterion validity for psychiatric diagnoses is to relate them to predictions of outcome. (Examples of this are discussed in detail later in this chapter.) Unlike content validity, which essentially depends on a consensus among experts, predictive validity is dependent on empirical results. *Predictive validity* refers to the empirical relationships between the instrument under study and external events or behaviors that can occur at three points in time: before, during, or after the instrument is used. In many studies, the empirical relationship is statistically estimated by a correlation if continuous data are used.

Post-dictive validity refers to correlating events/behaviors that have occurred in the past with the instrument one is presently using. These assessments are referred to as *retrospective*. For example, one might have a specific prediction about the early developmental history of patients, with a particular diagnosis that is being currently assessed with an instrument. Post-dictive validity entails correlating early history information with the diagnostic assessment currently obtained using the instrument under study.

Concurrent validity refers to correlating a measure and some criterion *at the same point in time*. This involves what are known as *cross-sectional assessments*. Thus, for example, if there were a laboratory test for diagnosing major depressive disorder, one could correlate the instrument used to diagnose the disorder with a laboratory test taken when the patient was interviewed.

The form of predictive validity most commonly referred to correlates a measure with a criterion that is assessed at some *future point in time*. This form of validity entails prospective assessments. A common use of predictive validity in psychiatry is to assess outcomes of a specific diagnostic group under study, under the assumption that certain diagnostic groups have worse or better outcomes than others (see examples below).

A fourth form of criterion validity is referred to as *discriminant validity*. Discriminant validity assesses whether certain external criteria (i.e., events or behaviors) are uncorrelated with the measure of interest compared with other criteria that are hypothesized to be related to the measure of interest. That is, is the measure of interest uncorrelated with events or behavior with which one expects it would be independent? This has also been referred to as *assessing the specificity* of the relationship between the measure of the concept of interest and the external criteria chosen to relate to the concept.

It is important to mention here that criterion validity is often assessed using correlations (when continuous data are involved). The strength of the correlation is often interpreted as the strength of the validity of the measure. However, the strength of the correlation depends not only on the variability and other characteristics of the measure of interest, including its reliability, but also on the choice, measurement, and reliability of the criterion.

Examples of Criterion Validity

For examples of applications of criterion validity, we turn to two recent studies in the psychiatric literature. The first study (Addington et al., 1993) provides a fairly typical example of the use of correlational techniques. At issue was whether a self-report instrument can be used in populations of schizophrenic patients to obtain valid ratings of depression. To examine this question, the authors compared self-report ratings obtained using the Beck Depression Inventory (BDI) with ratings of the Calgary Depression Scale (CDS), a semistructured interview designed to assess depression in schizophrenics. In this study, the CDS is the criterion because it makes use of informed judgements by trained clinicians, which form the current "gold standard" for identifying depression in clinical populations. BDI and CDS scores were compared by calculating the Pearson product-moment correlation coefficient (e.g., see Woolson, 1987), after creating scatterplots to examine the joint distribution of BDI and CDS scores as well as identifying any outliers. The latter step was essential because the presence of even a single outlier (i.e., an extreme and atypical value) could easily distort the product-moment correlation (e.g., see Simpson, 1982).

Another important methodologic step employed by Addington et al. (1993) was to compare correlations between the BDI and CDS in clinically distinct subgroups of schizophrenic patients: inpatients vs. outpatients, and (within these subgroups) patients who either did or did not require assistance in completing the self-report instrument. In this particular study, the correlation between the BDI and CDS was stronger among inpatients than outpatients, regardless of whether the patients required assistance ($r = 0.84$ vs. $r = 0.96$). However, the substantially greater percentage of inpatients requiring assistance (34% of inpatients vs. 12% of the outpatients) led the authors to conclude that "depressed affect can be assessed in schizophrenics by both self-report and structured interview, but the Beck Depression Inventory poses difficulties in use with inpatients" (Addington et al., 1993, p. 561).

For our purposes, however, the substantive findings of this study were less important than the fact that this study admirably illustrated the critical importance of selecting and describing validation samples that are clinically meaningful in the context of the measurement instrument of interest (Streiner, 1993). In particular, users of such instruments need to be aware that published validation studies might have used "samples of convenience" (e.g., university students) that do not approximate the clinical population the user has in mind and that the results of such studies do not necessarily generalize to other samples.

Our second example of criterion validity in psychiatric research (Somervell et al., 1993) also illustrates the critical importance of the validation sample. In this study, the validity of using a questionnaire (the Center for Epidemiologic Studies Depression Scale, or CES-D) (Radloff, 1977) as a case identification tool in studies of mood disorders among Native Americans was investigated. CES-D scores were compared with DSM-III-R diagnoses (American Psychiatric Association, 1987) based on a structured psychiatric interview (the Lifetime Version of the Schedule for Affective Disorders and Schizophrenia; Endicott and Spitzer, 1978). The authors had concerns about the cross-cultural applicability not only of the screening instrument but also of the criterion itself (e.g., DSM-III-R diagnoses of affective disorders). For purposes of the study, however, it was assumed that DSM-III-R diagnoses would be relevant among American Indians.

Although the CES-D, like the BDI in the above example, yields a numerical score, its proposed use as a screening instrument for depression was for the purpose of identifying not the degree of depression, but the presence of a particular clinical syndrome, namely, DSM-III-R major depression. The criterion was therefore a categorical (i.e., qualitative) rating rather than a numerical (i.e., quantitative) rating, making it inappropriate to use correlational procedures. Instead, to evaluate the validity of the instrument for case identification, the authors employed statistical methods that have been expressly developed for qualitative data, including sensitivity, specificity, and receiver operating characteristic (ROC) analysis.

Sensitivity and specificity are both calculated using data that have been summarized in a 2 × 2 table of frequencies (see Table 1 for definitions and computational formulas). In the example at hand, a 2 × 2 table was used to cross-classify the numbers of screened persons with and without the criterion (e.g., a DSM-III-R diagnosis of major depression) who either did or did not score above the cut-off for depression in the screening instrument, the CES-D. (ROC analysis was used to determine the optimal cut-off value for the CES-D.) As an illustrative finding, the sensitivity for DSM-III-R major depression was 100% (i.e., all three persons in the sample with a diagnosis of major depression scored

TABLE 1. Computation of Indices of Criterion Validity and Predictive Value[a]

| Rating | Criterion | | Total |
	Present	Absent	
Positive	a	b	a + b
Negative	c	d	c + d
Total	a + c	b + d	N

[a]a, b, c, d, and N are frequencies (e.g., numbers of persons rated). Sensitivity = a/(a + c); the probability of a positive rating among those possessing the criterion. Specificity = d/(b + d); the probability of a negative rating among those lacking the criterion. Positive predictive value = a/(a + b); the probability of having the criterion among those with positive ratings. Negative predictive value = d/(c + d); the probability that those with negative ratings will not have the criterion. Prevalence = (a + c)/N the base rate of the criterion in the validation sample.

above the cut-off on the CES-D). The corresponding value of specificity was 82% (i.e., 82% of those persons in the sample who did not have diagnoses of major depression scored below the CES-D cut off for depression). It follows directly from the reported specificity value of 82% that 18% (100% − 82%) of the persons in the sample with no psychiatric diagnoses or with DSM-III-R diagnoses other than major depression scored *above* the CES-D cutoff and would have been classified as depressed by that screening instrument.

Whether or not this degree of misclassification error (or invalidity) is considered to be an unacceptably high "false-positive rate" depends on the proposed use of the instrument and on the comparable "operating characteristics" of alternative instruments. For example, a higher CES-D cut-off value could be expected to decrease the false-positive rate (via increased specificity), but at the expense of sensitivity. In this particular study, a higher CES-D cut-off actually increased specificity without decreasing sensitivity, but this was probably attributable to the small number of cases with DSM-III-R diagnoses of major depression. In most studies there is a systematic trade-off between sensitivity and specificity, and for that reason both of these indices of criterion validity must be considered together in determining whether a particular instrument is more valid than the available alternatives. ROC analysis provides a useful framework for making such comparisons (e.g., see Murphy et al., 1987). In the present example, the non-negligible false-positive rate was consistent with the investigators' concerns (based on previous research by a number of researchers using other samples) that the CES-D might be reflecting symptoms of not only major depression but also increased levels of anxiety, demoralization, or even physical ill health (Somervell et al., 1993).

The study by Somervell et al. (1993) also illustrates the difference between criterion validity and the related, but nevertheless distinct, concept of predictive value. *Positive predictive value* is literally the predictive value of a positive rating, i.e., the probability of having the criterion of interest *given* a positive rating on the instrument under investigation. (Formulas for calculating positive predictive value, and the related index, negative predictive value, are given in Table 1.) Since the criterion (e.g., DSM-III-R major depression) is frequently of more direct clinical importance than the rating (e.g., a particular CES-D score), positive and negative predictive values are often more clinically meaningful than sensitivity and specificity. For example, most clinicians would probably be more interested in the usefulness of the CES-D for predicting major depression than the other way around. However, positive predictive value is a joint function of sensitivity, specificity, and prevalence, such that low prevalence values can severely constrain the values of positive predictive value that can be realistically attained, even with very high sensitivity and specificity values (Baldessarini et al., 1983; Glaros and Kline, 1988). (Negative predictive value is similarly constrained by high prevalence values.)

In the study by Somervell et al. (1993), the prevalence of major depression can be estimated from the rate of major depression in the sample as $3/120 = 0.025$. Using a cut-off value of 16 on the CES-D, the reported specificity value of 82.1% therefore corresponds to a positive predictive value of 0.125. In other words, even though sensitivity was perfect (100%) and specificity was very high, only one of every eight persons who scored above the CES-D cut-off of 16 would be expected actually to have major depression. Even increasing the CES-D cut-off to improve specificity would not dramatically change this result. Again, this is due to the constraint imposed by the low estimated prevalence of major depression in the study population. (With the CES-D cutoff set at 28, the reported specificity value of 96.6% corresponds to a positive predictive value of 0.429.) In conclusion, this example shows that even though an instrument may have excellent criterion validity as assessed using standard indices (namely, sensitivity and specificity), the actual predictive value of the instrument could be much more limited, depending on the prevalence of the disorder of interest, which in turn may vary with the composition of the validation sample.

Construct Validity

Of the three basic types of validity, *construct validity* involves the most complex process. Content validity and criterion validity used alone are limited in contributing to understanding the relationship between the theoretical (unobserved) concept and the empirical measure used to indicate it. In fact, content and criterion validity are considered part of the process of assessing construct validity. As first pointed out by Cronbach and Meehl (1955), construct validity is essential for all abstract concepts, since there is no criterion or entire content of a domain that is wholly adequate to define the concept of interest. Construct validity is thus defined in a theoretical context. It is the extent to which one's measure of interest is related to other theoretically related concepts that are also measured (Nunnally, 1978; Carmines and Zeller, 1979).

There are three steps to assessing construct validity (Carmines and Zeller, 1979). First, one must have an understanding of the theoretical relationships between related concepts. Second, one must estimate the empirical relationships between operational measures of these concepts. Finally, the empirical evidence must be interpreted within the theoretical context in which the concept of interest is embedded. In addition, findings from other studies must be related to one's current findings regarding the measure and the concept it is intended to indicate. The theoretical context allows one to make theoretical predictions that then lead to empirical tests using the operational measure of the concept of interest. One study cannot wholly validate a measure of a concept. Construct validity requires a pattern of consistent findings across studies involving different samples and different settings.

Cronbach and Meehl (1955) refer to the theoretical context as the *nomologic network*. The use of the nomologic network requires relating theoretical constructs to each other, theoretical constructs to empirical indicators, and empirical indicators to each other. The construct is not reduced to the empirical indicators; it is combined with other constructs in the nomological net that allow for predictions using the empirical indicators (Cronbach and Meehl, 1953, p. 290).

Application of Construct Validity to Psychiatric Diagnosis

In psychiatry, there are no known laboratory tests for wholly identifying a psychiatric case. In 1972, Robins and Guze established five criteria that have become standards for validating a diagnosis. Kendler (1990) recently reviewed these standards for psychiatric diagnoses and pointed out a number of potential limitations to this approach. For example, he discusses the frequent need to take "fundamentally nonempirical" matters into consideration in formulating and using psychiatric diagnoses. Such matters can include, for example, various clinical, historical, and administrative issues, needs, and imperatives. For purposes of this discussion, however, we consider only the empirical criteria originally proposed by Robins and Guze (1972).

The first criterion of Robins and Guze (1972) consists of establishing the clinical description of the disorder. This involves specifying the phenomenology or symptomatology, premorbid history, age at onset, sociodemographic distribution, and precipitating factors. The clinical description criterion thus involves issues of content validity. For example, what is the domain of symptoms chosen to represent the diagnosis? "On the face of it," do these symptoms reasonably represent the domain of interest? Furthermore, how would one construct an instrument to assess these symptoms? The clinical description criterion also involves criterion validity. For example, post-dictive validity would be relating premorbid history, age at onset, or precipitating factors to the measure of diagnosis.

The second criterion refers to the relationship of the diagnostic measure to laboratory tests. As mentioned earlier, this is a form of concurrent validity. Laboratory tests may include chemical, anatomic, physiologic, or psychological tests (Robins and Guze, 1972). In psychiatry, however, at present there are no laboratory "gold standards" for validating diagnoses.

The third criterion involves the use of family history to contribute to validation. The assumption behind the use of family history is that many psychiatric disorders run in families. Thus, an increased prevalence of the same disorder in family members can be used as an indicator that the diagnosis is a valid entity. Family history can be thought of as a concurrent validator (in reference to ill relatives who are currently alive) or as a post-dictive validator (in reference to relatives who were ill but who are now decreased).

The fourth criterion, commonly thought of as predictive validity in psychiatric research, relates the diagnosis of interest to outcomes, including treatment response. The assumption behind using this criterion is that individuals with the same diagnosis will have similar outcomes. Furthermore, it is sometimes assumed that certain diagnostic groups have particularly poor or good outcomes compared with other diagnostic groups. However, the use of outcome as a validating criterion is problematic because many psychiatric disorders have heterogeneous outcomes. This validating criterion will remain controversial unless more definitive knowledge regarding the specific outcomes of diagnostic groups can be elaborated.

The final criterion for validating a diagnosis involves assessing the specificity of the other criteria for a particular diagnosis. This can be referred to as *discriminant validity*. Although different diagnoses may share, for example, certain symptoms, laboratory test results, or outcomes, it is the role of discriminant validity to specify how a particular disorder is differentiated from other disorders. If it cannot be differentiated from other disorders, this becomes support for rejecting the validity of this particular diagnosis as a separate entity.

In summary, the assessment of the validity of a diagnosis cannot be accomplished in one study. As discussed with construct validity, it is an ongoing process that requires multiple studies, using different samples, across different settings. One must relate empirical evidence regarding the five criteria to each other, driven by a theory of how and why these findings "fit together" in predicted ways. The theory is the basis for developing appropriate empirical measures. The relationships between empirical measures of one's concepts of interest will contribute to testing empirically one's theory about the concept.

Threats to Construct Validity

There are a number of threats to construct validity. We will briefly mention three of the most important that are discussed in detail by Cook and Campbell (1979): inadequate theoretical conceptualization, mono-operations bias, and mono-methods bias. Inadequate theoretical conceptualization leads to the development of empirical measures that do not adequately assess one's concept of interest. An inadequate representation of the concept of interest may also result from the other two threats to construct validity. *Mono-operations bias* refers to the use of an inadequate number of empirical items used to measure a particular concept, e.g., if only one question was asked to measure the concept. *Mono-methods bias* refers to the inadequate use of methods to obtain empirical information on the criterion of interest. That is, the use of different methods to obtain empirical information on the same criterion will increase the reliability of that information and thus contribute to the validity of the use of that empirical data to measure the concept of interest. For example, to assess a research psychiatric diagnosis, the use of a standardized structured interview in combination with medical record review and informed clinical judgement may provide the most valid assessment of the diagnosis.

VALIDITY OF THE RELATIONSHIPS BETWEEN VARIABLES

The second use of the term *validity* that we discuss in this chapter refers to the "internal and external validity" of the empirical relationships between measures used to assess abstract concepts. Internal and external validity are discussed thoroughly by Cook and Campbell (1979) in relation to quasiexperimental design studies. They are also discussed in basic textbooks on epidemiology (MacMahon and Pugh, 1970; Susser, 1973).

Internal validity refers to the extent to which a relationship found to be statistically significant is a causal relationship. Internal validity is an empirical issue. That is, do the empirical measures used to assess concepts of interest relate to each other in a causal way? It is also a theoretical issue in that the presumed causal association between variables must be coherent with other empirical evidence and theory.

In epidemiology, there are five "criteria of judgement" that are used to aid in establishing a causal relationship (Susser, 1973): 1) the temporal (time) sequence of variables, 2) the consistency of associations on replication, 3) the strength of the association, 4) the specificity of association, and 5) the coherency of the explanation of the association. The *time sequence* refers to the temporal order of the variables of interest. The *consistency of the association* refers to its reliability. The strength of the association is measured empirically using relative risk, correlational, or nonparametric statistics. *Specificity* refers to what we previously discussed as discriminant validity. Finally, the *coherence criterion* refers to a more theoretical question of whether the explanation of the association between the variables of interest "fits" with pre-existing theory and evidence. These five criteria are then used to make judgements regarding whether the empirical association between variables has internal validity or causal plausibility.

The causal plausibility of a relationship may in part be dependent on the type of study design used to assess one's variables of interest. In a controlled experimental study, one may specifically manipulate the time order of variables and experimentally control for confounding factors that may be threats to internal invalidity. However, many epidemiologic studies are not experimental, but rather are observational and what has been called *quasiexperimental* (Cook and Campbell, 1979). In these types of studies, it may be more difficult to establish the internal validity of the relationship between variables. There are a number of threats to internal validity that may arise in using nonexperimental designs. They are discussed in detail by Cook and Campbell (1979; pp. 51–59) and briefly described here.

Suppose that in a treatment study one found that treatment "a" was significantly better for a specific diagnostic group than treatment "b," as measured by pre- and post-treatment measurements of symptomatology. However, suppose there was no random assignment to treatment; thus the study was not an experimental design. The following threats to the "internal validity" of the effect of treatment "a" may be operating and should be addressed. In general, threats to internal validity have to do with the possibility of *differential* effects of events on the treatment versus the control groups that are not due to the treatment of interest per se.

History effects refer to the influence of events outside of the control of the study that may differentially affect the outcomes of the groups being studied but have little relationship to the treatment of interest. *Maturation* involves the differential development of participants in each group that is not due to treatment effects. *Testing and instrumentation effects* refer, respectively, to the number of times a test is given resulting in differential learning effects and changes in instrumentation over time that differentially affects one's groups unrelated to treatment effects.

Statistical regression artifacts are especially difficult to control for. They can occur if the groups at pretreatment time are not equivalent, i.e., do not come from the same population. In a nonrandomized study, one attempts to match groups on certain pre-treatment variables. However, the matching variables may be unreliable themselves, resulting in unmatched groups at pretreatment assessment time. Respondents with high scores on unreliable pretreatment variables may score lower at post-treatment time, and the reverse may be true for respondent with low scores on unreliable pretreatment variables. The expected direction of the change in unreliable scores from pre- to post-treatment is always toward the population mean (Cook and Campbell, 1979). This is referred to as *regression to the mean*. Thus, the change in one's treatment groups would not be due to treatment, but rather to these regression artifacts. One way to control for these artifacts is to ensure that pretreatment matching variables are as reliable as possible. It is often difficult to match one's groups completely, and therefore using experimental designs in treatment studies is preferable, although not always possible.

A classic example of how regression artifacts can adversely affect results was the Westinghouse–Ohio University study of Head Start (preschool education) (Campbell and Erlebacher, 1970). In this study, the cases and controls were undermatched for socioeconomic status resulting in making Head Start look damaging to children. This occurred because controls were selected from a more able population than Head Starters. That is, the pretreatment or pretest matching variable, socioeconomic status, which includes educational status, was unreliable. When cognitive measures were assessed post–Head Start, the control group's cognitive scores regressed to their population mean, which were higher than those in the Head Start group. The population means of the two groups were different, because the controls were originally selected from a population that was educationally and cognitively more advanced than the Head Start group (Campbell and Erlebacher, 1970). When controls were appropriately selected for comparison with the Head Start children, the Head Start program was shown to have a significant impact on the cognitive functioning of the children who experienced the program.

Selection effects are related to regression artifacts. Selection becomes a threat to internal validity when the characteristics of one's groups are different, and this results in differential changes from pre- to post-treatment assessment between groups. For example, *mortality* can result in selection artifacts. *Mortality effects* refer to the differential dropout or refusal rates between the groups that may affect the group's post-treatment mean.

For example, if the more severely ill patients dropped out of treatment "a," then post-treatment assessment of symptoms among the treatment "a" group may look better due to the differential drop-out of severely ill patients in that group rather than to effects of treatment "a" on symptomatology.

Other threats to internal validity discussed by Cook and Campbell (1979, pp. 53–55) include differential social influences on the groups being compared. For example, communication between patients in the treatment and control groups about the treatment of interest may result in rivalry between the groups, "resentful demoralization" of the group receiving a less desirable treatment, or imitation of one group by the other.

The *external validity* of a significant result refers to the extent to which a finding is generalizable to and across persons, time periods, and settings (Cook and Campbell, 1979). Random sampling of one's groups from the population of interest contributes to the ability to "generalize to" the population of interest. *Generalizing across* populations refers to the identification of "to which" populations can the findings be attributed? That is, it refers to the extent of the generalization of findings to other populations aside from those that were directly studied or subpopulations among those studied. For example, most readers would be cautious about generalizing across males and females from a study of health services utilization based solely on a sample of males.

The threats to external validity can be thought of as interaction effects with the treatment of interest (Cook and Campbell, 1979). For example, differences in treatment response between the sexes or socioeconomic statuses will lower the generalizability across the population as a whole. There are three types of interaction effects that are threats to external validity: interactions of selection, setting, and history with treatment (Cook and Campbell, 1979, pp. 73–74). For example, selection interactions, or systematic recruitment artifacts, may result in findings being attributable only to those recruited into the study. The same can be said for interactions of treatment with setting and history. For example, using a university setting may limit one's generalizability across other settings. Conducting the treatment study during a particular historical period may not allow generalizability to future time periods. To minimize both of these threats, multiple studies would need to be implemented using different populations at different historical time periods.

SUMMARY

In summary, *validity* can have different meanings depending on the context in which it is used. It is applied to the measurement of concepts, called *construct validity*, and to the relationship between operational measures, called the *internal and external validity of a presumed causal relationship*. As applied to construct validity, it is an unending process in which one attempts to measure a concept of interest as accurately as possible. Thus, as discussed, validity involves a theoretical understanding of the concept as well as an empirical assessment of the criteria chosen to operationalize the concept. This chapter discussed three basic ways in which validity is assessed: content validity, criteria validity, and construct validity. Content and criterion validity can be thought of as part of the process of assessing construct validity. One study cannot wholly validate a measure of a concept. It requires a pattern of consistent findings across studies involving different samples and different settings.

The other way in which validity has been discussed in this chapter refers to the "internal and external validity" of empirical relationships between operational measures of the concepts of interest. *Internal validity* refers to the extent that a statistically significant relationship is a causal one. There are a number of ways in which causal plausibility is assessed, e.g., the five criteria of judgement used in epidemiologic studies (Susser, 1973). In addition, causal plausibility is dependent on the type of study design employed. As discussed, quasiexperimental designs are open to a number of threats to internal validity, e.g., regression artifacts, history and selection effects. Experimental study designs, in which one manipulates the time order of variables and controls for confounding factors, are less vulnerable to threats to internal validity. Finally, *external validity* refers to the extent that one can generalize the study findings to and across persons, time periods, and settings. To minimize threats to external validity, multiple studies are needed in which the study populations, the historical time periods, and the setting are varied.

ACKNOWLEDGMENTS

This chapter was written while Dr. Goldstein was supported by NIMH Scientist Development Award K21 MH00976.

REFERENCES

Addington D, Addington J, Maticka-Tyndale E (1993): Rating depression in schizophrenia: A comparison of a self-report and an observer scale. J Nerv Men Dis 181:561–565.

American Psychiatric Association (1987): "Diagnostic and Statistical Manual of Mental Disorders," 3rd ed, revised. Washington, DC: American Psychiatric Association.

Anastasi A (ed) (1976): "Psychological Testing," 4th ed. London: Macmillian.

Baldessarini RJ, Finklestein S, Arana GW (1983): The predictive power of diagnostic tests and the effect of the prevalence of illness. Arch Gen Psychiatry 40:569–573.

Campbell DT, Elebacher A (1970): How regression artifacts in quasiexperimental evaluations can mistakenly make compensatory education look harmful. In Helmuth J (ed): "Compensatory Education: A National Debate, vol 3, Disadvantaged Child." New York: Brunner/Mazel.

Carmines EG, Zeller RA (1979): In Sullivan JL (ed): "Reliability and Validity Assessment. Series Quantitative Applications in the Social Sciences." Beverly Hills, CA: Sage University Press.

Cloninger CR (1987): A systematic method for clinical description and classification of personality variants: A proposal. Arch Gen Psychiatry 44:573–588.

Cook TD, Campbell DT (eds) (1979): "Quasi-Experimentation Design and Analysis Issues for Field Settings." Chicago, IL: Rand McNally College Publishing Company.

Cronbach LJ (1971): Test validation. In Thorndike RL (ed): "Educational Measurement," 2nd ed. Washington, DC: American Council on Education.

Cronbach LJ, Meehl PE (1955): Construct validity in psychological tests. Psychol Bull 52(4):281–302.

Endicott J, Spitzer RL (1978): A diagnostic interview: The Schedule for Affective Disorders and Schizophrenia. Arch Gen Psychiatry 35:837–844.

Glaros AG, Kline RB (1988): Understanding the accuracy of tests with cutting scores: The sensitivity, specificity, and predictive value model. J Clin Psychol 44:1013–1023.

Kendler KS (1990): Toward a scientific psychiatric nosology. Strengths and limitations. Arch Gen Psychiatry 47:969–973.

Kim JO, Mueller CW (1978): "Factor Analysis: Statistical Methods and Practical Issues". Sage

University Paper Series on Quantitative Applications in the Social Sciences, 07-014. Beverly Hills, CA: Sage Publications.

MacMahon B, Pugh TF (1970): "Epidemiology: Principles and Methods." Boston: Little, Brown, and Co.

Murphy JM, Berwick DM, Weinstein MC, Borus JF, Budman SH, Klerman GL (1987): Performance of screening and diagnostic tests: Application of receiver operating characteristics analysis. Arch Gen Psychiatry 44:550–555.

Nunnally JC (ed) (1978): "Psychometric Theory," 2nd ed. New York: McGraw-Hill.

Radloff LS (1977): The CES-D Scale: A self-report depression scale for research in the general population. Appl Psychol Measurement 1:385–401.

Robins E, Guze SB (1970): Establishment of diagnostic validity in psychiatric illness: Its application to schizophrenia. Am J Psychiatry 126(7):983–987.

Robins LN, Helzer JE, Croughan J, Ratcliff KS (1981): The NIMH Diagnostic Interview Schedule: Its history, characteristics, and validity. Arch Gen Psychiatry 38:381–389.

Schwartz CC, Myers JK, Astrachan BM (1975): Concordance of multiple assessments of outcome in schizophrenia: On defining the dependent variables in outcome studies. Arch Gen Psychiatry 32:1221–1227.

Simpson JC (1982): Amino acid levels in schizophrenia and celiac disease: Another look. Biol Psychiatry 17:1353–1357.

Somervell PD, Beals J, Boehnlein J, Leung P, Manson SM (1993): Criterion validity of the Center for Epidemiologic Studies Depression Scale in a population sample from an American Indian village. Psychiatry REs 47:255–266.

Streiner DL (1993): A checklist for evaluating the usefulness of rating scales. Can J Psychiatry 38:140–148.

Susser M (ed) (1973): "Causal Thinking in the Health Sciences. Concepts and Strategies of Epidemiology." London: Oxford University Press.

Takeuchi M, Yoshino A, Kato M, Ono Y, Kitamura T (1993): Reliability and validity of the Japanese version of the Tridimensional Personality Questionnaire among university students. Comp Psychiatry 34:273–279.

Woolson RF (1987): "Statistical Methods for the Analysis of Biomedical Data." New York: John Wiley and Sons.

CHAPTER 11

How to Choose Among the Riches: Selecting a Diagnostic Instrument

LEE N. ROBINS

Washington University School of Medicine, St. Louis, MO 63110

INTRODUCTION

The last 30 years have seen the end of the homemade psychiatric interview. In the old days, a researcher into the causes of psychiatric illness decided what psychiatric illness meant to him and wrote or selected questions from older instruments to match his definition. Such an approach seems as bizarre nowadays as if an investigator into tuberculosis were to decide for himself what tuberculosis is and then create his own patch test. But specification of the criteria by the researcher was necessary in those days, even if he or she preferred using "official" definitions.

For example, when I did my first study (Robins, 1974), I needed criteria to detect "Sociopathic Personality Disturbance, Antisocial Reaction", the term in the recently published (1952) first edition of the *Diagnostic and Statistical Manual for Mental Disorders* for what became *Antisocial Personality* in DSM-II and thereafter. I found it impossible to translate DSM's definition into questions. *DSM-I* had been published by the American Psychiatric Association to be used by mental hospitals, replacing the *Statistical Manual for the Use of Hospitals for Mental Diseases* published by the National Committee for Mental Hygiene (now the National Association for Mental Health). A mere 33 pages of text defined all its terms. The section on Sociopathic Personality Disturbance, Antisocial Reaction contained four sentences, only two of which listed criteria. Those two sentences conveyed the then current view of the disorder, based primarily on Cleckley's *The Mask of Sanity* (1955), but provided little guidance to the would-be author of a structured interview.

What was this Antisocial Reaction a reaction to? Should the phrase "individuals who were *always* in trouble" be taken literally? Did one trouble-free day exclude the diagnosis? If sociopaths had "no *real* loyalties," how could one detect the fact that their loyalties were false? To demonstrate that they had "an ability to rationalize their behavior so that it appears warranted, reasonable, and justified," would the interviewer have to believe their explanations, or would the interviewer have to establish that others had been taken in by

Textbook in Psychiatric Epidemiology, Edited by Tsuang, Tohen, and Zahner
ISBN 0-471-59375-3   © 1995 Wiley-Liss, Inc.

it (but not the interviewer)? To meet diagnostic criteria, did a respondent need all of the traits listed, or would fewer do? For how long did these traits have to last? Unable to answer these questions, I asked my husband, an academic psychiatrist greatly concerned with nosologic issues, what he thought the criteria should be. His responses were much easier to implement in question form than those ambiguous sentences of DSM-I, so I used them. His criteria, recorded in my volume, *Deviant Children Grown Up* (Robins, 1974), the first influenced the criteria for antisocial personality in *DSM-III* (American Psychiatric Association, 1980), a newer edition of the official manual that was dedicated to making criteria so explicit that they would be comparatively easy to operationalize.

Today things are vastly different when it comes to carrying out studies that require psychiatric diagnoses. The heart of the interview will generally be one of the already available diagnostic interviews. Selecting which one to use is rather like buying a motor vehicle; the instruments have different advantages and disadvantages, but, like vehicles that were warranted to meet automotive standards as of the time of manufacture, each enables the user to match the criteria of one or more standard diagnostic systems. However, as buying older motor vehicles can result in owning one that fails to meet modern standards for fuel efficiency, safety, and emissions, older interviews generally cannot match all the criteria of new diagnostic systems. If being up to date diagnostically is important to the researcher, he or she must use only the newest products or revise the older ones appropriately.

The analogy to purchasing a vehicle holds also in other respects. While use of any interview, like driving a car, requires some skill and knowledge of basic rules, there are instruments that require special expertise to administer, as tractor-trailers and taxis may not be driven by those who qualify only for general purpose driver's licenses. Also as choice of a vehicle affects future upkeep costs, the choice among instruments has continuing cost consequences for users. If it needs clinicians to administer it, if the training required is extensive, if its administration is lengthy, if respondents' responses must be corroborated by outside informants and medical records, if there are open-ended questions that must be coded for content, if there are no data entry, cleaning, and scoring programs available on computer, if the copyright prohibits photocopying, then the interview will be expensive to use. If the study is to be supported by a research grant, a choice of instruments must be made early to estimate these future costs when constructing the budget.

Interviews differ not only in the systems they serve, the expertise needed to administer them, and their operational costs, but also in their product. They produce different levels of information—from screening to complete diagnosis, with or without subtyping, from description of status in the last week or two to coverage of the lifetime.

An excellent review of the diversity of instruments as of a few years ago can be found in Thompson's *The Instruments of Psychiatric Research* (1989). Of course, it omits the most recent products. Table 1 presents those in greatest current use and shows their diagnostic coverage, their degrees of structure, their time spans, whether they allow skip outs, and what systems they serve. Further details can be found in their manuals.

My task in the current chapter is to help researchers become more aware of the consequences of choosing among the instruments listed in Table 1 or others they might consider. There is no one "best" instrument. The choice should depend on the particular goals of a study and the resources one has. One might assume that it is obvious that one should pick the newest instrument because it will serve the current diagnostic system. However, there are also arguments in favor of a well-established instrument even if it does not

TABLE 1. Current Broad-Range Adult Diagnostic Instruments

	Fully Structured	Subclinical (No Skip Outs)	Time Span	System(s)	References
AXIS I[a]					
SADS	No	No	Current/previous	RDC	Spitzer and Endicott (1977a)
SADS-L	No	No	Ever		Spitzer and Endicott (1977b)
PSE-9	No	No	Last month	ICD-8	Wing et al. (1974)
DIS-III	Yes	Yes	Life, last year, 6 mo, 1 mo, 2 wk	Feighner, RDC, DSM-3	Robins et al. (1981)
DIS-IIIA				3 above +	Robins and Helzer (1985)
DIS-IIIR				DSM-3R	Robins et al. (1989)
SCID-P	No	Yes	Last month, previous	DSM-3R	Spitzer et al. (1991a)
SCID-NP					Spitzer et al. (1991c)
CIDI	Yes	Yes	Same as DIS	DSM-3R ICD-10	WHO (1993)
SCAN	No	No	Current, worst	DSM-3R ICD-10	WHO (1992b)
AXIS II[b]					
SIDP	No		Last 5 years	DSM-III	Pfohl et al. (1982)
SIDP-R				DSM-III-R	Pfohl et al. (1989)
PDE	Yes	Yes	Current year, before age 25, lasted 5 years	DSM-III-R	Loranger (1988)
IPDE	Yes	Yes	Same as PDE	DSM-3R, ICD-10	WHO (1992a)
SCID-II	No	Optional	Current, lasted 5 years	DSM-3R	Spitzer et al. (1991b)

[a]These cover some psychoses, affective disorders, anxiety disorders, and somatization. All except SADS, PSE, and SCID cover chronic brain syndromes; all except PSE cover substance abuse and eating disorders.

[b]These cover all disorders on axis II of DSM-III-R and/or ICD-10 specific personality disorders (F60).

Note: The DIS, SCID, SCAN, and IPDE are being revised to cover DSM-IV (1994).

cover the most recent version of DSM or ICD: When an instrument has been widely used previously, more is known about its properties, it may be more readily accepted by those reviewing a grant proposal or deciding whether to publish a paper, and one's results can be compared with results obtained in previous studies.

I begin with issues that vary with specific studies.

STUDY-SPECIFIC CRITERIA

Coverage of Disorders of Interest

As shown in Table 1, interviews differ with respect to which diagnoses they cover, in which diagnostic systems, and for which time frames. Obviously, it is vital to choose an instrument that evaluates the diagnoses of interest in the diagnostic system of interest. If the study does not require all the diagnoses available, instruments organized in modular form generally allow dropping disorders that are not of interest to the current study. Interviews organized by topic rather than diagnosis make such a reduction in the interview extremely difficult.

Instruments that measure only current status, and do not cover the whole lifetime, evaluate syndromes rather than diagnoses, because diagnosis requires a knowledge of the psychiatric history. If diagnosis is needed, a longitudinal perspective is essential.

Another aspect of coverage that may be critical is the degree of detail provided for the diagnoses of interest. Interviews that terminate the exploration of a disorder's symptoms as soon as it can be ascertained that criteria for the disorder will not be met, for example, do not provide a total symptom profile or a profile of all criteria met. Interviews that assess disorders in most of the major diagnostic groups in the manual served have often sacrificed making distinctions between diagnostic subtypes (e.g., the various schizophrenias) to achieve that breadth.

Instruments also differ in how much information they provide about the course of disorders. Only some provide the age at which the first symptom appeared, the age at which the disorder would first have been diagnosable, the most recent date at which symptoms were present, the most recent date at which sufficient symptoms were present to justify diagnosis, and whether the symptoms of the disorder were discussed with a physician. None of the interviews now available provides a complete natural history.

A study that requires symptom profiles and some information about course for certain disorders, but needs only the presence or absence of other disorders, may be best served by an instrument that exists in both a complete and a screening version, because sections of the two can be interwoven to allow assessing some disorders in detail and others in screening form.

If there are plans to follow the sample at a later time to measure change in psychiatric status, interviews that ascertain symptoms only for a time period close to the point of interview will miss episodes that occurred and resolved earlier in the follow-up interval. On the other hand, instruments using lifetime formats are also unsatisfactory for repeated administration, because they provide information redundant with that previously obtained and fail to determine whether newly reported disorders actually first occurred since the last interview or had merely been overlooked previously. For repeated diagnostic assessments, modification of the interview will probably be necessary, whichever interview is selected. This was successfully done with the DIS to study effects of exposure to floods (Robins et al., 1983).

Appropriateness to the Study Sample

Standardized interviews have been used in studies of all sorts of samples, from general populations of diverse ethnic backgrounds to homogeneous clinic populations. In general, interviews requiring clinician interviewers have been used primarily in clinical settings, in part because a shortage of clinical manpower makes it impractical to use these interviewers in large epidemiologic studies, where interviewers must travel to respondents' homes.

For ethnically and culturally diverse samples, interviews that have been translated into all the relevant languages and that avoid criteria satisfied only by problems unique to western industrialized cultures (for example, auto accidents when drinking for alcohol abuse and fear of flying or elevators for phobias) would be most appropriate. The CIDI and SCAN, sponsored by WHO for international comparisons, have had particular attention focused on cross-cultural applicability.

Appropriateness to the Study Resources

Selecting an instrument has important financial implications. As noted above, if administration can be done only by clinicians, if the training period is long, if computer programs for data entry, data cleaning, and scoring of diagnoses must be produced by the user, costs will be high. Such requirements can also substantially lengthen the duration of a research project.

Survey costs are lowest when a computerized version of the interview is available that can be self-administered by a sample that is both literate and willing to come to a central location. Although there will be an initial investment in personal computers, a single interviewer can supervise data entry by several respondents simultaneously, the interviewer's training can be considerably less extensive, and there are no data entry costs.

Telephone interviewing comes next in economy. It too is typically carried out with a computerized version of the interview, whose questions the interviewer reads to the respondent. While clearly inappropriate for cultures in which telephones are not common, telephone interviews may be reasonable for industrialized nations where only the poorest are lost to the sample because they have no telephone. The consequences of this loss (or the cost of supplementing the telephone sample with face-to-face interviews for persons with no telephone) must be judged against the advantage of being able to do simple random sampling of those with a telephone rather than having to use the clustered samples traditional in face-to-face area sampling, with a concomitant decrease in effective sample size. Telephone interviews can also be carried out without computer, of course. However, both self-administered and telephone interviews require the sacrifice of observation of the respondent.

UNIVERSAL DESIDERATA

A researcher may discover that more than one of the available interviews is appropriate to the study's coverage, sample, and resources. If so, more universalistic criteria can be applied in selecting among them. An instrument can be chosen on the basis, first, of its efficiency; second, because the format promotes error-free recording of responses; third, because its diagnostic algorithms are easily understood; fourth, because it is known to be acceptable to respondents or interviewers; fifth, because it is well supported by its developers; finally, because it is thought to be reliable and valid.

INTERVIEW EFFICIENCY

Only fully structured interviews can be adequately compared with respect to their efficiency because only these specify all the questions to be used and the order in which topics are covered. An interview should be easy to give and easy to understand. It is easy to give if it is short, if the questions follow each other in a sequence that feels like a natural conversation to both the respondent and the interviewer, and if the flow is logical, so that the interviewer does not need to retrace his steps through material already covered as a result of information received from asking an earlier question.

Interviews are as short as possible when questions that do not contribute to diagnosis are few, when no unnecessary diagnostic questions are included, and when questions ask for no more detail than is needed by the scoring system. A few questions or introductory remarks that are not used for diagnosis may be necessary to build rapport or prepare a respondent for questions that will follow. A general principle, although there will be exceptions, is that all questions should prove that they are essential either by appearing in a diagnostic computer statement or by defining who is eligible to be asked a question that appears in a diagnostic computer statement.

There are more subtle criteria for interview efficiency, but applying them requires data analysis that is not widely available. It would be ideal to be able to show that an interview contains no highly intercorrelated symptom questions and that every positive response to a symptom question significantly increases the likelihood of a positive diagnosis. This would demonstrate that there is no redundancy.

Interviews are easy to understand by respondents with a wide range of education and from different subcultures if the language is limited to everyday, nonjargon terms and is without idioms that are specific to certain locations, age groups, or lifestyles. Tests developed to grade the reading level of written text can be applied to interview questions to assess their difficulty. Another way of testing comprehensibility is to pretest the interviews with subjects similar to the intended sample and ask them to paraphrase questions. If the paraphrase captures the meaning of the questions, one can assume the questions were understood.

Format of the Interview

Interviewer Instructions. Interviews are often accompanied by manuals and "question-by-question specifications" to be used in training interviewers. These documents advise interviewers about the intention of questions, about how to ask questions that differ from the standard format, and about how to probe atypical responses. While these manuals and specifications are very useful for study by interviewers-in-training, their details are often forgotten during the field period. To increase the chances that the directions given during training will be followed in the field, as many of these instructions as possible should be incorporated into the body of the interview, where interviewers will see them at the time they need to implement them. Instructions should be in distinctive type to separate them from questions to be asked.

Coding Blanks. Coding blanks should be on the same document as the questions, so that the answer is placed next to the question to which it applies. They should be in the same position on each page, and codes for common responses like "Yes," "No," and "Don't know" should be consistent throughout the interview. These features minimize the chance that interviewers will enter the wrong code or place it in the wrong position.

When the range of appropriate answers is known, all acceptable answers should be printed, to be circled or checked off. When the answer required is a number, coding blanks should indicate the appropriate number of digits.

Provision should have been made for all possible replies, including respondent refusal, lack of knowledge, responses not foreseen, and responses that straddle two or more codes provided.

Transparency of Computer Programs

The researcher should not have to take the accuracy of an interview's diagnostic output on faith. Understanding the diagnostic algorithms is facilitated when the interview question number is used as the name of its response entry variable in computer programs, making it easy to link program statements to the questions that provided the data and when the program creates a category for each criterion listed in the official manual and names it with the number or letter that identifies that criterion in the manual. Disorders should be clearly labeled with the name and numeric code in the manual to clarify the level of subtyping.

Acceptability

Acceptability of the interview to both respondents and the interviewers will affect the study's completion rate and the accuracy of diagnosis. Acceptability is best judged by others' experience with an interview in previous studies. Publications usually report the proportion of the target population interviewed, but this is not very helpful because refusals occur before the respondent is exposed to the questions. More valuable is knowing the frequency of "break offs," i.e., interviews started but not completed, the average number of questions refused in completed interviews, the proportion of respondents who agreed to be reinterviewed in a second wave, and, in "snow-ball" sampling (where a respondent is asked for names of friends or relatives to be invited to be interviewed), how many respondents were willing to provide names. Unfortunately, these figures are not routinely published, but could be requested from study directors who have used the interview.

There is even less information available about interviewers' satisfaction. Audio tapes of fully structured interviews reveal whether interviewers could not resist modifying questions, although trained to ask them as written, and whether they rushed subjects through the interview or indicated relief when respondents' answers to certain key questions saved them from having to pursue some sections of the interview. Most threatening of all would be low interviewer productivity and high interviewer turnover rates.

Supports Available

Instruction manuals, data entry programs, data cleaning programs, and diagnostic scoring programs are all important assets in using diagnostic interviews. Also valuable are well-planned schedules training for interviewers and supporting videotapes and other audiovisual tools to be used in training. During the field and analysis periods, it is useful for the researcher to have access to the developer's staff to answer questions that may arise.

Reliability of the Interview

The usual study of an interview's reliability either has an observer score the interview while the interviewer also scores it and then compares the two scorings to see whether they agree (inter-rater reliability) or has the interview repeated at a later time by a different interviewer to see whether the same results are attained (test–retest reliability).

Neither method provides very satisfactory measures of reliability. Even if inter-rater reliability is high, there is no assurance that the same answers would have been given to a different interviewer. Also, the observer may have elevated the interview's apparent reliability by scoring it as he guessed the interviewer would score it whether or not he agreed with that rating. In the test–retest method, the respondent cannot be blind to the previous answers given. The respondent may either attempt to reproduce them, increasing apparent reliability, or avoid repetition, exaggerating the unreliability. If the interval between repeated interviews is so long that the respondent will have forgotten the previous answers, his or her psychiatric status may have changed and a difference in response should not be assumed to indicate unreliability. In any case, respondents, for unknown reasons, appear generally to give fewer positive responses in second interviews, no matter whether the instrument used is the SADS (Bromet et al., 1986), the DIS (Robins et al., 1982), or the SCID (Williams, 1992). As Williams (1992) notes, the degree of agreement in a reliability test may be a function not only of the interview itself, but also of the reliability of the diagnostic criteria being evaluated, the characteristics of the interviewers, the characteristics of the subjects, and the study method.

Fortunately, there are a few other measures in the literature that can be added to improve our judgment of reliability. If replication of a study in a new sample from the same population produces very similar results, if responses remain similar despite changes in the interview procedures—e.g., telephone instead of face-to-face interview—if the history of earlier episodes is unaffected by the presence or absence of current symptoms, then the interview would have to be reasonably reliable.

Validity of the Interview

Common practices for evaluating validity have been recognized as unsatisfactory as well. Usually the interviewer's results are compared with results of a clinician's free-form interview or with diagnoses in medical records, which represent the past judgment of one or more clinicians who also used free-form assessment methods. The problem is that clinicians' judgments are known to be unreliable, as shown by lack of agreement between them when diagnosing the same patient.

Again there are several alternative assessment methods. The most straightforward is evaluating the interview's face validity. Do its questions appear to elicit the symptoms listed in the manual? Are the responses combined according to an algorithm that closely matches the manual's? Is every criterion assessed? A clear, well-written, well-documented computer program is a great help in making these judgments.

A second method is to judge whether the level of severity required to assess disorders seems appropriate. This is particularly important for instruments used in epidemiologic studies, where appearance in the sample does not depend on the presence of disorder, as it usually does in patient samples. Unfortunately, diagnostic interviews include few measures of impairment, but the studies in which they are used have usually collected at least treatment and demographic data. If diagnosis is associated with treatment seeking, prolonged unemployment, or inability to form lasting marriages, it is more likely that those identified as cases actually have a disorder. Not every case need have evidence for disability, nor must every noncase be fully employed, married only once, and without mental health consultations, but the overall rate of treatment and disability should clearly be elevated among those considered positive.

However, finding elevated rates of disability among those affected does not indicate that the correct *specific* diagnosis was made. This would be better judged by the frequency with which clinical interviewers or the editors for lay interviewers were satisfied that the examples and elaborations of symptoms, requested in all of the interviews in Table 1, were appropriate to the intention of the questions. This evaluation is a particular feature of the PSE and SCAN, where it is referred to as *cross-examination*. Unfortunately, the contents of these examples and elaborations have not been published to allow judging the clarity of the questions.

Thus establishing the relative validity of these interviews can be only partially solved. For both reliability and validity, it is probably advisable to use multiple methods of assessment, since no single one is entirely satisfactory.

SUMMATION

A variety of standardized interviews are now available that allow making specific psychiatric diagnoses according to one or more of the official diagnostic nomenclatures. The number of interviews to choose among is likely to continue to grow. It is not always obvious which instrument would be best for a particular study. This chapter offers criteria that should be considered both in judging the appropriateness of an instrument for the special needs of a particular study and, when more than one would serve, in making a choice based on more general criteria.

ACKNOWLEDGMENTS

This work was presented at the Festschrift for Ben Locke, 1992, and also appears in a special issue of the *International Journal of Methods in Psychiatric Research* devoted to papers from that Festschrift.

REFERENCES

American Psychiatric Association (1952): "Diagnostic and Statistical Manual." Washington, DC: American Psychiatric Association.

American Psychiatric Association: "Diagnostic and Statistical Manual," 3rd ed (1980). 3rd ed rev (1982), 4th ed (1994). Washington, DC: American Psychiatric Press.

Bromet EJ, Dunn LO, Connell MM, Dew MA, Schulberg HC (1986): Long-term reliability of diagnosing lifetime major depression in a community sample. Arch Gen Psychiatry 43:435.

Cleckley H (1955): "The Mask of Sanity." St. Louis: Mosby.

Loranger AW (1988): "Personality Disorder Examination (PDE) Manual." Yonkers, NY: DV Communications.

Pfohl B, Blum N, Zimmerman M, Stangl D (1989): Structured Interview for DSM-III-R Personality (SIDP-R)." Iowa City: University of Iowa.

Pfohl B, Stangl D, Zimmerman M (1982): "Structured Interview for the DSM-III Personality Disorder (SIDP)." Iowa City: University of Iowa Department of Psychiatry.

Robins LN (1974): "Deviant Children Grown Up: A Sociological and Psychiatric Study of Sociopathic Personality." Baltimore: Williams & Wilkins, 1966. Reprinted by Robert E. Krieger, Huntington, New York, 1974.

Robins LN, Helzer JE (1985): "The Diagnostic Interview Schedule," Version III-A. St. Louis: Mosby.

Robins LN, Helzer JE, Cottler L, Goldring E (1989): "The Diagnostic Interview Schedule," Version III-R. St. Louis: Mosby.

Robins LN, Helzer JE, Croughan JL, Williams JBW, Spitzer RL (1981): "The NIMH Diagnostic Interview Schedule," Version III. Public Health Services (HSS) ADM-T-42-3 (5-81, 8-81). Washington, DC: NIMH.

Robins LN, Helzer JE, Ratcliff KS, Seyfried W (1982): Validity of the Diagnostic Interview Schedule, Version II: DSM-III diagnoses. Psychol Med 12:855–870.

Robins LN, Smith EM, Cottler LB, Fischbach RL, Goldring E (1983): "The Diagnostic Interview Schedule Disaster Supplement." St. Louis: Mosby.

Spitzer RL, Endicott J (1977a): "Schedule for Affective Disorders and Schizophrenia." New York: New York State Psychiatric Institute.

Spitzer RL, Endicott J (1977b): "Schedule for Affective Disorders and Schizophrenia—Life-time Version (SADS-L)." New York: New York State Psychiatric Institute.

Spitzer RL, Williams JBW, Gibbon M, First MB (1991a): Structured Clinical Interview for DSM-III-R: Patient Edition." Washington, DC: American Psychiatric Association.

Spitzer RL, Williams JBW, Gibbon M, First MB (1991b): "Structured Clinical Interview for DSM-III-R-Personality Disorder (SCID-II)." Washington, DC: American Psychiatric Association.

Spitzer RL, Williams JBW, Gibbon M, First MB (1991c): "Structured Clinical Interview for DSM-III-R: Non-patient Edition." Washington, DC: American Psychiatric Association.

Thompson C (1989): "The Instruments of Psychiatric Research." Chichester: John Wiley & Sons.

WHO (1992a): "International Personality Disorder Examination." Geneva: WHO.

WHO (1992b): "Schedule for Clinical Assessment in Neuropsychiatry (SCAN)." Geneva: WHO.

WHO (1993): "The Composite International Diagnostic Interview (CIDI)." Geneva: WHO.

Williams JBW (1992): The structured clinical interview for DSM-III-R (SCID). II. Multisite test–retest reliability. Arch Gen Psychiatry 49:630–636.

Wing J, Cooper JE, Sartorius N (1974): "The Measurement and Classification of Psychiatric Symptom." Cambridge: Cambridge University Press.

CHAPTER 12

Diagnostic Schedules and Rating Scales in Adult Psychiatry

JANE M. MURPHY

Department of Psychiatry, Massachusetts General Hospital, Harvard Medical School, and
Department of Epidemiology, Harvard School of Public Health, Boston, MA 02115

INTRODUCTION

This chapter concerns assessment of the psychiatric status of adults by means of systematic questions. For generic reference, a set of such questions along with preestablished categories for response is often called an *instrument* or a *test*. Instruments tend to be of two main types.

One type is focused on a dimension of psychopathology and is often described as a *scale*. Other ways of referring to this type of instrument include *screening instrument*, *symptom inventory*, and *questionnaire*, the latter usually being reserved for a paper/pencil test. The other type deals with one or more diagnostic categories and is often referred to as a *schedule*, or sometimes as an *examination*.

Most instruments are known by an acronym standing for its full name or by the name of an author. These abbreviations regularly appear in published reports. The following is the list of instruments discussed in this chapter along with a reference for each that describes its construction and basic attributes. For ease of discourse, the instruments are referred to in the text by the abbreviation.

"Beck"	Beck Depression Inventory (Beck et al., 1961)
CES-D	Center for Epidemiologic Studies Depression Scale (Radloff, 1977)
CIDI	Composite International Diagnostic Interview (Robins et al., 1988)
CMI	Cornell Medical Index (Brodman et al., 1949)
CSI	Cornell Selectee Index (Weider et al., 1944)
DIS	Diagnostic Interview Schedule (Robins et al., 1981)
GHQ	General Health Questionnaire (Goldberg, 1972)
"Gurin"	Gurin Scale (Gurin et al., 1960)
HOS	Health Opinion Survey (Macmillan, 1957)

Textbook in Psychiatric Epidemiology, Edited by Tsuang, Tohen, and Zahner
ISBN 0-471-59375-3   © 1995 Wiley-Liss, Inc.

HSCL   Hopkins Symptom Checklist (Parloff et al., 1954; Derogatis et al., 1974)
ISPI   Iowa Structured Psychiatric Interview (Tsuang et al., 1980)
MMPI   Minnesota Multiphasic Personality Inventory (Dahlstrom et al., 1972)
MPI   Maudsley Personality Inventory (Eysenk, 1947)
MSS   Mental Status Schedule (Spitzer et al., 1967)
NSA   U.S. Army's Neuropsychiatric Screening Adjunct (Star, 1950)
PERI   Psychiatric Epidemiology Research Instrument (Dohrenwend et al., 1986)
PSE   Present State Examination (Wing, 1961; Wing et al., 1974)
PSS   Psychiatric Status Schedule (Spitzer et al., 1970)
SADS   Schedule for Affective Disorders and Schizophrenia (Endicott and Spitzer, 1978)
SCID   Structured Clinical Interview for DSM-III-R (Spitzer et al., 1992)
SCL-90   Symptom Checklist: 90 Items (Derogatis and Cleary, 1977)
SF-36   Short Form (36 Items) Health Survey (Ware and Sherbourne, 1992)
"Zung"   Zung Depression Scale (Zung, 1963)
22IS   Twenty-Two Item Scale, sometimes known as the "Langner" Scale (Langner, 1962)

This selection of instruments should not be thought of as exhaustive but rather as giving background and examples for discussion in this chapter (Murphy, 1986, 1990). Specifically excluded are rating scales for use by observers rather than as a means of asking direct questions. The Hamilton (1960) Rating Scale for Depression is an example of a well-known instrument excluded on this basis. For a full appreciation of the number, variety, and history of such instruments, the *Mental Measurements Yearbook* (Buros, 1992) should be consulted. In addition, other volumes give overviews that cover instruments not included here (McDowell and Newell, 1987; Thompson, 1989).

BACKGROUND AND RELATIONSHIPS

The question/answer mode of inquiry regarding psychopathology emerged during the 1930s in psychology, with the MMPI often being thought of as "the grandfather" of such efforts. In this chapter, primary attention is given to the proliferation of instruments that has taken place since the Second World War. This period has involved continuing research by *psychometricians* and increasing participation on the part of *sociologists*, who bring expertise in survey methodology, and, more recently, of *psychiatrists*, who bring clinical experience and expertise in nomenclature.

Figure 1 presents this historical period in terms of the times and places where instruments have been developed. Each new instrument has been influenced to some degree by prior instruments. Some examples of such influence involve the evolutionary approaches taken by particular groups of researchers. As Spitzer and colleagues at Columbia improved their schedule, they changed the name with each new generation (MSS, PSS, SADS, SCID). A similar evolutionary sequence is shown for the PSE, now in its ninth revision based on the work of Wing and his coworkers at the British Medical Research Council (BMRC). The improvements leading to the SCID and PSE-9 mainly involved in-

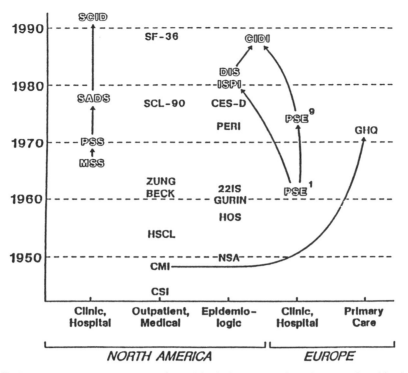

FIGURE 1. Time, place, and purpose of Psychiatric Instrument Development. Psychiatric scales are shown in bold letters, diagnostic schedules in outlined letters. Names of the scales and schedules are given in the text. Arrowed lines refer to influence from one instrument to another. Vertical lanes refer to geographic locations and to the types of populations for which instruments were designed (psychiatric clinics and mental hospitals; psychiatric outpatient, general medical, primary care; epidemiologic populations).

terests within clinical psychiatry as consensus criteria for diagnoses became more highly specified.

Another sequence involved the work of Wolff and his collaborators at Cornell when they changed the CSI, a wartime psychiatric screening instrument, into the CMI, as a comprehensive medical inquiry. The expansion was based on the goal of assessing both physical and psychologic states in order to understand their relationships. Psychosomatic theory had formative influence on the direction taken by this instrument. A recent scale designed for assessing both physical and psychiatric status is the SF-36. This scale has been used in the Medical Outcomes Study (Tarlov et al., 1989).

A group at Hopkins carried out what Derogatis et al. (1974) have called a *programmatic sequence* of instrument improvement. This particular line of influence is not visible in Figure 1 for reasons of simplicity. A set of questions called the *Discomfort Scale* (a name that was not perpetuated) served as the basis for the HSCL, which in turn is the progenitor of the SCL-90. Many of the improvements embodied in the SCL-90 derive from a psychometric tradition of using factor analysis to clarify the dimensional properties of psychopathology.

The Beck and Zung scales were constructed by psychiatrists to deal exclusively with depression. They reflect the growing attention given to this disorder as psychotropic medications were developed and marketed. While a number of the earlier instruments had names that do not immediately indicate their psychiatric content (*Sympton Checklist, Health Opinion Survey*), the Beck and Zung scales influenced later instruments in the direction of using explicit names to indicate the purpose and content of the inquiry.

It can be seen that several developmental sequences were carried out at a given institution (BMRC, Columbia, Cornell, Hopkins). Other lines of influence cut across institutions and geographic areas. For example, the GHQ, developed in Britain, was designed specifically to overcome problems that had come to light in using the American CMI in a London study of psychiatric illness in general practices (Shepherd et al., 1966). One such problem was that the CMI was found to have high test–retest performance, suggesting that it measured stable personality traits rather than the episodes of psychiatric illness, which were thought to be the primary concern in general medical settings. The GHQ was strongly influenced by the concept of an "episode" as a reaction to the CMI.

The link between the PSE and the ISPI is another example of cross-national influence. The PSE was used in the U.S./U.K. Study of Diagnosis (Cooper et al., 1972) and in the International Study of Schizophrenia (World Health Organization, 1973) both of which dealt with hospitalized psychotics. The PSE served as a model for the ISPI, which was designed for the Iowa 500 Study (Tsuang and Winokur, 1975), in which not only hospitalized psychotics were followed for interview but also normal controls and family members were studied. Thus the ISPI represents the types of influence by which one model was used to construct an adaptation for a different purpose. In this case, a clinical instrument served as a model for a psychiatric epidemiologic instrument.

A more recent example of a similar influence is the CIDI. The World Health Organization sponsored the CIDI in 1988 as an amalgamation of the best features of the PSE and the DIS. By this time the PSE, which started out as a clinical instrument, had been used in epidemiologic studies of Camberwell in London (Bebbington et al., 1981) and of Canberra, Australia (Henderson et al., 1981). The DIS had been used in the National Institute of Mental Health (NIMH) Epidemiologic Catchment Area (ECA) program (Robins and Regier, 1991). The joining of the two traditions in the CIDI involved technical improvements and wider applicability across cultures.

EPIDEMIOLOGIC APPLICATIONS

Prior to the ISPI, DIS, and CIDI, most epidemiologic investigations in North America had used psychiatric *scales*. The NSA, for example, was designed as a psychiatric screening test during the Second World War. Its development and use in the final month of the War is extensively reported in *The American Soldier* (Stouffer et al., 1950).

In the early 1950s, questions from the NSA were incorporated into the data-gathering methods for both the Midtown Manhattan Study (Srole et al., 1962) from which the 22IS was derived and the Stirling County Study (Leighton et al., 1963) for which the HOS was designed. These studies were among the first in which samples of adults selected to represent typical community populations were interviewed face to face about psychiatric symptoms. The site of the Midtown Study is a highly urbanized U.S. locale and that of the Stirling Study is a rural county in Atlantic Canada.

During the 1960s and 1970s further work with psychiatric scales was carried out with national samples in the United States. An adaptation of the HOS, with some questions from the 22IS, was used in *Americans View Their Mental Health* (Gurin et al., 1960) and in the longitudinal repetition of this national sample study reported in *The Inner American* (Veroff et al., 1981) and in *Mental Health in America* (Veroff et al., 1981). Although these studies involved large samples of the U.S. population, neither was strictly an epidemiologic study, since they did not use the results of asking questions about psychiatric symptoms to estimate prevalence rates.

The PERI incorporates many features of the HOS and the 22IS but covers a larger portion of the psychiatric spectrum. It has been used in a number of methodologic studies that have been interpreted to mean that instruments such as the NSA, HOS, and 22IS actually measure a phenomenon called *demoralization* rather than true psychiatric illness (Dohrenwend et al., 1980; Link and Dohrenwend, 1980). The PERI has also been used in a substantive investigation of psychiatric disorder and social status in Israel (Dohrenwend, 1989; Dohrenwend et al., 1992).

The CES-D was designed by the NIMH Center for Epidemiologic Studies and was first used in a comparative study of Kansas City, MO, and Washington County, MD (Markush and Favero, 1974; Comstock and Helsing, 1976). The CES-D has continued to be used in studies where assessment of the current level of depressed mood is needed. It has been replaced, however, by the DIS and CIDI for epidemiologic research where lifetime rates of psychiatric disorders are sought.

During the 1980s, an initiative in psychiatric epidemiology of unprecedented scale was undertaken. The U.S. President's Commission on Mental Health (1978) established the directive through which NIMH Epidemiologic Catchment Area (ECA) Program was put into operation. The development of criteria for diagnosis, which were ultimately embodied in DSM-III (American Psychiatric Association, 1980), laid the foundation for producing a new type of data-gathering instrument.

The DIS was designed by Lee Robins. Its most direct progenitor was the Renard Diagnostic Interview (Helzer et al., 1981), which had been developed and used in the Department of Psychiatry at Washington University in St. Louis, Missouri. Under the headship of Eli Robins, this department had taken the lead in developing explicit criteria for different diagnostic categories. The first set was known as the Feighner criteria (Feighner et al., 1972), Feighner being the first author of the publication in which the criteria were described. Subsequently the Washington University group collaborated with the group at Columbia under Spitzer to produce an improved set of criteria known as the *Research Diagnostic Criteria* (RDC) (Spitzer et al., 1978). The development of DSM-III drew on these earlier efforts and represented a wide level of consensus when adopted by the American Psychiatric Association.

The DIS was ready for use in 1980 when research was started in the first of the five sites of the ECA program. The sites included areas of New Haven, CT, Baltimore, MD, Durham, NC, St. Louis, MO, and Los Angeles, CA. When the samples were combined the number of subjects was almost 20,000 (Robins and Regier, 1991). By the end of the decade, the DIS had been used in numerous investigations located elsewhere in North America as well as in Europe and Asia (Helzer and Canino, 1992).

On the basis of increasingly well-defined questions, a new NIMH effort was undertaken in the 1990s: the National Comorbidity Study (NCS), which used the CIDI as a data-gathering instrument. This study was based on a national sample of the United States rather than a five-site design as in the ECA. A primary goal was to investigate further the ECA evidence that one individual is often found to have a multiplicity of psychiatric diagnoses (Kessler et al., 1994). This work is being conducted through the Michigan Institute of Social Research, which had carried out the 1956 and 1976 national sample studies using the Gurin scale.

PSYCHIATRIC SCALES

Psychiatric scales usually involve a short series of questions concerning symptoms. The term *item* is often used to refer to an individual question in a scale. The scales used in outpatient or medical settings are often in the form of a paper/pencil test that a patient can take while waiting to see a doctor. Those used in epidemiologic research are administered verbally when an interviewer visits the home of a person selected at random to represent a given community.

With very few exceptions, the scales shown in Figure 1 are limited to symptoms in the domains of anxiety and/or depression. The types of symptoms queried for depression are dysphoric mood along with disturbances of sleep, appetite, energy, concentration, and self-esteem as well as ideation involving death and suicide. The questions for anxiety concern frightened mood along with concomitants of autonomic hyperactivity (such as palpitations and cold sweats) and of motor tension (such as trembling and muscle twitches).

Each question is asked of each subject and specific categories of response are spelled out in advance. Sometimes the response categories refer simply to the presence or absence of a symptom as, for example, "yes" or "no." In others, presence or absence is expanded to cover frequency of occurrence as in "almost all the time" to "never" or to the degree the symptom bothers the subject as in "very distressing" to "not distressing at all."

Responses are given numerical values that are added together to form a score. Sometimes each symptom positively endorsed is given the value of one; other times the value is weighted for frequency or distress. Each scale has a score range and has usually been published with a recommended "threshold score" or "cutting point" for separating psychiatric cases from noncases.

By and large, two types of procedures have been used to select symptoms for scales. With many scales, the selection is based on consulting the clinical literature or on studying earlier instruments that have been used in psychiatric studies. For example, the MMPI and the MPI have been sources for the questions asked in many of the more recently designed instruments.

Other scales, especially the NSA, the HOS, and the GHQ, were produced through a procedure called *calibration*. Calibration is based on administering a long set of questions to a known ill group and to a known (or presumed) well group. The questions that produce responses that statistically discriminate between the two groups are considered to be the best indicators of the type of psychopathology exhibited by the known ill group.

The calibration procedures carried out by the U.S. Army for the NSA produced a set of questions that indicate anxiety. The HOS was calibrated for both men and women of a much broader age range, and its questions are a mixture of anxiety and depression indicators. The GHQ was produced by a more elaborate procedure for identifying levels of severity as well as making a division between cases and noncases. It lacks the autonomic equivalents of anxiety but has numerous items about depression. Presumably related to its focus on levels of severity, the GHQ includes a longer section on thoughts of death and suicide than appears in the clinical instruments that have focused specifically on depression. Thus, while the GHQ is named "General Health Questionnaire," it actually contains several pathognomonic indicators of severe depression.

Many of the scales reflect influence from psychometric theory and survey methodology. In fact, psychologists and sociologists were more prominent as their designers than were clinical psychiatrists. One of the psychometric influences on scales concerns ways for controlling "response styles" or "response biases."

The response styles that concerned scale designers dealt with "acquiescence," "social desirability," "lying," and the "error of central tendency," to name a few (Guilford, 1936; Nunnally, 1978). *Response style* refers to social or personality attributes that interfere with the subject's ability to understand the question adequately, consider it thoughtfully, interpret it meaningfully, and answer it truthfully.

A voluminous literature exists on response style from the early 1930s through the 1960s (Rorer, 1965). Thereafter psychometric interest in the topic dwindled. Nunnally (1978) attributes the disappearance of this interest to the fact that response styles had been found to account for very little variance. Also procedures for reducing the effects of such styles introduced unnecessary complexity.

Nevertheless, concern about response styles continued to influence the design of scales throughout the 1970s. One method thought to reduce error by holding the subject's attention was to reverse the wording of selected questions so that the pathologic response was sometimes "yes" and sometimes "no." This method, called *balancing*, is especially prominent in the GHQ and CES-D.

It was also thought that a simple "yes" versus "no" response pattern as used in the CSI and CMI was more likely to foster "acquiescence" than would a set of categories requiring more discrimination on the part of the subject. A trichotomous response pattern, as used in the NSA, HOS, and most of the 22IS, was thought to promote the "error of central tendency" in which subjects would automatically and without thinking much about it choose the middle category rather than either extreme. Every scale developed after these early ones had at least a four-category response pattern. The earliest version of the HSCL, the Discomfort Scale, for example, drew heavily on the psychiatric sections of the CMI, but the response categories were expanded from two to four.

It can be appreciated that if a widespread tendency exists for people to respond on the basis of middle-category preference, the distribution of scores for a three-category scale would form a bell-shaped curve. There is no evidence, however, that such is the case. The common pattern of response using the HOS, for example, is that 7% of the time subjects say they "often" experience a symptom, 23% of the time "sometimes," and 70% of the time "never".

Where evidence about score distribution has been published or can be calculated, marked skewness appears. For the CES-D, skewness is 1.5 (Radloff, 1977); for the 22IS, 1.4 (Langner, 1962); for the HOS, based on calculations across several samples in the Stirling County Study, it is 1.2 (Murphy, 1992); and for the NSA, it is 1.2 (Star, 1950). This means that in a general population, the majority of people report that they do not have any psychiatric symptoms, or have only a few, and a minority of people report many symptoms. This pertains across instruments that have used different numbers of response categories and other forms of reducing the influence of response styles.

It is a solid fact of the history of psychiatric scales that the shape of score distributions is the pattern one would expect with an indicator of abnormal pathologic process. Psychiatric symptoms are *not* distributed normally the way height, weight, and some social attitudes are. It is not a matter of everybody having an average amount of psychiatric symptomatology, with some people having more and some less.

Evaluation of the reliability of a scale has usually involved a statistical assessment of internal consistency and test−retest performance. Measures of internal consistency tend to be 0.80 to 0.85. Test–retest correlation coefficients are more variable. They point to another major change in the history of scale development. This change concerns the conceptualization of illness as necessarily being episodic.

It was said above that the GHQ was constructed to overcome the fact that the CMI appeared to measure stable personality traits as indicated in a 1-year test–retest correlation coefficient of 0.89. The theoretical orientation of the GHQ is that illness is a break from the subject's usual state and that illness is packaged in time-discrete episodes. Thus, a prominent difference between these two instruments is that the CMI asks about symptoms that the patient *usually* experiences without specifying a time frame, while the GHQ asks about symptoms that are experienced *more than usual* or *less than usual* in the recent few weeks.

The focus of the GHQ on unusual symptoms had a marked influence on test–retest reliability. For example, a readministration of the GHQ after 1 week produced a low correlation of 0.44 (Duncan-Jones and Henderson, 1978). This correlation can be compared with a coefficient of 0.72 for a readministration of the HSCL after 6 months (Rickels et al., 1971). While the HSCL focuses on the recent week, it does not require that the symptoms reported reflect a break from the normal state, and thus it seems to identify both acute and chronic symptomatology. It is possible that a strong emphasis on an episode of unusual symptoms contributes to unreliable reporting.

In regard to the validity of scales, numerous factor analytic studies have been carried out in order to compare the empirical clustering of symptoms with clinical syndromes. By and large, the results have been promising, especially when such studies have been repeated several times on different populations as with the HSCL and SCL-90. In addition, virtually all of the scales shown in Figure 1 have been correlated with each other, and all have been found to be related. This evidence of convergent validity is probably due to their common focus on depression and anxiety.

Most of the scales have also been validated using a comparison either between presumed normals and psychiatric patients or between the scale results and those based on a subsequent blind assessment in which a psychiatrist used one or another of the diagnostic schedules. As with factor analysis, the results have tended to be good, especially if the timing of the validation interview was well adjusted to the time frame of the scale. For example, in several studies where the validation interview occurred promptly after the GHQ administration, sensitivity and specificity values have been close to or above 90%.

DIAGNOSTIC SCHEDULES

Diagnostic schedules are more comprehensive in psychiatric coverage than are the scales. All of them deal with depression and anxiety disorders as well as psychotic disorders such a schizophrenia and manic-depressive psychosis. The British PSE stands alone in that it does not include substance abuse disorders nor does it contain reference to any of the personality disorders. Most of the U.S. schedules include these latter disorders.

Another important difference between PSE and the other schedules is the fact that the PSE is exclusively concerned with the "present state," as indicated in its title. The reason for this focus is that the PSE was originally developed for patients at the time of admission into hospitals or clinics where description of the current clinical status is of primary significant. Most U.S. schedules, on the other hand, are lifetime in orientation.

As an instrument for use with patients, the SCID opens with questions about current symptomatology in given diagnostic categories but then asks for information regarding earlier episodes relevant to the same category. The DIS, as an epidemiologic instrument for use in populations where many subjects do not have psychiatric disorders, asks about episodes that have *ever* occurred in the life of the subject up to the time of interview. The emergence of a lifetime approach in epidemiologic studies relates to the need for population norms in family genetic studies where the lifetime experience of disorders among family members is compared with the lifetime disorders of the index cases.

It is helpful in understanding the lifetime schedules to consider the concept of an "episode." Building on what was said above about the GHQ, an episode is typically described as a "fluorescence of symptoms" that has a particular "time of occurrence" and a "duration." DSM-III makes use of this concept, in part or in whole, for many diagnostic categories. Especially prominent are requirements for a minimum duration of symptomatology. Major depression, for example, is considered to be an episodic disorder for which 2 weeks is a minimum duration.

The diagnostic schedules were originally intended to be used as guides for a face to face interview. None was developed in a paper/pencil format. At the present time, however, considerable experimentation is going on regarding the use of interactive computer methods for the administration of such schedules (Blouin et al., 1987).

Some of the schedules are *not* amenable to such computer administration, however, because they are designed for interviewers who have clinical training and so can apply clinical judgment during the interview. For example, the PSE uses standard questions, but the subject is not asked to respond in predetermined categories. Rather, it is the responsibility of the interviewer to decide whether the severity of the symptom justifies it being taken into account for diagnosis.

The requirements of epidemiologic research for studying large numbers of subjects often makes it impossible to employ interviewers who have had previous clinical training. Thus instruments such as the DIS and CIDI are administered by "lay" interviewers trained specifically for this task. The training may take as long as 2 weeks and involve carrying out practice interviews and reliability checks in addition to didactic presentation of the principles underlying the schedule and how they relate to the clinical manifestations of psychiatric disorders.

Because the DIS has been used in numerous epidemiologic studies, it will serve to illustrate many features of a schedule. Its content and format are linked to DSM-III in which the steps of the diagnostic process are spelled out. Usually DSM-III emphasizes syndrome recognition in terms of essential feature and associated symptoms. As said above, duration of symptomatology is taken into account in most categories. Some categories also give consideration to impairment in everyday functioning.

The DIS is organized as a series of sections, each of which concerns a particular diagnosis. For some diagnoses, the section opens with a "stem" question concerning the "essential feature" of that diagnosis. For some sections, the rest of the questions can be skipped ("skip outs") if a negative response is given to the initial inquiry about the essential feature. For other sections, skip outs occur at other places.

The depression section begins with a stem question concerning the essential feature and its durational requirements: "In your lifetime, have you ever had 2 weeks or more during which you felt sad, blue, depressed, or when you lost all interest and pleasure in things that you usually cared about or enjoyed?" Following a question for dysthymia, there are eight groups of questions concerning the associated symptoms. After completing the latter, the interviewer reviews the section in order to count the number of associated symptoms. If the number does not reach the criterion threshold of three, the rest of the section is skipped.

If the section is continued, questions are asked for ruling out simple bereavement and establishing that the essential feature and associated symptomatology coexisted in time. Information is also gathered about the number of episodes, age of onset, and various features of the worst episode.

The depression section requires that the interviewer use a "probe flow chart" for most of the associated symptoms. The purpose in using the chart is to ensure that positive symptoms are "psychiatric" in meaning. The question, "Has there ever been a period of 2 weeks or more when you felt worthless, sinful, or guilty?" does not require the chart because it is assumed that such feelings are inherently psychiatric. On the other hand, the questions about appetite, fatigue, sleep, and so forth, require further "probing" in which the subject is asked if a doctor was told about the symptom and if so what the doctor's diagnosis was. If the symptom was, in the doctor's view or by default in the subject's view, always caused by taking drugs or alcohol or by a physical illness or injury, the response does not count toward reaching the criterion threshold.

It can be appreciated that the DIS is a different kind of interview from one based on a psychiatric scale. It is much more demanding since it requires keeping one's whole life in mind and continual review for discrete time periods of given durations when symptoms were present in specified clusters.

The section most like the psychiatric scales concerns alcohol abuse and dependence. These questions tend to be simpler, as in "Did you ever think that you were an excessive drinker?" and the response categories are limited to "yes/no." Sixteen questions must be asked of all subjects except teetotallers before a skip out can be used.

Commenting on the grammar of diagnosis and the problems of translating diagnostic criteria into questions, Robins (1989) indicates that it was easier to write questions for the alcohol section than for some of the others. She also points out that the results of this section have stood up particularly well in assessments of validity and reliability, especially in comparison with the depression section.

Reliability testing for the DIS and other schedules is different from that for psychiatric scales. The tests have concerned whether or not all of the diagnostic criteria were met in each retest (Robins, 1985; Dohrenwend, 1989). It is a dichotomous rather than a scaled approach to reliability and can be thought of as "hard" compared with the "soft" reliability of the correlation coefficient. A troublesome aspect of reliability for the DIS is that second administrations of the schedule have regularly been found to show a lower report of symptoms than the first (Robins, 1985)

Studies of the validity of the DIS have been carried out at the Baltimore site of the ECA (Anthony et al., 1985) and in St. Louis (Helzer et al., 1985). In each case interviews conducted by psychiatrists served as the "gold standard." The results have been variable, not only according to site but also by diagnostic category. Robins (1985) has suggested that a major problem continues to be the absence of an acceptable "gold standard." To illustrate inadequacies of the validation standard, she points out that prevalence rates based on the interviews by psychiatrists varied markedly by site, while prevalence rates based on the DIS were comparable for the two sites.

In studying large samples of residents of places like Baltimore and St. Louis, it can reasonably be expected that accurate prevalence rates will be comparable. Thus in terms of such expectation, it is possible that the DIS was a better "gold standard" than was the psychiatric validation procedure.

CRITICISMS AND LIMITATIONS

These instruments are predicated on the idea that useful information for understanding and diagnosing psychiatric disorders can be obtained by asking questions about symptoms. It cannot be overemphasized that "questions" and "symptoms" are central to the approach described in this chapter.

This approach has not always commanded the interest of the psychiatric community nor has it been accepted as equally pertinent to all kinds of psychiatric disorders. In the early phases of this history, the psychiatric community was opposed to the symptom-oriented, question–answer approach to assessment on the assumption that the important features for diagnosis are not the symptoms of which a patient is aware but rather the intrapsychic processes of which the patient is unconscious.

It was largely due to this assumption that the Midtown Study gave American psychiatric epidemiology in its early period a reputation for being antidiagnostic. The Midtown Study is recognized as a pioneer effort in using "questions" about "symptoms" in face-to-face interviews with a large sample of adults. At the same time, recognition of the importance of intrapsychic processes in clinical psychiatry at that time led the Midtown Study to use "mental health ratings" rather than "psychiatric diagnoses."

The results of the Midtown interviews were read and evaluated by psychiatrists in order to place each subject on a linear dimension of psychiatric impairment. The rationale for this was that "symptomatic information offered the psychiatrists no firm perceptual footing to discern intrapsychic dynamics" and that intrapsychic dynamics were thought to be the "sine qua non of operable data for diagnosis within psychiatry's rapidly evolving nosological framework" (Srole et al., 1962, p. 134).

Disinterest on the part of clinical psychiatry was not due only to the issue of intrapsychic dynamics. Equally important was skepticism about the face validity of the scales. Such reservations were fostered by the absence of agreement about diagnostic criteria and by the lack of a nomenclature for communicating clearly about diagnostic categories.

The NSA illustrates the origins of the criticism about face validity. The large number of questions used in the calibration from which the NSA was produced included several items about early life experiences and potentially unconscious conflicts. These questions were congruent with the dominant interests of dynamic psychiatry at that time. The 15 items that did the best job of discrimination, however, were those contained in a scale named *Psychosomatic Complaints.*

Looking back at the scale, aided by language that has now become standard, it is clear that the scale measures "panic." It asks about nervousness and registers all the physiologic signals that accompany intense fear in a panic disorder: racing heart, choking, dizziness, and, in the earliest version, uncontrollable incontinence. There is probably no psychiatric syndrome more likely to interfere with a nonpsychotic soldier's ability to function in combat than "panic." If this had been recognized in the NSA, the next two decades of asking psychiatric questions might have been considerably more untrammelled than they actually were.

Later in this history, several researchers took the position that it was not only face validity that was absent from these scales but also construct and criterion validity. For example, the test–retest coefficient of 0.44 for an administration of the GHQ after 1 week led Duncan-Jones and Henderson (1978) to suggest that what the GHQ measures is not "true illness" but rather "transient reactions to disturbing experiences."

Commenting on the validity of the HOS, Tousignant et al. (1974, p. 250) noted that "if we define mental illness by the permanence and irreversibility of the symptoms, we can wonder how an instrument covering a range from mild to moderate symptoms can indicate a disabling mental disorder."

The Dohrenwends also saw clinical psychiatric disorder as having the hallmark of intractability and persistence of symptomatology. Evidence of poor congruence between some of the scales and psychiatric assessment led them to suggest that these scales measure "demoralization" or "nonspecific psychological distress' in contrast to specific diagnosable mental disorders (Dohrenwend and Dohrenwend, 1965, 1982).

Despite this criticism, several of the scales have continued to be used, either as the sole means of gathering information or in conjunction with a schedule. It has become increasingly clear that the reconstruction of the lifetime history of disorders is influenced by the current clinical state (Bromet et al., 1986). Thus scales that direct attention to the current week or month, as with the CES-D, the HSCL, and the GHQ, have been found to play a useful role as an adjunct to a schedule, especially for depression and anxiety.

While criticism has been voiced about diagnostic schedules, numerous advances are to be noted. For example, there was a time when it was thought that subjects would not answer questions about socially unacceptable behaviors such as drunkenness, violence, and pathologic gambling. The DIS experience suggests that this apprehension has not been borne out and that, if the interview is set up as a professional inquiry conducted by a stranger, most people appear to be willing to describe behaviors of these types if they pertain.

An important criticism of the DIS, however, is that the section on depression has not borne up to reliability and validity testing as well as the alcohol abuse section has. Since both disorders are common in a general population, there is need to rethink the special needs for depression and to develop a diagnostic grammar for it that makes fewer demands on subjects.

Where the psychoses are concerned, there is a difference between using a schedule in a clinical setting and using it in an epidemiologic study. There is ample demonstration from the PSE and the SCID that useful information can be gathered from psychotic patients. It is not equally clear, however, that a highly structured schedule administered by a lay interviewer is the best means of identifying people with psychotic disorders in an epidemiologic study. Systematic means of adding third-party information and observation of behaviors may be needed.

In recent years, interest has been expressed in estimating the prevalence of cognitive impairment as an indicator of dementia. The Mini-Mental Status Examination (Folstein et al., 1975) is an example of a test used for this purpose. It differs from the symptom-oriented approaches in that it consists of a series of mental tasks. Nevertheless, it does involve the question–answer format and has been successfully added on to the DIS as part of the interviews carried out in the ECA and other studies.

CONTROVERSIES

While both scales and schedules deal with symptoms, controversies continue regarding the relative merits of dimensional versus diagnostic measurement. Dimensional assessments usually employ a quantitative gradient based on continuous scoring of items on a particular qualitative theme. The qualitative themes involve depressive mood, anxious apprehension, paranoid ideation, and hallucinatory tendencies. Those who favor dimensional approaches argue that most psychiatric disorders involve more than one dimension. A schizophrenic patient often suffers from depression. If only the category of schizophrenia is used, information about the depressive quality is lost.

Diagnostic measurement implements a categorical approach in which effort is made to discover which syndromal pattern best describes the subject's disorder. Much of the criticism of this approach relates to the fact that under the influence of hierarchical classification, effort was made to use one and only one diagnostic category. Inherent in the hierarchical approach was the goal of using the most informative of all the possible categories that pertain. For example, if a patient exhibited four syndromal patterns (schizophrenia, alcohol abuse, depression, and anxiety), it was customary to use only schizophrenia to describe this patient. A major achievement of the ECA was demonstration of the pervasiveness of multiple categories (Boyd et al., 1984) and with this recognition of the need to relax exclusion criteria that hide such comorbidity.

Thus it is possible that controversies about dimensional and diagnostic approaches can be resolved through procedures that allow keeping a record of the fact that a given subject displays several dimensions through the availability of several categories.

In addition, it is important to recognize that *continuous* and *categorical* may involve a false dichotomy. Psychiatric scales involve continuous measurement, but they are routinely converted to categorical statements by the application of a cutting point. Also categorical measurement, insofar as it involves algorithmic steps, almost always involves some dimensional assessments.

EXPERIMENT IN MEASUREMENT

Based on the view that *continuous* and *categorical* are not necessarily incompatible, an experiment in analyzing a psychiatric scale by means of a diagnostic algorithm can be described. This experiment took place as part of the Stirling County Study, for which the HOS was designed. As part of an effort to provide longitudinal findings that would be as interpretable as possible by contemporary diagnostic standards, a computer program was written and named DPAX, DP standing for depression and AX for anxiety (Murphy et al., 1985). The program involves diagnostic principles that have been used throughout the study and that bear considerable similarity to those later spelled out in DSM-III.

In Figure 2, Receiver Operating Characteristic (ROC) analysis is shown for purposes of comparing continuous scoring of the HOS with the scoring system developed for the same data but embodied in the DPAX program (Murphy et al., 1987). The standard for assessment consists of psychiatrist decisions about who should be counted as a case of depression and/or anxiety and who not after reading the results of the research protocol.

ROC analysis produces a curve based on the calculation of all possible sensitivity and specificity values as the threshold is moved across the score range. A value called *area under the curve* (AUC) is a statistical assessment of the congruence between the test and the standard. If the sensitivity and specificity values track across the line of no information, it means that the test is unable to discriminate the ill from the well. The more the curve arches toward the upper left corner, the better the test.

It can be seen that the continuous scoring of the HOS agreed well with the psychiatrist's decisions. With a low score of only two symptoms, everyone who was judged to be

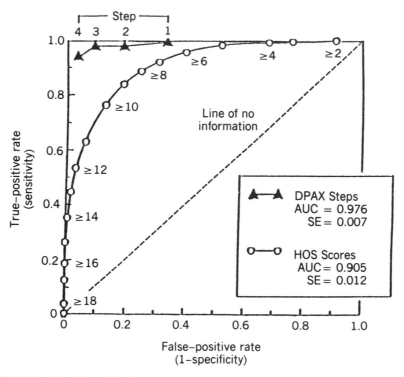

FIGURE 2. Receiver Operating Curve (ROC) analysis: continuous and categorical scoring Assessment. DPAX (DP standing for depression and AX for anxiety) is a computer program consisting of four steps that implement a categorical algorithm for diagnosis (Murphy et al., 1985). HOS (Health Opinion Survey) is a continuously scored psychiatric scale (Macmillan, 1957). ROC analysis of these scoring procedures was first reported by Murphy et al. (1987).

a case has been identified and sensitivity is perfect. As the threshold is moved from low to high scores, sensitivity deteriorates while specificity becomes perfect. When the threshold is set at the highest possible score, everybody who was judged not to be a case has been excluded.

While the AUC value for the continuous scoring of the HOS is significantly different from the line of no information, it needs to be emphasized that there is a constant relationship between sensitivity and specificity in this kind of continuous scoring. If the threshold is raised to improve specificity, there is an automatic loss in sensitivity.

The ROC curve for the DPAX program involves four steps. The first step is the application of discriminant function coefficients that were tested in split-half designs and by application to samples other than the test sample. Because this first step uses all of the questions, it can be thought of as capturing everybody who has any significant amount of associated symptomatology. The second step establishes that the essential features are present; the third applies criteria for impairment and duration; and the fourth establishes that the symptoms are sufficiently frequent in occurrence to suggest a clinical level of intensity.

The curve indicates that the first step casts a wide net intended to identify everyone who could possibly be a case, and then with each successive step the mesh is narrowed by the application of more criteria. Accordingly the algorithm begins with high sensitivity at the first step and then improves specificity without serious loss of sensitivity. By the fourth step, the program has 92% sensitivity and 98% specificity.

DIRECTIONS FOR THE FUTURE

Psychiatric measurement has taken several different directions during the years since the Second World War. In the following five points, suggestions are offered regarding ways in which past and present approaches might be blended to improve the products of measurement in the future.

1. Interdisciplinary collaboration. Clinical criteria, psychometric principles, and survey methodology constitute a troika of resources for improved measurement.

2. The "simplicity principle". Psychometric theory and survey experience (Nunnally, 1978; Choi and Comstock, 1975) suggest that the best ways of reducing carelessness and misunderstanding on the part of the subject and of decreasing error and variability on the part of interviewers is to a) prepare clear instructions, b) use simple language in the questions; and c) reduce the number of response categories

3. Alcohol abuse and depression. Measurement of alcohol abuse and depression should be equally reliable and valid. The simplicity of the alcohol abuse section in the DIS could serve as a model for improving the reliability and validity of the depression section.

4. "Essential features" and "associated symptoms". The increasing explicitness of clinical criteria has emphasized that syndrome recognition requires a division between features that must be present and associated symptoms that only need to be reasonably well represented. Experimentation suggests that a computer program can bear much of the burden of making the complex differentiations necessary for syndrome recognition, thereby relieving both subjects and interviewers of some of this burden.

5. Lifetime orientation and episode demarcation. Further exploration is needed regarding reliability. One direction would be experimentation to see if improvement is introduced by beginning inquiry with the present and moving backward in time as contrasted to asking whether the subject *ever* had the symptoms of interest. Of special importance is further investigation of the concept of "episode," indicating a boundary in historical time that separates illness from wellness. Major depression in DSM-III and the DIS is assumed to be an episodic disorder, and this assumption underlies the formulation of questions. This assumption needs scrutiny, as does also existing durational criteria. Lastly, consideration should be given to the question of whether it is realistic to expect people to recall their lives in packages of 2 weeks.

ACKNOWLEDGMENTS

This chapter is based on the course titled "Psychiatric Screening and Diagnostic Tests" taught in the Department of Epidemiology at the Harvard School of Public Health from 1987 to the present. It also draws on a report prepared for the National Institute of Mental Health under contract

80M014280101D titled "Psychiatric Instrument Development for Primary Care Research: Patient Self-Report Questionnaire," 1981. Extensions of that report have been prepared and published by Murphy (1986, 1990). In addition, the chapter draws on materials from the Stirling County Study, a longitudinal investigation in psychiatric epidemiology (Murphy, 1992).

REFERENCES

American Psychiatric Association (1980): "Diagnostic and Statistical Manual of Mental Disorders," 3rd ed. Washington, DC: American Psychiatric Association.

Anthony JC, Folstein M, Romanoski AJ, Von Korff MR, Nestadt GR, Chahal R, Merchant A, Brown CH, Shapiro S, Kramer M, Gruenberg EM (1985): Comparison of the lay Diagnostic Interview Schedule and a standardized psychiatric diagnosis: Experience in eastern Baltimore. Arch Gen Psychiatry 42:667–675.

Bebbington P, Hurry J, Tennant C, Sturt E, Wing JK (1981): Epidemiology of mental disorders in Camberwell. Psychol Med 11:561–579.

Beck AT, Ward CH, Mendelsohn M, Mock J, Erbaugh J (1961): An inventory for measuring depression. Arch Gen Psychiatry 4:561–571.

Blouin AG, Perez EL, Blouin JM (1987): Computerized administration of the Diagnostic Interview Schedule. Psychiatry Res 23:335–344.

Boyd JH, Burke JD, Gruenberg E, Holzer CE, Rae DS, George LK, Karno M, Stoltzman R, McEvoy L, Nestadt G (1984): Exclusion criteria of DSM-III: A study of co-occurrence of hierarchy-free syndromes. Arch Gen Psychiatry 41:983–989.

Brodman K, Erdmann AJ, Lorge I, Wolff HG (1949): The Cornell Medical Index: An adjunct to Medical Interview. JAMA 140:530–534.

Bromet EJ, Dunn LO, Connell MM, Dew MA, Schulberg HC (1986): Long-term reliability of diagnosing lifetime major depression in a community sample. Arch Gen Psychiatry 43:435–440.

Buros OK (ed) (1992): "Mental Measurements Yearbook." Lincoln: University of Nebraska Press.

Choi IC, Comstock GW (1975): Interviewer effect on responses to a questionnaire relating to mood. Am J Epidemiol 101:81–92.

Comstock GW, Helsing KJ (1976): Symptoms of depression in two communities. Psychol Med 6:551–563.

Cooper JE, Kendell RE, Gurland BJ, Sharpe L, Copeland JRM, Simon R (1972): "Psychiatric Diagnosis in New York and London." London: Oxford University Press.

Dahlstrom WG, Welsh GS, Dahlstrom LE (1972): "An MMPI Handbook, vol I, Clinical Interpretation." Minneapolis: University of Minnesota Press.

Derogatis LR, Cleary PA (1977): Confirmation of the dimensional structure of the SCL-90: A study in construct validation. J Clin Psychol 33:981–989.

Derogatis LR, Lipman RS, Rickels K, Uhlenhuth EH, Covi L (1974): The Hopkins symptom checklist (HSCL): A self-report symptom inventory. Behav Sci 19:1–15.

Dohrenwend BP (1989): "The problem of validity in field studies of psychological disorders" revisited. In Robins LN, Barrett JE: "The Validity of Psychiatric Diagnosis." New York: Raven Press, pp 35–55.

Dohrenwend BP, Dohrenwend BS (1965): The problem of validity in field studies of psychological disorder. J Abnorm Psychol 70:52–69.

Dohrenwend BP, Dohrenwend BS (1982): Perspectives on the past and future of psychiatric epidemiology: The 1981 Rema Lapouse Lecture. Am J Public Health 72:1271–1279.

Dohrenwend BP, Levav I, Shrout PE (1986): Screening scales from the Psychiatric Epidemiology

Research Interview (PERI). In Weissman MM, Myers JK, Ross CE (eds): "Community Surveys of Psychiatric Disorders." New Brunswick, NJ: Rutgers University Press, pp 349–375.

Dohrenwend BP, Levav I, Shrout PE, Schwartz S, Guedalia N, Link BG, Skodol AE, Stueve A (1992): "Socioeconomic status and psychiatric disorders: The causation-selection issue." Science 255:946–952.

Dohrenwend BP, Shrout PE, Egri G, Mendelsohn FS (1980): Nonspecific psychological distress and other dimensions of psychopathology. Arch Gen Psychiatry 37:1229–1236.

Duncan-Jones P, Henderson S (1978): The use of a two-phase design in a prevalence survey. Social Psychiatry 13:231–237.

Endicott J, Spitzer RL (1978): A diagnostic interview: The Schedule for Affective Disorders and Schizophrenia. Arch Gen Psychiatry 35:837–844.

Eysenk HJ (1947): "Dimensions of Personality." London: Routledge and Kegan Paul Ltd.

Feighner JP, Robins E, Guze SB, Woodruff RA, Winokur G, Munoz R (1972): Diagnostic criteria for use in psychiatric research. Arch Gen Psychiatry 26:57–63.

Folstein MF, Folstein SE, McHugh PR (1975): "Mini-Mental State": A practical method for grading the cognitive state of patients for the clinician. J Psychiatr Res 12:189–198.

Goldberg DP (1972): "The Detection of Psychiatric Illness by Questionnaire: A Technique for the Identification and Assessment of Non-Psychotic Psychiatric Illness." London: Oxford University Press.

Guilford S (1936): "Psychometric Methods." New York: McGraw-Hill.

Gurin G, Veroff J, Feld S (1960): "Americans View Their Mental Health: A Nationwide Interview Survey," Monograph No. 4, Joint Commission on Mental Illness and Health. New York: Basic Books, Inc.

Hamilton M (1960): A rating scale for depression. J Neurol Neurosurg Psychiatry 23:57–62.

Helzer JE, Canino GJ (eds) (1992): "Alcoholism in North America, Europe, and Asia." New York: Oxford University Press.

Helzer JE, Robins LN, Croughan JL, Weiner A (1981): Renard Diagnostic Interview: Its reliability and procedural validity with physicians and lay interviewers. Arch Gen Psychiatry 38:393–398.

Helzer JE, Robins LN, McEvoy LT, Spitznagel EL, Stoltzman RK, Farmer A, Brockington IF (1985): A comparison of clinical and Diagnostic Interview Schedule Diagnoses: Physician reexamination of the lay-interviewed cases in the general population. Arch Gen Psychiatry 42:657–666.

Henderson S, Byrne DG, Duncan-Jones P (1981): "Neurosis and the Social Environment." Sydney: Academic Press.

Kessler RC, McGonagle KA, Shanyang Z, Nelson CB, Hughes M, Eshleman S, Wittchen HU, Kendler KS (1994): Lifetime and 12-month prevalence of DSM-III-R psychiatric disorders in the United States: results from the National Comorbidity Survey. Arch Gen Psychiatry 51:8–19.

Kessler R et al (1994): National Comorbidity Study. Arch Gen Psychiatry (in press).

Langner TS (1962): A twenty-two item screening score of psychiatric symptoms indicating impairment. J Health Hum Behav 3:269–276.

Leighton DC, Harding JS, Macklin DB, Macmillan AM, Leighton AH (1963): "The Character of Danger: The Stirling County Study of Psychiatric Disorder and Sociocultural Environment," vol III. New York: Basic Books, Inc.

Link B, Dohrenwend BP (1980): Formulation of hypotheses about the true prevalence of demoralization in the United States. In Dohrenwend BP, Dohrenwend BS, Gould MS, Link B, Neugebauer R, Wunsch-Hitzig R: "Mental Illness in the United States: Epidemiological Estimates." New York: Praeger Press, pp 114–132.

Macmillan AM (1957): The Health Opinion Survey: Technique for estimating prevalence of psychoneurotic and related types of disorders in communities. Psychol Rep 3:325–339.

Markush RE, Favero RV (1974): Epidemiologic assessment of stressful life events, depressed mood, and psychophysiological symptoms—A preliminary report. In Dohrenwend BS, Dohrenwend BP (eds): "Stressfull Life Events: Their Nature and Effects." New York: John Wiley & Sons, pp 171–190.

McDowell I, Newell C (1987): "Measuring Health: A Guide to Rating Scales and Questionnaires." New York: Oxford University Press.

Murphy JM (1986): Diagnosis, screening, and 'demoralization': Epidemiologic implications. Psychiatr Dev 2:101–133.

Murphy JM, Berwick DM, Weinstein MC, Borus JF, Budman SH, Klerman GL (1987): Performance of screening and diagnostic tests: Application of receiver operating characteristic (ROC) analysis. Arch Gen Psychiatry 44:550–555.

Murphy JM (1990): Depression screening instruments: History and issues. In Attkisson CC, Zich JM (eds): "Depression in Primary Care: Screening and Detection." New York: Routledge, Chapman and Hall, pp 65–83.

Murphy JM (1992): Measurement and design in a longitudinal epidemiologic study: Depression and anxiety in a general population. In Fava M, Rosenbaum JF (eds): "Research Designs and Methods in Psychiatry." Amsterdam: Elsevier Science Publishers B.V., pp 127–143.

Murphy JM, Neff RK, Sobol AM, Rice JX, Olivier DC (1985): Computer diagnosis of depression and anxiety: The Stirling County Study. Psychol Med 15:99–112.

Nunnally JC (1978): "Psychometric Theory," 2nd ed. New York: McGraw-Hill.

Parloff MB, Kelman HC, Frank JD (1954): Comfort, effectiveness, and self-awareness as criteria of improvement in psychotherapy. Am J Psychiatry 111:343–351.

President's Commission on Mental Health (1978): "Report to the President," vol I. Washington, DC: United States Government Printing Office.

Radloff LS (1977): The CES-D Scale: A self-report depression scale for research in the general population. Appl Psychol Measurement 1:385–401.

Rickels K, Garcia CR, Fisher E (1971): A measure of emotional distress in private gynecologic practice. Obstet Gynecol 38:139–146.

Robins LN (1985): Epidemiology: Reflections on testing the validity of psychiatric interviews. Arch Gen Psychiatry 42:918–924.

Robins LN (1989): Diagnostic grammar and assessment: Translating criteria into questions. Psychol Med 19:57–68.

Robins LN, Helzer J, Croughan J, Ratcliff KS (1981): The NIMH Diagnostic Interview Schedule: It's history, characteristics and validity. Arch Gen Psychiatry 38:381–389.

Robins LN, Regier DA (eds) (1991): "Psychiatric Disorders in America: The Epidemiologic Catchment Area Study." New York: The Free Press.

Robins LN, Wing JK, Wittchen HU, Helzer JE, Babor TF, Burke J, Farmer A, Jablenski A, Pickens R, Regier DA, Sartorius N, Towle LH (1988): The Composite International Diagnostic Interview: An epidemiologic instrument suitable for use in conjunction with different diagnostic systems and in different cultures. Arch Gen Psychiatry 45:1069–1077.

Rorer LG (1965): The great response-style myth. Psychol Bull 63:129–156.

Shepherd M, Cooper B, Brown AC, Kalton G (1966): "Psychiatric Illness in General Practice." London: Oxford University Press.

Spitzer RL, Endicott J, Fleiss JL, Cohen J (1970): The Psychiatric Status Schedule: A technique for evaluating psychopathology and impairment in role functioning. Arch Gen Psychiatry 23:41–55.

Spitzer RL, Endicott J, Robins E (1978): Research Diagnostic Criteria: Rationale and reliability. Arch Gen Psychiatry 35:773–782.

Spitzer RL, Fleiss JL, Endicott J, Cohen J (1967): Mental Status Schedule: Properties of factor-analytically derived scales. Arch Gen Psychiatry 16:479–493.

Spitzer RL, Williams JB, Gibbon M, First MB (1992): The Structured Clinical Interview for DSM-III-R (SCID): I: History, rationale, and description. Arch Gen Psychiatry 49:624–629.

Srole L, Langner TS, Michael ST, Opler MK, Rennie TAC (1962): "Mental Health in the Metropolis: The Midtown Manhattan Study." New York: McGraw-Hill.

Star SA (1950): The screening of psychoneurotics in the Army: Technical development of tests. In Stouffer SA, Guttman L, Suchman EA, Lazarsfeld PF, Star SA, Clausen JA: "The American Soldier: Measurement and Prediction," vol IV. Princeton: Princeton University Press, pp 486–547.

Stouffer SA, Guttman L, Suchman EA, Lazarsfeld PF, Star SA, Clausen JA (1950): "The American Soldier: Measurement and Prediction," vol IV. Princeton: Princeton University Press.

Tarlov AR, Ware JE, Greenfield S, Nelson EC, Perrin E, Zubkoff M (1989): The Medical Outcomes Study: An application of methods for monitoring the results of medical care. JAMA 262:925–930.

Thompson C (ed) (1989): "The Instruments of Psychiatric Research." New York: John Wiley & Sons.

Tousignant M, Denis G, Lachapelle R (1974): Some considerations concerning the validity and use of the Health Opinion Survey. J Health Soc Behav 15:241–252.

Tsuang MT, Winokur G (1975): The Iowa 500: Field work in a 35-year follow-up of depression, mania, and schizophrenia. Can Psychiatr Assoc J 20:359–365.

Tsuang MT, Woolson RF, Simpson JC (1980): The Iowa Structured Psychiatric Interview: Rationale, reliability and validity. Acta Psychiatr Scand 283(Suppl):1–58.

Veroff J, Douvan E, Kulka RA (1981): "The Inner American: A Self-Portrait From 1957 to 1976." New York: Basic Books, Inc.

Veroff J, Kulka RA, Douvan E (1981): "Mental Health in America: Patterns of Help-Seeking From 1957 to 1976." New York: Basic Books, Inc.

Ware, JE, Sherbourne CD (1992): The MOS 36-item short-form health survey (SF-36): 1. Conceptual framework and item selection. Med Care 30:473–483.

Weider A, Mittelmann B, Wechsler D, Wolff HG (1944): The Cornell Selectee Index: A method for quick testing of selectees for the armed forces. JAMA 124:224–228.

Wing JK (1961): A simple and reliable subclassification of chronic schizophrenia. J Ment Sci 107:862–875.

Wing JK, Cooper JE, Sartorius N (1974): "Description and Classification of Psychiatric Symptoms." London: Cambridge University Press.

World Health Organization (1973): "International Pilot Study of Schizophrenia." Geneva: World Health Organization.

Zung WWK (1963): A self-rating depression scale. Arch Gen Psychiatry 12:63–70.

CHAPTER 13

DSM-IV and Psychiatric Epidemiology

ALLEN FRANCES, AVRAM H. MACK, MICHAEL B. FIRST, TOM WIDIGER,
STEVE FORD, NANCY VETTERELLO, and RUTH ROSS

Department of Psychiatry, Duke University Medical Center, Durham, N.C. 27710 (A.F., S.F., A.H.M.,
R.R.); New York State Psychiatric Institute, New York, N.Y. 10032 (M.B.F.); Department of
Psychology, University of Kentucky, Lexington, KY 40506 (T.W.); and American Psychiatric
Association, Washington, DC (N.V.)

INTRODUCTION

A major purpose of psychiatric epidemiology is to determine the prevalence of psychiatric disorders. Among DSM-IV's many purposes, one of its most important is the facilitation of such research. The availability of a widely accepted and reliable diagnostic system is an essential prerequisite to psychiatric epidemiology. Epidemiologic research is impossible without clear and consistent methods of classifying and diagnosing psychiatric disorders. Before DSM-III, psychiatric epidemiology was severely constrained by the lack of a reliable system of diagnosis and assessment that could be applied in community studies. The availability of DSM-III, and the subsequent development of formal structured interviews based on it, was necessary to the Epidemiological Catchment Area (ECA) Study and to other recent studies of the prevalence of psychiatric disorders in the community. It is hoped that DSM-IV, in its turn, will also be helpful to psychiatric epidemiology by introducing an updated, yet conservative, set of diagnostic criteria for the various mental disorders. The purpose of this chapter is to explore the ways in which the decisions made in DSM-IV may impact on the methods and results of epidemiologic studies. We first review the development of DSM-IV and then describe its relation to psychiatric epidemiology.

THE DEVELOPMENT OF DSM-IV

DSM-IV was developed over a 5 year period and involved more than 1,000 mental health experts, including psychiatrists, psychologists, social workers, and members of

The opinions expressed in this chapter are those of the authors and do not necessarily represent the position of the American Psychiatric Association and its Task Force on DSM-IV. We find ourselves writing on DSM-IV so often and for so many different audiences that some repetition of previous papers has been inevitable.

Textbook in Psychiatric Epidemiology, Edited by Tsuang, Tohen, and Zahner
ISBN 0-471-59375-3   © 1995 Wiley-Liss, Inc.

various other medical specialties (Frances et al., 1989). A substantial number of the participants and consultants were expert in the field of psychiatric epidemiology. The 27 Task Force members were experienced in the different areas of mental health, including epidemiologic research. Their decisions were based on the recommendations of the 13 Work Groups, each of which consisted of 5–10 experts in a particular domain of psychopathology. Each Work Group regularly received input from 50–100 advisors. In this way, the decisions of the DSM-IV Task Force reflect a consensus in the mental health field and are fully informed by data that have emerged from epidemiologic studies.

The most innovative aspect of DSM-IV was the three-stage process of empirical review employed by the Task Force in deciding whether any given change would be made (Pincus et al., 1992). This process was outlined early in the DSM-IV process at a series of methods conferences (Widiger et al., 1991; Frances et al., 1989). The consensus of the participants of these meetings was to follow the guidelines suggested by the meta-analysis literature for conducting systematic, comprehensive, and explicit reviews (Cooper, 1984; Light and Pillemer, 1984; Rosenthal, 1984; Bangert-Drowns, 1986).

The three-stage process served as the organizational backbone of the investigations of the Work Groups. The first stage consisted of comprehensive and systematic reviews of the published literature. This was followed by reanalyses of already collected but not previously analyzed data. The third stage consisted of field trials.

Literature Reviews

Each Work Group identified which questions were most pertinent regarding each diagnosis. The 150 literature reviews that resulted each made specific recommendations that were presented to the Task Force, and then to the field, in the DSM-IV Options Book (American Psychiatric Association [APA], 1991). The requirement that decisions have empirical support ensured that everyone was working from a common and consensually accepted database. This resulted in a less passionate and more objective discourse and facilitated the development of consensus among individuals who often started from quite opposite positions (Frances et al., 1989; Widiger et al., 1990). Optimally, the decisions reached by the DSM-IV Work Groups were those that would have been reached by a "consensus scholar," with no preconceptions (Cooper, 1984). The epidemiologic literature was very helpful in this first phase of the DSM-IV process as it was also in the second phase.

Data Reanalyses

The literature reviews revealed that there were a number of diagnostic questions of considerable importance for which there were very few answers available in the published literature. Fortunately, for many of these questions data had been collected by various investigators but had not been analyzed or reported in a fashion that would be informative to the Work Group deliberations. A method of data reanalysis was devised to allow the Work Groups to benefit from these collected, but unpublished data. Questions would be framed for data sets collected at multiple sites. Data that had been collected in epidemiologic studies were used in a number of the reanalyses that were performed. Supported by grants from the John D. and Catherine T. MacArthur Foundation, these analyses also helped to develop and refine suggested new criteria items that could then be studied in field trials (Widiger et al., 1991).

Field Trials

Field trials fill the gap between clinical research and practice. They assess the acceptability, feasibility, coverage, generalizability, reliability, and construct validity of the criteria sets and their diagnostic algorithms in settings and using methods that more closely approximate general practice (Burke, 1988). The DSM-IV field trials addressed these concerns through two methodologies: 1) surveys and 2) focused field trials. Although convenient and economical, surveys are easily biased by sampling methods, differential response rates, and/or the particular ordering and phrasing of questions. It is also never clear whether the survey participants are sufficiently aware of the issues, literature, or data to offer an informed opinion about a proposed diagnosis. Several surveys were conducted as part of the DSM-IV process, but these had relatively little impact on the final decisions that were made (Frances et al., 1991).

There were 12 DSM-IV field trials, which were sponsored by the National Institute of Mental Health (NIMH) in conjunction with the National Institute on Drug Abuse (NIDA) and the National Institute on Alcohol Abuse and Alcoholism (NIAAA). The field trials were intended to give the DSM-IV Work Groups the chance to test the advantages and disadvantages of the different criteria sets that were being considered for inclusion in DSM-IV. The alternatives tested included the criteria sets presented in DSM-III, DSM-III-R, and ICD-10 and new criteria items that were recommended by the work groups based on their literature reviews and data reanalyses. To ensure generalizability, many different sites were chosen. They reflected geographic, socioeconomic, cultural, and ethnic diversity, and, in some instances, included randomly selected community samples. Each trial compared the options at 5–10 sites, using approximately 100 subjects at each site (Widiger et al., 1991).

The DSM-IV decision-making process emphasized conservatism and almost always sought to maintain the same definition of caseness and the same prevalence rates as in previous systems. It is hoped that DSM-IV will minimally disrupt the conduct of epidemiologic studies and allow for the comparability of results collected over time and across differing diagnostic systems. The DSM-IV *Sourcebook* (APA, 1994b), containing the results of the literature reviews, data reanalyses, and field trials, will outline in much greater detail the rationale for decisions made in this process.

METHODOLOGICAL ISSUES

There were a number of issues addressed in the work on DSM-IV that have had an impact on the way in which it was developed and on its applications to epidemiologic studies.

Thresholds

Most disorders in DSM-IV are diagnosed when a patient exhibits a certain proportion of the criteria listed. In this sense, most DSM-IV diagnoses are polythetic rather than monothetic. The threshold number of criteria required for the disorder to be diagnosed will determine its prevalence in epidemiologic studies. The restrictiveness of a threshold depends on how many criteria are offered in the definition of the disorder and what fraction must be present to make the diagnosis. The particular cutoff number of criteria required for any DSM-IV diagnosis has been set in an effort to maximize an optimal balance between specificity and sensitivity. Setting a low threshold provides for good sensitivity and few false negatives, but at the expense of lower specificity and many false positives. In contrast, setting a high threshold provides good specificity (few false positives) but low sensitivity (many false negatives). In many instances, alternative thresholds using different cut offs perform equally well or almost equally well. The number of criteria chosen as a threshold for making the diagnosis (and the number of items in the criteria set) may have a great impact on the prevalence of any psychiatric category. The fact that the particular thresholds chosen in DSM-IV are usually not supported by robust external validators suggests that prevalence data gathered in epidemiologic studies using this diagnostic system should be approached with appropriate caution and an awareness of the limitations of the diagnostic method.

Definitions

The specific wording of the criteria sets for the disorders in DSM-IV will likewise have an appreciable effect on the definition of "caseness" and therefore on the prevalence of disorders in community samples. The DSM-IV Work Groups were well aware that if a criteria set were to be reworded (even slightly to improve stylistic or grammatic correctness), this might alter the prevalence of the item so that prevalence rates of the diagnosis might be affected. As discussed above, another issue in selecting items for criteria sets was whether to focus on sensitivity (i.e., those items that emphasize the core symptoms most characteristic of the disorder) or to focus on specificity (i.e., those items that best differentiate the given disorder from its near-neighbor disorders). The greater the emphasis on specificity, the lower will be its prevalence, and the less likely it is that the definition of the diagnosis will create artifactual comorbidity. By being conservative with respect to making changes from DSM-III-R, the Task Force hoped to reduce disruptions for the makers and users of assessment instruments and to maintain a consistency with results generated across research studies and at different times.

Reliability

Reliability for most DSM-IV categories is generally satisfactory or better, but there is considerable variability in the reliability achieved by the various diagnoses throughout the system. Moreover, reliability is much more satisfactory for the major sections of disorders than for the specific categories themselves (e.g., the reliability for the section Mood Disorders is greater than the reliability for the single category Major Depressive Disorder). Most reliability studies have been conducted by expert raters and may not be generalizable to the average clinician in the average clinical setting or to lay interviewers making assessments in community settings. It must also be recognized that the reliability a diagnosis will achieve in a given study will depend on the base rate of the disorder in the given sample. Since base rates of psychiatric disorders are expected to be much lower in epidemiolgic studies than in clinical studies, reliability is also likely to be much lower in epidemiologic studies (Spitzer and Fleiss, 1974).

Validity

It is, of course, desirable to have clear-cut, externally valid standards for establishing a criteria set and for making a diagnosis (Kendell, 1975). Unfortunately, such gold standards were not yet readily available as a guide for most DSM-IV decisions. The Task Force had to balance the various kinds of available validation. An important question faced in the DSM-IV process was what respective weight was to be given to clinical versus epidemiologic studies, considering that each may generate different findings and results. DSM-IV is first and foremost a clinical document, but epidemiologic studies were also given considerable weight. It must also be realized that the prevalence rates reported in studies of psychiatric epidemiology refer to descriptive presentations. Psychiatric epidemiology will become more precise and valuable as we gradually develop a more profound understanding of disease and more powerful methods of diagnoses.

Clinical Significance

There is a requirement that the mental disorders in DSM-IV cause clinically significant distress or impairment. Indeed, according to the Cautionary Statement in DSM-IV: "The specified diagnostic criteria for each mental disorder are offered as guidelines for making diagnoses, since it has been demonstrated that the use of such criteria enhances agreement among clinicians and investigators. The proper use of these criteria requires specialized clinical training that provides both a body of knowledge and clinical skills" (APA, 1994a). It is important to note that individuals may experience the symptoms included in the DSM-IV criteria and sets and yet not have a mental disorder. For example, an individual may meet the specific definitional criteria for a major depressive episode, but this would not be sufficient to make the diagnosis unless there is also significant psychiatric distress or impairment associated with the symptom presentation. To reiterate, one must evaluate not only the presence of items that define the criteria set but also whether they cause clinically significant distress or impairment in making a diagnosis.

To make a diagnosis, one must not only evaluate the presence or absence of diagnostic criteria but must also determine that they cause clinically significant distress and/or impairment. The attention to clinically significant distress or impairment is especially crucial in determining the prevalence of those disorders that are at the boundary with normality, a boundary that has particular relevance to the epidemiologic study of community samples. Patients presenting in clinical settings are usually more severely impaired or distressed and have self-defined themselves as distressed or impaired. Clinicians working in these settings are trained to assess the amount of distress and impairment caused by the symptoms. It must be remembered that epidemiology is a study of psychiatric disorders, not just the presence of symptom constellations. The judgment about clinically significant impairment is inherently easier for clinicians to make in clinical settings than for lay interviewers evaluating community samples. However, for reasons of feasability and cost, epidemiologic studies generally cannot use clinical interviewers and must usually rely on lay interviewers.

There is a limited, but growing, literature attempting to evaluate empirically whether there is satisfactory reliability in diagnostic assignment between lay and clinical interviewers. Inter-rater reliability between clinicians and lay interviewers is most difficult to achieve for those diagnoses that in their less severe manifestations, are likely to be confused with normality (e.g., specific phobia, major depressive disorder, obsessive/compulsive disorder). In many criteria sets, this issue has been emphasized by including the statement that the symptoms must "cause clinically significant distress or impairment in social, occupational, or other important areas of functioning." This caveat is especially difficult for lay interviewers to evaluate, both because they lack the clinical experience necessary to evaluate the question and because the question of clinically significant impairment is inherently more difficult to answer with respect to people who do not self-identify by resorting to clinical environments.

Splitting vs. Lumping

DSM-IV has ended the recent trend toward a rapidly increasing number of categories included in the diagnostic system. The threshold for including a new disorder in DSM-IV was set high. Very few new diagnoses were added to DSM-IV despite the fact that nearly 100 new categories were suggested for inclusion. Many of these suggested new diagnoses were at the border between psychopathology and normality (e.g., minor depression, mixed anxiety/depression, minor cognitive disorder). Undoubtedly many of these would have had a high prevalence were they included in the system. For example, rates of mood disorder in the community might have doubled if minor depression were included as a separate category in DSM-IV. DSM-IV has an expanded Appendix B of "Criteria Sets and Axes Provided for Further Study." Appendix B provides criteria sets and texts for new suggestions in the hope that research will be aided by their specification. Such research will determine their fate in future manuals.

Comorbidity

Although the DSM system retains an emphasis on differential diagnosis, since DSM-III there has also been a much greater emphasis on multiple diagnosis (APA, 1980; Spitzer et al., 1980). This tendency was extended still further in DSM-III-R, which eliminated many diagnostic hierarchies and increased rates of multiple diagnosis and comorbidity (APA, 1987). Several factors in the DSM system have resulted in the recent greatly increased interest in comorbidity and resulting concerns that it may be artifactually elevated. These factors include 1) narrowly defined criteria sets, 2) the increased number of diagnoses, 3) the explicit diagnostic criteria, 4) the use of structured interviews, and 5) the removal of diagnostic hierarchies (First 1990; Frances 1990).

CONCLUSION

The results obtained in epidemiologic studies will be influenced by the methods that have been used in developing DSM-IV. The DSM-IV reliance on empirical documentation and conservative standards for change should help to facilitate continuity in research studies and the interpretation of results generated through different diagnostic systems. DSM-IV is a descriptive system and for the most part not based on any gold standard. As we obtain more knowledge about the underlying diseases, we may have more reliable and valid diagnostic methods, leading to more precise knowledge of the prevalence of disease and its risk factors.

The design of any system of psychiatric diagnosis to be used in epidemiologic studies must be approached carefully to ensure accurate prevalence rates. Thresholds must be calibrated to balance specificity and sensitivity. Definitions must accurately reflect the symptoms of the disorder and balance the presentation of the core pathology with items that are most discriminating with near-neighbor disorders. One must be aware of the requirement that disorders cause clinically significant distress or impairment when using the manual in order to allow for generalization across clinical and epidemiologic studies and to reduce inflated prevalences in epidemiologic studies. Finally, it is particularly relevant to epidemiology that information gained through lay interviews be compared with, and not immediately taken as equivalent to, that based on data from clinical settings. The DSM-IV is the product of a great deal of empirical research, much of which used epidemiologic data. Careful and thoughtful use of DSM-IV by the epidemiologic community will pave the road for DSM-V.

REFERENCES

American Psychiatric Association (1980): "Diagnostic and Statistical Manual of Mental Disorders," 3rd ed. Washington DC: American Psychiatric Association.

American Psychiatric Association (1987): "Diagnostic and Statistical Manual of Mental Disorders," 3rd ed, revised Washington DC: American Psychiatric Association.

American Psychiatric Association (1991): "Diagnostic and Statistical Manual of Mental Disorders, 4th ed, Options Book." Washington, DC: American Psychiatric Association.

American Psychiatric Association (1994a): "Diagnostic and Statistical Manual of Mental Disorders," 4th ed. Washington, DC; American Psychiatric Association.

American Psychiatric Association (1994b): "Diagnostic and Statistical Manual of Mental Disorders," 4th ed, Sourcebook." Washington, DC: American Psychiatric Association.

Bangert-Drowns R (1986): Review of the developments in meta-analytic method. Psychol Bull 99:388–399.

Cooper HM (1984): "The Integrative Research Review. A Systematic Approach," vol. 2. Beverly Hills, CA: Sage Publications.

First M, Spitzer RL, Williams J (1990): Exclusionary principles and comorbidity of psychiatric diagnoses: A historical review and implications for the future." In Maser JD, Cloninger CR (eds): "Comorbidity of Mood and Anxiety Disorders." Washington, DC: American Psychiatric Association, pp 83–109.

Frances A, Davis WW, Kline M, et al. (1991): The DSM-IV field trials: Moving toward an empirically derived classification. Eur Psychiatry 6:307–314.

Frances A, Widiger T, Fyer M, (1990): The influence of classification methods on comorbidity. In Maser JD, Cloninger CR (eds): "Comorbidity of Mood and Anxiety Disorders." Washington, DC: American Psychiatric Association, pp 41–59.

Frances A, Widiger T, Pincus H (1989): The development of DSM-IV. Arch Gen Psychiatry 46:373–375.

Kendell RE (1975): "The Role of Diagnosis in Psychiatry." London: Blackwell.

Light RL, Pillemer DB (1984): "Summing Up. The Science of Reviewing Research." Cambridge: Harvard University Press.

Pincus HA, Frances AJ, Davis WW, et al. (1992): DSM-IV and new diagnostic categories: Holding the line on proliferation. Am J Psychiatry 149:112–117.

Rosenthal R (1984): "Meta-Analytic Procedures for Social Research." Beverly Hills, CA: Sage Publications.

Spitzer RL, Fleiss JL (1974): A reanalysis of the reliability of psychiatric diagnosis. Br J Psychiatry 125:341–347.

Spitzer RL, Williams JBW, Skodol AE (1980): DSM-III: The major achievements and an overview. Am J Psychiatry 137:151–164.

Widiger TA, Frances AJ, Pincus HA, et al. (1991): Towards an empirical classification for the DSM-IV. J Abnorm Psychol 100:280–288.

Widiger TA, Frances AJ, Pincus HA, Davis WW (1990): The DSM-IV literature reviews: Rationale, process, and limitations. J Psychopathol Behave Assess 12:189–202.

PART IV

EPIDEMIOLOGY OF MAJOR PSYCHIATRIC DISORDERS

CHAPTER 14

Epidemiology of Psychosis With Special Reference to Schizophrenia

EVELYN J. BROMET, MARY AMANDA DEW, and WILLIAM EATON

Department of Psychiatry and Behavioral Science, State University of New York, Stony Brook, NY 11794 (E.J.B.); Department of Psychiatry, Epidemiology, and Psychology, University of Pittsburgh, Pittsburgh, PA 15260 (M.A.D.); Department of Mental Hygiene, The Johns Hopkins University, Baltimore, MD 21218 (W.E.)

INTRODUCTION

Psychotic disorders, such as schizophrenia, schizoaffective disorder, psychotic depression, bipolar disorder with psychotic features, and delusional disorder, are among the most debilitating and persistent diseases known to humankind. It is estimated that the annual cost for treatment of schizophrenia in the United States is 7 billion dollars (National Advisory Mental Health Council, 1988). Epidemiologic contributions to research on psychosis have focused primarily on schizophrenia and involve descriptive studies of incidence, prevalence, and risk factors associated with disease occurrence, as well as longitudinally designed analytic studies of etiology and course. Many comprehensive reviews of the descriptive epidemiology of schizophrenia have appeared, including contributions by the current authors (e.g., Bromet et al., 1988; Eaton et al., 1988) and by other eminent investigators (e.g., Beiser and Iacono, 1990; Cooper, 1978; Jablensky, 1986; Turner, 1972). This chapter extends the scope of review by considering not only descriptive research on rates and risk factors but also analytic research on etiology and course. We begin with a brief overview of the history of epidemiologic contributions to schizophrenia and then review descriptive and analytic findings. Lastly, we consider target areas for future epidemiologic research. Since relatively little research has been conducted on other psychotic conditions, we argue that such work is needed both to characterize these disorders in their own right and to improve our understanding of schizophrenia itself.

HISTORICAL OVERVIEW

Three types of epidemiologic research on the occurrence of schizophrenia, distinguished by differences in sampling and case definition, have evolved. Similar to Dohrenwend and

Textbook in Psychiatric Epidemiology, Edited by Tsuang, Tohen, and Zahner
ISBN 0-471-59375-3 © 1995 Wiley-Liss, Inc.

TABLE 1. Types of Research Methods Applied to Epidemiologic Research on Schizophrenia

Study Population	Source of Diagnosis	
	Medical Record	Structured Interview
Patients	A	B
Community residents	N/A	C

Dohrenwend's historical perspective (1982) on the development of psychiatric epidemiologic research, the first type of study (A in Table 1), conducted prior to world War II primarily, relied on key informants' reports and agency/hospital records for case ascertainment. The earliest prevalence study of this sort was the classic census on the "insane" conducted in nineteenth century Massachusetts that enumerated approximately 3,600 "lunatics" and "idiots" in family, private, or public care (Jarvis, 1971). Faris and Dunham (1939), using Illinois state mental hospital records, were the first investigators to apply the ecologic method to research on mental disorders. This research showed that, unlike patients with other diagnoses, hospitalized schizophrenic patients were most likely to come from inner-city areas of Chicago (46%) and least likely to have lived in suburban areas outside the city with better socioeconomic conditions (13% in the outermost district). Although aggregated data such as these could not be used to test causal hypotheses, they clearly supported an association between lower social class and the occurrence of schizophrenia, a finding later confirmed in other ecologic studies of Chicago (Levy and Rowitz, 1970) and elsewhere (e.g., Giggs, 1986). This association was subsequently supported by nonecologic studies of treated (e.g., Goldberg and Morrison, 1963; Hollingshead and Redlich, 1958) and randomly selected (Dohrenwend and Dohrenwend, 1969) community populations.

In addition to establishing prevalence rates, another focus of research in this first category was on treatment outcome patterns. Although the introduction of phenothiazines in the 1950s ushered in dramatic changes in discharge patterns, earlier studies clearly showed that the rates of discharge started to decrease during the first half of the twentieth century (Ram et al., 1992). Factors predicting discharge in these earlier reports bore a striking similarity to predictors of better outcome in the phenothiazine era. For example, Locke (1962) identified factors predicting probability of discharge in 5,781 Ohio state mental hospital patients admitted from 1948 to 1952 and followed over a period of 5 years; significant predictors included being 15–34 years old at the time of first admission, married, well educated, and employed in a higher status job. Except for age, these variables proved to have prognostic significance in longitudinal outcome studies following the introduction of phenothiazines and have been interpreted as indicators of better premorbid functioning (Ram et al., 1992).

Research falling under the first category, which continues to this day, relies on medical record diagnosis. In contrast, the second type of research on the epidemiology of psychosis grew out of the recognition that diagnostic practices varied in different countries and across institutions in the United States. In fact, by the 1970s, differences in diagnostic practices, amplified by the absence of explicit operational criteria, were viewed as major impediments to progress in research on the epidemiology of schizophrenia (Cooper,

1978). The problem reached a crescendo with the publication of the findings from the United States/United Kingdom (U.S./U.K.) project (Cooper et al., 1972). Prior to this project, higher rates of schizophrenia in hospitalized patients were reported in studies in the United States than in the United Kingdom, while relatively elevated rates of affective disorders, such as manic depressive disorder, were reported in the United Kingdom. The U.S./U.K. project, for the first time, trained psychiatrists in two countries in a structured diagnostic interview (the Present State Examination) and applied a common set of diagnostic criteria. The results showed that the proportions of U.S. and U.K. patients with schizophrenia and affective disorder were similar, indicating that previously observed variations in the rates of these disorders were a function of diagnostic practices rather than of true differences in morbidity patterns.

The introduction of modern nosologic systems, following the U.S./U.K. study, such as the Research Diagnostic Criteria (RDC) (Spitzer et al., 1978) and DSM-III (American Psychiatric Association, 1980), led to renewed interest in epidemiologic research on schizophrenia, using structured interviews and formal diagnostic systems. Thus the second type of study (B in Table 1) is characterized by a focus on treated populations using psychometric advances in diagnosis. The most noteworthy epidemiologic research in this category is the world Health Organization's (WHO's) program, particularly the Determinants of Outcome of Severe Mental Disorders study. In this project, 1,379 psychotic individuals aged 15–54 years were identified after making their first lifetime contact with services in catchment areas in 10 countries. They were then followed annually over a 2 year period (Jablensky et al., 1992; Sartorius et al., 1986). Findings on incidence are reported below. In North America, several recent studies of first-admission patients have also addressed incidence (Beiser et al., 1988), as well as etiology (Pulver et al., 1981) and course (Beiser et al., 1989; Bromet et al., 1992; Tohen et al., 1992), in heterogeneous samples of psychotic patients diagnosed using systematic criteria. These studies are distinct from other clinical studies of psychotic disorders in their attention to representative sampling, use of structured diagnostic interview schedules, and focus on first-admission patients, as opposed to consecutive admission with varying treatment histories.

The third type of epidemiologic study of schizophrenia combines modern community sampling techniques with structured interview approaches to case identification (C in Table 1). The earliest studies using this design were conducted by psychiatrists in European towns and villages before World War II (Jablensky, 1986). In the United States, the first large-scale community study of this sort was the Epidemiologic Catchment Area (ECA) study conducted in the early 1980s. However, the lay interviewers' diagnosis of schizophrenia, using the Diagnostic Interview Schedule (DIS), was not congruent with psychiatrists' classifications. In the Baltimore site, for example, the DIS identified only 20% of the cases of schizophrenia that a psychiatrist identified in an independent examination (Anthony et al., 1985). Thus, the ECA is not a suitable source of information on the rates of schizophrenia.

To provide more reliable and valid estimates of the rates of schizophrenia and other psychoses in the United States, Kessler et al. (1993) used a two-stage procedure for case identification in the National Comorbidity Survey, a study of a national probability sample aged 15–54 years. Clinicians reinterviewed by telephone all individuals endorsing psychotic symptoms during the lay structured interview (the University of Michigan refinement of the Composite International Diagnostic Interview, or UM-CIDI). The telephone interview was a modified version of the Structured Clinical Interview for DSM-III-R (SCID) Spitzer et al., 1992; Williams et al., 1992). Classification was thus based on the additional clinical information rather than on the lay interview material exclusively as was done in the ECA.

Much of the descriptive epidemiologic findings on schizophrenia, thus, emanate from these three methods of sampling and case identification, that is, patients with a medical chart diagnosis of schizophrenia, patients rediagnosed using research interviews and standardized diagnostic criteria, and community residents receiving structured diagnostic interviews administered by clinicians. In the next sections, we summarize findings on the incidence and prevalance of schizophrenia, factors associated with the occurrence of the disorder, and variables linked to better or worse course.

PREVALENCE AND INCIDENCE

Definition of Disorder

The essential features of schizophrenia are the presence of specific psychotic symptoms (delusions, hallucinations, thought disorder) during the active phase of illness; a decline in social or occupational functioning below the highest level achieved or expected; and a 6 month duration of illness, including the prodromal and residual phases (American Psychiatric Association, 1987). In addition, there may be a loss of motivation or drive, flat or blunted affect, and odd psychomotor behaviors, such as catatonic posturing or strange gestures (Bellack and Blanchard, 1993). Only a minority of patients with schizophrenia are believed to have a benign course (Ciompi, 1980), with 50%–80% of initially discharged patients eventually being rehospitalized (Eaton et al., 1992b; Westermeyer and Harrow, 1988).

Rates

Prevalence. In 1988, Eaton et al. published a comprehensive review of the prevalence and incidence rates of schizophrenia. Prevalence studies were included if their samples contained at least 2,500 persons and the study diagnosis was made by a psychiatrist. A total of 25 suitable studies published from 1960 to 1983 were reviewed, most of which were conducted prior to the introduction of the DSM-III. As shown in Table 2, the median point prevalence rate across the 13 studies reporting this rate was 3.2 per 1,000 (range 0.6–8.3). The median lifetime prevalence rate across the five relevant studies was 2.7 per 1,000 (range 0.9–3.8). Finally, the median period prevalence rate (not shown) across seven studies was 4.4 per 1,000 (range 1.7–7.0). Interestingly, there was considerable overlap in rates among the types of prevalence measures, presumably because schizophrenia has a low incidence and a chronic, usually nonfatal course. It should also be noted that when studies smaller than those required by Eaton et al. (1988) are considered, differences within and across prevalence measures are considerably greater (De Salvia et al., 1993).

Two recent epidemiologic studies of untreated samples based their diagnoses on the structured assessments of clinicians. The first was Dohrenwend's two-phase study of mental disorders in an Israeli cohort born between 1949 and 1958 (Levav et al., 1993). In the first phase, the Psychiatric Epidemiology Research Interview was administered to 4,914 native Israeli subjects. For the second phase, all screened positives and one-fifth of the screened negatives—2,741 altogether—were interviewed by psychiatrists with a He-

TABLE 2. Overview of Prevalence Rates of Schizophrenia

Source	Diagnostic System	Rate/1,000
Eaton et al. (1988) review		
Median lifetime prevalence	pre-DSM-III[a]	2.7
Median point prevalence	pre-DSM-III[a]	3.2
Levav et al. (1993)		
6 Month prevalence (Israel)	SADS/RDC	0.7
Kessler et al. (1993)		
U.S. National Comorbidity		
Survey clinical diagnosis	SCID/DSM-III-R	0.1

[a]The vast majority of the 25 studies reviewed by Eaton et al. utilized medical record diagnoses.

brew translation of the lifetime version of the Schedule for Affective Disorders and Schizophrenia (Endicott and Spitzer, 1978). The 6-month prevalence of RDC schizophrenia was approximately 0.7%, and an additional 0.1% were categorized with schizoaffective disorder.

The second epidemiologic study is the National Comorbidity Survey described earlier, in which all lay-interviewed cases evidencing symptoms of psychosis were reinterviewed by a psychiatrist with the SCID. The lifetime and 12 month clinician-based prevalence rates for all DSM-III-R nonaffective psychoses combined (schizophrenia, schizophreniform disorder, schizoaffective disorder, delusional disorder, and atypical psychosis) were 0.69% (SE = 0.12) and 0.52% (SE = 0.11), respectively, but the lifetime rate for schizophrenia alone was only 0.14% (SE = 0.05) (R. Kessler, personal communication, 1993). These rates are lower than those found in the Israeli cohort and substantially lower than those reported in the ECA (1.3% lifetime and 0.8% 6 month) based only on lay interview data (Regier et al., 1988). It must be emphasized that, although the prevalence rates are low, the public health importance of schizophrenia is substantial as more than four-fifths of schizophrenics receive psychiatric treatment (Link and Dohrenwend, 1980) and the majority of patients are repeatedly hospitalized (Eaton et al., 1992b; Westermeyer and Harrow, 1988).

Incidence. The review of Eaton et al. (1988) included 23 incidence studies with psychiatrist-diagnosed classifications published between 1950 and 1986, including 11 studies from case register data bases, eight WHO sites from the Determinants of Outcome study, and four community studies. The median annual incidence rate per 1,000 for the case register studies, which emanated primarily from Europe, was 0.20 (range 0.11–0.70). For the eight WHO sites, the median was 0.22 (Dublin and Nottingham; range from 0.16 in Hawaii to 0.42 in rural Chandigarh, India). Interestingly, a recent study of two slums in Madras, India, reported a similar incidence rate (0.35 per 1,000) to that of Chandigarh (Rajkumar et al., 1993). Finally, the median rate for the four community studies was 0.35 per 1,000. An important finding from the WHO research is that the frequency of schizophrenia was similar across the various sites (Jablensky et al., 1992).

RISK FACTORS

Cooper (1978) grouped the factors associated with the distribution of schizophrenia into three categories: demographic characteristics (social class, age, gender, marital status), predisposing factors (season of birth, pregnancy and birth complications, rheumatic disease, substance abuse, genetic background), and precipitating factors (environmental conditions, stress) (Table 3). We briefly review the findings in each of these areas.

Demographic Characteristics

Social Class. One of the most consistent epidemiologic findings is an inverse relationship between social class and schizophrenia (Dohrenwend and Dohrenwend, 1969). Eaton et al. (1988) concluded that the difference in rates between the lowest and highest class is approximately 3 to 1. Since the publication of Faris and Dunham's study in 1939, two hypotheses to explain the association with social class have been tested. One hypothesis is that environmental conditions in poor neighborhoods precipitate the onset of schizophrenia. The specific conditions responsible for onset and believed to be more prevalent in lower class areas include infectious agents, occupational hazards, poor quality maternal and obstetric care leading to higher risk of fetal injury, and increased psychosocial stress.

In contrast, the second hypothesis, termed the *selection-drift hypothesis,* is that schizophrenia-prone individuals are either prevented from attaining higher social class levels (selection) or move progressively downward (drift). This is thought to result because illness onset is most frequently insidious and often has its origin in adolescence, when social and occupational skills are learned. In support of this hypothesis, Turner and Wagenfeld (1967) showed that in Monroe County, New York, schizophrenic males were less upwardly mobile from their fathers than were their peers in the general population. Similarly, in a study of young, male schizophrenic patients, Goldberg and Morrison (1963) found less than expected upward mobility from their fathers as well as downward drift af-

---

TABLE 3. Risk Factors Studied in Epidemiologic Research on Schizophrenia

Demographic characteristics
    Social class
    Age
    Gender
    Marital status
Predisposing factors
    Season of birth
    Pregnancy and birth complications
    Rheumatic disease
    Substance abuse
    Genetic background
Precipitating factors
    Environmental conditions
    Stress

ter the initial appearance of psychotic symptoms. More recently, Jones et al. (1993) confirmed both findings of Goldberg and Morrison in a sample of schizophrenics. They also showed that patients with affective psychosis suffered a decline in occupational performance after diagnosis; unlike schizophrenics, these patients were not underachievers compared with their fathers.

Since one of the cardinal features of schizophrenia is the failure ever to achieve one's potential or, once diagnosed, never to return to one's best premorbid level of functioning, the selection-drift hypothesis to explain the social class distribution has the most adherents. On the other hand, if schizophrenia is indeed a heterogeneous disease (Bellack and Blanchard, 1993), then both hypotheses may have merit in different subgroups of schizophrenic patients.

Gender and Age. As we mentioned above, findings about rates and risk factors depend on case definition. Earlier studies with less systematic diagnostic criteria concluded that the prevalence of schizophrenia was equal in males and females (Dohrenwend et al., 1980). However, treated prevalence samples have limited usefulness in understanding this finding since there are gender differences in patterns of mental health service utilization and in long-term course (Angermeyer et al., 1989). Several recent incidence studies based on first-admission schizophrenic cases reported higher rates in males than females (see Riecher et al., 1991, for a review) although this gender difference may be partially confounded by the fact that relatively more male than female patients are *hospitalized* for schizophrenia (Munk-Jorgensen, 1985). Jablensky et al. (1992) found that in the WHO sites, in which cases were identified at their first contact with any type of mental health provider, the gender difference was specific to patients under 35 years of age. In contrast, women predominated in the age group 35–54. The male excess was also found in the Markers and Predictors of Schizophrenia Project (MAPS), a study of the incidence and course of first-episode psychosis conducted in Vancouver, Canada. Neither methodologic issues nor diagnostic artifacts explained the gender finding, suggesting that the morbidity rate is indeed higher in males than in females (Iacono and Beiser, 1992).

An additional difference linked to gender pertains to age of onset. Since the writings of Kraepelin, psychiatry textbooks have consistently asserted that males develop schizophrenia at an earlier age than females, with the rates of onset occurring in the early twenties in males and in the late twenties to early thirties in females, a 5–10 year difference (Lewine, 1988). This conclusion, however, is typically based on studies that use age at first hospitalization to define age of onset and also contain many limitations in sampling and diagnosis (Riecher et al., 1991). In the MAPS study, Beiser et al. (1993) utilized three other definitions of onset: age at first noticeable symptom, age of first prominent psychotic symptom, and age at initiation of treating seeking. Unlike studies defining onset by first hospitalization, they found the same age of onset for males and females, early twenties, with these definitions. Moreover, the average age of onset was younger for the schizophrenic than for the psychotic depressed and bipolar cases.

Examination of age and gender effects has continued to be an important topic of research. To the extent that there are gender differences in age at onset, questions arise about the disease process itself. If schizophrenia has an earlier onset in males, and this onset tends to be more insidious than in females, then what biologic factors might account for this difference? Identification of these factors might provide clues about etiologic agents or disease-promotion mechanisms.

Marital Status. The findings for marital status are as consistent as those for social class. Eaton et al. (1988) previously noted that the risk ratio for nonmarried individuals to married persons varied from 2.6 to 7.2. In our current study of first-admission patients, only 26% of cases diagnosed with schizophrenia had ever married (Bromet, 1993). Several studies have found that female schizophrenics are more likely to be married than male schizophrenics. Riecher et al. (1991) found that in Mannheim and Denmark, 31% and 29% of first-admission schizophrenic females were married, respectively, compared with 13% and 9% of males. To some extent, this is accounted for by the older age of females at the time of admission. These findings also suggest that females may have better premorbid social competence than males. It may also be the case that females are more likely to have a milder form of the disease and/or that they are better able to adapt to their illness than are males.

Predisposing Characteristics

Season of Birth. A number of studies have reported that the proportion of schizophrenics born during the winter months is approximately 5%–15% higher than that at other times of the year (Torrey et al., 1993) and that this winter excess cannot be discredited on methodologic grounds (Pulver et al., 1990; Watson, 1990). Pulver et al. (1991) found the effect to be more pronounced in females than in males. In addition, it appears to be related to family psychiatric history: A recent study from Dublin of 616 patients reported that schizophrenics with *no* family history of psychiatric disorder were significantly more likely to be born in the winter than schizophrenics with a positive family history (O'Callaghan et al., 1991). Compared with the general population, only those without a family history showed an excess of winter births. While these findings are based on medical record information and need to be confirmed using the family study methodology, they nevertheless suggest that season of birth is associated with schizophrenia in some "nongenetic" cases.

How important a role to assign to season of birth is open to debate. Angst (1991), in fact, commented that the relative contribution of this variable is the lowest of all potential risk factors examined to date. If season of birth is important, hypotheses about the mechanisms that might explain its association will inevitably be complex, potentially involving social class, parental age, maternal viral infections, use of medications, diet, or many other variables that might adversely affect fetal development, particularly during the second trimester (for thoughtful reviews of this issue, see Hare, 1988, and Sham et al., 1992).

Pregnancy and Birth Complications. It has been repeatedly hypothesized that pregnancy and birth complications (PBCs) might be risk factors for schizophrenia. These complications occur frequently in mild form (approximately 20% of births) and not too rarely in more severe form (approximately 5% of births). A variety of specific complications have been studied; one common pathway might be lack of oxygen. Retrospective evidence from recall by the mother is weak since the mother may be striving for an explanation for the sickness of her child. Done et al. (1991) reviewed 12 studies, in which 10 revealed some sort of positive association between pregnancy and/or obstetric factors and risk for schizophrenia. The strongest study was the British Perinatal Study Follow-up (Done et al., 1991), which revealed a relative odds of 1.4. The risk was in the expect direction but not statistically significant. An unusual study of a famine in Holland revealed a statistically significant effect in the expected direction (Susser and Lin, 1992). Studies of obstetric complications and abnormal brain structures (especially enlarged ventricles) in samples limited to schizophrenics only show a strong positive association (Murray et al., 1988). Overall, the evidence indicates that a subgroup of schizophrenics exists for which PBCs are a risk factor of moderate strength. The trick for the future will be to identify the subgroup.

PBCs may be important as a mediator of other risks. For example, it may be that the genetic risk for schizophrenia is expressed by higher risk for PBCs, in which case the increase in PBCs should occur more strongly in familial schizophrenics than in nonfamilial schizophrenics. In the Danish High Risk Cohort, individuals with schizophrenia had a higher rate of PBCs than the general population controls, as expected. What was somewhat surprising was that individuals in the high-risk cohort with schizophrenia spectrum disorder, but not full-blown schizophrenia, had a lower rate of PBCs than the normal controls (Parnas et al., 1982). This finding suggests that PBCs are a potentiator of schizophrenia among genetically vulnerable persons.

PBCs may be an indicator of viral infection of the fetus. The theory of viral infection as a cause of schizophrenia is circumstantially supported by the season of birth effect, since many viruses differ in their potency by season; by evidence for changes in the rate of schizophrenia over the past 200 years, since viral epidemics may take similar forms (Hare, 1979); and by several studies showing higher rates of schizophrenia among births occurring during flu epidemics (e.g., O'Callaghan et al., 1991). However, direct evidence of person-to-person contagion, or of the presence of higher levels of viral antibodies in the blood of schizophrenics than of normals, has not been demonstrated despite repeated attempts.

Rheumatoid Arthritis. A repeated finding in the epidemiologic literature is the apparent protective effect of schizophrenia on rheumatoid arthritis. Several studies have shown that individuals with schizophrenia contract rheumatoid arthritis at about one-fifth the level of comparison populations (Eaton et al., 1992a). The finding does not appear to be an artifact of medication use, or hospitalization, but there is no obvious explanation for it. It may be that schizophrenia involves a lowering of immunologic capability, which is associated with a weakened autoimmune response and, thereby, lessened risk for the disease.

Substance Abuse. An active area of current research concerns whether the rate of substance abuse in general, as well as use of specific substances (e.g., alcohol, cocaine), is greater in schizophrenic patients than in the general population. A 15 year follow-up study of 45,570 Swedish army recruits showed that those consuming *Cannabis* on more than 15 occasions were six times more likely to develop schizophrenia than less frequent or nonusers (Andreasson et al., 1987). There is also debate as to whether substance-abusing schizophrenics are clinically different from schizophrenics without such a history. Substance-abusing schizophrenics have been described as more difficult to manage clinically and to have a poorer course (Lieberman and Bowers, 1990). However, Mueser et al. (1990) found that stimulant abusers did not differ clinically from nonabusing schizophrenic patients. Similarly, Kovasznay et al. (1993) found no significant clinical differences between first-admission schizophrenics according to their substance abuse history. More research in first-admission psychotic samples is needed to address the role of substance abuse as a risk factor in the onset of schizophrenia.

Genetic Studies. Gottesman and Shields (1982, p. 84) commented in *Schizophrenia: The Epigenetic Puzzle* that "the overwhelming majority of all relatives of schizophrenics are not themselves schizophrenic." Nevertheless, most studies have shown that first-degree relatives have a significantly elevated risk of schizophrenia. The data presented by Gottesman and Shields (1982, p. 85) indicated that the morbid risk among first-degree relatives ranges from 5.6% in the parents of schizophrenics, to 12.8% in the children of one schizophrenic parent, and to 46.3% in the children of two schizophrenic parents. Kendler (1988) concluded that, in family studies using blind diagnoses, control groups, personal interviews and operationalized diagnostic criteria, the risk for schizophrenia in close relatives of schizophrenics is 5–15 times greater than in the general population. The risk for other psychotic and schizophrenia spectrum disorders is also higher in the first-degree relatives of schizophrenic patients. Furthermore, Kendler (1988, pp. 450–451) concluded from his review of twin and adoption research that "the heritability of liability of schizophrenia is probably between 60 and 70%. By contrast, if present, environmental familial factors appear to account for less than 20% of the variance in liability." Current research is attempting to integrate environmental, biologic, and genetic risk factors and to understand the mode of transmission of the genetic liability itself in an effort to uncover the etiology of schizophrenia (Stabenau and Pollin, 1993).

Precipitating Factors

Environmental Variables. Two geographic areas have yielded unusually high rates of schizophrenia, the Istrian peninsula in Yugoslavia and the western coast of Ireland. The study of residents of the Istrian peninsula was conducted jointly by faculty from the Johns Hopkins University and the Institute of Public Health in Zagreb, using hospital statistics as well as community interviews. The relative risk was greater than 2 for the target area compared with a control site and was most pronounced for women and for those over 40 years of age (Lemkau et al., 1980). Similarly, the west coast of Ireland was also believed to be a high-rate area (Walsh et al., 1980), although recent incidence data cast some doubt on this finding.

Another geographic variable that has been examined is an urban–rural difference in rate of schizophrenia. In their classic review of this topic, Dohrenwend and Dohrenwend (1974) concluded that the crude prevalence of schizophrenia per se was similar in rural and in urban areas. However, Eaton (1974) subsequently presented age-specific rates of first hospitalization for rural, suburban, and urban Maryland and found the urban rate to be 2.17 times higher than the rural rate (0.60 vs. 0.23 per 1,000), with the suburban rate falling in between (0.30). The higher rate in urban areas was recently confirmed using a quasiprospective design in Sweden (Lewis et al., 1992). Like other macro or ecologic variables, urban versus rural residence combines a host of differences under a single rubric. Thus, differences in illness severity and comorbidity, service availability, selective migration to urban versus rural areas, social and physical environmental parameters, to name a few, are all subsumed within the overall dichotomy.

Stress. Attempts to link social stressors to the onset of schizophrenia have been fraught with methodologic difficulties (Norman and Malla, 1993). Of greatest concern is the difficulty of separating cause and effect, because the onset of schizophrenia is insidious and sometimes impossible to date with precision. Nevertheless, it has been hypothesized that social stress plays a triggering role in vulnerable individuals and may be conceptualized as a precipitating variable in the onset of schizophrenia. Careful review of the evidence from first-admission studies, however, finds mixed support for this contention. Several British researchers have found support for the notion that social environmental stressors play a precipitating role in triggering psychotic episodes (e.g., Birley and Brown, 1970; Brown and Birley, 1968; Bebbington et al., 1993). On the other hand, Chung et al. (1986) examined recent life events in a British first-admission sample and, interestingly, found a significant relationship to onset of schizophreniform disorder although not to schizophrenia. By contrast, Jacobs and Myers (1976) assessed retrospectively a small sample of first-admission schizophrenics in New Haven. Although schizophrenics reported more life events than controls during the year prior to onset, life events that were judged truly independent of the illness were not differently distributed. If, as some have argued, the overall contribution of stress to episodes of schizophrenia is negligible (Dohrenwend and Egri, 1981), it may well be the case, as Zubin suggested, that, in vulnerable individuals with a predisposition to psychosis and inadequate social buffers, stress can function as a precipitant of psychotic episodes (Zubin and Spring, 1977; Zubin et al., 1983).

COURSE AND ITS PREDICTORS

Cohen and Cohen (1984) commented that the perception that schizophrenia has a chronic, often deteriorating, course is biased by clinical illusions from patients who stay in or return to treatment. Indeed, almost all longitudinal studies of schizophrenia and other psychoses, especially affective disorders, focus on the course and outcome of samples consecutively admitted to treatment facilities—samples that include varying proportions of chronic patients. The failure to design studies with patient cohorts that are homogeneous with respect to illness stage reflects, in our opinion, the lack of input from epidemiologists into research on course even though this research area represents one of the cardinal purposes of epidemiology (Morris, 1975). Fortunately, significant work is now underway in the form of longitudinal studies designed with epidemiologic principles in mind, such as the WHO Determinants of Outcome Study, the Vancouver First-Episode Project (MAPS), the McLean Study, and the Suffolk County project. Each of these studies assembled heterogeneous, quasirepresentative samples of first-admission psychotic patients, used structured diagnostic assessments combined with medical information to formulate the diagnosis, and contained systematic follow-up assessments.

The 5 year outcome study of Shepherd et al. (1989) illustrates the importance of studying first-admission patients. Of the 107 schizophrenic patients in their sample, 49 were first-admission patients and 58 had had previous hospitalizations. Twenty-two percent of the first-admission patients experienced no relapse throughout the follow-up period, 35% had one or more relapses with no/minimal impairment at the time of the 5 year follow-up, and 43% remained impaired throughout. By contrast, in the rehospitalized group, only 10% displayed no impairment and had no further episodes during the follow-up period, while 29% had multiple episodes with no/minimal impairment, and 60% were impaired with no return to normality (Mantel-Haenszel $X^2$4.194; df $= 1$; $p = 0.041$). Even more striking, the total time spent hospitalized during the 5 year follow-up was 26.2 weeks for the first-admission subgroup compared with 76.2 weeks for those with prior hospitalizations. Thus, recovery rates must be evaluated in cohorts who enter the study during their first hospitalization or, even better, at the start of their first episode of illness.

Ram et al. (1992) reviewed three sets of first-admission follow-up studies: statistical reports from state hospitals, long-term follow-back studies, and recent prospective studies. Overall, about one-third of patients across the 13 prospectively designed studies had a benign course during the first 2 years, but two-thirds relapsed or were readmitted to the hospital. (Of course, definitions employed for course or outcome status will affect recovery rates reported.) In the Vancouver study, 40/72 psychotic patients were described as "incapacitated" at 18 months follow-up (Beiser et al., 1988). These findings reaffirm the pernicious nature of this disorder.

Schizophrenic patients do more poorly over time than psychotic patients with affective disorders (Beiser et al., 1989). Among affectively ill patients with psychosis, findings on the relationship of diagnosis to course are mixed. In one study, 37% of psychotic depressed subjects compared with 58% of bipolar subjects had one or more relapses during a 2 year follow-up period (Jablensky, 1987). In contrast, compared with bipolar patients, 68% of whom achieved a functional recovery at 6 months follow up, fewer depressives (23%) in the McLean study recovered by 6 months (Tohen et al., 1992).

Some of the variables associated with the occurrence of schizophrenia are also predictive of poor course, including being male, being unmarried, having a family history of schizophrenia, and living in a stressful environment. In consecutive admission samples, high "expressed emotion"—criticism and hostility directed toward the patient—is significantly related to poorer course, but, when measured at the time of the first episode, the association with early course is considerably weaker (Westermeyer and Harrow, 1988; Ram et al., 1992).

Other prognostic variables that have frequently been associated with poorer outcome are lower intelligence level, poor premorbid social competence, longer duration between illness onset and receiving neuroleptic treatment, relatively fewer positive symptoms (active delusions and hallucinations) and more negative ones (flat or blunted affect, alogia), and noncompliance with medication treatment (Westermeyer and Harrow, 1988). Of all the variables noted above, the most neglected by epidemiologists, even though it is one of the few that may be open to modification, is medication compliance. As Kane et al. (1986, p. 4) noted: "Given the overall enormous impact of antipsychotic drug treatment on relapse rates in schizophrenia, when we attempt to explore outcome predictors it is critical that we attend to pharmacological treatment factors in order to eliminate potential confounding of effects and to explore potential interactions." The case for the importance of phenothiazines is clear, but the relative importance in unbiased samples—individuals not necessarily involved in clinical trials—has rarely been studied. Future naturalistic follow-up studies of first-admission patients need to document and evaluate carefully the relative contribution of medication usage to course and outcome.

Another important finding, recently uncovered by WHO researchers, is that patients in developing countries have a more benign course than patients in developed countries (Leff et al., 1992). Many factors may contribute to this finding, including differences in the nature of the illness (since schizophrenia is a heterogeneous disease) and in the physical and sociocultural environments.

Only a few studies have examined the predictors of outcome in first-admission patients with psychotic disorders other than schizophrenia. The National Institute of Mental Health Collaborative Depression Study included a small group of first-admission patients with psychotic features (Coryell et al., 1990a,b). Among the depressed group, being unmarried, having had poorer adolescent social functioning, and having mood-incongruent psychotic delusions were associated with poorer outcome; among the bipolar patients, longer duration of the index episode, poorer adolescent social functioning, and temporal dissociation between psychotic and affective symptoms were associated with poorer functioning. Tohen et al. (1992) also found that in bipolar patients followed over a 4 year period, mood-incongruent delusions were associated with poorer outcome, defined as shorter time in remission. These findings suggest that some prognostic indicators associated with adolescent functioning may not be specific to schizophrenia. Research is needed to test the relative prognostic utility of these variables in diagnostically mixed samples of psychotic patients ascertained initially at similar stages of their illness.

TARGET AREAS FOR FUTURE EPIDEMIOLOGIC RESEARCH

There are three cardinal methodologic requirements that distinguish epidemiologic from clinical research: a representative sample, a valid and reliable diagnosis, and specification of time of onset. In schizophrenia and other psychotic disorders, there has been progress with all three, but they nevertheless remain methodologic target areas.

Obtaining a representative sample through two-stage procedures is extremely costly, and we therefore need to design better methods for sampling treated cases. In the Suffolk County project, for example, we attempted to deal with this issue by involving all of the treatment facilities in the county in recruiting first-admission psychotic patients for the study (Bromet et al., 1992). However, some patients seek treatment outside the county or from nontraditional sources and thus are missed by our net. To our knowledge, in North America, only the MAPS project has been able to identify a representative, treated sample.

The second issue, pertaining to a valid and reliable diagnosis, is to some extent ameliorated by systematic criteria currently available, along with structured interviews, such as the SCID and the recent Diagnostic Interview for Genetics Studies (DIGS). However, when these instruments are used without supplementary medical record and significant other corroboration, important symptoms may be missed. Retrospective information from cross-sectional interviews is also not ideal for formulating a differential diagnosis in first-admission patients. Interview information is inconsistent over time and is influenced by current state (Bromet et al., 1986). Moreover, in first-admission samples, the illness may still be evolving when the researcher first interviews the patient. The decision as to whether the patient has schizophrenia or some other psychotic disorder cannot always be made with retrospective information. Therefore, multimethod, longitudinal approaches to data collection need to be incorporated in epidemiologic research on all psychotic disorders.

The third issue, which is perhaps the most difficult after the illness has come to medical attention, is establishing the time of onset. Beiser et al. (1993, p. 1349) commented that there are "no standardized, replicable methods for establishing illness onset." Yet this variable is crucial for etiologic research attempting to identify causal factors. With the exception of the high-risk longitudinal studies, we are faced with obtaining this information retrospectively. Multiple sources of information, combined with consensus meetings to make as accurate an estimate as possible, would enable us to get beyond clinical judgment in determining this crucial set of variables.

From a substantive viewpoint, several elegant vulnerability models have been proposed to explain the onset of schizophrenia (see Eaton et al., pp. 190–194). Zubin and colleagues (Zubin and Spring, 1977; Zubin et al., 1983) attempted to integrate six etiologic models—genetic, internal environment, ecologic, neurophysiologic, developmental, and learning theory—into a single vulnerability model. They likened schizophrenia to an allergic condition that develops only when triggered by a stimulus and therefore hypothesized that, when stress exceeds the vulnerability threshold, a crisis develops and an episode ensues. Likewise, when the stress wears off, the individual returns to his or her pre-episode level of functioning. The vulnerability markers are derived from each of the six etiologic models. Thus, Zubin and colleagues advocate for the need to determine the vulnerability markers and to follow vulnerable individuals over time to identify the factors that trigger psychotic episodes.

This and other models entail studies incorporating longitudinal biologic and psychosocial data that can begin to test these models. To our knowledge, only the Vancouver study has the potential to address these hypotheses with a representative sample and to compare the value of the model for other psychotic disorders. Explicit testing of these models vis-à-vis etiology and illness course of psychotic disorders represents the next major challenge for epidemiologists.

REFERENCES

American Psychiatric Association (1980): "Diagnostic and Statistical Manual of Mental Disorders, "3rd ed." Washington, DC: American Psychiatric Association Press.

American Psychiatric Association (1987): "Diagnostic and Statistical Manual of Mental disorders," 3rd ed. Revised Washington, DC: American Psychiatric Association Press.

Andreasson S, Allebeck P, Engstrom A, Ryberg U (1987): *Cannabis* and schizophrenia: A longitudinal study of Swedish conscripts. Lancet 2(8574):1483–1486.

Angermeyer M, Goldstein J, Kuehn L (1989): Gender differences in schizophrenia: Rehospitalization and community survival. Psychol Med 19:365–382.

Angst J (1991): Epidemiology of schizophrenia: Discussion. In Hafner H, Gattaz WF (eds): "Search for the Causes of Schizophrenia." Berlin: Springer-Verlag, pp 48–53.

Anthony JC, Folstein M, Romanoski AJ, Von Korff M, Nestadt G, Chahal R, Merchant A, Brown H, Shapiro S, Kramer M, Gruenberg E (1985): Comparison of lay DIS and a standardized psychiatric diagnosis: Experience in Eastern Baltimore. Arch Gen Psychiatry 42:667–675.

Bebbington P, Wilkins S, Jones P, Foerster A, Murray R, Toone B, Lewis S (1993): Life events and psychosis: Initial results from the Camberwell Collaborative Psychosis Study. Br J Psychiatry 162:72–79.

Beiser M, Erickson D, Fleming J, Iacono W (1993): Establishing the onset of psychotic illness. Am J Psychiatry 150:1349–1354.

Beiser M, Iacono W (1990): An update on the epidemiology of schizophrenia. Can J Psychiatry 35:657–668.

Beiser M, Iacono WG, Erickson D (1989): Temporal stability in major mental disorders. In Robins LN, Barrett JE (eds): "The Validity of Psychiatric Diagnosis." New York: Raven Press, pp 77–98.

Beiser M, Jonathan AE, Fleming MB, Iacono WG, Lin T (1988): Refining the diagnosis of schizophreniform disorder. Am J Psychiatry 145:695–700.

Bellack A, Blanchard JJ (1993): Schizophrenia: Psychopathology. In Bellack A, Hersen M (eds): "Psychopathology in Adulthood." Boston: Allyn and Bacon, pp 216–233.

Birley J, Brown GW (1970): Crisis and life changes preceding the onset of relapse of acute schizophrenia: Clinical aspects. Br J Psychiatry 16:327–333.

Bromet E (1993): Premorbid and onset characteristics as predictors of short-term course of psychosis: A comparison of first-admission patients with schizophrenia and affective psychosis. Presented at the World Psychiatric Association Section on Epidemiology and Community Psychiatry, Groningen, Holland, September 1–3.

Bromet E, Davies M, Schulz SC (1988): Basic principles of epidemiologic research in schizophrenia. In Tsuang MT, Simpson JC (eds): "Handbook of Schizophrenia, vol 3, Nosology, Epidemiology and Genetics." Amsterdam: Elsevier Science Publishers BV, pp 151–168.

Bromet E, Dunn L, Connell M, Dew MA, Schulberg H (1986): Long-term reliability of diagnosing lifetime major depression in a community sample. Arch Gen Psychiatry 43:435–440.

Bromet E, Schwartz JE, Fennig S, Geller L, Jandorf L, Kovasznay B, Lavelle J, Miller A, Pato C, Ram R, Rich C (1992): The epidemiology of psychosis: The Suffolk County Mental Health Project. Schiz Bull 18:243–255.

Brown GW, Birley JLT (1968): Crises and life changes and the onset of schizophrenia. J Health Soc Behav 9:203–214.

Chung RK, Langeluddecke P, Tennant C (1986): Threatening life events in the onset of schizophrenia, schizophreniform psychosis and hypomania. Br J Psychiatry 148:680–685.

Ciompi L (1980): Catamnestic long-term study on the course of life and aging of schizophrenics. Schiz Bull 6:606–618.

Cohen P, Cohen J (1984): The clinician's illusion. Arch Gen Psychiatry 41:1178–1183.

Cooper B (1978): Epidemiology. In Wing JK (ed): "Schizophrenia: Towards a New Synthesis." New York: Grune and Stratton, pp 31–51.

Cooper R, Kendell RE, Gurland BJ, Sharpe L, Copeland JRM, Simon R (1972): "Psychiatric Diagnosis in New York and London: A Comparative Study of Mental Hospital Admissions." Institute of Psychiatry, Maudsley Monographs, No. 20. London: Oxford University Press.

Coryell W, Keller M, Lavori P, Endicott J (1990a): Affective syndromes, psychotic features, and prognosis, I: Depression. Arch Gen Psychiatry 47:651–657.

Coryell W, Keller M, Lavori P, Endicott J (1990b): Affective syndromes, psychotic features, and prognosis, II: Mania. Arch Gen Psychiatry 47:658–662.

De Salvia D, Barbato A, Salvo P, Zadro F (1993): Prevalence and incidence of schizophrenic disorders in Portogruaro: An Italian case register study. J Nerv Ment Dis 181:275–282.

Dohrenwend BP, Dohrenwend BS (1969): "Social Status and Psychological Disorder: A Causal Inquiry." New York: John Wiley & Sons.

Dohrenwend BP, Dohrenwend BS (1974): Psychiatric disorders in urban settings. In Caplan G (ed): "American Handbook of Psychiatry," 2nd ed, vol 2. New York: Basic Books, pp 424–447.

Dohrenwend BP, Dohrenwend BS (1982): Perspectives on the past and future of psychiatric epidemiology: The 1981 Rema Lapouse lecture. Am J Public Health 72:1271–1279.

Dohrenwend BP, Dohrenwend BS, Gould MS, Link B, Neugebauer R, Wunsch-Hitzig R (eds) (1980): "Mental Illness in the United States: Epidemiological Estimates." New York: Praeger.

Dohrenwend BP, Egri G (1981): Recent stressful life events and episodes of schizophrenia. Schiz Bull 7:12–23.

Done EJ, Johnstone EC, Frith CD, Golding J, Shepherd PM, Crow TF (1991): Complications of pregnancy and delivery in relation to psychosis in adult life: Data from the British perinatal mortality survey sample. Br Med J 302:1576–1580.

Eaton WW (1974): Residence, social class, and schizophrenia. J Health Soc Behav 15:289–299.

Eaton WW (1991): Update on the epidemiology of schizophrenia. Epidemiol Rev 13:320–328.

Eaton WW, Day R, Kramer M (1988): The use of epidemiology for risk factor research in schizophrenia: An overview and methodologic critique. In Tsuang MT, Simpson JC (eds): "Handbook of Schizophrenia, vol 3, Nosology, Epidemiology and Genetics." Amsterdam: Elsevier Science Publishers BV, pp 169–204.

Eaton WW, Hayward C, Ram R (1992a): Schizophrenia and rheumatoid arthritis: A review. Schiz Res 6:181–192.

Eaton WW, Preban BM, Herrman H, Freeman H, Bilker W, Burgess P, Wooff K (1992b): Long-term course of hospitalization for schizophrenia: Part 1. Risk for rehospitalization. Schiz Bull 18:217–228.

Endicott J, Spitzer R (1978): A diagnostic interview: The schedule for affective disorders and schizophrenia. Arch Gen Psychiatry 35:837–844.

Faris R, Dunham H (1939): "Mental Disorders in Urban Areas: An Ecological Study of Schizophrenia and Other Psychoses." Chicago: University of Chicago Press.

Giggs JA (1986): Mental disorders and ecological structure in Nottingham. Soc Sci Med 23:945–961.

Goldberg E, Morrison S (1963): Schizophrenia and social class. Br J Psychiatry 109:785–802.

Gottesman I, Shields J (1982): "Schizophrenia: The Epigenetic Puzzle." Cambridge: Cambridge University Press.

Hare EH (1979): Schizophrenia as an infectious disease. Br J Psychiatry 135:468–473.

Hare E (1988): Temporal factors and trends, including birth seasonality and the viral hypothesis. In Tsuang MT, Simpson JC (eds): "Handbook of Schizophrenia, vol 3, Nosology, Epidemiology and Genetics." Amsterdam: Elsevier Science Publishers BV, pp 345–377.

Hollingshead A, Redlich F (1958): "Social Class and Mental Illness." New York: John Wiley & Sons.

Iacono W, Beiser M (1992): Where are the women in first-episode studies of schizophrenia? Schiz Bull 18:471–480.

Jablensky A (1986): Epidemiology of schizophrenia: A European perspective. Schiz Bull 12: 52–73.

Jablensky A (1987): Prediction of the course and outcome of depression. Psychol Med 17:1–9.

Jablensky A, Sartorius N, Ernberg G, Anker M, Korten A, Cooper JE, Day R, Bertelsen A (1992): Schizophrenia: Manifestations, incidence and course in different cultures: A World Health Organization Ten-Country study. Psychol Med, Monograph Suppl 20. Cambridge, England: Cambridge University Press.

Jacobs SC, Myers JK (1976): Recent life events and acute schizophrenic psychosis: A controlled study. J Nerv Ment Dis 162:75–87.

Jarvis E (1971): "Insanity and Idiocy in Massachusetts." Cambridge, MA: Harvard University Press.

Jones PB, Bebbington P, Foerster A, Lewis S, Murray R, Russell A, Sham P, Toone B, Wilkins S (1993): Premorbid social underachievement in schizophrenia: Results from the Camberwell Collaborative Psychosis Study. Br J Psychiatry 162:76–71.

Kane J, Woerner M, Lieberman J (1986): Historical predictors of relapse in schizophrenia. In Lieberman R, Kane J (eds): "Predictors of Relapse in Schizophrenia." Washington, DC: American Psychiatric Press, pp 1–13.

Kendler KS (1988): The genetics of schizophrenia. In Tsuang MT, Simpson JC (eds): "Handbook of Schizophrenia, vol 3, Nosology, Epidemiology and Genetics." Amsterdam: Elsevier Science Publishers BV, pp 437–462.

Kessler R, McGonagle K, Zhao S, Nelson C, Hughes M, Eshleman S, Wittchen H-U, Kendler K (1994): Lifetime and 12-month prevalence of DSM-III-R psychiatric disorders in the United States: Results from the National Comorbidity survey. Arch Gen Psychiatry 51:8–19.

Kovasznay B, Bromet E, Schwartz J, Ram R, Lavelle J, Brandon L (1993): Substance abuse and onset of psychotic illness. Hosp Comm Psychiatry 44:567–571.

Leff J, Sartorius N, Jablensky A, Korten A, Ernberg G (1992): The International Pilot Study of Schizophrenia: Five-year follow-up findings. Psychol Med 22:131–145.

Lemkau P, Kulcar Z, Kesic B, Kovacic L (1980): Selected aspects of the epidemiology of psychoses in Croatia, Yugoslavia. Am J Epidemiol 112:661–674.

Levav I, Kohn R, Dohrenwend BP, Shrout PE, Skodol AE, Schwartz S, Link BG, Naveh G (1993): An epidemiological study of mental disorders in a 10-year cohort of young adults in Israel. Psychol Med 23:691–707.

Levy L, Rowitz L (1970): The spatial distribution of treated mental disorders in Chicago. Soc Psychiatry 5:1–11.

Lewine RRJ (1988): Gender and schizophrenia. In Tsuang MT, Simpson JC (eds): "Handbook of Schizophrenia, vol 3, Nosology, Epidemiology, and Genetics." Amsterdam: Elsevier Science Publishers BV, pp 379–397.

Lewis G, David A, Andreasson S, Allebeck P (1992): Schizophrenia and city life. Lancet 340:137–140.

Lieberman JA, Bowers JB (1990): Substance abuse comorbidity in schizophrenia. Schiz Bull 16:29–30.

Link B, Dohrenwend BP (1980): Formulation of hypotheses about the ratio of untreated to treated cases in the true prevalence studies of functional psychiatric disorders in adults in the United States. In Dohrenwend BP, Dohrenwend BS, Gould MS, Link B, Neugebauer R, Wunsch-Hitzig R (eds): "Mental Illness in the United States: Epidemiological Estimates." New York: Praeger, pp 133–149.

Locke B (1962): Outcome of first hospitalization of patients with schizophrenia. Pub Health Rep 77:801–805.

Morris JN (1975): "Uses of Epidemiology," 3 ed. London: Churchill-Livingstone.

Mueser K, Yarnold P, Levinson D, Singh H, Bellack A, Kee K, Morrison R, Yadalam K (1990): Prevalence of substance abuse in schizophrenia: Demographic and clinical correlates. Schiz Bull 16:31–56.

Munk-Jorgensen P (1985): The schizophrenia diagnosis in Denmark. A register-based investigation. Acta Psychiatr Scand 72:266–273.

Murray RM, Lewis SW, Owen MJ (1988): The neurodevelopmental origins of dementia praecox. In Bebbington P, McGuffin P (eds): "Schizophrenia: The Major Issues." London: Heinmann, pp 90–106.

National Advisory Mental Health Council (1988): "A National Plan for Schizophrenia Research." Washington, DC: U.S. Government Printing Office, DHHS Publication No. (ADM) 88-1571.

Norman RMG, Malla A (1993): Stressful life events and schizophrenia II: Conceptual and methodological issues. Br J Psychiatry 162:166–174.

O'Callaghan E, Gibson T, Colohan H, Walshe D, Buckley P, Larkin C, Waddington J (1991): Season of birth in schizophrenia: Evidence for confinement of an excess of winter births to patients without a family history of mental disorder. Br J Psychiatry 158:764–769.

Parnas J, Schulsinger R, Teasdale TW, Schulsinger H, Feldman PM, Mednick SA (1982): Perinatal complications and clinical outcome within the schizophrenia spectrum. Br J Psychiatry 140: 416–420.

Pulver A, Moorman C, Brown CH, McGrath J, Wolyniec P (1990): Age-incidence artifacts do not account for the season-of-birth effect in schizophrenia. Schiz Bull 16:13–15.

Pulver A, Sawyer JW, Childs B (1981): The association between season of birth and the risk of schizophrenia. Am J Epidemiol 114:735–749.

Rajkumar S, Padmavati R, Thara R, Menon MS (1993): Incidence of schizophrenia in an urban community in Madras. Indian J Psychiatry 35:18–21.

Ram R, Bromet E, Eaton W, Pato C, Schwartz J (1992): The natural course of schizophrenia: A review of first-admission studies. Schiz Bull 18:185–207.

Regier D, Boyd JH, Burke JD, Rae DS, Myers JK, Kramer M, Robins LN, George LK, Karno M,

Locke BZ (1988): One-month prevalence of mental disorders in the United States based on five epidemiologic catchment area sites. Arch Gen Psychiatry 45:977–986.

Riecher A, Maurer K, Loffler W, Fatkenheuer B, An Der Heiden W, Munk-Jorgensen P, Stromgren E, Hafner H (1991): Gender differences in age at onset and course of schizophrenic disorders. In Hafner H, Gattaz WF (eds): "Search for the Causes of Schizophrenia." Berlin: Springer-Verlag, pp 14–33.

Sartorius N, Jablensky A, Korten A, Ernberg G, Anker M, Cooper JE, Day R (1986): Early manifestations and first-contact incidence of schizophrenia in different cultures. Psychol Med 16:909–928.

Sham P, O'Callaghan E, Takei N, Murray G, Hare E, Murray R (1992): Schizophrenia following pre-natal exposure to influenza epidemics between 1939 and 1960. Br J Psychiatry 160: 461–466.

Shepherd M, Watt D, Falloon I, Smeeton N (1989): "The Natural History of Schizophrenia: A Five-year Outcome and Prediction in a Representative Sample of Schizophrenics." Cambridge: Cambridge University Press.

Spitzer R, Endicott J, Robins E (1978): Research diagnostic criteria: Rationale and reliability. Arch Gen Psychiatry 35:773–782.

Spitzer R, Williams J, Gibbon M, First MB (1992): The Structured Clinical Interview for DSM-III-R (SCID) I: History, rationale, and description. Arch Gen Psychiatry 49:624–629.

Stabenau J, Pollin W (1993): Heredity and environment in schizophrenia, revisited: the contribution of twin and high-risk studies. J Nerv Ment Dis 181:290–297.

Susser E, Lin S (1992): Schizophrenia after prenatal exposure to the Dutch hunger winter of 1944–1945. Arch Gen Psychiatry 49:983–988.

Tohen M, Stoll AL, Strakowski SM, Faedda GL, Mayer PV, Goodwin DC, Kolbrener ML, Madigan AM (1992): The McLean First-Episode Psychosis Project: Six-month recovery and recurrence outcome. Schiz Bull 18:273–282.

Tohen M, Tsuang M, Goodwin D (1992): Prediction of outcome in mania by mood-congruent or mood-incongruent psychotic features. Am J Psychiatry 149:1580–1584.

Torrey EF, Bowler AE, Rawlings R, Terrazas A (1993): Seasonality of schizophrenia and stillbirths. Schiz Bull 19:557–562.

Turner RJ (1972): The epidemiological study of schizophrenia: A current appraisal. J Health Soc Behav 13:360–369.

Turner RJ, Wagenfeld MO (1967): Occupational mobility and schizophrenia: An assessment of the social causation and social selection hypotheses. Am Soc Rev 32:104–113.

Walsh D, O'Hare A, Blake B, Halpenny J, O'Brien P (1980): The treated prevalence of mental illness in the Republic of Ireland: The three county case register study. Psychol Med 10:465–470.

Watson C (1990): Schizophrenic birth seasonality and the age-incidence artifact. Schiz Bull 16:5–12.

Westermeyer JF, Harrow M (1988): Course and outcome in schizophrenia. In Tsuang MT, Simpson JC (eds): "Handbook of Schizophrenia, vol 3, Nosology, Epidemiology and Genetics." Amsterdam: Elsevier Science Publishers BV, pp 205–244.

Williams JBW, Gibbon M, First MB, Spitzer RL, Davies M, Borus J, Howes MJ, Kane J, Pope HG, Rounsaville B, Wittchen H-U (1992): The structured clinical interview for DSM-III-R (SCID): II. Multisite test-retest reliability. Arch Gen Psychiatry 49:630–636.

Zubin J, Magaziner J, Steinhauer SR (1983): The metamorphosis of schizophrenia from chronicity to vulnerability. Psychol Med 13:551–571.

Zubin J, Spring B (1977): Vulnerability—a new view of schizophrenia. J Abnorm Psychol 86: 103–126.

CHAPTER 15

Epidemiology of Bipolar Disorder

MAURICIO TOHEN and FREDERICK K. GOODWIN

Bipolar and Psychotic Disorders Program and Epidemiology Laboratory, McLean Hospital, Belmont, MA, Department of Psychiatry, Harvard Medical School, and Department of Epidemiology, Harvard School of Public Health, Boston, MA 02115 (M.T.); The Center on Neuroscience Behavior & Society, George Washington University Medical Center, Washington, DC 20037 (F.K.G.)

INTRODUCTION

Epidemiology is the study of the causes and distribution of illnesses. It is, therefore, a discipline that permits an accurate understanding of a disorder. The basic principles of epidemiologic research remain unchanged since John Snow identified the course of cholera in the City of London 100 years ago; we still observe, count, and compare. To understand bipolar disorder, we observe the condition, count its incidence and prevalence, and compare its outcome depending on risk factors.

Disease in human populations develops through complex interactions of competing factors, including genetics, demographic variables, and psychosocial factors. Epidemiologic observational studies are conducted with large groups of individuals. This chapter will try to describe, count, and compare features of bipolar disorder in order to unravel the complexity of this condition.

To count, one first needs to observe and describe. To describe and compare findings from time to time and from place to place, case definition must be established. This represents a problem with bipolar disorder, since there has been an ongoing evolution in the case definition of the condition.

Not unlike other psychiatric disorders, diagnostic criteria in bipolar illness have changed across different time periods, significantly affecting the case definition. In addition, until recently, the definition of a case was not clearly operationalized, causing a great degree of variability in the assessment of cases.

More than two decades ago, the U.S./U.K. diagnostic study (Cooper et al., 1972) highlighted the variability of diagnosis in patients with psychotic disorders. The study demonstrated that when clear operational criteria are not utilized, the differential diagnosis of manic-depressive illness or schizophrenia may be uncertain. In spite of the use of operationalized diagnostic criteria, inconsistencies of diagnosis may persist due to poor reliability in the method of assessment or in the collection of symptoms.

Textbook in Psychiatric Epidemiology, Edited by Tsuang, Tohen, and Zahner
ISBN 0-471-59375-3 © 1995 Wiley-Liss, Inc.

To diminish such variability, standardized diagnostic instruments have been developed for different diagnostic classifications. Examples are the Renard Diagnostic Interview (Helzer et al., 1981), which utilizes Feighner criteria (Feighner et al., 1972); the Schedule for Affective Disorders and Schizophrenia (SADS) (Spitzer et al., 1978), which utilizes Research Diagnostic Criteria (RDC) (Spitzer et al., 1978); the Present State Examination (PSE) (Wing et al., 1974), which elicits International Classifications of Disease (ICD) diagnosis; and the Diagnostic Interview Schedule (DIS) (Robins et al., 1981), which permits the identification of DSM-III-R criteria. More recently, other new diagnostic instruments have appeared on both sides of the Atlantic, including the Structured Clinical Assessment for Neuropsychiatric Disorders (SCAN) (Wing et al., 1990), the Structured Clinical Interview for the DSM-III-R (SCID) (Spitzer et al., 1990), and the Diagnostic Instrument for Genetic Studies (DIGS) (Nurnberger et al., 1994). The failure of most epidemiologic studies of bipolar disorder conducted prior to 1980 to use a structured instrument or diagnostic criteria make their results difficult to interpret.

NOSOLOGY

Manic-depressive illness was probably first described by Aretaeus of Cappadocia in 30 AD (Adams, 1990). In contemporary history, it was Falret (1854) in the midnineteenth century who first described the condition and called it *folie circulaire*. Kraepelin (1921) further defined the concept by separating it from *dementia precox* or schizophrenia. According to Kraepelin, manic-depressive illness is characterized by a periodic course with good prognosis and mood symptoms in the acute phase. For Kraepelin, course of illness was the major distinction. He, therefore, included under the category of manic-depressive illness other periodic affective disorders, including "involutional melancholia," producing an overestimation of the disorder in the early literature.

On the other hand, there was also an underestimation, as most studies did not consider Bipolar II Disorder (hypomania and depression) as part of the bipolar spectrum. During the first half of the twentieth century, interest in psychiatric nosology diminished, particularly in North America due to the influence of psychoanalysis.

The second half of the century has witnessed what has been described as a "renaissance" of psychiatric nosology (Krauthammer and Klerman, 1979). The advent of new treatments, especially psychopharmacologic, has invigorated the field's interest in differentiating the diagnoses of manic-depressive illness and schizophrenia. Baldessarini (1970) emphasized that the appearance of phenothiazines in the early 1950s biased the diagnosis of schizophrenia over manic-depressive illness. More recently investigators from McLean Hospital (Stoll et al., 1994) reported that in six major North American teaching hospitals from 1972 to 1991 the rate of admissions for affective disorder has increased as the rate of admission of schizophrenic disorders has decreased. Several factors have influenced this change, including the more narrow definition of schizophrenia and parallel broadening of the category of affective disorders. Also, as new drugs for the treatment of affective disorders have been developed, clinicians may be influenced toward the diagnosis of affective disorders, causing a "treatment-oriented" diagnostic bias. The authors also speculate that third-party reimbursement rates may have favored patients given the diagnosis of an affective disorder. A number of reports (Klerman and Weissman, 1989; Cross National Collaborative Group, 1992) have suggested that the incidence of affective disorders has increased worldwide.

CASE DEFINITION OF BIPOLAR DISORDER

According to the *Diagnostic and Statistical Manual of Mental Disorders,* 4th edition, revised (DSM-IV) (American Psychiatric Association [APA], 1994), the essential feature of mood disorders is disturbance of mood that is defined as a "sustained emotion that colors the perception of the world." Although elevated mood may be considered the characteristic of a manic episode, the predominant mood may also be irritability. Patients with mania have inflated self-esteem, which may range from unusual self-confidence to grandiose delusions. Decreased need to sleep is associated with hyperactivity, where the individual remains awake during long periods of the night, involved in new projects, or making numerous telephone calls, and in some cases the individual wakes up several times during the night full of energy and "ready to go." The speech is usually pressured and at times difficult to interrupt. Flight of ideas may be present. Other symptoms include hypersexuality and impulsivity. The disturbance must be severe enough to cause marked impairment in social activities, occupational functioning, and interpersonal relationships or to require hospitalization to prevent harm to self.

Types of mood disorders are determined by their longitudinal pattern. They are subdivided into bipolar and depressive disorders. To meet Bipolar I Disorder criteria, there must have been at least one manic episode. Hypomania is a less severe presentation of mania without impairment of social or occupational functioning or the need for hospitalization. Bipolar II Disorder is characterized by hypomanic and full major depressive episodes. In cyclothymia a number of hypomanic episodes intermingle with major depressive symptoms. An episode may be subclassified as mild, moderate, or severe with or without psychotic features. Psychotic features may also be specified as mood congruent or mood incongruent. Mood congruent psychotic features are defined as being consistent with "typical manic themes of inflated worth, power, knowledge, identity, or special relationship to a deity or famous person." On the other hand, mood-incongruent psychotic features are "delusions or hallucinations whose content does not involve the typical manic themes" (APA, 1994). Psychotic features considered to be mood incongruent include persecutory delusions (not directly related to grandiose) and the so-called schneiderian first-rank symptoms (Schneider, 1959).

A significant change with the recently published DSM-IV criteria (APA, 1994) is that manic episodes precipitated by somatic antidepressant treatment such as electroconvulsive therapy or medication are not considered part of a Bipolar I Disorder but instead would be classified as substance induced mood disorder. The five-digit codes remain the same as in DSM-III-R. A significant improvement from DSM-III-R includes specific criteria for hypomanic episodes and for cyclothymic disorder. In addition, DSM-IV provides criteria for subtypes of Bipolar I Disorder, including the single manic episode where there should be the presence of only one manic episode and no past major depressive episodes. Another improvement includes the description of the most recent episode, which may be hypomanic, manic, mixed, or depressed, or the residual category of unspecified. Furthermore, DSM-IV includes the new term *Bipolar II Disorder.* It also includes *bipolar disorder not otherwise specified;* examples include a history of recurrent hypomanic episodes without any recurrent depressive symptoms or manic episodes superimposed on Psychotic Disorder NOS, residual schizophrenia, or a delusional disorder. DSM-IV also includes the category Mood Disorder due to a general medical condition.

Another new feature of DSM-IV is cross-sectional symptom features, which includes melancholic features, atypical features, or catatonic features. In addition, the course of mood disorders may be defined with "course specifiers," which include 1) rapid cycling, 2) seasonal pattern, and 3) postpartum onset. Furthermore, DSM-IV provides a description for the longitudinal course for Bipolar I Disorder, which includes 1) with full interepisode recovery, defined as "if no prominent mood symptoms between two most recent manic or major depressive episodes"; and 2) without full interepisode recovery, defined as "if prominent mood symptoms between two most recent manic or major depressive episodes." There are, now, a number of options to define the longitudinal course, which include 1) single episode with no cyclothymic disorder; 2) single episode superimposed on cyclothymic disorder; 3) recurrent with full interepisode recovery with no cyclothymic disorder; 4) recurrent without full interepisode recovery with no cyclothymic disorder; 5) recurrent with full interepisode recovery superimposed on cyclothymic disorder; and 6) recurrent without full interepisode recovery superimposed on cyclothymic disorder.

MAJOR STUDIES

Epidemiologic Catchment Area (ECA) Program

The 1978 report on the President's Commission on Mental Health made a number of recommendations that led to the creation of The Epidemiologic Catchment Area (ECA) Program in psychiatric epidemiology (Regier et al., 1984). Recommendations included the need to determine prevalence rates for mental disorders defined by contemporary diagnostic criteria, including community and institutionalized populations, and to obtain longitudinal data to identify new (incident) cases, as well as recurrence rates. The commission also underscored the need to identify mental health and general medical services in the U.S. population. In this chapter, we only review the findings related to bipolar disorder. For further review of the ECA project, see Chapter 5, this volume).

The ECA program collected data on bipolar disorder according to the DSM-III criteria with the use of the Diagnostic Interview Schedule (DIS) (Robins et al., 1981). With the exception of the study conducted by Weissman and Myers (1978), it is the first study in this country that has obtained prevalence rates for bipolar disorder utilizing structured diagnostic instruments. Using a probability sample, the ECA project obtained prevalence data for bipolar I and bipolar II disorders, but did not obtain information on cyclothymic disorder. In addition to obtaining prevalence rates of bipolar I and II disorders, an estimate of specific manic symptoms was also obtained (Weissman et al., 1991). The A criteria for a manic episode consisting of elevated, expansive, or irritable mode for at least 1 week duration had a lifetime prevalence of 2.7%. The most frequent manic symptom reported was hyperactivity (9.3%), followed by decreased need for sleep (7.5%), and distractibility (7.2%). Not surprisingly, manic symptoms were more frequent in the age group 18–29 years and also in men more than in women. Blacks were also more likely to present manic symptoms, especially hyperactivity, in 12.3% compared with 9% in whites and 1% in Hispanics; and decreased need for sleep, with 9.8% in blacks, 7.3% in whites, and 6.2% in Hispanics. Men were more likely than women to present hyperactivity, inflated self-esteem, distractibility, and involvement in risky activities; females were more likely to experience racing thoughts and distractibility. For all symptoms, the ages 18–29 had the highest prevalence rate.

The lifetime prevalence rate of a manic episode was 0.8% (Robins et al., 1984). The age group with the highest lifetime prevalence rate was 30–44 years, in contrast to manic symptoms for which the highest prevalence was in the 18–29 year group. There was no

**TABLE 1. ECA Lifetime Prevalence (Percent) of
Bipolar Disorder Subtypes by Age, Sex, and Ethnicity**[a]

	Bipolar I	Bipolar II
Total	0.8	0.5
Age (years)		
18–29	1.1***	0.7**
30–44	1.4	0.6
45–64	0.3	0.2
65+	0.1	0.1
Sex		
Male	0.7	0.4
Female	0.9	0.5
Ethnicity		
White	0.8	0.4
Black	1.0	0.6
Hispanic	0.7	0.5

[a]Variation within groups, controlling for age, sex, or ethnicity:
**$p < 0.01$, ***$p < 0.001$.
SOURCE: Weissmann et al. (1991).

difference by sex or ethnic group. Bipolar II disorder was present in 0.5% of the population. Table 1 presents data on lifetime prevalence for Bipolar I and bipolar II disorders stratified by age group, gender, and ethnicity. It demonstrates that all age groups show a difference in prevalence rates, but there was no difference in gender or ethnicity. There was also a difference for bipolar I across different sites, with New Haven showing a 1.2% and St. Louis 1.0% in contrast to 0.6% for Baltimore and Los Angeles and 3.4% for Durham. The rates for bipolar II disorders were also inconsistent across sites, ranging from 0.4% in Durham to 0.6% in Baltimore. The 1 year prevalence of bipolar I disorder showed, again, only a difference in age, with the highest rate (1.2%) in the age group 30–44 years.

One month prevalence for manic episodes (Regier et al., 1988) ranged in the five sites from as low as 0.1% in Los Angeles to 0.6% in St. Louis. The highest prevalence for males concentrated in the 25–44 year age group, where it was 0.5%, and for females in the 18–24 year age group, where it was 0.8%. Regier et al. (1993) recently estimated a 1 year prevalence of 1.2%, which translates to 1,908,000 people suffering from bipolar disorder.

Weissman et al. (1988) reported that the mean age of onset of bipolar disorder in the ECA data was 21 years old. The mean age of onset across the five sites was 21.2 years, adjusting for the age distribution at each site. The range was 17.9 years for the Los Angeles site compared with 26.3 for the Baltimore site.

New Haven Community Sample

In 1978, Weissman and Myers published the first epidmiologic survey using research diagnostic criteria. The authors utilized the Schedule for Affective Disorders and Schizophrenia and the Diagnostic Research Criteria (SADS-RDC) (Spitzer et al., 1978). Weissman and Myers sampled 1,095 households and identified a lifetime prevalence rate of

0.8% for mania and 0.8% for hypomania. They found that bipolar disorders cluster in the higher socioeconomic classes, with 4.6% in Hollingshead and Redlich's classes 1 and 2 (1958), 1% in class 3, 0.9% in class 4, and no cases in class 5.

The Amish Study

More than a decade ago, Egeland and Hostetter (1983) reported their epidemiologic study of affective disorders among the Amish. It was a 6 year study of affective disorders among the Old Order Amish, which is an ultraconservative Protestant religious sect. This study was conducted in one of their settlements in Lancaster County, Pennsylvania, with approximately 11,000 residents. The investigators have stressed that the Amish are a culturally and genetically homogenous group where alcohol and drug abuse are essentially not found. One of the major goals of the Amish study was to explore the genetic aspects of affective disorders. The prevalence of bipolar I and II disorders in the population aged 15 years and older was 0.46%.

The National Comorbidity Survey

The National Comorbidity Survey (NCS) (Kessler et al., 1994) is based on a probability sample of individuals aged 15–54 from noninstitutionalized populations from 48 states. It utilized the University of Michigan version of the Composite International Diagnostic Instrument (UM-CIDI). A total of 8,098 individuals were interviewed. It builds upon the experience of the ECA but expands into a more comprehensive assessment on risk factors (Kessler et al., 1994).

The NCS reported a lifetime prevalence of 1.6% for a manic episode compared with only 0.6% for nonaffective psychosis (schizophrenia, schizophreniform disorder, schizoaffective disorder, delusional disorder, and atypical psychosis). The 1 year prevalence for a manic episode was 1.3% (Kessler et al., 1994). It should be mentioned, however, that the diagnosis of nonaffective psychosis was based on a clinical interview using the SCID while the diagnosis for mania was based only on the UM-CIDI.

Substance Use Disorder Comorbidity and Bipolar Disorders

Kessler (see Chapter 7, this volume) recently reviewed the comorbidity of different psychotic disorders in the NCS and in the ECA. In both surveys, mania was accompanied by a comorbid disorder in more than 50% of the cases. Goodwin and Jamison (1990) argued that comorbidity in bipolar patients has not been studied as comprehensively as it has in major depressive disorder and stressed the importance of studying the effects of comorbidity in illness course. They summarized the existing literature and estimated a 35% prevalence of bipolar illness and alcohol abuse. They also raised the issue of determining the chronologic sequence of the onset of each disorder and the lack of much needed empirical information in this area.

The ECA study (Regier et al., 1990) reported that the bipolar I group had a prevalence of substance abuse of 60.7%. The ECA investigators suggested that a high degree of comorbidity in bipolar disorders greatly complicates treatment. Interestingly, the ECA Study (Helzer and Pryzbeck, 1988) reported that the prevalence of comorbid alcoholism in mania was three times that in major depression. Furthermore, the likelihood (odds ratio) of an individual with bipolar disorder having a substance use disorder was 6.6 greater than that of the general population. The only diagnosis that had a higher ratio than mania was antisocial personality disorder.

Non–North American Studies

In addition to the ECA study, a number of population-based prevalence studies using structured diagnostic instruments and modern diagnostic criteria have recently been conducted outside North America and have included the diagnosis of bipolar disorder. We describe some of those studies.

Notably, in the community surveyed in Florence, Italy, by Faravelli, et al. (1990), DSM-III diagnoses were obtained with interviews conducted by psychiatrists in a community sample of 1,000 people. The 1 year prevalence for bipolar I disorder was 1.86% for females and 0.65% for males. For bipolar II disorder, the overall prevalence was 0.2%. In a study in Taiwan, Hwu and collaborators (1989) conducted a multistage random sampling of 5,005 residences from metropolitan Taipei, 3,004 from small towns, and 2,995 from rural villages. They utilized the DIS and found a prevalence for manic episode of 1.6% for Taipei, 0.7% for small towns, and 1.0% for rural villages. Another study that utilized the DIS was conducted in Puerto Rico by Canino and collaborators (1987). The lifetime prevalence for manic episode was 0.7% for males and 0.4% for females. The 6 month prevalence was 0.3% for males and 0.3% for females. Bland et al. (1988) conducted a prevalence study in Alberta, Canada, from a community sample of 3,258, also utilizing the DIS. The lifetime prevalence for manic episode was 0.7% for males and 0.4% for females.

Different studies have utilized other diagnostic instruments. A study conducted in the Netherlands (Hodiamont et al., 1987) utilized PSE, which uses the International Classification of the Diseases (ICD) system. For manic episodes, the prevalence was 0.1% for both genders.

Incidence Data

Boyd and Weissman (1981) have reported incidence data for bipolar disorders in Scandinavian countries. The annual incidence rate for bipolar disorders varied from 9.2 to 15.2 cases per 100,000 subjects in males and from 7.4 to 32.5 cases per 100,000 in females. Leff and collaborators (1976), using the PSE, obtained first-admission rates for patients hospitalized with mania in London, England, and Aarhus, Denmark. The prevalence rate was 2.6 per 100,000 individuals in both sites. The ECA Project has also provided incidence data (Eaton et al., 1989; Regier et al., 1993). In a recent publication, Regier et al. (1993) reported new cases during a 1 year period (annual incidence rates). The project, known as Wave 2 of the ECA study, was conducted on approximately 20% of the initial population. This prospective follow up permitted the estimation of new cases as well as of relapses. For bipolar disorder, the annual cumulative rate was 0.5% ± 0.1%.

RISK FACTORS

Age

In the textbook by Goodwin and Jamison (1990), the mean age of onset is estimated to be 30 years. There is some evidence that in some recent studies age of onset in bipolar disorder is lower. This may be due in part to increased awareness of the diagnosis among child psychiatrists. The range of age of onset goes as low as 12–13 years old, but may also be present in the over-65 age group. A recent study by Tohen and collaborators (1994) suggested that many first-episode bipolar cases in the elderly are associated with a comorbid cerebrovascular disorder.

There is also a recent interest in secular trends in bipolar disorder. Klerman and Weissman (1989) noted an increased rate for major depression in cohorts born after 1940. The same has been found for bipolar disorder (Gershon et al., 1987). Gershon and collaborators (1987) published birth cohort changes in patients with mania in a cohort of relatives of bipolar and schizoaffective patients. Utilizing life table analysis, the investigators reported higher rates of bipolar disorder in the cohorts born after 1940, suggesting that the cumulative hazard for bipolar disorder in a given age group was greater in those born after 1940. The authors found that for individuals born in the 1940s, the prevalence for bipolar I was 6.0%, and for those born in the 1950s it was 8.6%, in contrast to individuals born in the 1920s, for whom the rate was 3.4%, and for those born in the '30s, at 2.5%. The authors speculate that the cohorts with high rates of affective illness seem to have been born in decades during which there was a major war, accompanied by extensive use of alcohol and illicit drugs. Lasch et al. (1990) also reported birth cohort changes in prevalence rates for mania utilizing data from the ECA study. The authors identified 17,827 individuals and divided them into different cohorts separated by decades. They found a high risk of developing mania in those born after 1935. The authors also suggested that environmental and historical events may have increased the rates, suggesting a gene–environment interaction.

Urban Versus Rural

In the ECA St. Louis site (Weissman et al., 1991), the rate in the urban population was 1.5% compared with 0.5% in the rural population, with an odds ratio of 2.25 adjusted for sex, age, and ethnicity ($P = 0.001$). For the Durham site (Blazer et al., 1985), again there was a higher rate in the urban population, with 0.8% compared with 0.2% in the rural population and an adjusted odds ratio of 3.78 ($p = 0.05$). Not surprisingly, the rate of bipolar illness was higher in institutionalized individuals living in prisons or nursing homes, with a 9.7% prevalence rate for individuals living in nursing homes and 5.4% for those living in prisons. The odds ratio comparing nursing home residents with those living in households was 10.8, adjusted for sex, age, and ethnicity, and 5.75 for those living in prison ($p = 0.05$).

Gender

Most studies have noticed no gender difference in the prevalence of bipolar disorder. Both the ECA and Amish studies found a 1 to 1 female/male ratio.

Social Class

Most studies published before 1980 found a higher prevalence in the upper socioeconomic classes. This finding may be attributed to a bias assessment of researchers and clinicians in diagnosing subjects from lower socioeconomic status as schizophrenic and psychotic subjects from upper socioeconomic status as bipolar. In contrast, more recent epidemiologic studies have not found a significant difference of bipolar disorder related to social class. However, the New Haven Community Sample (Weissman and Myers, 1978) found higher rates in upper socioeconomic groups. On the other hand, the ECA program found higher rates of mania in adults with fewer years of education (Weissman et al., 1991). Individuals with less than 12 years of education had a prevalence of 1.1% compared with 0.9% in those with more than 12 years of education. The odds ratio after adjusting for sex, age, and ethnicity was 1.93 ($p = 0.01$).

Race

The ECA program found no significant race difference. Jones et al. (1981) suggested that in previous studies where an ethnic difference was reported, blacks were more likely to be diagnosed as schizophrenic and whites as bipolar, with a consequent underdiagnosing of bipolar illness in black patients.

Marital Status

The ECA study (Weissman et al., 1991) found that individuals who are cohabiting, divorced, or never married are more likely to suffer from bipolar disorder than married individuals. The ECA data estimated that the 1 year prevalence of suffering from bipolar disorder was 3.2% in subjects who are cohabitating compared with 1.3% in the never married and 0.2% in the married. The odds ratio for those cohabitating compared with the married/never divorced was 8.3 adjusting for sex, age, and race. Similarly, Boyd and Weissman (1981) found that more single and divorced individuals suffer from manic-depressive illness.

Cultural Factors

Since the turn of the century, Kraepelin noted that certain cultures may show high rates of manic-depressive illness. Whether this is secondary to the genetic load or to cultural factors still needs to be determined. specifically, Kraepelin noted a higher incidence of manic-depressive illness in some Indonesian groups. Other societies in which manic-depressive illness appears to be particularly high include the Hutterities in North American (Eaton and Weil, 1955). Similarly, higher rates of manic depressive illness have been identified in Jews of European background than in those of North African background (Miller, 1967; Gershon and Liebowitz, 1975). Emigration has also been considered a risk factor of bipolar illness (Hemsi, 1967; Pope et al., 1983). It is not clear if individuals predisposed to a bipolar illness are more likely to emigrate or if the migration process in itself precipitates the condition in otherwise predisposed individuals.

Homelessness

Koegel et al. (1988), utilizing the DIS, found very high rates for manic episode among the homeless across different ethnic groups. Prevalence rates were 10.7% for whites, 11.7% for African-Americans, and 8.5% for Hispanics.

UTILIZATION OF HEALTH AND MENTAL SERVICES

The ECA study (Weissman et al., 1991) reported that individuals suffering from bipolar disorder are high users of health services; 38.5% will receive outpatient psychiatric treatment within a 1 year period, and 9.6% will receive inpatient treatment within a 6 month period. Approximately 79.2% received treatment in a medical outpatient facility, and 29.5% received treatment in a medical inpatient facility (6 month period).

Regier et al. (1993) described the de facto U.S. mental and addictive disorders service system as composed by general medical physicians, other human services professions, and the voluntary support sector; the latter includes self-support groups, family and friends. For bipolar disorder, 60.9% received one of those services with overlap among sectors. Professional services were received by 58.9% of bipolar (I and II) patients. Specialty mental health was provided by general medical (32.4%) and other human service (10%) professionals. The voluntary support network provided 9.6% of services. Narrow et al. (1993) reported used of services by individuals with different disorders. Of the 1.9 million individuals suffering from bipolar disorder, 1.1 million received care during a 1 year period. The services included 16 million outpatient visits (Table 2), including 23.7% of them by mental health specialists in private practice and 19% by a general medical physician. The average number of visits per treated person per year in ambulatory services was 14.7 (Table 2), including 13.9 by mental health specialists and 16.3 by the voluntary support network. Bipolar patients received inpatient treatment in a variety of settings (Table 3), including 34.4% in a VA hospital psychiatric unit and 33.4% in a general hospital psychiatric unit.

FAMILIAL TRANSMISSION

The NIMH Collaborative Program on the Psychobiology of Depression (Rice et al., 1987) estimated the morbid risk of bipolar disorder in family members of bipolar patients. Rates varied depending on the familial relationship. For children, the risk was 1.5%, with 6% for brothers, 4.1% for mother, and 6.4% for father.

GENETIC STUDIES

A century after psychoanalysis revolutionized psychiatry, genetics promises to do the same at the turn of the twenty-first century. The evidence that many psychiatric conditions are genetically based appears pretty solid. However, the field is not yet advanced to the point of unraveling the web of psychiatric genetics. The hope is that at some point genetics will help to develop new strategies for prevention and treatment of psychiatric disorders.

A national meeting held at the National Institute of Mental Health concluded that the evidence from family, adoption, and twin studies supports the evidence that bipolar disorder is genetically transmitted (Blehar et al., 1988). Nevertheless, 5 years later, the questions raised at the meeting have not been answered, including the mode of transmission and its genetic relationship to other affective disorders. Different investigative teams have looked at linkage studies. Linkage is the phenomenon of alleles of different chromosomal loci being inherited together (Baron et al., 1990). It is assumed that when two alleles are

TABLE 2. Ambulatory Mental Health Services for Bipolar Patients[a]

	Percentage Treated	Percentage Distribution of Visits	Average No. of Visits per Treated Person per Year
Psychiatric hospital outpatient clinic	2.7	2.3	12.3
MH center outpatient clinic	9.5	8.6	13.2
General hospital outpatient clinic	9.0	5.7	9.3
VA Hospital outpatient clinic	4.7	1.3	3.9
Alcohol/drug unit outpatient clinic	2.0	0.7	4.9
MH specialist in health/plan/clinic	6.5	6.8	15.4
MH specialist in private practice	25.8	23.7	13.5
Crisis center	0.9	0.1	1.0
SMA subtotal	51.8	49.0	13.9
General hospital emergency dept.	5.7	0.9	2.3
GM physician	52.3	19.1	5.4
GM subtotal	55.9	20.0	5.2
Health systems subtotal	88.5	69.0	11.5
Family/social service agency	2.7	2.3	12.4
Clergy/religious counselor	7.3	2.7	5.5
Natural therapist	1.1	0.2	2.0
Other HS	7.7	7.9	15.1
HS subtotal	16.7	13.1	11.6
Professional subtotal	96.6	82.1	12.5
Self-help group	4.8	9.9	30.4
Friend/relative	11.3	8.0	10.3
VSN subtotal	16.1	17.9	16.3
Total	1,092.000 patients treated	16,046.000 visits	14.7 visits per person

[a]ADM, alcohol, drug, or mental; MH, mental health; VA, Veterans Affairs; SMA, Specialty mental and addictive services; GM, general medical; HS, human services; and VSN, voluntary support network.
SOURCE: Modified from Narrow et al. (1993).

close together on the same chromosome, it is more likely that they will be inherited together.

The NIMH meeting concluded that a major problem in linkage analysis that follows a single gene hypothesis is the lack of identification of sufficient chromosomal markers covering the entire genome. In recent years molecular genetics has made progress in mapping the entire genome. In spite of this, the search continues. In addition to issues in

TABLE 3. Percentage of Bipolar Patients Treated in an Inpatient Setting[a]

Setting	Percent
General hospital (psychiatric unit and scatterbed)	33.4
State and county mental hospitals	13.4
Residential supportive care	3.1
Community mental health center	0.0
Private mental hospital	19.5
VA hospital psychiatric unit	34.4
Alcohol/drug treatment unit	0.0
Nursing home	1.3

[a]Total = 144,000 patients admitted.

SOURCE: Modified from Narrow et al. (1993).

molecular genetics, other aspects of genetic epidemiology require close attention, including the identification of informative families, the precision of diagnostic methods, and the criteria utilized in studying family members. Other aspects that still need to be resolved are the relationships between bipolar and other conditions such as schizophrenia, unpolar depression, and personality disorders. Linkage analysis is more likely to yield positive findings in conditions that have a single gene mode of transmission, which may not be the case with bipolar disorder, where a multifactional mode of transmission is more likely.

In a meeting organized by the MacArthur Foundation in 1989, linkage studies in bipolar disorder were reviewed (Merikangas et al., 1989). The consensus was that the major problems with the linkage approach included 1) the complexity of bipolar disorders, 2) comorbidity with other disorders, 3) nonrandom mating, 4) cohort effects, and 5) the poor diagnostic validity of bipolar disorder. The investigators concluded that most successes in molecular genetics have been with disorders with a mendelian mode of inheritance, where a phenotype is easily defined for example in Huntington's disease, while the success is less clear with conditions where the mode of transmission is nonmendelian, such as with diabetes, hypertension, or psychiatric disorders. Existing data suggest that the genetic transmission of bipolar disorder follows a nonmendelian pattern.

To date there has been no replication of linkage of any particular gene in bipolar disorder. Notable examples are the X-linkage initially suggested by Baron et al. (1990) and chromosome 11 suggested by the Amish studies. Difficulties in linkage analysis in bipolar disorder include the complexity of the condition, such as the tendency for assortative mating, which is a tendency for spouses to have similar phenotypic traits. Assortative mating makes linkage analysis difficult due to the bilineal transmission of the condition, where genes are inherited on both maternal and paternal sides. Secular trends such as an increased prevalence of bipolar disorder in recent cohorts, if not properly analyzed, will also complicate linkage analysis. Other problems with linkage analysis include the lack of stability of diagnosis in bipolar disorder, which may be corrected by longitudinal diagnostic assessments.

Merikangas et al. (1989) emphasized the importance of replicating results. Pardes et al. (1989) suggested that psychiatry is undergoing a revolution with genetic research, which at some point will make it possible to develop novel approaches to the prevention and treatment of psychiatric disorders.

REFERENCES

Adams F (1990): "The Extant Works of Aretaeus, the Cappadocian." London: The Syndenham Society, 1856. Reprinted in the Classics of Medicine Library Series. Birmingham, AL: Gryphon Editions, Inc.

American Psychiatric Association (1994): "Diagnostic and Statistical Manual of Mental Disorders," 4th ed. Washington, DC: The American Psychiatric Association.

Andreasen NC, Rice J, Endicott J, Coryell W, Grove WM, Reich T (1987): Familial rates of affective disorder. Arch Gen Psychiatry 44:461–469.

Baldessarini RJ (1970): Frequency of diagnoses of schizophrenia versus affective disorders from 1944 to 1968. Am J Psychiatry 127:759–763.

Baron M, Endicott J, Ott J (1990): Genetic linkage in mental illness: Limitations and prospects. Br J Psychiatry 157:645–655.

Bland RC, Newman SC, Orn H (eds) (1988): Epidemiology of psychiatric disorders in Edmonton. Acta Psychiatr Scand 77(Suppl 338).

Blazer DG, George LK, Landerman R, Pennybacker M, Melville ML, Woodbury M, Manton KG, Jordan K, Locke B, (1985): Psychiatric disorders: A rural/urban comparison. Arch Gen Psychiatry 42:651–656.

Blehar MC, Weissman MM, Gershon ES, Hirschfeld MA (1988): Family and genetic studies of affective disorders. Arch Gen Psychiatry 44:289–292.

Boyd JH, Weissman MM (1981): Epidemiology of affective disorders: A re-examination and future directions. Arch Gen Psychiatry 38:1039–1046.

Canino GJ, Bird HR, Shrout PE, Rubio-Stipec M, Bravo Milagros, Sesman M, Guevara LM (1987): Prevalence of specific psychiatric disorders in Puerto Rico. Arch Gen Psychiatry 44:727–735.

Cooper JE, Kendell RE, Gurland BJ, Sharpe L, Copeland JRM, Simon R (1972): "Psychiatric Diagnosis in New York and London." London: Oxford University Press.

Cross-National Collaborative Group (1992): The changing rates of major depression. Cross-national comparisons. JAMA 268:3098–3105.

Eaton JW, Weil RJ (1955): "Culture and Mental Disorders: A Comparative Study of the Hutterites and Other Populations." New York: Free Press.

Eaton WW, Kramer M, Anthony JC, Dryman A, Shapiro S, Locke BZ, (1989): The incidence of specific DIS/DSM-III mental disorders: Data from the NIMH Epidemiologic Catchment Area Program. Acta Psychiatr Scand 79:163–178.

Egeland JA, Hostetter AM (1983): Amish study, I: Affective disorders among the Amish, 1976–1980. Am J Psychiatry 140:1, 56–61.

Falret JP (1854): Memoire sur la folie circulaire, forme de maladie mentale caracterisee per la reproduction successive et reguliere de l'etat maniaque, de l'etat melancolique, et d'un intervalle lucide plus ou moins prolonge. Bull Acad Med 19:382–415.

Faravelli C, Degl'Innocenti BG, Aiazzi L, Incerpi G, Pallanti S (1990): Epidemiology of mood disorders: A community survey in Florence. J Affect Disord 20:135–141.

Feighner JP, Robins E, Guze SB (1972): Diagnostic criteria for use in psychiatric research. Arch Gen Psychiatry 26:57–63.

Gershon ES, Hamovit JH, Guroff JJ, Nurnberger JI (1987): Birth-cohort changes in manic and depressive disorders in relatives of bipolar and schizoaffective patients. Arch Gen Psychiatry 44:314–319.

Gershon ES, Liebowitz JH (1975): Sociocultural and demographic correlates of affective disorders in Jerusalem. J Psychiatr Res 12:37–50.

Goodwin FK, Jamison KR (1990): "Manic-Depressive Illness." New York: Oxford University Press.

Helzer JE, Pryzbeck TR (1988): The co-occurrence of alcoholism with other psychiatric disorders in the general population and its impact on treatment. J Study Alcohol 49:219–224.

Helzer JE, Robins LN, Croughan JL, Welner A (1981): Renard diagnostic interview: Its reliability and procedural validity with physicians and lay interviewers. Arch Gen Psychiatry 38:393–398.

Hemsi LK (1967): Psychiatric morbidity of West Indian immigrants. Soc Psychiatry 2:95–100.

Hodiamont P, Peer N, Syben N (1987): Epidemiological aspects of psychiatric disorder in a Dutch health area. Psychol Med 17:495–505.

Hollingshead AB, Redlich FC (1958): Social Class and Mental Illness. New York: John Wiley.

Hwu HG, Yeh EK, Chang LY (1989): Prevalence of psychiatric disorders in Taiwan defined by the Chinese Diagnostic Interview Schedule. Acta Psychiatr Scand 79:136–147.

Jones BE, Gray BA, Parson EB (1981): Manic-depressive illness among poor urban blacks. Am J Psychiatry 138:654–657.

Kessler RC, McGonagle KA, Zhao S, et al. (1994): Lifetime and 12-month prevalence of DSM-III-R psychiatric disorders in the United States. Arch Gen Psychiatry 51:8–19.

Klerman GL, Weissman MM (1989): Increasing rates of depression. JAMA 261:2229–2235.

Koegel P, Burnam A, Farr RK (1988): The prevalence of specific psychiatric disorders among homeless individuals in the inner city of Los Angeles. Arch Gen Psychiatry 45:1085–1092.

Kraepelin E (1921): "Manic-depressive insanity and paranoia." Edinburgh: E&S Livingstone.

Krauthammer C, Klerman G (1979): The epidemiology of mania. In Shopsin B (ed): "Manic Illness." New York: Raven Press, pp 11–28.

Lasch K, Weissman MM, Wickramaratne PJ, Bruce ML (1990): Birth cohort changes in the rates of mania. Psychiatry Res 33:31–37.

Leff JP, Fischer M, Bertelsen A (1976): A cross-national epidemiological study of mania. Br J Psychiatry 129:428–442.

Merikangas KR, Spence A, Kupfer DJ (1989): Linkage studies of bipolar disorder: Methodologic and analytic issues. Arch Gen Psychiatry 46:1137–1141.

Miller L (1967): The social psychiatry and epidemiology of mental ill health in Israel. Top Prob Psychiatr Neurol 6:96–137.

Narrow WE, Regier DA, Rae DS, Manderscheid RW, Locke BZ (1993): Use of services. Findings from the National Institute of Mental Health Epidemiologic Catchment Area Program. Arch Gen Psychiatry 50:95–107.

Pardes H, Kaufmann CA, Pincus HA, West A (1989): Genetics and psychiatry: Past discoveries, current dilemmas, and future directions. Am J Psychiatry 146:4, 435–443.

Pope HG Jr, Ionescu-Pioggia M, Yurgelun-Todd D (1983): Migration and manic-depressive illness. Comp Psychiatry 24:158–165.

President's Commission on Mental Health (1978): "Report to the President from the President's Commission on Mental Health," Stock No. 040-000-00390-8, vol 1. Washington, DC: U.S. Government Printing Office.

Regier DA, Boyd JH, Burke JD, Rae DS, Myers JK, Kramer M, Robins LN, George LK, Karno M, Locke BZ (1988): One month prevalence of mental disorders in the US—based on the five epidemiologic catchment area sites. Arch Gen Psychiatry 45:977–986.

Regier DA, Farmer ME, Rae DS, et al. (1990): Comorbidity of mental health disorders with alcohol and other drug abuse. JAMA 264:2511–2518.

Regier DA, Myers JK, Kramer M, Robins LN, Blazer DG, Hough RL, Eaton WW, Locke BZ (1984): The NIMH epidemiologic catchment area program. Arch Gen Psychiatry 41:934–941.

Regier DA, Narrow WE, Rae DS, Manderscheid RW, Locke BZ, Goodwin FK (1993): The de Facto U.S. Mental and Addictive Disorders Service System. Epidemiologic Catchment Area prospective 1-year prevalence rates of disorders and services. Arch Gen Psychiatry 50:85–94.

Rice J, Reich T, Andreasen NC, Endicott J, Van Eerdewegh M, Fishman R, Hirschfeld RMA, Klerman GL (1987): The familial transmission of bipolar illness. Arch Gen Psychiatry 44:441–447.

Robins LN, Helzer JE, Croughan J, Ratcliff KS (1981): National Institute of Mental Health Diagnostic Interview Schedule: Its history, characteristics, and validity. Arch Gen Psychiatry 38:381–389.

Robins LN, Helzer JE, Weissman MM, Orvaschel H, Gruenberg E, Burke JD Jr, Regier DA (1984): Lifetime prevalence of specific psychiatric disorders in three sites. Arch Gen Psychiatry 41:949–958.

Schneider K (1959): "Clinical psychopathology." (M.W. Hamilton, translator.) New York: Grune & Stratton.

Shapiro S, Skinner EA, Kessler LG, Von Korff M, German PS, Tischler GL, Leaf PJ, Benham L, Cottler L, Regier DA (1984): Utilization of health and mental health services. Arch Gen Psychiatry 41:971–978.

Spitzer RL, Endicott J (1978): "Schedule for Affective Disorders and Schizophrenia." New York: Biometric Research, Evaluation Section, New York State Psychiatric Institute.

Spitzer RL, Endicott J, Robins E (1978): "Research Diagnostic Criteria." New York: Biometrics Research, Evaluation Section, New York State Psychiatric Institute.

Spitzer RL, Williams JBW, Gibbon M (1990): "Structured Clinical Interview for DSM-III." New York: Biometric Research, New York State Psychiatric Institute.

Stoll AL, Tohen M, Baldessarini RJ, Goodwin DC, Stein SM, Katz SM, Swinson RP, McGlashan T (1994): Shifts in the diagnostic frequencies of schizophrenia and affective disorders from 1972 through 1988: A combined analysis from four North American Psychiatric Hospitals. Am J Psychiatry 151:1642–1645.

Tohen M, Shulman KI, Satlin A (1994): First-episode mania in late life. Am J Psychiatry 151:130–132.

Weissman MM, Bruce ML, Leaf PJ, Florio LP, Holzer C (1991): Psychiatric disorders in America. In Robins L, Regier D (eds). New York: Free Press, pp 53–81.

Weissman MM, Leaf PJ, Tischler GL, Blazer DG, Karno M, Bruce ML, Florio LP (1988): Affective disorders in five United States communities. Psychol Med 18:141–153.

Weissman MM, Myers JK (1978): Affective disorders in a U.S. urban community: The use of Research Diagnostic Criteria in an epidemiological survey. Arch Gen Psychiatry 35:1304–1311.

Wing JK, Cooper JE, Sartorius N (1974): "Measure and classification of psychiatric symptoms: An instructional Manual for the PSE and CATEGO Programs." Cambridge: Cambridge University Press.

Wing JK, Babor T, Brugha T, Burke J, Cooper JE, Giel R, Jablenski A, Regier D, Sartorius N (1990): SCAN: schedules for clinical assessments in neuropsychiatry. Arch Gen Psychiatry 47:589–593.

CHAPTER 16

Epidemiology of Depression and Anxiety Disorders

EWALD HORWATH and MYRNA M. WEISSMAN

College of Physicians and Surgeons of Columbia University and Intensive Care Unit, Washington Heights Community Service, New York State Psychiatric Institute, New York, NY 10032 (E.H.); College of Physicians and Surgeons of Columbia University and Division of Clinical and Genetic Epidemiology, New York State Psychiatric Institute, New York, NY 10032 (M.M.W.)

INTRODUCTION

The epidemiologic study of depression and anxiety has a long history. The community surveys of the 1950s and 1960s are relevant to our current understanding of depression and anxiety insofar as they adopted the methodology of direct interview in the community, paid close attention to psychosocial variables, and documented significant levels of impairment due to psychiatric symptoms. However, these studies defined mental health and illness along a continuum and intentionally failed to establish rates of specific psychiatric disorders. They also assumed the social etiology of mental illness as a given. For these reasons, the findings of these studies had limited applications as research on the genetics, neuroscience, and psychopharmacology of psychiatric disorders emerged in the 1970s and 1980s.

In this chapter, we limit our review to epidemiologic studies of the 1980s that used standardized interview instruments, operationalized diagnostic criteria, and reported data on widely agreed upon diagnostic categories, such as those in the *Diagnostic and Statistical Manual of Mental Disorders,* 3rd edition (DSM-III) (American Psychiatric Association [APA], 1980) and the *International Classification of Diseases,* 9th revision, (ICD-9) (World Health Organization, 1978). We focus on two categories of affective disorder, major depression and dysthymia; and on five anxiety disorders, panic disorder, agoraphobia, social phobia, generalized anxiety disorder, and obsessive-compulsive disorder. Readers interested in the epidemiologic survey data prior to 1980 are referred to reviews by Boyd and Weissman (1982) and Charney and Weissman (1988).

Textbook in Psychiatric Epidemiology, Edited by Tsuang, Tohen, and Zahner
ISBN 0-471-59375-3   © 1995 Wiley-Liss, Inc.

MAJOR DEPRESSION

Definition

The DSM-III diagnosis of major depression requires a 2 week period of dysphoric mood or loss of interest or pleasure and at least four other symptoms, which may include significant weight loss or gain, appetite disturbance, insomnia or hypersomnia, psychomotor agitation or retardation, fatigue or loss of energy, feelings of worthlessness, inappropriate guilt, impaired concentration, recurrent suicidal ideas, or a suicide attempt (APA, 1980).

Rates

Table 1 shows the sample sizes and Table 2 shows the 6 month, 1 year, and lifetime prevalence rates per 100 of major depression based on community surveys using DSM-III criteria in the U.S.; Edmonton, Canada; Puerto Rico; Florence, Italy; Seoul, Korea; Taiwan; and Zurich, Switzerland. The 6 month rate of major depression across five sites in the Epidemiological Catchment Area (ECA) study was 2.2, ranging from 1.5 in Durham to 2.8 in New Haven. The 1 year five site prevalence in the ECA study was 2.7, with a range from 1.7 in Durham to 3.4 in New Haven. Lower annual rates were reported from Taiwan, while higher rates were reported from Florence (5.2), New Zealand (5.3), and Zurich (7.0).

The ECA five site lifetime rate per 100 was 4.4, with a range from 2.9 in Baltimore to 5.8 in New Haven. Rates were similar in Puerto Rico (4.6) and Seoul (3.4), but considerably higher in New Zealand (12.6) and in Edmonton, Canada (8.6), and, again, lowest in Taiwan.

TABLE 1. Epidemiological Community Surveys of Psychiatric Disorders Using DSM-III

Place	n	Age (Years)	References
U.S. ECA	18,572	18+	Weissman et al. (1988a,b)
New Haven	5,034		
Baltimore	3,481		
St Louis	3,004		
Durham, NC	3,921		
Los Angeles	3,132		
Edmonton, Canada	3,258	18+	Bland et al. (1988)
Puerto Rico	1,551	17–64	Canino et al. (1987)
Florence, Italy	1,110	15+	Faravelli et al. (1989, 1990)
Seoul, Korea	5,100	18–65	Lee et al. (1987, 1990a,b)
Taiwan	11,004	18+	Hwu et al. (1989)
Urban	5,005		
Small towns	3,004		
Rural villages	2,995		
New Zealand	1,498	18+	Joyce et al. (1989, 1990)
Zurich, Switzerland	6,193	19–24	Angst and Dobler-Mikola (1984, 1985)
U.S. National Survey	3,161		Uhlenhuth et al. (1983)

SOURCE: Paykel (1992).

TABLE 2. Prevalence Rates Per 100 for Major Depression Based on Community Surveys Using DSM-III Diagnosis

Place	Rate/100[a]		
	6 Month	1 Year	Lifetime
U.S. ECA	2.2	2.6	4.4
New Haven	2.8	3.4	5.8
Baltimore	1.7	1.9	2.9
St Louis	2.3	2.7	4.4
Durham, NC	1.5	1.7	3.5
Los Angeles	2.6	3.2	5.6
Edmonton, Canada	3.2	—	8.6
Puerto Rico	3.0	—	4.6
Florence, Italy	—	5.2	—
Seoul, Korea	—	—	3.4
Taiwan			
Urban	—	0.6	0.9
Small towns	—	1.1	1.7
Rural villages	—	0.8	1.0
New Zealand	5.3	5.3	12.6
Zurich, Switzerland	—	7.0	—

[a]Rates rounded off to one decimal place in most cases.

SOURCE: Paykel (1992).

A significant question is whether these cross-national differences are related to true cross-cultural variation in risk factors or to methodologic differences across studies. By far the lowest rates of major depression were reported in Taiwan even though, on the basis of diagnostic criteria, measurement, and sampling methods, the Taiwanese studies are comparable to the ECA and other cited studies. This suggests that the reported differences may represent true differences in rates of major depression or that there is a culturally mediated tendency to experience or report depression differently in Taiwan than in the West. This interpretation of the data is suggested by the fact that substance abuse/dependence and major depression are the most prevalent disorders in the ECA study, while psychophysiologic disorders are most prevalent in Taiwan. In Korea, which is more westernized than Taiwan, the lifetime prevalence per 100 of major depression was 3.4, more comparable with the five site ECA rate of 5.4 than the low Taiwanese rates.

Several investigators have reported on incidence data from the ECA study (Eaton et al., 1989; Anthony and Petronis 1991; Horwath et al., 1992a). Annual incidence of first-onset major depression was 1.6 per 100 across four sites (New Haven was excluded) (Eaton et al., 1989). Although incidence data are particularly valuable in studying risk factors that may improve our understanding of disease etiology, community epidemiologic surveys rarely provide such data because large prospectively observed samples are required in order to generate accurate estimates of incidence. We will comment further on the ECA incidence data in the discussion of specific risk factors for major depression.

Table 3 shows sample sizes and Table 4 shows point prevalence rates of depression based on community surveys using PSE, CATEGO (D,R,N), and ICD-9 (296.2/300.4). The rates range from a low of 4.6/100 in Finland to a high of 7.4/100 in Athens, Greece.

TABLE 3. Recent Epidemiological Studies Using PSE and ICD-9

Place	No. Sampled	No. Interviewed 2nd Stage	Age (Years)	References
Nijmegen,the Netherlands	3,245	775	18–64	Hodiamont et al. (1987)
Camberwell (UK)	800	310	18–64	Bebbington et al. (1981)
Canberra, Australia	756	170	18+	Henderson et al. (1979)
Santander, Spain	1,223	452	18+	Vazquez-Barquero et al. (1986)
Two districts, Finland	747	—	30+	Lehtinen et al. (1990
Athens, Greece	487	—	18+	Mavreas and Bebbington (1988)
Greek Cypriots in UK	285	—	18+	Mavreas and Bebbington (1988)

SOURCE: Paykel (1992).

The rates for these ICD-9 depression categories tend to be higher than those reported for the DSM-III studies. This may be accounted for by the inclusion of neurotic depression, a category that is broader than DSM-III major depression and may overlap with DSM-III dysthymic disorder.

Subtypes of Major Depression

Several studies of the ECA data have found evidence supportive of the validity of major depression with psychotic features and major depression with atypical features as subtypes. Johnson et al. (1991) found that 14% of major depressions were accompanied by psychotic features, and that these cases, when compared with nonpsychotic depression, had a more severe course, as reflected in increased risk of relapse, persistence over 1 year, suicide attempts, hospitalization, comorbidity, and financial dependency. These findings, based on a community sample, are consistent with reports from clinical samples and provide epidemiologic support for the validity and clinical significance of psychotic depression and for its continued inclusion as a distinct subtype in DSM-IV.

Horwath et al. (1992b), also reporting on ECA data, found that major depression with atypical features (defined as overeating and oversleeping), when compared with major depression without atypical features, was associated with a younger age of onset, more

TABLE 4. Point Prevalence Rates Per 100 for Depression by Sex-Based on Community Surveys Using PSE, CATEGO (D,R,N) , and ICD-9 (296.2/300.4)

Place	Male	Female	Total
Nijmegen,the Netherlands	4.3	7.7	5.4
Camberwell (UK)	4.9	9.2	7.1
Athens, Greece	4.3	10.2	7.4
Greek Cypriots in Camberwell	4.2	7.1	5.6
Canberra, Australia	4.3	7.7	6.1
Santander, Spain	4.3	5.5	4.6
Two districts, Finland	3.6	5.5	4.6
Edinburgh, Scotland	—	4.3	—

SOURCE: Paykel (1992).

psychomotor slowing, and more comorbid panic disorder, drug abuse or dependence, and somatization disorder. These differences could not be explained by differences in demographic characteristics or symptom severity. Prior treatment studies by Quitkin and colleagues found that atypical depression preferentially responds to monoamine oxidase inhibitors. Together, the evidence from epidemiologic and treatment studies suggests that major depression with atypical features constitutes a distinct and valid subtype of major depression.

Risk Factors

Sex Ratios. Clinical and epidemiologic studies in the Western world have consistently documented an increased risk for major depression in women. Studies reporting differential rates of major depression by sex and proposed explanations for this difference have been reviewed by Weissman and Klerman (1977, 1985), who concluded that the difference is not simply due to a tendency for women to report distress or to seek help more readily than men. This conclusion is supported by the observation that rates of bipolar disorder are similar in men and women and by the fact that rates of major depression are elevated for women even in community studies that report on both treated and untreated cases.

Consistently higher rates of major depression in women were reported in community studies using DSM-III (Table 5) and in all the ICD-9 surveys (Table 4). The ratios of rates of major depression in females to males were about 2:1, with a range from 1.4:1 in urban Taiwan to 2.7:1 in the ECA.

Simply relying on prevalence rates would leave open the possibility that this sex ratio could be explained, in part, by women having more persistent or recurrent courses of major depression, accounting for more active cases at any one point in time or better recall for lifetime rates. However, the increased risk of major depression was also seen in the incidence data from four sites of the ECA in which the annual incidence rate was almost

TABLE 5. Rates of Major Depression by Sex in Community Surveys Using DIS and DSM-III Diagnoses

Place	Female	Male	Sex Ratios Female/Male
Lifetime rates/100			
U.S. ECA	7.0	2.6	2.7
Edmonton, Canada	11.4	5.9	1.9
New Zealand	16.3	8.8	1.9
Taiwan			
Urban	1.0	0.7	1.4
Small towns	2.5	1.0	2.6
Rural villages	1.4	0.6	2.3
Seoul, Korea	4.1	2.4	1.6
Puerto Rico	5.5	3.5	1.6
Annual incidence rate/100			
U.S. ECA	1.98	1.10	1.8

[a]Four sites—New Haven excluded.

SOURCE: Paykel (1992).

twice as great in women as in men. This suggests that the higher prevalence rates in women reflect a truly increased risk of first onset of major depression.

The reports of a higher risk of major depression in women are remarkably consistent across cultures and persistent over time. The elevated rates for women appear in studies with a variety of sampling and measurement methods. Several recent studies have suggested a decreasing sex difference in rates among those persons born after World War II (see section on secular changes for further discussion of this). Although the increased risk of major depression in women is a firmly established and widely accepted finding, the reason for this increased risk remains unclear.

Secular Changes.   Recently, evidence from both epidemiologic and family studies has suggested that important temporal changes are occurring in the rates of major depression. Whereas previously depression was viewed as an illness of middle-aged and elderly persons, it is increasingly evident that this is no longer accurate. In a review of studies relevant to temporal trends in depression, Klerman and Weissman (1989) found evidence for an increase in the rates of major depression in cohorts born after the Second World War, a decrease in the age of onset, and an increase in rates of depression for all ages during the period between 1960 and 1975. Although a persistent gender effect was observed, with a two to three times greater risk for women than men across all ages, there was evidence for a narrowing of this differential risk to men and women due to a greater increase in the risk of depression among young men than young women.

Secular or temporal effects on rates of major depression are variations in rates over time and can be separated into age, period, or cohort effects. *Age effects* refer to age-specific stages in life during which persons are at higher risk of illness onset. The risk of schizophrenia onset, for example, rises sharply during late adolescence and young adulthood. *Period effects* refer to variations in rates of illness associated with a specific time period. The epidemic of AIDS during the 1980s is an example. *Cohort effects* usually refer to changes in rates of illness among groups of people born in the same year or decade. These temporal changes may occur separately or may interact with one another.

Evidence has been found of both period and birth-cohort effects for major depression. Hagnell (1986), in a 25 year follow-up of 2,500 inhabitants of Lundby, Sweden, found an increased risk for depression among both sexes in cohorts born after 1937. Lavori et al. (1987) described both a post-1930 birth cohort effect among siblings of depressed patients and a strong 1965–1975 period effect for all birth cohorts. In an analysis of the ECA data, Wickramaratne et al. (1989) found a similar combination of a 1935–1945 birth cohort effect and a 1960–1980 period effect.

More recently, the Cross-National Collaborative Group (1992) reported similar changes in the rate of major depression based on evidence from approximately 39,000 subjects in nine community surveys and 4,000 relatives from three family studies conducted in the 1980s in North America, Puerto Rico, Western Europe, the Middle East, Asia, and the Pacific Rim. Analyses of data from these studies showed an increase in the cumulative lifetime rates of major depression with each successive younger birth cohort at all sites with the exception of the Hispanic samples. Although the overall trend was toward increasing rates of depression over time over all countries, there were significant variations in the magnitude of the increase and in short-term fluctuations by country.

Klerman and Weissman (1989) have reviewed various explanations for these period and cohort effects, including potential artifactual causes, such as memory loss with increasing age, selective mortality or institutionalization, selective migration, and reporting bias of subjects. Although several studies have failed to support a diminishing recall hypothesis (Farrer et al., 1989; Lavori et al., 1987), the explanation for these secular trends remains controversial. Various environmental causes, including biologic, cultural, and economic factors, have been proposed as mediators of these temporal rate changes. The Cross-National Collaborative Group concluded that the variations in short-term trends for major depression by country was evidence that these rates were sensitive to changing historical, social, economic, or biologic environmental conditions.

Race Ethnicity. In comparing rates of major depression by race and ethnic group, both the similarities and differences are of interest. In the five ECA study sites, prevalence rates of major depression showed no consistent differences between African-American and white subjects (Somervell et al., 1989). Rates of major depression in Puerto Rico did not differ significantly from the rates in the ECA study, except that no significant birth-cohort differences were found in Puerto Rico (Canino et al., 1987; Cross-National Collaborative Group, 1992).

The results for Hispanics at the Los Angeles site of the ECA were somewhat inconsistent. Lifetime prevalence of major depression was lower among Hispanics in Los Angeles (Burnam et al., 1987), while the incidence rate was higher (Horwath et al., 1992a). A birth-cohort effect was not found for the Hispanic sample in Los Angeles (Cross-National Collaborative Group, 1992). The reasons for these differences are not clear.

The study from Taiwan (Hwu et al., 1989) showed much lower rates of major depression than did the Western studies. This finding is interesting in light of the work of Kleinman (1977), who suggests that depression may take on a different, more somatic and less psychologic, form in Chinese culture. Based on collaborative research with the Hunan Medical College in the People's Republic of China, Kleinman (1982) found that Chinese psychiatrists diagnosed one-third of their patients as having "neurasthenia," which is thought of as a functional disorder of the neurologic system characterized by weariness, irascibleness, difficulty in concentrating, and unstable and depressed mood. When 100 Chinese neurasthenic patients were interviewed using the Schedule for Affective Disorders and Schizophrenia (SADS), 87% were found to meet DSM-III criteria for major depressive disorder.

This cross-cultural research suggests that culturally mediated values and views of symptoms may influence the expression of psychiatric disorder. Although the use of standard interview techniques and methodologies across cultures may mitigate these effects to some extent, the sharply lower rates of depression in Taiwan as compared with the West suggest that cultural factors may play an important role in the expression of depression.

That culturally mediated factors may exert differential effects across diagnoses is suggested by the fact that psychophysiologic disorders were most common in Taiwan, while rates of depression were much lower than in the West. Similarly, comparisons between Greeks living in Athens and British Greek Cypriot immigrants living in Camberwell showed higher rates of anxiety disorders among both Greek groups than native Camberwell subjects, while rates of depression were comparable (Mavreas and Bebbington, 1988).

Socioeconomic Status. No association was found between socioeconomic status and major depression in the ECA study, although rates of major depression were higher among the unemployed. Men and women who had been unemployed at least 6 months in the last 5 years had a threefold higher risk for an episode of major depression in the past year. The causal direction of this association is unclear. Certainly, job loss and inability to find a job contribute to psychologic, social, and economic stress, which may predispose to depression. On the other hand, depressed individuals may be impaired in their ability to find or hold a job.

The New Haven survey by Weissman and Myers (1978) found current rates of major depression to be higher among lower social classes and lifetime rates higher among the upper classes. It was hypothesized that these differences reflected a longer persistence of symptoms in the lower social class as compared with the upper social class.

Urban–Rural Residence. The secular trend of increasing rates of major depression in successive birth cohorts raises questions about potential environmental causes of this effect. One hypothesis is that living in urban and suburban areas, where populations have been growing steadily since World War II, may be associated with factors that predispose to major depression. Community studies in the United States, Puerto Rico, Taiwan, and South Korea permitted urban–rural comparisons that could test such a hypothesis. In fact some differences were found.

The ECA study found significant differences between urban and rural rates of major depression at the Durham, NC, and at the St. Louis, MO, sites. In Durham, the 1 year prevalence of major depression was more than twice as high in the urban than the rural sample, while in St. Louis major depression was more prevalent in the rural sample. These sites were different, however, in that the Durham rural area sampled was remoted and isolated from the urban center, while in St. Louis the large urban center was more transitionally connected by suburban sprawl to the rural area.

In Taiwan, the small town samples showed trends toward higher major depression rates than the "rural village" or "metropolitan Taipei" samples (Hwu et al., 1989). The Puerto Rico study found trends toward higher prevalence rates among urban than rural residents. The study from South Korea (Lee et al., 1987) found no difference in rates of major depression between urban and rural Seoul. The cause of these differences is unclear, but one may hypothesize that factors in urban or transitional places of residence may predispose to depression. Hwu and colleagues suggested that conflicts in values between industrialized metropolitan areas and traditional rural areas might account for the rural–urban contrasts in their study.

Marital Status. Marital history exerted significant effects on rates of major depression in the ECA study. Married and never-divorced persons had the lowest 1 year prevalence, while divorced persons had the highest rates, controlling for sex, age, and race/ethnicity. Persons who were currently separated or divorced had a risk for major depression two to three times higher than those in any other marital status. The results of the ECA and Edmonton, Canada, studies were similar in the higher prevalence rates for separated/divorced persons and low, comparable rates of depression among never-married or continuously married persons.

Causal inferences regarding the nature and direction of the association between rates of major depression and separation/divorce are problematic. Episodes of major depression are often followed by marital maladjustment, which can persist for years after the acute depressive episode (Bothwell and Weissman, 1977; Rounsaville et al., 1980). The stresses of separation and divorce, however, could also predispose to the onset of depression.

Other Psychiatric Disorder. As a study with a large community sample and a longitudinal design, the ECA provided diagnostic and other data on predictors of first-onset major depression. Using a logistic regression model controlling for the effects of age, race, marital status, sex, and ECA site, Horwath and colleagues (1992a) found that DSM-III dysthymic disorder was associated with a five-fold increase and schizophrenia was associated with an almost threefold increase in the risk for first-onset major depression. Moreover, persons with a history of two symptoms of major depression of 2 weeks duration at any time in their lives had a greater than fourfold increased risk for a first episode of major depression.

Although the occurrence of dysthymic disorder and schizophrenia prior to onset of major depression had been observed previously in clinical settings, clinical studies of comorbidity are often skewed by the tendency of persons with more than one illness to preferentially seek treatment, a phenomenon referred to as Berkson's bias (1946). The ECA findings, based on community respondents and prospectively observed first episodes of major depression, suggest that dysthymic disorder and schizophrenia may be true risk factors for the development of first-onset major depression.

Family History. Investigators have noted for some time the tendency of major depression to cluster in families. Family studies have shown a two- to threefold increased risk of major depression among first-degree relatives of probands with major depression as compared with relatives of normal controls (Winokur and Morrison, 1973; Weissman et al., 1982, 1993; Maier et al., 1991). A genetic contribution to this increased risk of major depression among relatives is suggested by twin studies, which have shown higher concordance rates of major depression among monozygotic than dizygotic twin pairs (27% vs. 12%) (Torgersen 1986).

Attributable Risk. While estimates of relative risk have often been used in epidemiologic studies, the attributable risk, a useful measure to document the burden of risk to a community, has been used infrequently in published psychiatric studies. Attributable risk depends both on the magnitude of relative risk and on the prevalence of the risk factor in the population. Using longitudinal data from the ECA study, Horwath and colleagues (1992a) found that more than 50% of cases of first-onset major depression were associated with the earlier presence of two concurrent depressive symptoms for 2 weeks. This population attributable risk of greater than 50% was due to the substantial relative risk (5.5) associated with prior depressive symptoms and because of their high prevalence in the community.

The high attributable risk of depressive symptoms for first-onset major depression has implications for the development of preventive interventions for major depression. Heuristically, attributable risk may be thought of as the proportion of disease occurrence that would be prevented if exposure to a given risk factor were prevented. For example, the proportion of cases of lung cancer attributable to smoking is approximately 90% (Chyou et al., 1992). This implies that 90% of cases of lung cancer could be prevented if smoking were totally eliminated.

In a public health effort outside of psychiatry, the finding that *carcinoma in situ* of the cervix was predictive of more advanced and invasive stages of cervical carcinoma led to mass screening of cervical cytology in young women and the virtual elimination of invasive cervical carcinoma in regularly screened women. With additional study and public education, early identification of depressive symptoms may be a first step toward the prediction and prevention of major depression.

Any preventive intervention program that seeks to identify cases with depressive symptoms prior to the onset of the full syndrome would need to take into account the fact that most early cases will be false positives, i.e., will not develop major depression. Similarly, most smokers do not develop lung cancer, and most women with abnormal cervical cytology do not develop invasive cervical carcinoma, yet public health interventions, such as education about the risks of smoking and cervical cytologic screening, have been enormously successful in reducing morbidity and mortality from lung and cervical carcinoma. Hopefully, similar preventive efforts could be developed for major depression.

Summary

Rates of major depression are considerably higher than for bipolar disorder and somewhat more variable by site. The lifetime prevalence of DSM-III major depression varied from 2.9/100 to 12.6/100. As with bipolar disorder, prevalence rates of major depression in Taiwan were considerably lower. The more variable rates of major depression, as compared with the narrower range of rates for bipolar disorder, may be due to greater clinical heterogeneity of major depression.

The ECA study has provided evidence supportive of the validity of major depression with psychotic features and major depression with atypical features (overeating and oversleeping) as subtypes. This epidemiologic evidence is consistent with clinical findings.

The community studies provided data on a number of risk factors for major depression. Female gender was a clear and consistent risk factor across all community studies, using either DSM-III or ICD-9 diagnosis, and for the first time incidence data showed that the increased risk for women applied to first-onset cases. There is convincing evidence from the cross-national data of an increase in the cumulative lifetime rates of major depression with each successive younger birth cohort.

The ECA study showed few racial differences in rates of major depression when education and social class were controlled. The Taiwan study found substantially lower rates of major depression than other community studies.

The ECA study found that marital status was strongly associated with rates of major depression, with continuously married persons showing the lowest prevalence and divorced person showing the highest rates.

The ECA longitudinal data showed that a prior history of other psychiatric disorder or depressive symptoms was strongly predictive of the first-onset of major depression. Dysthymic disorder increased the relative risk of first-onset major depression fivefold; a 2 week period of two concurrent depressive symptoms increased the risk more than fourfold; and schizophrenia increased the risk almost threefold.

The ECA study found that depressive symptoms have significant public health implications for the onset of major depression. More than 50% of cases of first-onset major depression were attributable to a prior episode of 2 weeks of two concurrent depressive symptoms. These findings may have implications for the prediction and prevention of major depression.

Family studies have shown a clear and consistent increased risk for major depression among first-degree relatives of probands with major depression. This increased familial risk appears to be limited to cases of early-onset major depression.

DYSTHYMIC DISORDER

Definition

The essential feature of dysthymic disorder is a chronically depressed mood associated with appetite disturbance, insomnia or hypersomnia, low energy or fatigue, low self-esteem, impaired concentration or indecisiveness, or feelings of hopelessness, but not sufficient to meet criteria for major depression.

Rates

Lifetime rates of DSM-III dysthymic disorder are shown in Table 6. The five site rate of dysthymic disorder in the ECA study was 3.0/100, and almost half (42%) of the cases had a lifetime history of major depression as well. The lifetime prevalence of dysthymic disorder per 100 varied from 2.1 in Baltimore to 4.2 in Los Angeles.

Similar to the ECA findings, Bland et al. (1988) reported a prevalence of 3.7 per 100 in Edmonton, Canada. Apart from Taiwan, other studies found fairly comparable rates per 100, ranging from 2.2 in Korea and 2.3 in Italy (reported as 1 year prevalence by Faravelli and Incerpi, 1985) to a high of 4.7 in Puerto Rico, where a particularly high prevalence (7.6%) was noted among women. As with other disorders. Taiwan had the lowest rates of dysthymic disorder, ranging from 0.9 to 1.5 per 100 in the different sites.

Risk Factors

The study of risk factors for dysthymic disorder is somewhat complicated by the unresolved question of whether it is a mood disorder distinct from major depression. Clinical

TABLE 6. Rates of Dysthymic Disorder by Sex in Community Surveys Using DIS and DSM-III Diagnoses

Place	Lifetime Rates/100			Sex Ratios Female/Male
	Female	Male	Total	
U.S. ECA	4.1	2.2	3.0	1.9
New Haven	—	—	3.2	—
Baltimore	—	—	2.1	—
St. Louis	—	—	3.8	—
Durham, NC	—	—	2.3	—
Los Angeles	—	—	4.2	—
Edmonton	5.2	2.2	3.7	2.4
Puerto Rico	7.6	1.6	4.7	4.8
Florence	—	—	2.3	—
Taiwan				
Urban	1.1	0.7	0.9	1.6
Small towns	1.6	1.4	1.5	1.1
Rural villages	1.4	0.6	0.9	2.6
Seoul	2.8	1.6	2.2	1.7

SOURCE: Paykel (1992).

observation of depressed patients over time suggests that dysthymic disorder may be pro-dromal to or a residual state of major depression. Epidemiologic evidence indicates that individuals with dysthymic disorder, when compared with controls, are at a greater than fourfold increased risk for major depression (Horwath et al., 1992a). However, even those persons with the uncomplicated form of dysthymic disorder, when compared to individu-als with no psychiatric disorder, have significantly elevated rates of medical and psychi-atric treatment utilization, and suicide thoughts and attempts (Weissman et al., 1988a). Therefore, although the boundary between dysthymic disorder and major depression re-mains unclear, the evidence that uncomplicated dysthymic disorder predicts psychosocial morbidity and first-onset major depression suggests its continued utility as a separate di-agnostic category.

Sex. All of the community studies reporting separate male and female rates of dys-thymic disorder found an excess of cases among women. With the exception of small towns in Taiwan, where rates were similar, the ratios of female:male rates of dysthymic disorder ranged from 1.6:1 in urban Taiwan, 1.7:1 in Korea, and 1.9:1 in the ECA study to a high of 4.8:1 in Puerto Rico. As with major depression, and unlike bipolar disorder, dysthymic disorder is associated with an excess risk among women.

Age. Unlike the situation for major depression, in which the highest prevalence was found in younger groups, the lifetime rates of dysthymic disorder in the ECA tended to increase in the 30–65 age group and then drop dramatically in those over 65 years of age. South Korea and Edmonton, Canada, also found an increasing prevalence with age. As in the ECA, the Edmonton study showed a steep drop in prevalence over age 65 years, but Korea did not sample those over 65. It is not clear why the age effects are different for major depression and dysthymic disorder. The variations by age may reflect true differ-ences between these disorders, but an understanding of these differences is complicated by the high comorbidity between major depression and dysthymic disorder and by the fact that these are comparisons between the chronic disorder of dysthymia and major de-pression, which may range in duration from a brief to a chronic condition.

Race. The ECA study showed no significant differences in rates of dysthymic disorder when comparing African-Americans and whites. However, rates of dysthymic disorder were higher among Hispanics than those of African-Americans or whites, which is con-sistent with the higher rate in Puerto Rico. As with major depression, rates of dysthymic disorder were markedly lower in Taiwan than in the West, while the prevalence in Korea was comparable with that in the West.

Marital Status. Dysthymic disorder was more prevalent among unmarried than married persons under the age of 65 years in the ECA study. In Edmonton, divorced or widowed persons had higher rates than married persons, who had higher rates than the never mar-ried. As is the case with major depression, the direction of causality in these associations between age and prevalence of dysthymic disorder is not clear.

Urban–Rural. Puerto Rico showed a significantly higher rate of dysthymic disorder among urban than rural dwellers (5.5 per 100 vs. 3.3 per 100). In Taiwan, urban and rural rates were similar, but the small town rates were somewhat higher, as was the case for major depression.

Summary

Dysthymic disorder, a milder but more chronic form of depression than major depression, appears to share some of the characteristics of major depression. In terms of risk factors, dysthymic disorder, like major depression, had higher rates among women than men and higher rates among divorced than married persons. Although almost half of the persons with dysthymic disorder also had episodes of major depression, those persons with uncomplicated dysthymic disorder, when compared with individuals with no psychiatric disorder, had substantial evidence of morbidity, such as treatment seeking and suicide attempts. Whether dysthymic disorder is distinct from major depression remains unclear.

ANXIETY DISORDERS

Anxiety has been recognized as a symptom ever since the writings of Freud. However, it was only recently, with the incorporation into DSM-III and DSM-III-R of Klein's conceptualization of panic as a separate entity, that anxiety states began to be subdivided into distinct disorders such as panic, phobias, and generalized anxiety disorders.

In a review of five population studies conducted in the United States, the United Kingdom, and Sweden prior to the development of specified diagnostic criteria, Marks and Lader (1973) found that anxiety states were fairly common (about 2.0/100–4.7/100 current prevalence) and more prevalent in women, particularly younger women between 16 and 40 years of age. In a separate epidemiologic review, Weissman (1985) identified nine additional community studies of anxiety states that showed rates in the range reported by Marks and Lader (1973) and also showed that rates were higher in women than in men.

Our focus in this section is on the more recent epidemiologic studies in which anxiety disorders are subdivided on the basis of DSM-III criteria.

PANIC DISORDER

Definition

The key feature of panic disorder is the occurrence of three or more panic attacks within a 3 week period. These attacks cannot be precipitated only by exposure to a feared situation and must be accompanied by at least 4 of the following symptoms: dyspnea, palpitations, chest pain, smothering or choking, dizziness, feelings of unreality, paresthesias, hot and cold flashes, sweating, faintness, trembling, or shaking (APA, 1980).

Rates

Table 7 shows prevalence rates of panic disorder from community studies using DSM-III criteria. The 6 month prevalence of panic disorder ranged from 0.6/100 in New Haven, CT, to 1.1/100 in Puerto Rico, representing a remarkable level of consistency across sites. The highest reported prevalence was the 1 year rate of 3.1/000 from the Zurich survey, but this may reflect methodologic differences in that this study used a different instrument (SPIKE interview) and constructed a definition of panic that only approximated that of DSM-III. When diagnostic hierarchies are applied (i.e., precedence is given to a diagnosis

TABLE 7. Prevalence Rates Per 100 of Panic Disorder Using RDC/DSM-III Criteria

Place	Rate/100[a]		
	6 Month	1 Year	Lifetime
ECA			
New Haven, CT	0.6		
Baltimore, MD	1.0		
St Louis, MO	0.9		
Piedmont, NC	0.7		
Los Angeles, CA	0.9		
Zurich survey		3.1	
National survey[b]		1.2	
Edmonton, Canada	0.7		1.2
Puerto Rico	1.1		1.7
ECA, five site			1.6
New Zealand			2.2
Florence, Italy			1.4
Korea			1.7
Taiwan			
Urban			0.20
Small towns			0.34
Rural			0.13

[a]Rates rounded off to one decimal place in most cases.
[b]Panic with agoraphobia.
SOURCE: Roth et al. (1988).

of depression in comorbid cases) in the Zurich study, the 1-year prevalence rate of panic disorder was much lower, 0.2/100.

Lifetimes rates of panic disorder showed good agreement, with prevalence varying from 1.2/100 in Edmonton, Canada, to 2.2/100 in New Zealand. The exception to this narrow range of lifetime rates was Taiwan, where panic disorder occurred at rates from 0.13/100 in rural areas to 0.34/100 in small towns.

Risk Factors

Sex. Comparing lifetime prevalence rates, all of the studies reporting on panic disorder showed higher rates for women than for men. With the exceptions of Puerto Rico and Taiwan, the higher lifetime risk for women was statistically significant in all of the community studies. Of interest Eaton et al. (1989) analyzed incidence rates from the ECA study and found a twofold increased odds of incident panic disorder in women compared with men.

Age. In the ECA and Edmonton studies, older persons (65 and over) had the lowest lifetime prevalence rates of panic disorder. This pattern was quite different for Hispanics in the ECA and in the Puerto Rican study. In Puerto Rico and in Hispanic women in the ECA, the lifetime prevalence tended to increase with age. For Hispanic men in the ECA, the lifetime rate drops with each age group, reaching 0 in the group over 65 years of age. The reason for these differences is not clear. The drop in lifetime prevalence with increasing age may be due to a recall or reporting artifact, decreased survival to old age (e.g., increased cardiovascular mortality), or a cohort effect.

Race/ethnicity. In the ECA study, there were no significant differences in prevalence rates between African-American, Hispanic, and white groups (Horwath et al., 1993; Eaton et al., 1991). Comparisons of other studies are more remarkable for the cross-cultural similarities in rates of panic disorder, with the exception of the Taiwan study, which had the lowest rates of panic. As with major depression, Korean prevalence rates of panic disorder were comparable with those in the West, while Taiwan's were much lower. These differences may be due to the more industrialized nature of Korea or to methodologic artifacts.

Summary

The prevalence of panic disorder was fairly uniform, with higher risks for women and persons under the age of 65 years. As with most other disorders, Taiwan found much lower rates of panic disorder.

AGORAPHOBIA

Definition

DSM-III agoraphobia is defined as a fear and avoidance of being in places or situations from which escape might be difficult or in which help might not be available in the event of sudden incapacitation (APA, 1980). As a result of such fears, the agoraphobic person avoids travel outside the home or requires the accompaniment of a companion when away from home. Moderate cases may cause some construction in lifestyle, while severe cases of agoraphobia may result in the person being completely housebound or unable to leave home unaccompanied.

Rates

Table 8 shows prevalence rates of agoraphobia from community studies using DSM-III criteria. In the ECA study, 6 month prevalence rates ranged from 2.7/100 in St. Louis to 5.7/100 in Baltimore. Comparable 6 month and 1 year prevalence rates were found in Zurich and Puerto Rico. Lifetimes rates of agoraphobia showed considerable variation, from a low of 1.1/100 in urban Taiwan to a high of 6.9/100 in Puerto Rico. Some of this variation may have been due to the use of a translated Diagnostic Interview Schedule (DIS) (Robins et al., 1981). If one considers only the studies carried out in primarily English-speaking countries, the lifetime prevalence rates vary over a narrower range, from 2.9/100 in Edmonton, Canada, to 5.6/100 in the ECA data from four sites.

Risk Factors

Lifetime rates of agoraphobia were significantly higher for women than for men in each of the community studies. This is consistent with the gender differences found for panic disorder and major depression.

In the ECA study, lifetime prevalence of agoraphobia was higher among African-Americans than among whites or Hispanics. The effects of race/ethnicity and gender

TABLE 8. Prevalence Rates Per 100 of Agoraphobia Using DSM-III Criteria

Place	Rate/100[a]		
	6 Month	1 Year	Lifetime
ECA			
New Haven, CT	2.8		
Baltimore, MD	5.8		
St Louis, MO	2.7		
Piedmont, NC	5.4		
Los Angeles, CA	3.2		
Puerto Rico	3.9		6.9
Zurich survey	2.5		
ECA, four site			5.6
New Zealand			3.8
Florence, Italy			1.3
Edmonton, Canada			2.9
Korea			2.7
Taiwan			
Urban			1.1
Small towns			1.5
Rural			1.3

[a]Panic with agoraphobia.
SOURCE: Roth et al. (1988).

combined to produce a considerable range in lifetime prevalence, from 2.9/100 in white males to 12/100 in African-American women (Eaton et al., 1991).

Two studies reported significant urban rural differences in rates of agoraphobia, but they were in opposite directions. Puerto Rico found a significantly higher lifetime prevalence for the urban area, while Korea reported a higher rural rate. The reason for this is not clear.

Relationship Between Agoraphobia and Panic

In DSM-III, agoraphobia was considered a separate phobic disorder that may or may not be accompanied by panic attacks. Largely due to the influence of Klein's argument that agoraphobia is a conditioned avoidance response to the aversive stimulus of spontaneous panic attacks, the diagnostic view of agoraphobia changed considerably in DSM-III-R, in which panic disorder is viewed as primary, with or without the secondary development of agoraphobia. An important factor in this change was the observation by Klein and others that, in clinic settings, agoraphobia rarely occurs without preceding spontaneous panic attacks or limited symptom attacks.

Considerable controversy continues regarding the nature of the relationship between agoraphobic avoidance and panic attacks. Marks (1987) and other European investigators have questioned the temporal precedence and casual role of panic attacks in the development of agoraphobia.

Contributing to the controversy are the large differences between clinic and community studies in their estimates of the relative prevalence of agoraphobia with or without panic attacks. Table 9 shows the results of published community and clinical studies that have reported data permitting calculation of the proportion of agoraphobics with a history of panic attacks.

TABLE 9. Reported Frequency of Agoraphobia Without Panic Attacks

References	Date	No. Agoraphobics w/o Panic Attacks	Total No. Agoraphobics	Percent
Community studies				
Thompson	(1989)[a]	88	104	85
Angst and Dobbler-Mikola	(1985)	15	22	68
ECA		656	961	68
Wittchen	(1986)	13	26	50
Joyce et al.	(1989)	35[b]	76	46
Faravelli et al.	(1989)	4	14	29
Clinic studies				
Torgersen	(1983)[c]	8	26	31
Thyer and Himle	(1985)	20[d]	115	17
Argyle and Roth	(1986)	5	42	12
Garvey and Tuason	(1984)	1	13	8
Aronson and Logue	(1987)	2	36	6
Pollard et al.	(1989)	61[e]	993	6
Uhde et al.	(1985)	1	32	3
Barlow	(1988)	1[f]	42	2
DiNardo	(1983)	0	23	0
Breier	(1986)	0	54	0
Noves	(1986)	0	67	0
Kleiner	(1987)	0	50	0
Thyer et al.	(1985)	0	28	0

[a]Thompson study reported on agoraphobia without panic disorder.
[b]Joyce et al. study: 10 of 35 subjects reported limited symptom attacks.
[c]Torgersen study reported on agoraphobia without panic diosrder.
[d]Thyer and Himle study: These subjects "often suffered from unpredictable somatic symptoms . . . functional equivalent to panic attacks."
[e]Pollard et al study: Some subjects had limited symptom attacks.
[f]Barlow study: Subject had limited symptom attacks.

The population-based surveys found that a substantial proportion of subjects with agoraphobia reported no history of panic attacks. In these studies, 80% of the subjects were interviewed by lay persons using the DIS. In contrast, clinic-based studies, using less structured interviews administered by clinicians, almost invariably found much lower rates of agoraphobia without panic.

Several explanations for this discrepancy have been suggested. One explanation is that treated samples of persons with any illness have high rates of comorbidity (Berkson, 1946). An alternative explanation is that population studies may have overestimated the rate of agoraphobia without panic disorder.

In a reanalysis of the ECA data on agoraphobia without panic (Horwath et al., 1993), 22 community cases of agoraphobia without panic were clinically reappraised and only a single case of probable agoraphobia without panic was found. The diagnostic reappraisal found that 19 (87%) of the cases had simple or social phobias rather than agoraphobia or had no DSM-III phobia at all. The reappraisal also identified six cases of panic disorder, panic attacks, or limited symptom attacks that had been missed by the DIS interview. The authors concluded that community studies using the DIS may have overestimated the prevalence of agoraphobia without panic attacks in the community.

Summary

Prevalence rates of agoraphobia based on the DIS and DSM-III varied considerably. These rates and their variations by study are difficult to interpret for two reasons. First, the diagnostic view of agoraphobia has changed considerably since these studies were done. Second, a clinical reappraisal study of ECA cases of agoraphobia without panic attacks suggested that studies using the DIS may have overestimated rates of agoraphobia without panic. This overestimate may have been due to missed cases of panic disorder, panic attacks, and limited symptom attacks and to difficulty differentiating the boundary between agoraphobia and simple phobias.

In spite of the problems suggested above, the community studies consistently found higher rates of agoraphobia among women than men, and the ECA study found higher rates among African-Americans than among whites or Hispanics.

SOCIAL PHOBIA

Definition

The central feature of social phobia is the persistent, irrational fear of situations in which a person may act in a humiliating or embarrassing way while under the scrutiny of others (APA, 1980). Common social phobic situations involve speaking or eating in public, urinating in public lavatories, or writing in front of others.

Rates

Table 10 shows the lifetime prevalence of social phobia from studies using DSM-III criteria. Lifetime rates of social phobia varied considerably, with a low of 0.4/100 in rural Taiwan and a high of 3.9/100 in New Zealand. It is not clear whether these contrasting rates

TABLE 10. Lifetime Prevalence Rates/100 of Social Phobia Using DSM-III Criteria

Community Survey	Rates/100
ECA	2.4
Baltimore, MD	3.1
St Louis, MO	1.9
Durham, NC	3.2
Los Angeles, CA	1.8
Edmonton, Canada	1.7
Puerto Rico	1.6
New Zealand	3.9
Florence, Italy	1.0
Korea	0.6
Taiwan	
Urban	0.6
Small towns	0.5
Rural	0.4

SOURCE: Roth et al. (1988).

reflect true cross-cultural differences or are due to differences in methodology or translation of the DIS. The lifetime prevalence rates of social phobia vary over a somewhat narrower range—from 1.7/100 in Edmonton, Canada, to 3.9/100 in New Zealand—when comparing rates from English speaking countries.

Risk Factors

In an analysis of the ECA data from four sites (the New Haven site used a version of the DIS that did not include social phobia items), Schneier et al. (1992) found that lifetime prevalence rates of social phobia were highest among women and persons who were younger (aged 18–29 years), less educated, single, and of lower socioeconomic class. A significantly higher prevalence of lifetime social phobia was also found among women in Korea and urban Taiwan, while no significant gender differences were found in Edmonton, Puerto Rico, or small town or rural areas of Taiwan.

GENERALIZED ANXIETY DISORDER

Definition

The DSM-III criteria for generalized anxiety disorder (GAD) require the presence of unrealistic or excessive anxiety and worry, accompanied by symptoms from three of four categories: 1) motor tension, 2) autonomic hyperactivity, 3) vigilance and scanning, and 4) apprehensive expectation. The anxious mood must continue for at least 1 month, and the diagnosis is not made if phobias, panic disorder, or obsessive-compulsive disorder are present or if the disturbance is due to another physical or mental disorder, such as hyperthyroidism, major depression, or schizophrenia (APA, 1980). By this definition, GAD is treated primarily as a residual category after the exclusion of the other major anxiety disorders. DSM-III-R narrowed the definition further by requiring a minimum duration of 6 months.

Rates

Table 11 shows the prevalence of GAD from community studies using DSM-III criteria. One year prevalence rates of GAD varied from a high of 6.4/100 in the National survey to a low of 2.7/100 in the ECA study (GAD was not included in the first two ECA sites). These variations are probably due to methodologic differences. The National and Zurich surveys used different diagnostic instruments from the ECA, and the Zurich survey used a somewhat different definition of the syndrome. In the ECA study, hierarchical diagnostic exclusion of panic disorder and major depression yielded the 1 year prevalence of 2.7/100, while dropping the exclusions resulted in a rate of 3.8/100 (Blazer et al., 1991).

Lifetime prevalence of GAD in the ECA study was quite consistent across three study sites, varying from 4.1/100 in Los Angeles to 6.6/100 in Durham and St. Louis. Lifetime prevalence varied considerably more in the Taiwan study, from 3.7/100 in Taipei to 10.5/100 in small town areas of Taiwan.

The Florence study provides an interesting example of the effects of requiring the longer 6-month duration of DSM-III-R. For DSM-III, the point and lifetime rates were 2.8/100 and 5.4/100, respectively, while the narrower DSM-III-R definition resulted in the lower respective rates of 2.0/100 and 3.9/100.

TABLE 11. Prevalence Rates Per 100 of Generalized Anxiety Disorder Using DSM-III Criteria

Place	6 Month	1 Year	Lifetime
		Rate/100*	
National survey		6.4	
Zurich survey		5.2	
Florence, Italy			5.4
Florence (DSM-III-R)			3.9
Taiwan			
Urban			3.7
Small towns			10.5
Rural			7.8
Korea			3.6
ECA, three sites			
No exclusions		3.8	
No panic, no MDD[a]		2.7	
ECA, three sites (no panic, no MDD)			
Durham			6.6
St. Louis			6.6
Los Angeles			4.1

[a]MDD, major depressive disorder.
SOURCE: Roth et al. 1988.

Risk Factors

Based on data combined from three ECA study sites, the 1 year prevalence of GAD, with or without diagnostic exclusions, was significantly higher in females, in African-Americans, and in persons under 30 years of age, but the differences were significant for age only without diagnostic exclusions and for race only when panic and depression were excluded (Blazer et al., 1991). The Taiwan study reported significantly higher rates for women than for men, but no gender differences were found in Korea.

OBSESSIVE-COMPULSIVE DISORDER

Definition

DSM-III obsessive-compulsive disorder (OCD) requires the presence of obsessions or compulsions that are sources of significant distress or impairment and are not due to another mental disorder. Obsessions are defined as recurrent, persistent thoughts, images, or impulses that are experienced as senseless and repugnant. Compulsions are excessively repetitive, stereotyped behaviors, such as repeatedly checking locked doors or gas jets or washing hands (APA, 1980.)

Rates

Table 12 shows prevalence rates of OCD from community studies using DSM-III criteria. Six month prevalence of OCD varied from 0.7/100 in Los Angeles to 2.1/100 in Piedmont, NC. Lifetime prevalence of OCD varied from 0.3/100 in rural Taiwan to 3.2/100 in

TABLE 12. Prevalence Rates Per 100 of Obsessive Compulsive Disorder Using DSM-III Criteria

| Place | Rate/100[1] | | |
	6 Month	1 Year	Lifetime
ECA			
New Haven, CT	1.4		
Baltimore, MD	2.0		
St Louis, MO	1.3		
Piedmont, NC	2.1		
Los Angeles, CA	0.7		
Puerto Rico	1.8		
Edmonton, Canada	1.6		
ECA, five sites			2.6
Florence, Italy			0.7
Korea			2.1
Edmonton, Canada			3.2
Puerto Rico			3.2
Taiwan			
Urban			0.94
Small towns			0.54
Rural			0.30

SOURCE: Roth et al. (1988).

Puerto Rico. The studies in English language sites showed excellent agreement, with lifetime prevalence of 2.6/100 in the ECA and 3.0/100 in Edmonton, Canada. Most remarkable about these rates is that they contradict the previous traditional view of OCD as a rare disorder on the basis of published clinical reports.

Risk Factors

As with other anxiety disorders, prevalence rates of OCD were higher among women than men in the ECA study. However, when gender comparisons were controlled for marital status, employment status, job status, ethnicity, and age, there were no remaining differences in prevalence rates for women compared with men (Karno et al., 1987, 1989).

SUMMARY

Affective Disorders

Epidemiologic data support the validity of two subtypes of major depression: 1) major depressive disorder with psychotic features and 2) major depressive disorder with atypical features (overeating and oversleeping). The community studies found that female gender, divorce, and prior histories of dysthymic disorder, schizophrenia, or depressive symptoms were risk factors for major depression. From a public health perspective, depressive symptoms were associated with a more than 50% population attributable risk of major depression.

Cross-national data showed an increase in the cumulative lifetime rates of major depression with each successive younger birth cohort and substantially lower rates in Taiwan than in the West. Family studies showed an increased risk for major depression among relatives, apparently limited to cases of early onset major depression.

Dysthymic disorder, like major depression, had higher rates among women than men and higher rates among divorced than married persons. There is evidence for psychiatric morbidity in uncomplicated dysthymia, but the boundary between dysthymic disorder and major depression remains unclear.

Anxiety Disorders

Lifetime prevalence rates of panic disorder were remarkably consistent across the community studies and across cultural, racial, and ethnic boundaries, with the exception of the much lower rates in Taiwan. Panic disorder was more common among women and much less common among those over 65 years of age, with the exception of the Hispanic sample of the ECA and the Puerto Rico study.

The epidemiologic data on agoraphobia show considerable variation in rates across studies and cross-culturally. A recent clinical reappraisal of the ECA data on agoraphobia without panic suggests that community studies relying on the DIS and DSM-III may have overestimated the prevalence of agoraphobia without panic. Therefore, the prevalence estimates from studies such as these should be regarded with caution until the accuracy of their prevalence figures on agoraphobia can be more thoroughly tested.

Analyses of relative risks showed higher rates of agoraphobia for women than men, just as with panic disorder. Unlike panic disorder, however, agoraphobia was associated with higher rates for African-Americans than whites or Hispanics. The differential effects of race on panic disorder and agoraphobia suggest that the factors that cause panic disorder are not the same as the factors that lead to the subsequent development of agoraphobia.

The ECA study found that lifetime prevalence rates of social phobia were highest among women and persons who were younger, less educated, single, and of lower socioeconomic class. GAD was also more prevalent among women and younger persons.

Based on community data, OCD turned out to be a much more prevalent disorder than suggested by previous clinical studies.

NATIONAL COMORBIDITY SURVEY

The National Comorbidity Survey (NCS) (Kessler et al., 1994) is a community study based on a probability sample of persons aged 15–54 years in the noninstitutionalized civilian population in the 48 contiguous states. The NCS reports on DSM-III-R diagnoses generated by a modified version of the Composite International Diagnostic Interview (CIDI), which was administered by trained lay interviewers. Kessler et al. (1994) reported rates of lifetime DSM-III-R major depressive episode (17.1%), dysthymia (6.4%), panic disorder (3.5%), and GAD (5.1%). With the exception of GAD, these lifetime prevalence rates are considerably higher than the DSM-III rates reported in the other studies reviewed in this chapter. The NCS investigators attribute the higher lifetime prevalence rates to several factors: secular trends toward increasing rates, a national population sample concentrating on a younger age range than previous surveys, the use of correction weights to adjust for nonresponse bias, and the use of memory probes that may have improved recall. Although the lifetime rates of disorder are higher in the NCS than other surveys, the risk factor results are for the most part consistent with previous investigations in finding more affective and anxiety disorders among women and declining rates of most disorders with age and higher socioeconomic status.

FUTURE DEVELOPMENTS

In this chapter we focused primarily on studies that used DSM-III or ICD-9 diagnostic criteria. As we write this chapter, the American Psychiatric Association and the World Health Organization are about to publish new diagnostic systems, DSM-1V and ICD-10, respectively. When these new systems are used in epidemiologic studies, the revised diagnostic criteria and categories will undoubtedly yield different results.

Based on a review of a draft of DSM-IV criteria, the definitions of major depression and dysthymic disorder will remain basically unchanged. A new category, minor depression, was considered for inclusion, but will be retained only in the appendix as a proposed diagnosis in need of further study. In the anxiety disorders section, the principal changes involve the panic disorder section. In DSM-IV, panic attacks are defined separately, with an emphasis on differentiating cued (situationally bound) and uncued (unexpected) panic attacks. Furthermore, the criteria for panic disorder will no longer require four attacks in 4 weeks, as in DSM-III-R, but will be revised to require recurrent unexpected panic attacks, at least one of which is followed by a month of anxiety, worry, or changed behavior related to the panic attack. The separate definition of panic attacks and dropping the frequency criterion (four attacks in 4 weeks) are in keeping with epidemiologic evidence that substantial morbidity, treatment utilization, and impairment are associated with infrequent panic attacks that do not meet DSM-III or DSM-III-R criteria for panic disorder (Horwath et al., 1994b). The differentiation between cued and uncued panic attacks and the requirement for uncued panic attacks in panic disorder are supported by community data that show that the lack of a situational cue for panic is predictive of a worse clinical outcome (Horwath et al., 1994a). These changes are likely to result in a greater emphasis on the epidemiologic study of recurrent unexpected panic attacks that would not have met DSM-III or DSM-III-R criteria for panic disorder. One effect will be the reporting of more cases and the likely finding of more extensive morbidity and impairment associated with panic attacks that was previously appreciated.

DSM-IV will also specify a generalized subtype of social phobia for persons whose social fears include most social situations. This will differentiate these individuals from persons with fears of one or two social situations, such as speaking or eating in public. This differentiation is supported by community data showing that the generalized type of social phobia is associated with significantly higher rates of treatment utilization than the discrete type (Horwath et al., 1994a). The separation of these types may yield differential results in studies that examine comorbidity with other disorders or treatment utilization.

ACKNOWLEDGMENTS

This chapter was adapted from chapters in "Handbook of Affective Disorders," ES Paykel, editor, 2nd ed., Guilford Press, New York, 1992, pp. 111–129; and "Handbook of Anxiety, vol 1; Biological, Clinical and Cultural Perspectives," M Roth, R Noyes Jr, and GD Burrows, editors, Elsevier Science Publishers B.V., Amsterdam, 1988, pp 83–100. The authors acknowledge the support of NIMH grant MH 28274, "Genetic Studies of Depressive Disorders"; NIMH grant MH 36197, "Children at High and Low Risk for Depression"; and an NARSAD Established Investigator Award, "The Continuity Between Childhood and Adult Depression: A Longitudinal Study of Children as Depressed Adults."

REFERENCES

American Psychiatric Association (1980): "Diagnostic and Statistical Manual of Mental Disorders," 3rd ed. Washington, DC American Psychiatric Association.

American Psychiatric Association (1987): "Diagnostic and Statistical Manual of Mental Disorders," 3rd ed., revised. Washington, DC. American Psychiatric Association.

Angst J, Dobler-Mikola (1984): The Zurich study: III. Diagnosis of depression. Eurp Arch Psychiatry Neurol Sci 234:30–37.

Angst J, Dobler-Mikola A (1985): The Zurich study: V. Anxiety and phobia in young adults. Eur Arch Psychiatr Neurol Sci 235: 171–178.

Angst, Dobler-Mikola, Binder J (1984): The Zurich study: A prospective epidemiological study of depressive, neurotic and psychosomatic syndromes: I. Problems and methodology. Eur Arch Psychiatry Neurol Sci 234:13–20.

Anthony JC, Petronis KR (1992): Suspected risk factors for depression among adults 18–44 years old. Epidemiology 2:123–132.

Argyle N, Roth M (1986): The relationship of panic attacks to anxiety states and depression. In Shagass C. (ed): "Abstracts of the World Congress of Biological Psychiatry." New York: Elsevier Science Publishers, pp 460–462.

Aronson TA, Logue CM (1987): On the longitudinal course of panic disorder. Comp Psychiatry 28:344–355.

Barlow DH (1988): "Anxiety and Its Disorders: The Nature and Treatment of Anxiety and Panic." New York: Guilford Press.

Bebbington P, Hurry J, Tennant C, Sturt E, Wing JK (1981): Epidemiology of mental disorders in Camberwell. Psychol Med 11:561–579.

Berkson J (1946): Limitations of the application of four fold table analysis to hospital data. Biomet Bull 2:47–53.

Bland RC, Newman SC, Orn H (eds) (1988): Epidemiology of psychiatric disorders in Edmonton. Acta Psychiatr Scand 77 (Suppl 338).

Blazer D, Hughes D, George LK, et al. (1991): Generalized anxiety disorder. In Robins LN, Regier DA (eds): "Psychiatric Disorders in America. The Epidemiologic Catchment Area Study." New York: The Free Press, pp 180–203.

Bothwell S, Weissman MM (1977): Social impairments 4 years after an acute depressive episode. Am J Orthopsychiatry 47:231–237.

Boyd JH, Weissman MM (1982): Epidemiology. In: Paykel ES (ed): "Handbook of Affective Disorders." New York: Guilford Press, pp 109–125.

Breier A, Charney DS, Heninger GR (1986): Agoraphobia with panic attacks: development, diagnostic stability, and course of illness. Arch Gen Psychiatry 43:1029–1036.

Burnam MA, Hough RL, Escobar JI, Karno M (1987): Six-month prevalence of specific psychiatric disorders among Mexican Americans and non-Hispanic whites in Los Angeles. Arch Gen Psychiatry 44:687–691.

Canino GJ, Bird HR, Shrout PE, Rubio-Stipec M, Bravo M, Martinez R, Sesman M, Guevara LM (1987): The prevalence of specific psychiatric disorders in Puerto Rico. Arch Gen Psychiatry 44:727–735.

Charney EA, Weissman MM (1988): Epidemiology of depressive and manic syndromes. In Georgotas A, Cancro R (eds): "Depression and Mania." New York: Elsevier Press, pp 45–74.

Chyou PH, Nomura AM, Stemmermann GN (1992): A prospective study of the attributable risk of cancer due to cigaratte smoking. Am J Public Health 82:37–40.

Cross-National Collaborative Group (1992): The changing rates of major depression. Cross-national comparisons. JAMA 268:3098–3105.

DiNardo PA, O'Brien GT, Barlow DH, et al. (1983): Reliability of DSM-III anxiety disorder categories using a new structured interview. Arch Gen Psychiatry 40:1070–1074.

Eaton WW, Dryman A, Weissman MN (1991): Panic and phobia. In Robins LN, Regier DA (eds): "Psychiatric Disorders in America. The Epidemiologic Catchment Area Study." New York: The Free Press, pp 155–179.

Eaton WW, Kramer M, Anthony JC, Dryman A, Shapiro S, Locke BZ (1989): The incidence of specific DIS/DSM-III mental disorders: Data from the NIMH epidemiologic Catchment Area Program. Acta Psychiatr Scand 79:163–168.

Faravelli C, Degg l'Innocenti BG, Aiazzi L, Incerpi G, Pallanti S (1990): Epidemiology of mood disorders: A community survey in Florence. J Affect Disord 20:135–141.

Faravelli C, Degl'Innocenti BG, Giardinelli L (1989): Epidemiology of anxiety disorders in Florence. Acta Psychiatr Scand 79:308–312.

Faravelli C, Incerpi G (1985): Epidemiology of affective disorders in Florence. Acta Psychiatr Scand 72:331–333.

Farrer LA, Floria LP, Bruce ML, Leaf PJ, Weissman MM (1989): Reliability and consistency of self-reported age at onset of major depression. J Psychiatr Res 23:35–47.

Garvey M, Tuason V (1984): The relationship of panic disorder to agoraphobia. Comp Psychiatry 25:529–531.

Hagnell O (1986): The 25-year follow-up of the Lundby study: Incidence and risk of alcoholism, depression, and disorders of the senium. In: Barret J, Rose RM (eds): "Mental Disorders in the Community: Findings From Psychiatric Epidemiology." New York: Guilford Press, pp 89–110.

Henderson S, Duncan-Jones P, Byrne DG, Scott R, Adcock S (1979): Psychiatric disorder in Canberra. Acta Psychiatr Scand 60:355–374.

Hodiamont P, Peer N, Syben N (1987): Epidemiological aspects of psychiatric disorder in a Dutch health area. Psychol Med 17:495–505.

Horwath E, Johnson J, Hornig CD, Weissman MM (1994a): Social phobia diagnostic subtypes and the relationship between social phobia, panic disorder and agoraphobia. In Frances A, Widiger T (eds): "DSM-IV Sourcebook," vol IV. Washington, DC: American Psychiatric Press.

Horwath E, Johnson J, Klerman GL, Weissman MM (1992a): Depressive symptoms as relative and attributable risk factors for first-onset major depression. Arch Gen Psychiatry 49:817–823.

Horwath E, Johnson J, Weissman MM, Hornig CD (1992b): The validity of major depression with atypical features based on a community study. J Affect Disord 26:117–126.

Horwath E, Lish J, Johnson J, Hornig CD, Weissman MM (1993): Agoraphobia without panic: Clinical re-appraisal of an epidemiologic finding. Am J Psychiatry 150:1496–1501.

Horwath E, Wolk SI, Leon A, Fyer A, Johnson J, Klerman G, Weissman MM (1994b): Reanalyses of the ECA data in order to assess the diagnostic criteria and symptom threshold for DSM-III panic disorder. In Frances A, Pincus H, Widiger TA (eds): "DSM-IV Sourcebook," vol IV. Washington, DC: American Psychiatric Press.

Hwu H-G, Yeh E-K, Chang L-Y (1989): Prevalence of psychiatric disorders in Taiwan defined by the Chinese Diagnostic Interview Schedule. Acta Psychiatr Scandin 79:136–147.

Johnson J, Horwath E, Weissman MM (1991): The validity of major depression with psychotic features based on a community study. Arch Gen Psychiatry 48:1075–1081.

Joyce PR, Bushnell JA, Oakley-Brown MA, Wells JE, Hornblow AR (1989): The epidemiology of panic symptomatology and agoraphobic avoidance. Comp Psychiatry 30:303–312.

Joyce PR, Oakley-Browne MA, Wells JE, Bushnell JA, Hornblow AR (1990): Birth cohort trends in major depression: Increasing rates and earlier onset in New Zealand. J Affect Disord 18:83–90.

Karno M, Golding JM, Burnam MA, Hough RL, Esobar JI, Wells KM, Boyer R (1989): Anxiety disorders among Mexican Americans and non-Hispanic whites in Los Angeles. J Nerv Ment Dis 177:202–209.

Karno M. Hough RL, Burnam MA, Escobar JI, Timbers DM, Santan F, Boyd JH (1987): Lifetime prevalence of specific psychiatric disorders among Mexican Americans and non-Hispanic whites in Los Angeles. Arch Gen Psychiatry 44:695–701.

Kessler RC, McGonagle KA, Zhao S, et al. (1994): Lifetime and 12-month prevalence of DSM-III-R psychiatric disorders in the United States. Results from the National Comorbidity Study. Arch Gen Psychiatry 51:8–19.

Kleiner L, Marshall WL (1987): The role of interpersonal problems in the development of agoraphobia with panic attacks. J Anxiety Disorders 1:313–323.

Kleinman A (1977): Depression, somatization, and the "new cross-cultural psychiatry." Soc Sci Med 11:3.

Kleinman A (1982): Neurasthenia and depression: A study of somatization and culture. Culture Med Psychiatry 6:117.

Klerman GL, Weissman MM (1989): Increasing rates of depression. JAMA 261:2229–2235.

Lavori PW, Klerman GL, Keller MB, Reich T, Rice J, Endicott J (1987): Age-period-cohort analysis of secular trends in onset of major depression: Findings in siblings of patients with major affective disorder. J Psychiatri Res 23–36.

Lee C-K, Han J-H, Choi J-O (1987): The epidemiological study of mental disorders in Korea (IX): Alcoholism anxiety and depression. Seoul J Psychiatry 12:183–191.

Lee CK, Kwak YS, Yamamonto J, Rhee H, Kim YS, Han JH, Choi JO, Lee YH (1990a): Psychiatric epidemiology in Korea. Part I: Gender and age differences in Seoul. J Nerv Ment Dis 178:242–246.

Lee CK, Kwak YS, Yamonto J, Rhee H, Kim YS, Han JH, Choi JO, Lee YH (1990b): Psychiatric epidemiology in Korea. Part II: Urban and rural differences. J Nerv Ment Dis 178:247–252.

Lehtien V, Lindholm T, Veijola J, Vaisanen E (1990): The prevalence of PSE-CATEGO disorders in a Finnish adult population cohort. Soc Psychiatry Psychiatric Epidemiol 25:187–192.

Marks IM (1987): "Fears, Phobias and Rituals." New York: Oxford University Press.

Marks I, Lader M (1973): Anxiety states (anxiety neurosis): A review. J Nerv Ment Dis 156:3.

Mavreas VG, Bebbington PE (1988): Greeks, British Greek Cypriots and Londoners: A comparison of morbidity. Psychol Med 18:433–442.

Noyes R, Crowe RR, Harris EL (1986): Relationship between panic disorder and agoraphobia. Arch Gen Psychiatry 43:227–232.

Paykel ES (ed) (1992): "Handbook of Affective Disorders," 2nd ed. New York: Guilford Press.

Pollard CA, Bronson SS, Kenney MR (1989): Prevalence of agoraphobia without panic in clinical settings. Am J Psychiatry 146:559.

Robins LN, Helzer JE, Croughan J, Ratcliff KS (1981): National Institute of Mental Health Diagnostic Interview Schedule. Arch Gen Psychiatry 38:381–389.

Roth M, Noyes R, Burrows GD (1988): "Handbook of Anxiety," vol 1, Amsterdam: Elsevier.

Rounsaville BJ, Prusoff BA, Weissman MM (1980): The course of marital disputes in depressed women: a 48 month follow-up study. Compr Psychiatry 21:111–118.

Schneier FR, Johnson J, Hornig CD, Liebowitz MR, Weissman MM (1992): Social phobia: Comorbidity and morbidity in an epidemiological sample. Arch Gen Psychiatry 49:282–288.

Somervell PD, Leaf PJ, Weissman MM, Blazer DG, Bruce ML (1989): The prevalence of major depression in black and white adults in five United States communities. Am J Epidemiol 130:725–735.

Thompson AH, Bland RC, Orn HT (1989): Relationship and chronology of depression, agoraphobia, and panic disorder in the general population. J Nerv Ment Dis 177:456–4633.

Thyer BA, Himle J (1985): Temporal relationship between panic attack onset and phobic avoidance in agoraphobia. Behav Res Ther 23:607–608.

Thyer BA, Parrish RT, Curtis GC, Nesse RM, Cameron OG (1985): Ages of onset of DSM-III anxiety disorders. Comp Psychiatry 26:113–122.

Torgerson S (1983): Genetic factors in anxiety disorders. Arch Gen Psychiatry 40:1085–1089.

Torgersen S (1986): Genetic factors in moderately severe and mild affective disorders. Arch Gen Psychiatry 43:222–226.

Uhde TW, Boulenger JP, Roy-Byrne PP, Geraci MF, Vittone BJ, Post RM (1985): Longitudinal course of panic disorder. Prog Neuropsychopharmacol Biol Psychiatry 9:39–51.

Uhlenhuth EG, Balter MB, Mellinger GD, et al. (1983): Symptom checklist syndromes in the general population: Correlations with psychotherapeutic drug use. Arch Gen Psychiatry 40:1167–1173.

Vazquez-Barquero JF, Diez-Manriqe JF, Pena C, Quintanal G, Lopez LM (1986): Two stage design in a community survey. Br J Psychiatry 149:88–97.

Weissman MM (1985): The epidemiology of anxiety disorders: Rates, risks, and familial patterns. In Tuma AH, Maser JD (eds): Anxiety and the Anxiety Disorders. Hilldale, NJ.: Lawrence Erlbaum Associates, pp 275–296.

Weissman JJ, Adams PA, Lish J, Wickramaratne P, Horwath E, Charney D, Wood S, Leeman E, Frosch E (1993): The relationship between panic disorder and major depression: A new family study. Arch Gen Psychiatry 50:767–780.

Weissman MM, Bruce ML, Leaf PJ, Florio LP, Holzer C (1991): Psychiatric disorders in America. In Robins L, Regier D (eds): New York: Free Press, pp. 53–81.

Weissman MM, Klerman GL (1977): Sex differences in the epidemiology of depression. Arch Gen Psychiatry 34:98–111.

Weissman MM, Klerman GL (1985): Gender and depression. Trends Neurosci 8:416–420.

Weissman MM, Leaf PJ, Bruce ML, Florio L (1988a): The epidemiology of dysthymia in five communities: Rates, risks, comorbidity; and treatment. Am J Psychiatry 145:815–819.

Weissman MM, Leaf PJ, Tischler GL, Blazer DG, Karno M, Bruce ML, Florio LP (1988b): Affective disorders in five United States communities. Psychol Med 18:141–153.

Weissman MM, Myers JK (1978): Affective disorders in a U.S. urban community. Arch Gen Psychiatry 35:1304–1311.

Wickramaratne PJ, Weissman MM, Leaf PJ, Holford TR (1989): Age, period and cohort effects on the risk of major depression: Results from five United States communities. J Clin Epidemiol 42:333–343.

Winokur GW, Clayton PJ, Reich T (1969): "Manic Depressive Illness." St. Louis, CV Mosby.

Winokur GW, Morrison J (1973): The Iowa 500: Follow-up of 225 depressives. Br J Psychiatry 123:543–548.

World Health Organization (1978): "Mental Disorders: Glossary and Guide to Their Classification in Accordance With the 9th Revision of the International Classification of Diseases." Geneva: WHO.

Wittchen H-U (1986): "Natural Course and Spontaneous Remissions of Untreated Anxiety Disorders: Results of the Munich Follow-Up Study (MFS). Panic and Phobias," vol 2. Berlin: Springer-Verlag.

CHAPTER 17

Epidemiology of Alcohol Use, Abuse, and Dependence

NANCY L. DAY

Department of Psychiatry, University of Pittsburgh School of Medicine, Pittsburgh, PA 15213

INTRODUCTION

Alcohol use and abuse occupy unique positions within our culture and history, influencing our attitudes toward drinking and our definitions of alcoholism. In colonial days, alcohol was a major part of life, serving as food, medicine, social facilitator, and a safe substitute for frequently nonpotable water (Levine, 1973). It provided, as well, a major source of revenue. Drinking was acceptable to the colonials, who thought that people drank and got drunk by choice. Drunkenness was not proscribed; habitual drunkenness was considered an addiction, but an addiction to drunkenness, not to alcohol. It was conceptualized as a problem within the social and religious realms and punished with legal and religious sanctions.

Changes in social attitudes toward alcohol have created sweeping social movements throughout our history. The last of these resulted in the eighteenth amendment to the Constitution, Prohibition, which began in 1920 and was repealed in 1933. Some argue that there are signs that we may again be experiencing a return to prohibition sentiment (Room, 1991). What is less apparent but equally important is that, as a culture, we have maintained the earlier dual attitude toward alcohol, conceptualizing it as a positive benefit with restrained and appropriate use and a negative behavior when used to excess or harm. Similarly, we entertain at the same time the idea that alcoholism is a disease, or medical problem, and that alcoholism is a social problem related to excess consumption.

Two different research thrusts representing these differing approaches coexist within the field of alcohol studies. The sociologic approach has documented the prevalence of drinking, drinking patterns, and problems within the population. This approach studies the continuum from abstinence to problem drinking and focuses on the sociologic and environmental factors that affect position along this continuum. The medical approach has viewed alcoholism, or alcohol abuse and dependence, as a disease, focusing on biologic and genetic factors and clinical issues of diagnosis and treatment. Research covering both approaches is presented in this chapter since both are needed to describe the

Textbook in Psychiatric Epidemiology, Edited by Tsuang, Tohen, and Zahner.
ISBN 0-471-59375-3   © 1995 Wiley-Liss, Inc.

range of alcohol effects, as well as the breadth of alcohol research within the United States.

DRINKING AND DRINKING PRACTICES

Population-Based Estimates of Alcohol Use

On a population basis, there are several ways of estimating the amount of alcohol consumed. The most common is to estimate per capita alcohol consumption based on either alcohol production or sales. Apparent alcohol consumption, a measure derived by dividing the total quantity of alcohol sales by the total population in the United States aged 14 and older, was 2.46 gallons of absolute alcohol (approximately 50 six-packs) in 1990 (Williams et al., 1992). This is actually an underestimate of individual consumption, however, since abstainers were included in this calculation and illegal alcohol, home production, and duty-free purchases were not included in this estimate. In the United States, the highest levels of per capita consumption occurred in the West (2.7 gallons per capita) and the lowest occurred in the South (2.37 gallons) (Williams et al., 1992). When these data were corrected for the prevalence of abstainers in the population, the highest per capita rate was found in Washington, DC, at 11.14 gallons per drinker.

There has been a recent decrease in the consumption of alcoholic beverages, following a peak in the early 1980s (National Institute on Drug Abuse [NIDA], 1991; Williams et al., 1992). In a study that used data from the National Health Interview Survey, Williams and DeBakey (1992) found that, between 1983 and 1988, the rates of abstention increased among those who were married, at all levels of education, and among individuals with incomes above $10,000 per year. Among whites, both males and females increased their rates of abstention and decreased heavier drinking. African-American men and women and Hispanic men also showed decreases in heavy drinking, though they did not have increases in their rates of abstention.

These data, however, cannot give us individual patterns of use or the covariates of patterns of alcohol consumption. To do this, individual interviews are necessary to collect specific levels and patterns of consumption.

Measurement of Drinking

Drinking is a behavior that can be described by the quantity, frequency, and type of beverage consumed. Quantity, the number of drinks per occasion, is a measure of drinking style, while frequency, the number of occasions per unit time, is a measure of the role or the salience of alcohol in the individual's life style. The type of beverage also is a marker of the style of drinking as well as of social status. Interestingly, although the percent of absolute alcohol differs among the different beverages, the amount of absolute alcohol per served drink is roughly equivalent. That is, a 12 oz. can of beer, a mixed drink containing 1.5 oz. of spirits, and a 5 oz. glass of wine all contain about the same amount of absolute alcohol.

The different variations of quantity, frequency, and beverage type can be combined to describe a drinking pattern. In fact, these patterns are used within our culture as markers of social status. Contrast, for example, the descriptors that come to mind when you compare the drinking patterns of two people: the first person drinks a six-pack after work every night and two to three six-packs on weekend nights, while a second person drinks wine every night with dinner and on weekends either wine or a mixed drink before and with dinner. With high reliability, most readers will be able quickly to identify a gender, income, education, and occupational level for each of the individuals.

A number of scales have been developed that allow researchers to combine the various drinking parameters. The most common of these is average daily volume, an averaged estimate across all quantities, frequencies, and beverages. While this scale has the advantage that it is a continuous variable, it has the disadvantage that it ignores the diversity of drinking patterns. This diversity is important because, as noted above, drinking patterns correlate with other covariates of drinking, with consequences of drinking and with alcohol abuse and dependence. Other ways of combining the data have also been developed, including measures of binge, or clustered drinking, or frequent heavy drinking, the frequency of consuming five or more drinks per occasion. Other researchers have constructed typologies of drinking to describe different patterns. These measures usually focus on only one dimension of drinking behavior and therefore can only be used to explore the effects of a specific pattern of use.

At the top of the scale (the heaviest drinking levels) and the bottom (abstention and very light drinking) the concordance between scales is quite good. In the middle levels, there is considerable divergence, and in analyses that address more moderate levels of alcohol use the type of scale that is selected becomes important.

The Prevalence of Alcohol Use

The Alcohol Research Group assayed drinking practices and problems in a national sample in 1984 (Hilton, 1991a). This study was a national household probability sample with enhanced sampling to increase the number of African-American and Hispanic subjects. Data from this study demonstrated that a majority of the population, 69%, drank at least once a year: 76% of the men and 64% of the women (Hilton, 1991a). Overall, 7% of the population drank daily, though this was a more common behavior for men; 12% drank at this rate compared with women, among whom only 4% reported daily drinking. Men were also more likely to drink heavily. Twenty-four percent of the men drank five or more drinks on occasion at least weekly, and 8% drank eight or more drinks in a day at least weekly compared with 6% and 2% for women, respectively. A total of 3% of the population reported getting drunk at least weekly (5% of the men and 1% of the women). The beverage consumed most often was beer, followed by liquor and then wine.

Drinking and patterns of consumption changed with age (Hilton, 1991a). Among men, the younger (18–29 years of age) were less likely to be daily drinkers than were the older men. Younger men, however, had higher rates of frequent heavy drinking. One-third of the men aged 18–29 years reported drinking five or more drinks per occasion at least weekly compared with 26% of the men 40–49 years of age and 8% of the men aged 60 and over. Among women, similar patterns were found with respect to age, although the levels of consumption were much lower. However, it is not possible to know from these data whether this is an aging effect or a cohort effect.

In 1983, Stall (1986) followed up a group of men who had been interviewed in 1964. While stability was the mode, 25% of the men had decreased their intake while 15% increased their drinking over the 20 year time period. The decrease was greatest among the heavy and moderate drinkers (80%), and the stability was determined mostly by men who had been light drinkers in the base period. Quantity was more likely to decrease than frequency. Findings from another study using both men and women corroborated the Stall report (Adams et al., 1990). These data demonstrate that the decrease over time is not a cohort effect, but a behavioral change associated with aging.

White men (76%) and women (65%) were more likely to be drinkers than were African-American men (72%) or women (54%) (Hilton, 1991a). These differences disappeared at high levels of consumption, however. The rate of getting drunk at least weekly was 5% for both African-American and white men and 1% among women of both racial groups. Hispanic men were most likely to be drinkers, with a prevalence rate of 78%, and Hispanic women were least likely; only 54% reported any alcohol use in the past year. However, Hispanic men had the same prevalence of weekly drunkenness as African-American and white men. The rate for Hispanic women could not be estimated because of small numbers.

The prevalence of drinking increased with income (Hilton, 1991a). Among those with incomes less than $10,000 per year, 67% of the men and 49% of the women drank, compared with 91% and 81%, respectively, among those whose incomes were over $40,000. This pattern was also true for daily drinking and heavier drinking. Among men, 20% of those with incomes below $10,000/year drank five or more drinks per occasion at least weekly compared with 35% among those with incomes above $40,000. Comparable figures for women were 3% and 6%, respectively. At higher levels of consumption, however, the relationship changed and lower income men reported comparable levels of drinking eight or more drinks per day at least weekly and higher rates of weekly drunkenness.

Education level, like income level, was correlated with drinking patterns. Among both men and women, those with the most education were most likely to be drinkers. However, high school graduates were the most likely to report heavier drinking. For example, 11% of men who were high school graduates drank eight or more drinks per day at least weekly compared with 7% of men with less education and 4% of male college graduates.

Among both men and women, those who were never married and those who were divorced or separated were the most likely to drink and had the highest rates of heavy drinking.

Religion also predicted drinking patterns, both because of differing religious attitudes toward alcohol and because of the correlations between religion, ethnic identity, and socioeconomic status. Catholics and Jews were most likely to be drinkers (Hilton, 1991a). Among men, 89% of Catholics and 89% of Jews were drinkers, while 77% of Catholic women and 88% of Jewish women drank. Among Christians, Catholics were most likely to drink, followed by Liberal and then Conservative Protestants. High rates of drinking and heavy drinking were also found among those who specified no religious preference. People who were Jewish were least likely to be heavy drinkers, and those with no religious preference were most likely to drink heavily and to be drunk at least once a week.

Thus, drinking in the U.S. population followed traditional patterns determined by individual, demographic, and socioeconomic factors. People who were older or of higher social status were more likely to be drinkers, but they were less likely to drink heavily or report drunkenness. Those of lower income and education were less likely to drink. Also, younger, unmarried men and women were more likely to drink and to drink heavily.

Measurement of drinking in a population sample is, at best, difficult. Because our cultural attitudes toward alcohol are still ambivalent, drinking is usually underreported. In fact, comparisons of alcohol production to reported use find that only about half of all alcohol produced is accounted for by surveys of drinking behavior (Embree and Whitehead, 1993; De Lint, 1981). Although researchers have assumed that the amount of un-derreporting is not correlated with the actual drinking practices of the individual (Popham and Schmidt, 1981), this has not been demonstrated, and this inaccuracy could represent a significant bias.

DRINKING PROBLEMS

In addition to measuring the prevalence of drinking in the population, researchers have also focused on the consequences of alcohol use. These consequences are events such as accidents, family problems, and/or medical effects such as liver cirrhosis that may be at-tributed to drinking practices.

Definition of Drinking Problems

The measurement of drinking problems in survey research has a long history, extending back to the early national surveys on drinking and drinking problems (Clark, 1966; Keller, 1962), although considerable debate still exists regarding the list of eligible prob-lems and/or the definition of such problems. There are also problems with the assessment of these consequences. The first is the issue of attribution. Although the definition of these items assumes that the outcome was the result of alcohol use and would not have occurred in the absence of alcohol consumption, none of the consequences is unique to alcohol exposure, and this assumption is difficult to prove. Moreover, as alcohol con-sumption increases, the tendency to blame problems on alcohol may very well increase, confounding the relationship. In addition, there is a problem of negative labeling, as well as the process of denial, both of which may lead to a tendency to deny the role of alcohol in a given problem. The effect of these factors on the measurement of consequences is not known.

Hilton (1991b) divided drinking problems into three groups representing drinking pat-terns, consequences, and dependence. Consequences are variables such as fighting while intoxicated, problems with spouse, relatives, friends, job or finances, resulting from drinking. Health problems and accidents due to drinking are also included in the listing (Hilton, 1991b).

Dependence was defined by items such as loss of control and symptomatic behaviors such as tremors and blackouts. These symptoms parallel the diagnostic criteria for alcohol abuse and dependence, although the authors disavow this implication, arguing that they could reflect either a disease state or the immediate and short-term effects of too much drinking. This reflects a still-current argument within this area of research. While medical researchers and clinicians accept that the end product of alcohol exposure and negative symptoms and/or consequences from alcohol use is a phenomenon defined as alcoholism, or alcohol abuse and dependence, social researchers argue that this construct does not ap-ply as well in the general population (Clark, 1991).

Prevalence and Correlates of Drinking Problems

In the national survey, 72% of all drinkers reported no drinking problems, 10% reported one problem, and 14% reported three or more problems (Hilton, 1991c). These drinking problems were more common among men than women and were found at higher rates among younger people (Hilton, 1991b). Among current drinkers, African-American men had higher rates of drinking problems than did white men. Ten percent of African-American men reported high levels of dependence symptoms (four or more) and 13.2% reported high levels of consequences (four or more, but a weighted scale was used) compared with 5.1% and 6.6% for white men, respectively. White women had more dependence problems than African-American women, with rates of 2.7% and 2.3% respectively, but there was no difference in the rates of consequences. Among men, the rate of drinking problems was highest among divorced or separated men, 14.0% reported a high level of consequences, with widowed (12.5%) and never-married men (10.9%) next in order, compared with a low rate among married men (5.1%). Among women, however, never-married women were low (1.2% reported a high level of consequences), and the divorced/separated group had rates approximating the rates of the married women (2.5% and 2.7%, respectively).

Rates of problems were highest among low income groups and among those with the less education for both males and females. It was noted earlier that male high school graduates had higher levels of heavier drinking; they also report a higher level of drinking problems.

Jews, both male (0.8% for a high level of consequences) and female (0%), had the lowest rates of drinking problems. Within the Christian religion, Conservative Christians had the highest rates of drinking problems among current drinkers. Overall, the group that had no religion had the highest rates of drinking problems; 18.5% of the men and 3.9% of the women reported a high level of consequences.

A study by Fitzgerald and Mulford (1993) in a survey completed in Iowa in 1989 found that the most commonly reported consequence, a failure to fulfill responsibilities because of drinking, was reported by 2.8% of the population. Most other consequences had prevalence rates of less than 1%. By contrast, in the national survey reported above, on the average, each item was endorsed positively by 2.8% of the subjects (Hilton, 1991c). The relationship between problems was low. The average correlation coefficient between problems was 0.19 (SD = 0.10) for problems judged to be moderate level and 0.20 (SD = 0.09) for problems at a minimal level. There were higher correlations, on the level of 0.4, between loss of control, symptomatic behavior, and binge drinking. These three variables also tended to correlate more highly with other problems.

The highest rates of drinking problems, then, were found among men—those who were young, less educated, of lower income, and single. Moreover, the groups that had the highest rates of drinking problems also tended to be the groups that had the greatest proportion of abstainers. Drinking problems may be more prevalent among groups where drinking is less common and, perhaps, less approved.

As with drinking and heavy drinking, there were clear and significant correlations between sociodemographic factors and drinking problems. These predictors were, in general, the predictors of heavy drinking. It is important to separate these relationships, to determine whether heavy drinking mediates the relationship between these factors and drinking problems. Hilton (1991d) looked at the predictability of these factors within a group of frequent heavy drinkers and found that, after controlling for intake, few of the covariates contributed significant levels of explanation.

A separate analysis, using data from the National Household Survey on Drug Abuse, compared the rates of psychosocial consequences of alcohol and drug abuse between men and women (Robbins, 1989). This report found that while substance abuse was related more to intrapsychic problems among women and issues of social functioning among men, the majority of the differences by gender were explained by the greater frequency of heavy drinking among men. Therefore, in large part, the covariates of drinking problems were the predictors of heavy drinking.

It is difficult to make the transition from drinking problems, a concept from the survey and sociologic literature, to the diagnosis of alcoholism. These disparate approaches, as noted earlier, represent different conceptual models. Proponents of the disease concept of alcoholism point to the clear biologic elements in the development of alcoholism, the development of tolerance and withdrawal, and the genetic aspects of the disease. Those who support the sociologic model contend that there is no unitary phenomenon, pointing to the fact that there is a wide distribution in the types and the relationships between the symptoms that enter into the diagnosis (Clark, 1991; Tarter et al., 1991). The diagnostic criteria for alcoholism, in fact, bridge these arguments, since, like many chronic diseases, alcoholism is defined at the end of a continuum and the point between having symptoms and having a diagnosable disease is arbitrary. Moreover, it is the number of symptoms rather than a specific progression of symptoms that defines the disorder.

ALCOHOLISM OR ALCOHOL ABUSE AND DEPENDENCE

Definition and Diagnosis

Benjamin Rush (1785) categorized drunkenness as a progressive disease and noted that the body progressively adapts to the use of alcohol until the person becomes habituated. It was the first definition of both the disease state and tolerance. He proposed strikingly nonmedical treatments, including terrors, whippings, and shaming, and advocated temperance. Wine and beer were acceptable; the primary problem was spirits (liquor), particularly rum.

The use of the word *alcoholism* was proposed in Sweden in 1852 (Paredes, 1979) to remove the stigma of the term *drunkenness* and was defined as the biologic and behavioral symptoms resulting from the damage caused by excessive ingestion, an irresistible urge to drink, and a functional disturbance of the central nervous system. Jellinek (1960) laid the groundwork for current diagnostic thinking. He proposed that there were two types of alcoholics, those who suffered physical and physiologic changes resulting from prolonged use (chronic alcoholism) and others who had alcohol addiction, characterized by an urgent craving for alcohol.

There are as many different schemata for diagnosis as there are different names for the phenomenon. However, in general, the diagnoses include four concepts: tolerance to alcohol, withdrawal during abstinence, impaired control over alcohol consumption, and problems related to the use of alcohol (Beresford, 1991). These core factors that define the diagnosis, however, are only weakly correlated with each other (Cloninger, 1987).

Tolerance is defined as a physical dependence on alcohol and reflects the amount of physical habituation that the body has developed (Beresford, 1991). As tolerance increases, the effect of a given amount of alcohol will decrease. *Withdrawal* constitutes a set of symptoms that occur when a person is abstinent. The resulting symptoms can range from anxiety, nausea, and tachycardia to seizures and delirium tremens. Thus, tolerance and withdrawal are markers of the biologic effects of alcohol. *Impaired control* refers to the inability to control drinking once begun, to cut down, or to quit.

Social problems are problems that result directly from the use of alcohol. Driving or violence while intoxicated, neglect of responsibilities due to alcohol use, or failure to decrease alcohol use even in the face of physical problems caused by the exposure, such as cirrhosis, are all included in this category. This list parallels the list of consequences noted earlier and has been adapted from the studies of drinking problems. Accordingly, the same problems of attribution, labeling, and denial apply. Social consequences can be affected by a number of different drinking-related behaviors. They can result from the acute effects of intoxication, the effects of chronic drinking, or the prioritization of drinking over other roles and responsibilities.

These basic areas were combined into the diagnosis of alcohol abuse and dependence in the DSM-III (American Psychiatric Association [APA], 1980). The diagnosis of alcohol dependence required either tolerance or withdrawal and either loss of control or social or physical problems because of alcohol use. A separate category, alcohol abuse, required the presence of impaired control or social consequences in the absence of either tolerance or withdrawal. One weakness of the DSM-III system of classification for alcohol abuse and dependence was that there was no requirement that the symptoms occur together in time. Therefore, the estimates of lifetime prevalence may be considerably inflated as subjects experience symptoms over the course of their lifetime.

At the same time, Edwards (1986) developed a theoretical model, the alcohol dependence syndrome (ADS). This model focused more on the salience of drinking and alcohol-seeking behavior and less on social consequences. It was defined by seven criteria: narrowing the drinking repertoire, salience of alcohol-seeking behavior, increased tolerance, repeated withdrawal episodes, drinking to relieve or avoid withdrawal, subjective awareness of a compulsion to drink, and reinstatement of established drinking patterns following a period of abstinence.

In 1987, the DSM criteria were revised, incorporating the theoretical model of the ADS into the conceptualization of the DSM-III-R (APA, 1987). In the DSM-III-R, the diagnosis of alcohol dependence is made if three from a list of nine symptoms are present. Definitions of severity levels were also included in this revision, a recognition of the fact that alcohol dependence exists along a gradient. A diagnosis of alcohol abuse persists in the DSM-III-R and requires the presence of environmental problems due to alcohol use and recurrent use of alcohol when it is physically harmful.

A further revision, the DSM-IV, became official in 1994. The DSM-IV is based on the ADS, which was discussed above. To receive a diagnosis of alcohol dependence, a person must meet three of the following seven criteria: 1) tolerance; 2) withdrawal; 3) drinking in larger amounts or over a longer period than was intended; 4) a persistent desire to drink or unsuccessful efforts to cut down or control alcohol use; 5) spending a great deal of time obtaining, using, or recovering from the effects of alcohol; 6) giving up or reducing social, occupational, or recreational activities because of alcohol use; and 7) continued use even in the presence of physical or psychological problems caused or exacerbated by alcohol (APA, 1993). In the DSM-IV, the symptoms must occur within the same 12 month period, although they need not occur at the same time. As a result of this addition, the prevalence of alcohol dependence will be lower using the DSM-IV criteria than the DSM-III. The DSM-IV also allows the clinician to specify whether or not alcohol dependence includes physiologic dependence, either tolerance or withdrawal.

Alcohol abuse in the new system is diagnosed by the social effects of drinking, such as failure to fulfill major role obligations, use in situations in which drinking is physically hazardous, substance-related legal problems, and use despite problems caused by or exacerbated by drinking. In addition, dependence and abuse are now defined hierarchically, so that one cannot receive a diagnosis of abuse after meeting criteria for dependence. In the

DSM-III or DSM-III-R systems, it was possible to receive concurrent diagnoses of dependence and abuse. The hierarchical relationship in classification will reduce the number of cases of alcohol abuse.

A parallel diagnostic system, the International Classification of Diseases (ICD) is used internationally. The tenth revision of this system is based on the ADS (WHO, 1990) and therefore is similar to recent versions of the DSM system.

Although differences still exist with regard to the specific criteria for diagnosing alcohol abuse and dependence and the definitions of the variables included in the diagnosis, the availability of standardized diagnostic criteria has been invaluable in the development of epidemiologic studies of these disorders. In the absence of a standard case definition, research would have no external validity. In addition, this standardization enables the field of alcohol research to achieve reliability across studies so they can be compared. Further methodologic advances have included the development of structured and semi-structured instruments for interviewing, some of which are designed to be used by lay interviewers. These developments have made possible the general population surveys of psychiatric morbidity.

There are two factors that are unique in the diagnosis of alcohol abuse and dependence. First, substance abuse diagnoses require exposure to an outside agent as part of the causal sequence. Second, the diagnosis of alcoholism includes the effect of the disease on the environment as part of the diagnosis, a reflection of the unique history of alcohol.

Population Estimates

The Alcohol Epidemiologic Data System monitors data from the National Hospital Discharge Survey for discharges due to alcohol diagnoses (using the ICD-9 diagnostic criteria), including alcoholic psychoses, alcohol dependence syndrome, nondependent alcohol abuse, and liver cirrhosis (Caces et al., 1992). These data are from a sample of nonfederal, short-stay hospitals, and discharges are randomly sampled. In 1990, there were over 28,000,000 discharges; 1.3% had an alcohol diagnosis listed as the primary diagnosis, and an additional 3.6% had an alcohol diagnosis listed, though not as a primary diagnosis. Rates of alcohol diagnoses were higher for men than women, African-Americans than whites, highest for those aged 45–64, and lowest among those who were 15–24 years of age.

Another means of assessing the prevalence of alcoholism is to evaluate the distribution of deaths from liver cirrhosis. Jellinek (WHO, 1951) developed a formula for estimating the rate of alcoholism based on the rate of liver cirrhosis and the proportion of deaths from liver cirrhosis that can be attributed to alcoholism. Estimates are that between 41% and 95% of cirrhosis deaths are related to alcohol consumption (Day, 1977). In 1989, the age-adjusted mortality rate from cirrhosis of the liver was 9.1 per 100,000 persons in the United States (DeBakey et al., 1993), placing it as the ninth leading cause of death in the United States. Mortality from liver cirrhosis was more common among males and African-Americans.

There are a number of problems with the use of cirrhosis mortality as a surrogate for alcoholism. Although historically the rates of death from liver cirrhosis have responded quickly and dramatically to major changes in alcohol distribution, such as Prohibition or war (Terris, 1967), there was a 25% decrease in cirrhosis mortality between 1973 and 1983 in the absence of a comparable change in drinking practices (DeBakey et al., 1993). This could reflect the relative success of treatment programs, either for cirrhosis or for alcoholism, or changes in diagnostic practices and/or death certification. In addition, cirrhosis is more likely to occur with heavy daily drinking than with episodic or binge drinking (Smart and Mann, 1992) and with amounts above the range of 80 g of absolute alcohol per day (Savolainen et al., 1993), so many drinkers and drinking patterns are not represented by this measure. There are also biases in the determination and reporting of death from cirrhosis.

Prevalence and Correlates of Alcohol Abuse and Dependence

Two large recent surveys provide data on the prevalence of alcohol dependence and abuse in the United States, the Epidemiologic Catchment Area (ECA) study, a study conducted collaboratively at five sites throughout the United States, and the Alcohol Supplement to the National Household Interview Survey (NHIS).

The ECA study used standardized methods at all sites and diagnostic criteria from the DSM-III (Leaf et al., 1991). Data collection occurred between 1980 and 1984 across the separate sites. A structured diagnostic interview, the Diagnostic Interview Schedule (DIS), was developed and was administered by lay interviewers. Reliability studies of the diagnoses of alcohol abuse and dependence using this instrument are somewhat conflicting, and the reliability seems to be moderate (Anthony et al., 1985; Helzer et al., 1985).

The ECA study found high prevalence rates for alcoholism (defined by the authors as either abuse or dependence); 13.8% of all subjects met criteria for a lifetime diagnosis, and 6.3% met criteria in the year prior to interview (Robins et al., 1991). Alcohol disorders were second only to phobias in prevalence among psychiatric disorders. The disorders were more common in males; 23.8% of men and 4.6% of the women in the sample met criteria for a lifetime diagnosis of alcoholism (Helzer et al., 1991). The median age of onset was 21 years, and 90% of all subjects had experienced their first symptom before the age of 38 years.

Five percent of men and 0.9% of women met criteria for a diagnosis of alcoholism within the past month (Regier et al., 1993). Rates decreased across age categories, from 4.1% for those aged 18–24 to 0.9% among individuals over age 65. Rates were highest among Hispanics (3.6%), intermediate for African-Americans (3.4%), and lowest for whites (2.7%). People who were separated or divorced had the highest rate (5.9%) compared with a rate of 2.0% for married and 4.2% for single people.

The ECA project also surveyed institutionalized individuals, sampling residents of mental hospitals, nursing, convalescent, and rest homes, chronic hospitals, residential centers for alcohol and drug treatment, halfway houses, and correctional facilities (Leaf et al., 1991). Twelve percent of institutionalized individuals had alcoholism compared with 6% of household residents. Most commonly, these people were in correctional facilities (78%); 11% were in psychiatric facilities, and 11% were in chronic care facilities (Robins et al., 1991).

While the rate of alcoholism in the institutionalized and treatment population is high, the proportion of the general population with the diagnosis of alcoholism that receives treatment is very small. Of all of the subjects with a lifetime diagnosis of alcoholism, only 15% reported that they had ever mentioned their symptoms to a doctor. Furthermore, only 10% of those who currently had a diagnosis of alcohol abuse or dependence, in the absence of any comorbidity, received any mental health care (9% of the men and 14% of the women) (Robins et al., 1991).

In the ECA study, 49% of those who met criteria for a lifetime diagnosis of alcoholism reported a symptom within the recent year, while 51% of those with a lifetime diagnosis did not (Helzer et al., 1991). These findings have been confirmed by other researchers as well. Skog and Duckert (1993), for example, studied a treatment sample and found that heavy drinkers and alcoholics were as likely to decrease as to increase their consumption. These findings parallel reports from the drinking practices literature that demonstrate significant changes in heavy drinking over time among subjects (Clark, 1966) and challenge the assumption that alcoholism is a chronic and unremitting disorder.

Among remitted cases in the ECA study (symptom free for at least 1 year), 75% of the subjects reported no more than 11 years from first to last symptom (Helzer et al., 1991). These facts, combined with the stigma associated with seeking treatment for alcoholism, may explain the very low rates of treatment.

There were differing patterns in the prevalence of alcoholism by age, sex, and race in the ECA study (Helzer et al., 1991). The lifetime prevalence rate for alcoholism in white males increased from 26.6% to 27.9% between age groups 18–29 and 30–44, respectively, while the rate in white females decreased across the same ages from 6.9% to 5.5%. Thereafter, in both genders, the rates decreased with each age group. The decrease was greater for females, and the male to female ratio increased from 3.9 in the youngest age group to 9.1 in the oldest.

The prevalence of alcoholism among Hispanics had a pattern similar to that of white men and women with respect to age, but the prevalence rates were higher for Hispanic males (35.9% at ages 30–44) and lower for Hispanic females (3.7% at ages 30–44) compared with white males and females.

The pattern by age among African-Americans was different. For both males and females, the highest prevalence was found in the middle age groups, between ages 45 and 64, where the rate was 32.9% for males and 7.3% for females. Thus, although there was little difference in the overall rate of alcoholism between African-Americans and whites, there were quite different patterns in the distribution of prevalence rates by age.

There was an inverse relationship between alcoholism and educational level, and few of the identified alcoholics (9%) had a stable marriage (Helzer et al., 1991). Concordant with the findings on education, there was an inverse relationship between occupational level, income, and the prevalence of alcoholism. It is notable that these covariates are quite different from those that predict drinking and heavy drinking in the general population. They are similar, however, to those that predict drunkenness.

A second large national prevalence study was from the Alcohol Supplement to the National Health Interview Survey. This project surveyed 22,418 and 43,809 individuals in 1984 and 1988, respectively (Williams and DeBakey, 1992). In 1984, using DSM-III criteria, 8.6% of the respondents met diagnostic criteria for alcohol abuse and dependence within the past year (Grant et al., 1991). A second wave of data collection was carried out in 1988. This wave used DSM-III-R criteria and found a prevalence rate of 9% for alcoholism (Grant et al., 1991). These rates compare with the rate of 6.3% for the ECA sample using DSM-III criteria (Helzer et al., 1991).

The rate of alcoholism was 13.3% among males and 4.4% among females. Whites had a higher prevalence than African-Americans, 9.1% compared with 5.6%, respectively. Alcohol dependence was found in 6.2% and alcohol abuse among 2.4% of the total population. The 1988 NHIS survey also found that, at younger ages, more whites met criteria for alcohol abuse and dependence, while at older ages the ratio was tipped toward African-American respondents. As in the ECA project, the rates of diagnosis for males and females were most similar among the younger aged cohort and diverged sharply among the older subjects.

The rates found in the two NHIS surveys using DSM-III (8.6%) and DSM-III-R (9%) criteria were comparable. However, both of the rates were higher than the rate reported by the ECA project using DSM-III criteria (6.3%). The discrepancies in the data are mostly in the younger age groups, where the prevalence rates are much higher in the NHIS study, particularly among whites, than in the ECA study.

Alternative Models of Alcoholism

There are other formulations of the diagnostic spectrum of alcohol abuse and dependence, although few epidemiologic data exist for these proposed models. Cloninger (1987) has proposed a neurobiologic learning model of alcoholism, based on personality dimensions, that has two subtypes. Type I, or milieu-limited, alcoholics have a later onset, psychological rather than physiological dependence, and experience guilt over their use. Type II, or male-limited, alcoholics have problems at an earlier age, exhibit spontaneous alcohol-seeking behavior, and are socially disruptive when drinking. Zucker (1987), on the basis of developmental studies, has proposed a four-group subtype of alcoholism. Babor et al. (1992), using empirical clustering, have proposed two types of alcoholics based on premorbid risk factors, pathologic use of alcohol and other substances, and the chronicity and consequences of drinking. Other reviewers have questioned the validity of the conceptualization and have recommended a rethinking and reformulation of our ideas about alcoholism (Tarter et al., 1991).

All of these typologies have in common an attempt to combine the various effects of drinking, drinking patterns, social problems, predictors, including genetic background and environmental factors, and psychosocial variables into a pattern. Many were developed using clinical populations and thus reflect the biases inherent in such samples, including the preselection of subjects to a treatment facility for alcohol abuse and dependence.

Genetic Factors in Alcohol Abuse and Dependence

Family studies have demonstrated that the risk of alcoholism was much higher among first-degree family members of an alcoholic; on average, the risk was increased seven times (Merikangas, 1990). Studies of twin pairs also demonstrated a genetic influence, although the effect was moderated by gender and diagnosis. Concordance rates were higher for men than for women and for alcohol dependence than for alcohol abuse (Pickens et al., 1991).

Comorbidity

Alcohol and alcoholism are commonly associated with other disorders. In the ECA study (Helzer et al., 1991), 32% of all interviewees who had one diagnosis also had a second. Among those with a diagnosis of alcohol abuse and dependence, the proportion was 47%. The most common second diagnosis among alcoholics was drug abuse and dependence, but other diagnoses, including antisocial personality, mania, and schizophrenia were also highly associated with alcoholism. Although in clinical samples depression is the disorder most commonly associated with alcoholism, this phenomenon was not particularly notable among the general population study. Female alcoholics had the highest rates of co-morbidity, 65%, compared with 44% for the male alcoholics (Helzer et al., 1991).

Alcohol use and particularly drunkenness also contribute to morbidity and mortality rates for accidents, violence, cardiovascular disease, liver cirrhosis, and certain types of cancer (National Institute on Alcohol Abuse and Alcoholism [NIAAA], 1993). Further-more, alcohol use affects reproductive functioning among women (NIAAA, 1993), and use during pregnancy causes growth, morphologic, and neurologic deficits in the off-spring (Day, 1992).

SUMMARY

Drinking is the modal behavior in the United States. Overall, 70% of the population drinks at least once a year. Drinking behavior correlates with social and demographic sta-tus and is more prevalent among those who have higher levels of education and income. Heavy drinking and drunkenness are also frequent. Approximately 6% of the population reports drinking eight or more drinks in a day at least once a week, and 3% of respon-dents report being drunk as often as once a week. In contrast to drinking and heavy drink-ing, drunkenness is correlated with younger age, less education, and lower income.

Epidemiologic research in the area of drinking practices can make substantial contri-butions to the field in several areas. The first is in the measurement of drinking and drink-ing patterns. As noted above, general population estimates of drinking only account for a portion of the actual alcohol that is produced. It is necessary to explore new means of measuring alcohol use to develop new techniques of interviewing that may diffuse some of the social stigma associated with drinking and that will allow researchers to estimate more accurately the level of alcohol use and the pattern of use by demographic and social predictors and to identify the segments of the population that do not report their use accu-rately.

In addition, although we know what the correlates of the various drinking patterns are, we do not yet know what factors may predict the transition from one level of drinking to another. For example, although drinking is more prevalent among those who are better educated and have higher incomes, drunkenness is found among those who are less edu-cated and have lower incomes. We do not know what factors may trigger the transition from alcohol use to abuse and/or what it is about education and income (for example) that may predict this transition.

Six percent of the adult population reports current drinking problems at a high level, and 6%–9% of the general population of adults meet criteria for alcohol abuse and de-pendence within the year prior to interview. These rates are mirrored by the proportion of all hospitalized patients with alcohol diagnoses, 5%. The prevalence rates and the covari-ates are remarkably similar for heavy drinking, drinking problems, and alcohol abuse and dependence. We can conclude from this that while these approaches come from different conceptual models, they are evaluating the same symptoms and identifying equivalent proportions of the population.

To understand the relationship between drinking, drinking problems, and alcoholism will require the collection of data from both clinical and general population samples. A clearer view of the relationship between drinking problems and alcoholism will also al-low more definitive studies of the essential diagnostic elements of the disorder and allow better separation of the disease process from the consequences of alcohol misuse.

Thus, future directions of epidemiologic research on alcohol disorders will include further refinement of measurement techniques and exploration of the relationship between the social aspects of alcohol use, misuse, and alcoholism. This should allow more insight into the diagnosis of alcohol disorders, which in turn would allow us to develop a better understanding of the factors that affect the transition from drinking to alcoholism.

REFERENCES

Adams WL, Garry PJ, Rhyne R, Hunt WC, Goodwin JS (1990): Alcohol intake in the healthy elderly. Changes with age in a cross-sectional and longitudinal study. Am Geriatr Soc 38:211–216.

American Psychiatric Association (1980): "Diagnostic and Statistical Manual of Mental Disorders," 3rd ed. Washington, DC: American Psychiatric Association.

American Psychiatric Association (1987): "Diagnostic and Statistical Manual of Mental Disorder," 3rd ed, revised. Washington, DC: American Psychiatric Association.

American Psychiatric Association (1993): "DSM-IV Draft Criteria" (Task Force on DSM-IV). Washington, DC: American Psychiatric Association.

Anthony JC, Folstein M, Romanoski AJ, Von Korff MR, Nestadt GR, Chahal R, Merchant A, Brown CH, Shapiro S, Kramer M, Gruenberg EM (1985): Comparison of the lay Diagnostic Interview Schedule and a standardized psychiatric diagnosis: Experience in eastern Baltimore. Arch Gen Psychiatry 42:667–675.

Babor TF, Hofmann M, DelBoca FK, Hesselbrock V, Meer RE, Dolinsky ZS, Rounsaville B (1992): Types of alcoholics, I: Evidence for an empirically derived typology based on indicators of vulnerability and severity. Arch Gen Psychiatry 49:599–608.

Beresford TP (1991): The nosology of alcoholism research. Alcohol Health Res World 15:260–265.

Caces MF, Stinson FS, Noble J (1992): "Trends in Alcohol-Related Morbidity Among Short-Stay Community Hospital Discharges, United States, 1979–1990," (Surveillance Report No. 24). Washington, DC: U.S. Department of Health and Human Services, National Institute on Alcohol Abuse and Alcoholism.

Clark WB (1966): Operational definitions of drinking problems and associated prevalence rates. Q J Stud Alcohol 27:648–668.

Clark WB (1991): Conceptions of alcohol problems. In Clark WB, Hilton ME (eds): "Alcohol in America." Albany, NY: State University of New York Press, pp 165–172.

Cloninger CR (1987): Neurogenetic adaptive mechanisms in alcoholism. Science 236:410–416.

Day N (1977): "Alcohol and Mortality." Unpublished paper prepared for the National Institute on Alcohol Abuse and Alcoholism.

Day N (1992): The effect of alcohol use during pregnancy. In Zagon I, Slotkin T (eds): "Maternal Substance Abuse and the Developing Nervous System." Orlando: Academic Press, pp 27–44.

DeBakey SF, Stinson FS, Dufour MC (1993): "Liver Cirrhosis Mortality in the United States, 1970–1989" (Surveillance Report No. 25). Washington, DC: U.S. Dept of Health and Human Services, National Institute on Alcohol Abuse and Alcoholism.

De Lint J (1981): "Words and Deeds": Responses to Popham and Schmidt. J Stud Alcohol 42:359–361.

Edwards G (1986): The alcohol dependence syndrome: A concept as stimulus to enquiry. Br J Addict 81:171–183.

Embree BG, Whitehead PC (1993): Validity and reliability of self-reported drinking behavior: Dealing with the problem of response bias. J Stud Alcohol 54:334–344.

Fitzgerald JL, Mulford HA (1993): Alcohol availability, drinking contexts and drinking problems: The Iowa experience. J Stud Alcohol 54:320–325.

Grant BF, Harford TC, Chou P, Pickering R, Dawson DA, Stinson FS, Noble J (1991): Prevalence of DSM-III-R alcohol abuse and dependence, United States, 1988. Alcohol Health Res World 15:91–96.

Helzer JE, Robins LN, McEvoy LT, Spitznagel EL, Stoltzman RK, Farmer A, Brockington IF (1985): A comparison of clinical and Diagnostic Interview Schedule diagnoses. Arch Gen Psychiatry 42:657–666.

Helzer JE, Burnam A, McEvoy LT (1991): Alcohol abuse and dependence. In Robins LN, Regier DA (eds): "Psychiatric Disorders in America. The Epidemiologic Catchment Area Study." New York: The Free Press, pp 53–81.

Hilton ME (1991a): The demographic distribution of drinking patterns in 1984. In Clark WB, Hilton ME (eds): "Alcohol in America." Albany, NY: State University of New York Press, pp 73–86.

Hilton ME (1991b): The demographic distribution of drinking problems in 1984. In Clark WB, Hilton ME (eds): "Alcohol in America." Albany, NY: State University of New York Press, pp 87–104.

Hilton ME (1991c): A note on measuring drinking problems in the 1984 national alcohol survey. In Clark WB, Hilton ME (eds): "Alcohol in America." Albany, NY: State University of New York Press, pp 51–72.

Hilton ME (1991d): Demographic characteristics and the frequency of heavy drinking as predictors of self-reported drinking problems. In Clark WB, Hilton ME (eds): "Alcohol in America." Albany, NY: State University of New York Press, pp 194–212.

Jellinek EM (1960): "The Disease Concept of Alcoholism." Highland Park, NJ: Hillhouse Press.

Keller M (1962): The definition of alcoholism and the estimation of its prevalence. In Pittman D, Snyder C (eds): "Society, Culture and Drinking Patterns." New York: Wiley, pp 310–329.

Leaf PJ, Myers JK, McEvoy LT (1991): Procedures used in the epidemiologic catchment area study. In Robins LN, Regier DA (eds): "Psychiatric Disorders in America. The Epidemiologic Catchment Area Study." New York: The Free Press, pp 1–32.

Levine HG (1973): The discovery of addition: Changing conceptions of habitual drunkenness in America. J Stud Alcohol 39:143–174.

Merikangas KR (1990): The genetic epidemiology of alcoholism. Psychol Med 20:11–22.

National Institute on Drug Abuse (1991): "National Household Survey on Drug Abuse, Highlights 1990." Washington, DC: U.S. Department of Health and Human Services Publication Number (ADM) 1789–91.

National Institute on Alcohol Abuse and Alcoholism (1993): "Eighth Special Report to the U.S. Congress on Alcohol and Health." Washington, DC: U.S. Department of Health and Human Services.

Paredes A (1979): The history of the concept of alcoholism. In Tarter R, Sugarman A (eds): "Alcoholism—Interdisciplinary Approaches to an Enduring Problem." Reading MA: Addison-Wesley, pp 9–52.

Pickens RW, Svikis DS, McGue M, Lykken DT, Heston LL, Clayton PJ (1991): Heterogeneity in the inheritance of alcoholism. Arch Gen Psychiatry 48:19–28.

Popham RE, Schmidt W (1981): Words and deeds: The validity of self-report data on alcohol consumption. J Stud Alcohol 42:355–358.

Regier DA, Farmer ME, Rae DS, Myers JK, Kramer M, Robins LN, George LK, Karno M, Locke BZ (1993): One-month prevalence of mental disorders in the United States and sociodemographic characteristics: The Epidemiologic Catchment Area study. Acta Psychiatr Scand 88:35–47.

Robbins C (1989): Sex differences in psychosocial consequences of alcohol and drug abuse. J Health Social Behav 30:117–130.

Robins LN, Locke BZ, Regier DA (1991): An overview of psychiatric disorders in America. In Robins LN, Regier DA (eds): "Psychiatric Disorders in America. The Epidemiologic Catchment Area Study." New York: The Free Press, pp 53–81.

Room R (1991): Cultural changes in drinking and trends in alcohol problems indicators: Recent U.S. experience. In Clark WB, Hilton ME (eds): "Alcohol in America." Albany, NY: State University of New York Press, pp 149–164.

Rush B (1785): "An Inquiry Into the Effects of Ardent Spirits Upon the Human Body and Mind, With an Account of the Means of Preventing and of the Remedies for Curing Them" (8th ed, 1814). Reprinted in Keller M (1943): Classics of the alcohol literature. Q J Stud Alcohol 4:321–341.

Savolainen VT, Liesto K, Männikkö A, Penttilä L, Karhunaen PJ (1993): Alcohol consumption and alcoholic liver disease: Evidence of a threshold level for effects of ethanol. Alcohol Clin Exp Res 17:1112–1117.

Skog O, Duckert F (1993): The development of alcoholics' and heavy drinkers' consumption: A longitudinal study. J Stud Alcohol 54:178–188.

Smart RG, Mann RD (1992): Alcohol and the epidemiology of liver cirrhosis. Alcohol Health Res World 16:217–222.

Stall R (1986): Change and stability in quantity and frequency of alcohol use among aging males: A 19-year follow-up study. Br J Alcohol 81:537–544.

Tarter RE, Moss HB, Arria A, Mezzich AC, Vanyuko MM (1991): The psychiatric diagnosis of alcoholism: Critique and proposed reformulation. Alcohol Clin Exp Res 16:106–116.

Terris M (1967): Epidemiology of cirrhosis of the liver: National mortality data. Am J Public Health 57:2076–2089.

Williams GD, DeBakey SF (1992): Changes in levels of alcohol consumption: United States, 1983–1988. Br J Addict 87:643–648.

Williams GD, Stinson FS, Clem D, Noble J (1992): "Apparent Per Capita Alcohol Consumption: National, State and Regional Trends, 1977–1990" (Surveillance Report No. 23). Washington, DC: U.S. Department of Health and Human Services, National Institute on Alcohol Abuse and Alcoholism.

World Health Organization (1990): "Proposed 10th Revision of the International Classification of Diseases (ICD-10). Clinical Descriptions and Diagnostic Guidelines." Geneva: World Health Organization.

World Health Organization Expert Committee on Mental Health (1951): "Report on the First Session of the Alcoholism Subcommittee." Geneva: World Health Organization, Technical Report Series No. 42.

Zucker RA (1987): The four alcoholisms: A developmental account of the etiological process. In Rivers PC (ed): "Alcohol and Addictive Behavior." Lincoln, NB: University of Nebraska Press, pp 27–83.

CHAPTER 18

Epidemiology of Drug Dependence

JAMES C. ANTHONY and JOHN E. HELZER

Department of Mental Hygiene, School of Hygiene and Public Health, The Johns Hopkins University, Baltimore, MD 21205 (J.C.A.); Department of Psychiatry, School of Medicine, University of Vermont, Burlington, VT 05401 (J.E.H.)

INTRODUCTION

This is a chapter on the epidemiology of drug dependence and related psychiatric disturbances such as drug abuse. The chapter introduces the main clinical features of drug dependence and a set of contemporary case definitions now being used in clinical and epidemiologic research. It also provides an overview of recent basic epidemiologic evidence on drug dependence, with and without the related condition of drug abuse, including some coverage of adolescent drug use. The chapter offers several recommendations for future epidemiologic studies of drug dependence.

In this chapter, the term *drug* is used to encompass a set of internationally regulated substances such as marijuana and heroin, which generally are not available by medical prescription. This set of drugs also includes medicines more often available through legal channels, as well as illegal channels, of supply and distribution: cocaine and prescribed amphetamines; diazepam and other anxiolytic drugs; and flurazepam, secobarbital, and other sedative-hypnotic drugs. Tobacco (nicotine), coffee (caffeine), and alcohol (ethanol) also are drugs, although they are not subject to international controlled substances law. Tobacco dependence and caffeine dependence are discussed in this chapter, briefly. The epidemiology of alcohol dependence is the topic of a separate chapter.

There are many reasons to study drug-related problems by considering each drug compound or drug category, one at a time. Doing so, it is possible to take into account the individual pharmacologic and pharmacokinetic profile of each drug, which help to shape the biologic response to drug exposure, including the function of each drug as a reinforcer of human behavior. In turn, the biologic response to drug exposure and each drug's efficacy as a reinforcer help to determine, in part, whether drug dependence or other drug problems will occur within populations of drug users.

Textbook in Psychiatric Epidemiology, Edited by Tsuang, Tohen, and Zahner
ISBN 0-471-59375-3   © 1995 Wiley-Liss, Inc.

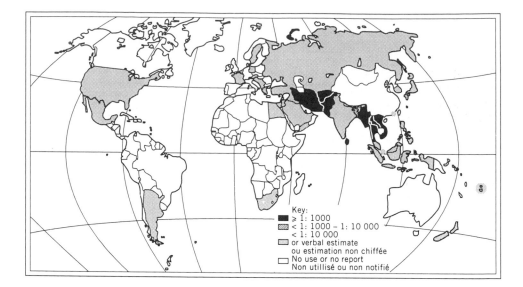

MAP 1. Opium. (From Hughes et al., 1983.) *NOTE:* For Maps 1 to 7, the key shows countries in which the prevalence of active cases is estimated to be greater than or equal to 1 per 1,000 persons, less than 1 per 10,000 persons, or intermediate.

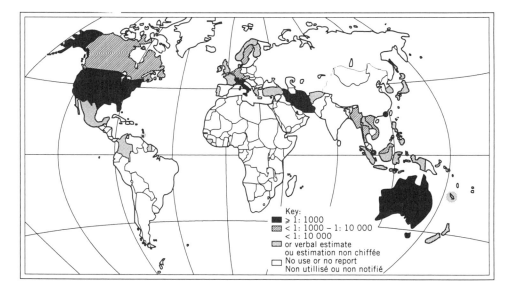

MAP 2. Heroin. (From Hughes et al., 1983.)

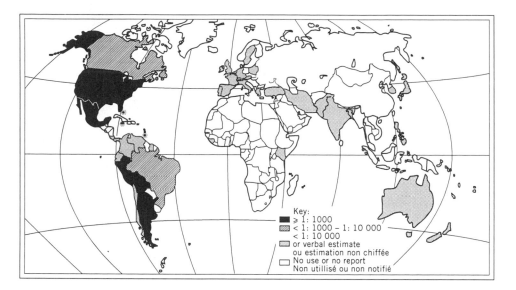

MAP 3. Cocaine and other coca derivatives. (From Hughes et al, 1983.)

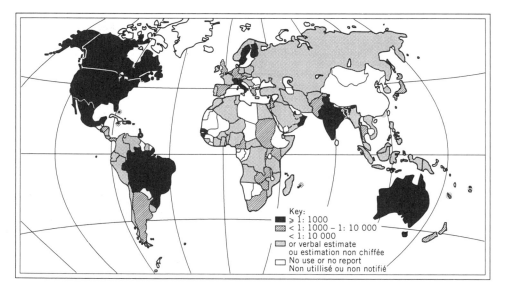

MAP 4. Cannabis. (From Hughes et al, 1983.)

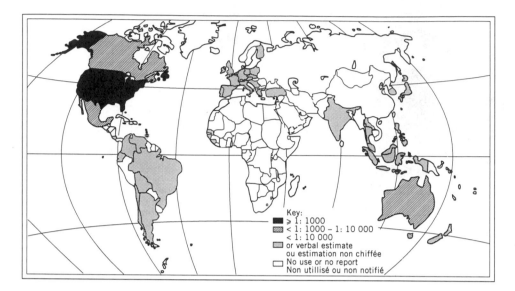

MAP 5. Hallucinogens. (From Hughes et al, 1983.)

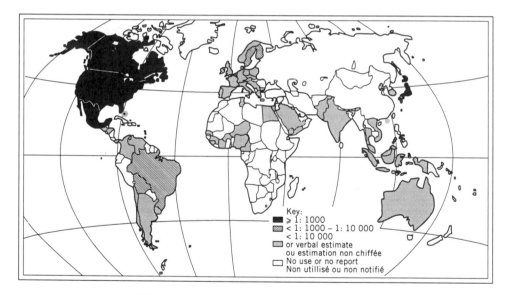

MAP 6. Amphetamines. (From Hughes et al., 1983.)

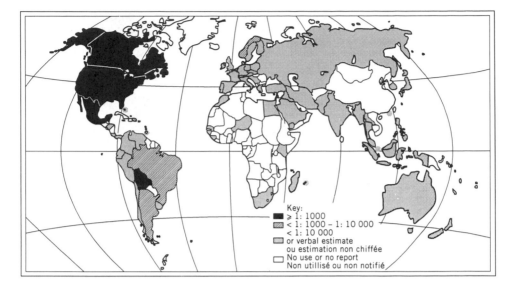

MAP 7. Barbituratures or other sedatives, and tranquilizers. (From Hughes et al, 1983.)

DISTRIBUTION OF DRUG-RELATED PROBLEMS IN SPACE AND TIME

Epidemiologic study of individual drugs and drug categories also reveals noteworthy variations in the global distribution of drug-related problems. Although recent estimates are not available for many parts of the world, problems associated with use of opium traditionally have been observed more often in South and Southeast Asia, where opium poppy cultivation is widespread (see Map 1). Heroin is derived from the opium poppy, but heroin problems have a substantially different global distribution (Map 2), related more to sites where heroin is refined from opium or morphine and to lines of supply and distribution from the clandestine heroin laboratories (Hughes et al., 1983).

By studying global maps of human drug experience such as these (Maps 1–7), the scholar interested in drug dependence will be led toward fascinating accounts of historical epidemiology, which add to our understanding of how drug-related problems are distributed in time as well as space. For example, since the middle of the twentieth century, the people of Japan seem to have been more affected by dependence on the psychostimulant amphetamine drugs than by other drugs, although in recent years problems associated with marijuana and other cannabis products (e.g., hashish) have become more prominent in Japan and elsewhere around the globe (Hughes et al., 1983). In the Americas, coca leaf chewing has been practiced for centuries, apparently with minimal health effects (Buck et al., 1968; Carroll, 1977). Nonetheless, after cocaine was extracted from the coca leaf in the last century, the U.S. population has experienced two epidemics of cocaine use and associated problems. The first American cocaine epidemic extended from the late nineteenth century into the early years of this century, and the second started in the mid-1970s, with a peak in the early 1980s, and a subsequent decline since then, as depicted in Table 1 (Petersen, 1977; Musto, 1990, 1991; Harrison, 1992; United States, 1993).

TABLE 1. One-Year Interval Prevalence Estimates From the NIDA National Household Survey on Drug Abuse, Depicting the Recent Epidemic of Cocaine Use in the United States[a]

Year of Survey	Estimate for Persons Aged 12–17 Years	Estimate for Persons Aged 18–25 Years	Estimate for Persons Aged 26 Years and Older
1972	1.5	NA	NA
1974	2.7	8.1	<0.5
1976	2.3	7.0	0.6
1977	2.6	10.2	0.9
1979	4.2	19.6	2.0
1982	4.1	18.8	3.8
1985	4.0	16.3	4.2
1988	2.9	12.1	2.7
1990	2.2	7.5	2.4
1991	1.5	7.7	NA
1992	1.1	6.3	NA

[a]Estimated prevalence of cocaine use in the past year (in percent) by year and age group at the time of the survey. Data are from the National Institute on Drug Abuse National Household Survey on Drug Abuse, 1972–1992.

PRESENTING CLINICAL FEATURES AND CASE DEFINITIONS

By comparison with typically more short-lived or acute problems such as drug intoxication, dependence on one of the internationally controlled drugs can be a chronic and debilitating mental and behavioral disorder. Dependence almost always develops insidiously over a time course of months or years, part and parcel with repeated bouts of drug intoxication. In the largest available epidemiologic sample of cases with a history of drug dependence and/or drug abuse, the median time from initial drug use to the initially recognized symptom was 2–3 years (Anthony and Helzer, 1991).

Contemporary case definitions for clinical practice and research on drug dependence are based primarily on neuropsychopharmacologic criteria (e.g., tolerance and withdrawal) and on behavioral criteria (e.g., drug seeking and drug taking). In some instances, the case definitions also refer to social maladaptation secondary to drug use; some stress a subjectively felt compulsion to take the drug, a craving, or some other similar disturbance in the mental life that can be linked to drug use. When attempts have been made to distinguish drug dependence from "drug abuse" and "harmful drug use" this typically has been accomplished by restricting the latter to socially maladaptive or harm-causing drug use without the complications implied by neuropsychopharmacologic criteria or by subjectively felt compulsions and craving (World Health Organization, 1992; Babor, 1992).

The neuropsychopharmacologic criteria of central importance to the diagnosis of drug dependence involve neuroadaptation that occurs secondary to drug exposure. Some aspects of neuroadaptation can be documented very early in the drug dependence process, for example, a pharmacologic tolerance manifest by change in the slopes or intercepts of dose–response curves upon repeated drug exposures. Other signs of neuroadaptation, such as the appearance of a drug withdrawal syndrome, are not readily apparent as clinical phenomena unless the drug dependence process is challenged by 1) administration of antagonists, such as the opioid antagonist naltrexone in the case of dependence on heroin or other opioids, or 2) an abrupt reduction in dosage or a complete cessation of drug use after drug-taking has been sustained for days or weeks.

In some cases, withdrawal symptoms appear several times daily and serve as a forerunner for subsequent drug-seeking and drug-taking behavior that can relieve the withdrawal symptoms for a time. In other cases, withdrawal symptoms are mild and infrequent and may escape clinical detection unless the drug-dependent patient is challenged under restrictive conditions.

Going beyond neuroadaptation, drug seeking and drug taking are represented among the criteria of drug dependence that tap its behavioral dimensions. Consistent with a description of the alcohol dependence syndrome first stated by Edwards and Gross (1976), these behavioral manifestations of drug dependence can be grouped under headings such as "salience" and "withdrawal avoidance." Salience of drug seeking or drug taking occurs together with the increasing time demands associated with drug use, concurrent with reduced commitment to social, occupational, and recreational activities and sometimes to a general narrowing in the behavioral repertoire unconnected to drug taking. Withdrawal avoidance implies drug taking in order to prevent or reduce the severity of drug withdrawal symptoms.

There is not yet a universal consensus that a subjectively felt compulsion to take a drug should be included as a sine qua non criterion in drug dependence case definitions. Nonetheless, this disturbance of the mental life has become prominent in some of the newer case definitions and diagnostic criteria for drug dependence. Neither compulsions to take drugs nor drug cravings were represented in dependence criteria written for the 1980 *Diagnostic and Statistical Manual of Mental Disorders*, 3rd ed (DSM-III; American Psychiatric Association, 1980). As shown in Table 2, drug-related desires and/or compulsions now appear in diagnostic guidelines written for the International Classification of Disease, 10th rev (ICD-10; World Health Organization, 1992), and for the revised DSM-III known as DSM-III-R (American Psychiatric Association, 1987). At the time of writing this chapter, a final version of DSM-IV had not been promulgated, but advance reports from the DSM-IV task force indicate that DSM-IV generally will resemble DSM-III-R in order to reduce unwarranted disruption in diagnostic practices (Woody et al., 1993).

Careful study of the diagnostic guidelines and criteria in Table 2, with comparison to DSM-111 and earlier criteria, will be repaid by a greater appreciation for how drug dependence case definitions are changing. The observable variations in these several diagnostic systems have emerged over a span of less than 15 years.

The history of the concept of opioid dependence suggests that we should expect continual refinement of the drug dependence diagnostic criteria for many years to come and possibly some radical changes coincident with new findings from laboratory, clinical, or epidemiologic studies. Emerging originally from primitive concepts of "customs," "habit," and "addiction" as a moral enslavement or a defect of human will, these contemporary case definitions now are among the accumulated results of more than 40 years of work by the World Health Organization's Expert Committee on Drug Dependence, task panels organized for the DSM-III and DSM-III-R, more recently the DSM-IV task panel, and by others. Until strengthened by a more confirmatory body of empirical evidence, the criteria most likely will continue to be changed every half-decade or so (e.g., see Sonnedecker, 1962; Eddy et al., 1965; Musto, 1987; Kosten and Kosten, 1991; Woody et al., 1993).

Of course, continual change in the drug dependence case definitions tends to compli-

TABLE 2. DSM-III-R and ICD-10 Case Definitions

DSM-III-R

Diagnostic criteria for psychoactive substance dependence

A. At least three of the following:
1. Substance often taken in larger amounts or over a longer period than the person intended
2. Persistent desire or one or more unsuccessful efforts to cut down or control substance use
3. A great deal of time spent in activities necessary to get the substance (e.g., theft), taking the substance (e.g., chain smoking), or recovering from its effects
4. Frequent intoxication or withdrawal symptoms when expected to fulfill major role obligations at work, school, or home (e.g., does not go to work because hung over, goes to school or work "high," intoxicated while taking care of his or her children), or when substance use is physically hazardous (e.g., drives when intoxicated)
5. Important social, occupational, or recreational activities given up or reduced because of substance use
6. Continued substance use despite knowledge of having a persistent or recurrent social, psychological, or physical problem that is caused or exacerbated by the use of the substance (e.g., keeps using heroin despite family arguments about it, cocaine-induced depression, or having an ulcer made worse by drinking)
7. Marked tolerance: need for markedly increased amounts of the substance (i.e., at least a 50% increase) in order to achieve intoxication or desired effect, or markedly diminished effect with continued use of the same amount

Note: The following items may not apply to cannabis, hallucinogens, or phencyclidine (PCP):
8. Characteristic withdrawal symptoms (see specific withdrawal syndromes under Psychoactive Substance-Induced Organic Mental Disorders)
9. Substance often taken to relieve or avoid withdrawal symptoms

B. Some symptoms of the disturbance have persisted for at least 1 month or have occurred repeatedly over a longer period of time.

Diagnostic criteria for psychoactive substance abuse

A. A maladaptive pattern of psychoactive substance use indicated by at least one of the following:
1. Continued use despite knowledge of having a persistent or recurrent social, occupational, psychological, or physical problem that is caused or exacerbated by use of the psychoactive substance
2. Recurrent use in situations in which use is physically hazardous (e.g., driving while intoxicated)

B. Some symptoms of the disturbance have persisted for at least 1 month or have occurred over a longer period of time

C. Never met the criteria for Psychoactive Substance Dependence for this substance

ICD-10

Diagnostic guidelines for the dependence syndrome due to psychoactive drug use

A definite diagnosis of dependence should usually be made only if three or more of the following have been experienced or exhibited at some time during the period year:

A. A strong desire or sense of compulsion to take the substance
B. Difficulties in controlling substance-taking behavior in terms of its onset, termination, or levels of use
C. A physiological withdrawal state when substance use has ceased or been reduced, as evidenced by the characteristic withdrawal syndrome for the substance or use of the same (or a closely related) substance with the intention of relieving or avoiding withdrawal symptoms

TABLE 2. DSM-III-R and ICD-10 Case Definitions (*Continued*)

D. Evidence of tolerance, such that increased doses of the psychoactive substance are required in order to achieve effects originally produced by lower doses (clear examples of this are found in alcohol- and opiate-incapacitate or kill nontolerant users)

E. Progressive neglect of alternative pleasures or interests because of psychoactive substance use; increased amount of time necessary to obtain or take the substance or to recover from its effects

F. Persisting with substance use despite clear evidence of overtly harmful consequences, such as harm to the liver through excessive drinking, depressive mood states consequent to periods of heavy substance use, or drug-related impairment of cognitive functioning; efforts should be made to determine that the user was actually, or could be expected to be, aware of the nature and extent of the harm.

SOURCES: American Psychiatric Association, 1987; World Health Organization, 1992.

cate research progress in this field. For example, in the United States, the two largest and most definitive epidemiologic studies of drug dependence have been the National Institute of Mental Health Epidemiologic Catchment Area (ECA) surveys with fieldwork conducted between 1980 and 1985, followed by the National Comorbidity Survey conducted between 1990 and 1992. The ECA Program was a multisite collaborative study, with an aggregate sample that included almost 20 thousand interviewed respondents aged 18–96 years, selected by probability sampling from households, prisons, mental hospitals, and other institutions and group quarters. The ECA Program has provided epidemiologic findings based on the DSM-III criteria for drug dependence as implemented by the Diagnostic Interview Schedule (DIS) method, which combined assessments by standardized interview with computer-assisted diagnostic procedures (Robins et al., 1985; Anthony and Helzer, 1991).

The National Comorbidity Survey (NCS), initiated less than 5 years after the end of data gathering for the ECA program, involved a national probability sample with 8,098 respondents 15–54 years of age, selected by probability sampling of household residents. The NCS assessment plan made use of a DIS-like method known as the Composite International Diagnostic Interview (CIDI), with standardized interview items and a computer program based on diagnostic criteria from DSM-III-R (Kessler et al., 1994).

According to results from population surveys in the five ECA sites, cocaine dependence was nonexistent among American adults in the early 1980s. By comparison, findings from the NCS showed that an estimated 2.7% of Americans aged 15–54 years qualify as currently active or former cases of cocaine dependence. While it is plausible that the prevalence of cocaine dependence actually increased between 1985 and 1990, concurrent with declines in the recent American epidemic of cocaine experimentation, this difference in findings from the two surveys is attributable entirely to a change in the drug dependence case definitions. The DSM-III did not include a category of cocaine dependence, and this by itself explains why no cases were detected or reported in the ECA survey.

However, the DSM-III-R had adopted a diagnostic category for cocaine dependence. When the NCS applied this case definition, some cocaine users were found to have become affected by this newly recognized form of drug dependence. This recent experience serves to illustrate that between-study comparisons depend heavily on constancy or at least rough similarity in case definitions and in the manner of making case definitions operational in each study's assessment plan (Anthony et al., 1994).

CASE ASCERTAINMENT METHODS

The ECA and NCS initiatives offer a good example of contemporary practice in epidemiologic studies of drug dependence, which now rely for the most part on interview-administered standardized questions on the manifestations of drug dependence. In general, these questions are directed toward the individual respondent, with no attempt to augment the information base by gathering data from collateral informants (e.g., spouses, supervisors, coworkers) or by drawing biologic specimens to test for recent drug exposure.

For clinicians familiar with denial of drug-related problems and other complicating features of drug dependence, this method of assessment may seem to leave something to be desired. Nonetheless, it is important to recognize that denial can be a fluctuating clinical characteristic of drug dependence, perhaps most readily apparent in clinical or judicial proceedings that provide the suspected case with no shelter from self-incrimination. In contemporary epidemiologic studies such as the ECA surveys and the NCS, the investigators made special efforts to develop a respondent's trust and rapport before broaching sensitive topics of illicit behavior and to provide special assurances of confidentiality so that the respondents would be protected from harm that otherwise might come from self-disclosure of drug dependence (e.g., see Robins, 1983; Eaton et al., 1984; Johnston, 1985; Anthony et al., 1994).

The actual translation of diagnostic criteria for drug dependence into standardized interview questions for case ascertainment and diagnosis is a topic of several papers (Boyd et al., 1985; Anthony and Helzer, 1991). The underlying concept is a simple one that can be illustrated without difficulty by considering the example of pharmacologic tolerance.

When the DIS and DSM-III-R criteria ask for evidence that pharmacologic tolerance has developed, the DIS and CIDI seek the respondent's answers to standardized questions such as the following:

> DIS: Did you find you needed larger amounts of these drugs to get an effect—or that you could no longer get high on the amount you used to use?
>
> CIDI: Did you ever find that you had to use more drug than usual to get the same effect or that the same amount had less effect on you than before?

Once the answers to questions of this type have been entered into an electronic database, the diagnostic computer program checks the respondent's data record and counts an affirmative answer toward the tolerance criterion of the dependence diagnosis. A corresponding process is followed for each of the diagnostic criteria for drug dependence; respondents who meet the required criteria are designated as cases, and all others are designated as noncases.

There is universal agreement that we need more studies on the reliability and validity of this form of standardized drug dependence diagnosis. Nevertheless, to date, the result of this approach to assessment in epidemiologic field studies has been a set of alcohol and drug dependence diagnoses with levels of reliability and validity that are appreciably better than corresponding diagnoses for other categories of mental disorders (e.g., see Wittchen, 1994). In relation to the issue of diagnostic validity, it is important to remember that individuals can be drug dependent even when bioassays show no recent drug exposure—to the extent that symptoms such as compulsion to take a drug remain present for some time after drug use. It also is important to remember that many individuals who test positive for recent drug use would not qualify as cases of drug dependence: Many drug users are not drug dependent (Anthony et al., 1994). For these reasons, drug dependence is evaluated on clinical grounds, and the validity of drug dependence diagnoses does not depend on agreement between a bioassay for recent drug use versus a clinical diagnosis of drug dependence.

PATHOGENESIS OF DRUG DEPENDENCE

Drug dependence will not occur, and the full syndrome of drug dependence cannot persist, in the complete absence of a drug. For this reason, it makes sense to think of each drug as an important etiologic agent in relation to the occurrence of dependence on that drug. Analogous to an agent of infectious disease that must be conveyed from its reservoir of origin toward effective contact with a human host, a drug must be conveyed to its users from the point or points of origin, which might include agricultural fields (e.g., for marijuana, opium poppy, or coca leaf) as well as chemistry laboratories (e.g., for a barbiturate sedative-hypnotic or for methamphetamine). Humans are the vectors that bring drugs out of their reservoirs and into contact with drug users (e.g., see Anthony, 1983); once drug taking begins, there is person-to-person diffusion of drug-taking behavior and drug dependence (e.g., see de Alarcon, 1969; Hanzi, 1976).

Working from the reservoir of drug supply toward the clinical case of drug dependence, it is possible to identify moments or intervals of exposure opportunity before which there is no chance of drug dependence. For many individuals, exposure opportunities are presented by members of their peer groups, and it appears that exposure opportunity may be determined in part by an individual's social class, level of paternal alcohol consumption, history of childhood misbehavior (e.g., truancy), low emotional control, and patterns of social interactions with peers and others. It follows that effective prevention and control of drug dependence depends in part on regulation of exposure opportunities and by attention to the determinants of these exposure opportunities (e.g., see Hawkins et al., 1992; Stenbacka et al., 1993; Crum et al., 1994).

Once an exposure opportunity has occurred, drug dependence cannot develop unless there is an effective contact manifest in some form of biologic response, for example, a drug intoxication state. As in the case of infective agents, effective contact with a drug also can be measured in the form of immune response to antigen. Current molecular biologic research supported by the National Institute on Drug Abuse and others holds promise for future development of improved immunoassays for drug exposure as well as possible immunizing agents that might modulate biologic responsivity once drug exposure occurs (e.g., see Landry et al., 1993).

A single effective contact is not sufficient for the development of drug dependence. Typically, drug dependence will not develop unless there are repeated bouts of drug intoxication over a span of days or weeks, signifying multiple effective contacts. The reinforcing function of drug taking may become apparent as early as the second occurrence of effective contact; multiple bouts of drug intoxication may serve as an indicator of the reinforcing efficacy of drug use. However, differences in availability of individual drugs can determine the frequency and duration of their use, notwithstanding a broad contrast in the laboratory evidence on relative reinforcement potential of these drugs. For example, in laboratory research it has been difficult to show that marijuana smoking is a powerful reinforcer; not so for cocaine (e.g., see Pickens et al., 1973). Nonetheless, in the United States, persistent marijuana users have outnumbered persistent cocaine users for more than two decades, most likely due to generally greater availability of marijuana (e.g., see Kandel, 1991, 1992; Harrison, 1992).

Neuroadaptation and the clinical features of drug dependence develop during the course of repeated bouts of drug intoxication. Whereas the diagnostic criteria and case definitions often imply a clear transition point before and after drug dependence, the more general experience is consistent with an insidious onset and there is no clear "first episode" of drug dependence, as is true for many other medical conditions (Beiser et al., 1993). For this reason, an "incident" case of drug dependence is one who is found upon assessment to meet the diagnostic criteria, against a background history of one or more prior assessments when full criteria have not been met (Eaton et al., 1989).

In general, retrospective data do not give a clear or distinct impression of when criteria were met for the first time, and prospective data on the timing of a first episode are no more fine-grained than the interval from one observation to the next. In this respect, drug dependence is no different from many other diseases with insidious onset that are studied routinely by epidemiologists. Research progress must be made by specifying sometimes arbitrary rules about when to date the age or time of initial onset, and age at first diagnosis sometimes is the only possibility.

Notwithstanding some notable exceptions, most of the scientific and clinical literature on the natural history of drug dependence actually concerns its clinical course in that the literature draws heavily on the experience of cases that have been treated or incarcerated (e.g., see Vaillant, 1966; Sells, 1977; McGlothlin, 1985; Anglin et al., 1986; Nurco et al., 1989). The result can be a distorted view of what happens "in nature" when drug dependence is left without intervention, as often is the case (e.g., see Smart, 1977; Anthony and Helzer, 1991; Robins, 1993).

The "clinical course" of drug dependence is its natural history modified by one or more experiences of clinical intervention. Under these circumstances, the course generally is portrayed as chronic and with few lasting remissions: Relapse is said to be the rule rather than the exception. Often, the course is complicated by legal problems connected to drug seeking or drug taking, as well as intervals of incarceration within the criminal justice system (e.g., see Haastrup, 1973; Nurco et al., 1989).

Mortality rates for drug-dependent cases have been observed to exceed those of age-matched controls, even when differences in gender and social class are taken into account. Although "drug dependence" is allowable as a recognized cause of death, many drug-dependent individuals die prematurely from other proximal causes, such as homicide, suicide, opportunistic infections secondary to drug injection practices, and drug overdosage (e.g., see Sapira et al., 1970; Sells, 1977). Of course, many of these premature deaths might be prevented if drug dependence were to be recognized, kept under medical surveillance, and treated as a chronic medical condition.

Given the overwhelming impression of a serious and chronic condition that does not respond well to treatment or to changes in environmental conditions, the experience of Vietnam veterans returning to the United States is noteworthy and deserves careful scrutiny (e.g., see Robins, 1977; 1993; Helzer, 1985). Consistent with evidence from recent epidemiologic surveys in the United States (e.g., see Anthony and Helzer, 1991; Anthony et al., 1994), the experience of these soldiers seems to suggest that it was relatively common to become drug dependent and then to return to nondependent periods of abstinence, without treatment. One of the pressing items on the research agenda for drug dependence is to clarify this difference between findings on the "clinical course" of drug dependence based on studies of treated or incarcerated cases versus findings on its "natural history" based on both treated and untreated cases.

THE OCCURRENCE AND FREQUENCY OF DRUG DEPENDENCE

In common with most mental disorders, drug dependence takes its toll during life and leaves very little trace after death. For this reason, mortality rates based on deaths attributed to drug dependence are an unstable foundation for epidemiologic inferences, and with no more than a few exceptions epidemiologists generally have turned to the field survey method in order to study the occurrence (incidence) and frequency (prevalence) of this condition in human populations.

The Occurrence (Incidence) of Drug Dependence

Incidence values are *rates* that deserve special attention because they help to convey the probability of *becoming* a case of drug dependence for the first time, among members of a defined population. An incidence estimate is one way to express the risk of developing drug dependence during some span of time. By comparing incidence or risk estimates for different subgroups of a population, it is possible to discriminate conditions of heightened risk and risk factors, as distinct from prevalence correlates that do not determine risk of drug dependence (e.g., see Anthony et al., 1994).

It is important to recognize that drug-taking can be conceptualized and measured in relation to an underlying dimension that runs from no drug use upward through increasing levels of drug involvement. Many strengths and benefits accrue by studying drug taking in this fashion (e.g., see Pandina et al., 1981). Nonetheless, when investigators specify dimensional drug taking as an outcome in their studies, they have abandoned the statistical concept of risk, and in a formal sense they no longer can gain a direct view of the risk factors for drug taking or drug dependence. Indeed, there is no compelling reason to think that a profile of risk factors for the transition from no use to initial drug use should be identical to the profile of risk factors for the transition from drug experimentation to fully developed drug dependence (e.g., see Robins, 1977; Anthony, 1991a; Glantz, 1992; Smart, 1992; Anthony et al., 1994).

To our knowledge, the ECA program has been the only epidemiologic study that has sought to estimate prospectively the incidence of drug dependence for a general population, using standardized diagnostic assessments in the context of an epidemiologic field survey. By means of a prospective study design and taking advantage of repeatedly administered DIS assessments, ECA surveys conducted in four American communities have provided evidence on the occurrence of drug dependence in adulthood, measured as a cumulative annual incidence estimate of 1.09% for the diagnostic category of drug dependence combined with drug abuse (Eaton et al., 1989). Approximately 40% of identified cases in the ECA surveys have been found to qualify for a diagnosis of drug abuse without drug dependence; the remaining 60% qualified for drug dependence with or without drug abuse (Anthony and Helzer, 1991). Thus, assuming generalizability of these estimates from the ECA sites to the nation as a whole, for adults living in the United States during the early 1980s, an estimated 0.6%, or 6 per 1,000, were found to become incident cases of drug dependence during a 1 year interval of observation.

By comparison with this approximate annual incidence value of 6 cases of drug dependence per 1,000 adults in the population, an estimated 6 per 1,000 American adults become incident cases of panic disorder each year, and an estimated 7 per 1,000 develop obsessive-compulsive disorder. For major depression and alcohol abuse/dependence syndromes, the estimated risk is slightly more than 15 incident cases per 1,000 per year. Phobic disorders among adults developed at an annual rate of 40 cases per 1,000 per year, and the other mental disorders were observed to occur too infrequently for suitable estimates, despite the unprecedented large size of the ECA sample within the field of psychiatric epidemiology (Eaton et al., 1989).

The Frequency (Prevalence) of Drug Dependence

Lifetime Prevalence. In contrast with incidence, prevalence values are *proportions* that communicate the probability of *being* affected by drug dependence within a defined population. Among persons who have survived to some specific time, the lifetime prevalence expresses the probability of being a currently active or a former case of drug dependence—that is, among these survivors, lifetime prevalence is the probability of having become a case during the span of life prior to assessment (Kramer et al., 1980).

When studying drug dependence, it is especially important to link the concept of survivorship with the concept of lifetime prevalence. To the extent that drug dependence accounts for excess mortality, a lifetime prevalence value can understate the cumulative probability of developing drug dependence. Furthermore, lifetime prevalence comparisons can give a distorted view of high-risk groups. That is, if two groups have equal risk of developing drug dependence, but different risks of dying from drug-related causes, then lifetime prevalence comparisons will suggest falsely that the group with long-surviving cases is at greater risk of drug dependence than the group whose cases die sooner (Kramer et al., 1980).

Because lifetime prevalence confounds the forces of becoming drug dependent together with the forces of mortality, our analyses of lifetime prevalence data generally cannot provide the definitive epidemiologic evidence required to discriminate risk factors or conditions of heightened risk from other correlates of prevalence. Nonetheless, lifetime prevalence estimates can help us to understand how commonly drug dependence has affected a population and may serve as a guide toward more definitive epidemiologic research on risk factors (Anthony et al., 1994).

No more than a handful of surveys have produced usable estimates for lifetime prevalence of drug dependence, separated from the condition of drug abuse. When a DIS-like method and DSM-III criteria were used in a survey of adults in Taiwan, an estimated 0.8% of metropolitan Taipei residents were found to have become drug dependent as compared with a prevalence estimate of 2.0% for residents of small towns. In the rural villages of Taiwan, no cases of drug dependence were found (Hwu et al., 1989).

In the United States between 1980 and 1985, the ECA surveys of adults aged 18 years and older found lifetime prevalence of drug dependence to be close to 3.0%, according to the DIS/DSM-III method. In 1990–1992, the NCS survey of 15–54-year-old American household residents applied the CIDI/DSM-III-R method and produced a lifetime prevalence estimate of 7.5%. This larger NCS value appears to be due primarily to changes in the diagnostic criteria for drug dependence from DSM-III to DSM-III-R, including the addition of a DSM-III-R cocaine dependence category. Another potential source of variation in survey estimates was a slightly different way of grouping the controlled substances for the NCS, and inclusion of a new category for dependence on inhalants such as glue and other volatile intoxicants (Anthony et al., 1994). In a later section of this chapter, there is a discussion of how different age compositions of the samples might have led to larger overall NCS prevalence values.

Grouping drug dependence with the syndrome of drug abuse, and applying the DIS/DSM-III method, epidemiologists studying adults in different geographic locations have produced lifetime prevalence estimates with a range from under 1% (Taiwan, Korea, and Puerto Rico) to 6.9% (Edmonton, Canada) and 7.6% (Los Angeles, CA). In Christchurch (New Zealand), and in ECA surveys of Baltimore, New Haven, and St. Louis, the lifetime prevalence estimates have been within the range from 5.6% to 5.9%. A lower value of 3.8% was found in the Durham-Piedmont ECA site, and in Munich (Germany) a modified DIS-like method was used for follow-up assessments of an adult population sample, yielding a lifetime prevalence value of 1.8%. Differences in sampling plans and samples (e.g., age composition) account for some unknown part of the variation in these estimates (Bland et al., 1988a; Hwu et al., 1989; Wells et al., 1989; Lee et al., 1990a,b; Anthony and Helzer, 1991; Wittchen et al., 1992; Canino et al., 1993).

The lifetime prevalence of alcohol dependence and/or abuse generally has been found to be roughly two to three times greater than the lifetime prevalence of the drug abuse/dependence syndromes. For example, lifetime prevalence estimates from the NCS are 14.1% for alcohol dependence and 7.5% for dependence on controlled substances (Anthony et al., 1994). However, to date, no ECA-like or NCS-like surveys have been conducted in a Moslem country, where the relative prevalence of these conditions might be reversed due to religious proscription of alcohol use.

By grouping alcohol abuse/dependence syndromes together with abuse/dependence syndromes involving internationally controlled substances, it is possible to gain a better appreciation for the magnitude of psychiatric disorders directly connected with the use of these psychoactive substances. By this standard, in the United States an estimated 17% of adults 18 years of age or older have become cases as identified by the DIS/DSM-III method (Anthony and Helzer, 1991). Using the CIDI/DSM-III-R method to study younger Americans aged 15–54 years, and combining the alcohol and other drug use disorders in a similar fashion, Kessler et al. (1994) reported that 26.6% had become cases of abuse and/or dependence. The corresponding estimate for Christchurch (New Zealand) and Edmonton (Canada) was 21%, while it was 13.5% according to the modified DIS-like method used in the Munich Follow-Up Study (Bland et al., 1988a; Wells et al., 1989; Helzer et al., 1990; Wittchen et al., 1992).

The ECA and NCS initiatives have provided a useful glimpse of drug-specific lifetime prevalence values, as depicted in Table 3. The lifetime prevalence of alcohol dependence was 14.1% in the NCS data, mentioned above. According to ECA estimates, some 13% had become cases of alcohol dependence and/or abuse (Helzer et al., 1991). Given that some 80%–90% of adult Americans have consumed alcohol, roughly 15%–20% of alcohol users had become cases (Anthony et al., 1994).

About 4% of the 15–54-year-old household population had become cases of cannabis dependence by NCS estimates. A corresponding value of 4.4% was obtained from the ECA surveys of all adults, which combined cannabis dependence with cannabis abuse. Among cannabis users, approximately 9%–20% had become cases (Anthony and Helzer, 1991; Anthony et al., 1994). By comparison, reporting on their valuable longitudinal sample of young men and women in New York State, Kandel and Davies (1992) have estimated that almost one-half of the young male marijuana users had started near-daily marijuana use by ages 28–29, and about 37% of the young female marijuana users had done so.

Close to 3% of adults had become cases of cocaine dependence by NCS estimates, and 0.2% qualified for cocaine abuse by ECA estimates; cocaine dependence was not assessed in the ECA study. Among cocaine users, slightly more than 15% had become cocaine dependent, and about 3% had qualified for the DSM-III cocaine abuse diagnosis (Anthony and Helzer, 1991; Anthony et al., 1994).

TABLE 3. A Comparison of Lifetime Prevalence Estimates for Drug Dependence Syndromes, Based on the National Comorbidity Survey (NCS) and the Epidemiologic Catchment Area (ECA) Surveys, Specific for Individual Drug Groups.[a]

Drug Group	NCS Estimate (%)	ECA Estimate (%)
Alcohol	14.1	13.0
Cannabis	4.2	4.4
Cocaine	2.7	NA
Heroin	0.4	<0.7
Stimulants[b]	1.7	1.7
ASH drugs[c]	1.2	1.2
Hallucinogens	0.5	0.4
Inhalants	0.3	NA

[a] The NCS surveyed U.S. household residents 15–54 years of age between 1990–1992, with CIDI/DSM-III-R assessment of the drug dependence syndromes. The ECA surveys were conducted between 1980 and 1984, encompassed both household and non-household residents age 18 years of age and older, and used Diagnostic Interview Schedule assessments of drug dependence and drug abuse, defined in terms of the DSM-III criteria.

[b] Here, the stimulant group includes methamphetamine and other amphetamines as well as methylphenidate and other psychostimulants, but does not include cocaine products.

[c] The ASH drugs are anxiolytic (tranquilizer), sedative, and hypnotic drugs, such as diazepam and other benzodiazepines marketed at the time of each survey, and the barbiturates.

SOURCES Anthony and Helzer, 1991; Anthony et al., 1994.

For other controlled substances, the NCS estimates for the dependence syndrome did not differ appreciably from the ECA estimates for the dependence syndromes combined with the category of drug abuse. Among heroin users, more than 20% had developed heroin dependence and/or abuse. Among users of stimulants (other than cocaine), more than 10% had become cases of stimulant dependence or abuse. Among users of sedative, hypnotic, or anxiolytic drugs, an estimated 10%–25% had developed dependence or abuse involving these drugs. For hallucinogens, the corresponding value was under 10% (Anthony and Helzer, 1991; Anthony et al., 1994).

It also is instructive to make a comparison to lifetime prevalence values for tobacco dependence, now available only for three locales. Using a DIS-like method and DSM-III criteria to study adults (aged 18–64) in urban and rural Korea, epidemiologists found that 20% of urban residents and 21% of rural residents had become tobacco dependent (Lee et al., 1990b). When the same methods were used in Taiwan, the lifetime prevalence of tobacco dependence was found to be 7.8% in metropolitan Taipei, 12.2% in small towns of Taiwan, and 13.6% in the rural villages of Taiwan (Hwu et al., 1989). The NCS estimate for lifetime prevalence of tobacco dependence, based on the CIDI/DSM-III-R method, was 24.1%. Among those who had used tobacco, roughly 32 percent had developed tobacco dependence, a value not too distant from a corresponding estimate of 27% based on a population sample of young adults living in the Detroit, Michigan area (Breslau et al., 1993).

This overview of lifetime prevalence estimates helps to substantiate a growing awareness in psychiatry and public health that many persons are affected by dependence on the internationally regulated drugs such as marijuana, cocaine, and heroin—particularly in nations of the Western world, where a general finding is that well over 1% of the adult population has become drug dependent. Moreover, there are some areas where an estimated 3%–8% of adults can be discovered to have a history of drug dependence (e.g., see Bland et al., 1988b; Wells et al., 1989; Anthony et al., 1994).

These forms of drug dependence occur against a background of somewhat higher lifetime prevalence values for alcohol and tobacco. To the extent that drug dependence is sustained by some of the same forces that give rise to high frequency of alcohol dependence and tobacco dependence, effective control of drug dependence may require coordinated action in relation to alcohol and tobacco as well.

Research to be conducted over the next decade quite likely will show that dependence on coffee and other caffeine-containing products is a widely prevalent condition in many countries of the world: If caffeine supplies were disrupted, symptoms of headache and other manifestations of caffeine withdrawal would affect many individuals. Nonetheless, it is not at all clear that caffeine dependence merits inclusion within diagnostic classifications for mental disorders. This issue now is under discussion (Hughes et al., 1992; Woody et al., 1993).

Point Prevalence and Interval Prevalence. Complementing the information from lifetime prevalence estimates, interval prevalence estimates can be used to express the probability of being a recently active case of drug dependence. For example, a 1-year prevalence value conveys the probability of being active within a 1 year interval prior to the assessment session (e.g., see Kessler et al., 1994).

The published literature includes 1 month and 6 month prevalence estimates, as well as 1 year prevalence estimates for drug dependence (Myers et al., 1984; Regier et al., 1988; Kessler et al., 1994). To our knowledge, no one has published estimates for point prevalence, that is, the proportion affected by drug dependence at some specific defined *point* in time.

In common with lifetime prevalence, interval prevalence is affected by survivorship of cases relative to noncases and does not give a clear view of the risk to become a case. In addition, interval prevalence is affected more generally by the duration of drug dependence, where duration can be influenced by factors such as availability and access to early intervention or treatment. That is, even when two groups have equal risk of developing drug dependence and equal risk of dying from drug-related causes, the probability of being an active case can be shown to depend on the duration of being an active case. For example, if the advantage of earlier or more effective intervention leads one group to have mainly short-duration cases relative to the longer-duration and more chronic cases in another less-advantaged group, then the two groups will differ in their 1 year prevalence values: Earlier and more effective intervention will lead to lower interval prevalence values (see Anthony et al., 1992, for a detailed discussion of this issue in relation to risk factor research on drug dependence syndromes).

Despite these complications, interval prevalence estimates are useful because they serve to tell us *how many* persons have recently been affected by drug dependence. As distinct from the former cases, these recently active cases represent the potential burden and caseload for current early intervention and treatment programs.

According to ECA 1 year prevalence estimates for the adult population of the United States, an estimated 2.7% ($\pm0.22\%$) were recently active cases of drug dependence and/or drug abuse with at least one symptom or drug-related problem occurring in the 1 year prior to assessment (Anthony and Helzer, 1991). In the small towns of Taiwan, the 1 year prevalence of drug dependence/abuse was 1.3%, but in metropolitan Taipei and in rural villages the survey found essentially no recently active cases (Hwu et al., 1989). For Christchurch (New Zealand), a comparable 6 month prevalence estimate was 1.5% (±0.4%), as reported by Oakley-Browne and colleagues (1989); in the Munich Follow-Up Study (Wittchen et al., 1992), it was 0.6% (±0.24%).

For many purposes, it can be useful to say that a case of drug dependence remains active until drug use stops: Among cases of drug dependence, continuing drug use may be taken as an indicator that the dependence process has not been interrupted. In some instances, this approach to dating the recency of drug dependence produces an increase in the number of active cases and in the 1 year prevalence estimate. For example, the 1 year prevalence of active drug dependence and/or abuse in the Baltimore ECA was 2.9% (±0.3%) when cases were defined as active if they had experienced at least one dependence symptom or drug-related problem within the year prior to assessment; the estimate was 4.0% (±0.4%) when cases were defined as active if they reported drug use within the year prior to assessment. In the Los Angeles ECA, the increase was from 2.9% (±0.3%) to 4.6% (±0.4%). Of course, this approach to prevalence estimation is available only when investigators assess recency of drug use in addition to recency of drug problems (Anthony and Helzer, 1991).

By the same token, an extremely conservative approach can be taken by requiring a case to meet *all* of the criteria for drug dependence in the recent past. Working along these lines, and focusing specifically on cases of DSM-III-R drug dependence who met the full criteria for dependence during the 1 year prior to assessment, the NCS has estimated that 1.8% of 15–54-year-old Americans (±0.2%) qualify as recently active drug dependence cases (Kessler et al., 1994). The group of recently active cases primarily was affected by marijuana dependence, cocaine dependence, and/or dependence on other psychostimulant drugs such as the amphetamines. The corresponding 1 year prevalence estimate for alcohol dependence, from the same source, was 4.4% (±0.4%).

Summary Overview

Currently available prospective data indicate that the risk of developing drug dependence is just under 1% per year for adults in the United States. There are no available incidence estimates for teenagers or for other countries of the world.

Recent estimates for the lifetime prevalence of drug dependence indicate a broad range from under 1% in some countries (e.g., Korea, Puerto Rico) to above 3% in other locales (e.g., Christchurch, New Zealand; Edmonton, Canada; Los Angeles, CA). The proportion of drug users who develop drug dependence seems to vary considerably from one drug category to another and most likely is determined by factors such as drug availability as much as by the reinforcing functions served by these drugs. For example, among alcohol users, the proportion who had become cases of alcohol dependence and/or abuse has been estimated to be 15%–20%, not too distant from that observed for users of cocaine but slightly greater than the proportion observed for cannabis users. For users of tobacco and users of heroin, the proportion appears to be higher, sometimes approaching or exceeding 30% (e.g., see Anthony et al., 1994).

In the United States, the 1 year prevalence of drug dependence is between 1.4 and 2.2

active cases per 100 persons aged 15–54 years. In other countries where comparable surveys have been taken, the 1 year prevalence of drug dependence is lower than this.

Based on these estimates for adults living in the United States, the 1 year prevalence of drug dependence is some two to four times the cumulative annual incidence of drug dependence. This relationship between 1 year prevalence and cumulative annual incidence is consistent with the concept of drug dependence as a persistent psychiatric disturbance with a duration of more than 1 year. For every newly developed incident case of drug dependence in the adult population at present, there are several other adults whose drug dependence started some years back and who continue to be burdened by its complications in their present lives.

SUSPECTED DETERMINANTS OF DRUG DEPENDENCE PREVALENCE

An important goal for epidemiologic research on drug dependence, beyond quantifying its occurrence and frequency, is to identify its determinants in human populations and to translate these research findings into practical strategies for public health work and preventive psychiatry. As discussed in the prior section of this chapter, prevalence is influenced not only by the conditions and processes out of which drug dependence develops but also by forces that extend or shorten the duration of drug dependence, including mortality rates.

In this context, mortality rates are important for two reasons. First, excess mortality associated with drug dependence will reduce the duration of drug dependence and the survivorship of cases, with a resulting downward impact on prevalence values. Second, mortality rates together with birth rates can affect the broad age structure of human populations, and certain changes in age structure can yield either dramatic increases or dramatic declines in the number of cases of drug dependence over spans of 10–20 years, even when there is no change in other factors that influence risk or duration of drug dependence. For example, as discussed in the following section on age-specific risk and prevalence of drug dependence, the number of cases of drug dependence in many countries will increase dramatically between 1990 and 2010 solely as a result of demographic shifts in the population of these countries, due largely to high birth rates and declining mortality rates. These increases will occur unless there are compensatory changes in the other determinants of prevalence, including such factors as more effective prevention or treatment initiatives (Anthony, 1992).

As in all of epidemiology, our capacity to translate drug dependence research findings into practical strategies rests in part on our discrimination of risk-modifying conditions and processes from duration-modifying conditions and processes. This capacity is impaired to the extent that our epidemiologic research on drug dependence has produced no more than prevalence estimates and has failed to shed light on incidence, risk, and risk factors (e.g., see Anthony, 1993). What follows is a summary overview of promising leads in relation to what might influence prevalence of drug dependence either by reducing risk or by shortening its duration. In many instances, our knowledge is constrained because we have many studies based on prevalent cases found in cross-sectional surveys but few estimates from good epidemiologic studies of incident cases of drug dependence.

The breadth of suspected determinants of prevalence ranges from the microscopic to the macroscopic, from maps of our human genome to maps of human social environments and group characteristics such as shared social values and customs. The current program of genome mapping will help to clarify possible genetic vulnerability to drug dependence by identifying specific candidate genes for drug dependence. New research on families headed by drug-dependent parents will shed light on impaired parenting practices, supportive community and school programs, and other suspected environmental determinants of drug dependence.

The search for these determinants is made more exciting and challenging by the prospect of interactions between various determinants, for example, the discovery of protective environmental factors that might modify what otherwise should be moderate or high risks linked to heredity or other family factors. Our plans for these discoveries can build from what has been observed about drug dependence in relation to demographic risk factors associated with sex and age—for which we have some risk estimates as well as prevalence estimates. Ultimately, it should be possible to develop more effective prevention and control strategies for public health work by drawing on new knowledge about the separate and inter-related contributions of social, psychological, and other biologic conditions that foster and sustain drug dependence in human populations.

Demographic Risk Factors: Sex and Age

Sex, Gender Roles, and Drug Dependence. Modern awareness of drug dependence emerged from a nineteenth century view of morphine addiction as a "soldier's disease," mainly affecting American Civil War veterans—men who had received morphine by injection for relief of pain due to wounds of battle and associated trauma. By the early twentieth century, clinical attention shifted somewhat, more in the direction of problems experienced by women who were taking large daily doses of nonprescription patent medicines and other products containing alcohol, tincture of opium, or morphine, or perhaps the newer products of a growing pharmaceutical industry: for example, heroin derived from the opium poppy; cocaine extracted from coca leaf; chloral hydrate or other drugs used to calm, sedate, or bring sleep. Some attention also was given to opium smoking, apparently practiced by Chinese of both sexes, but made notorious in the United States by popular stories of Chinese immigrant-laborers whose opium dens lured not only men but also women later entrapped into prostitution and slavery (Musto, 1987).

With enforcement of laws to regulate supply, distribution, and use of these drugs, including early twentieth century international treaties, the bulk of clinical and scientific attention shifted back to drug dependence among individuals—mainly men—who would break the law to sustain their drug taking. In part, this emphasis on men may have been due to creation in the late 1920s of a United States Public Health Service research program on drug addiction, which until the 1970s drew study subjects primarily from men incarcerated for drug-related federal offenses. However, from the late nineteenth century onward, there has been a continuing stream of clinical case reports and occasional sociologic or ethnographic studies featuring narrative descriptions of women who suffered from drug dependence. This early research set the stage for more contemporary epidemiologic studies of drug taking and drug dependence in various countries, which now generally show that both sexes are affected, men somewhat more than women (e.g., see Rae and Braude, 1989; Kandel, 1991).

Recent ECA estimates for annual incidence of drug dependence and/or drug abuse corroborate a general pattern of male preponderance among drug-dependent individuals. Based on ECA estimates for adult men, the risk of developing a drug dependence/abuse syndrome has been observed to be close to 1.7% per year; the corresponding value for adult women is lower, at about 0.7% per year (Eaton et al., 1989). Lifetime prevalence values for men have exceeded those for women in epidemiologic surveys conducted in New Zealand, Canada, the five ECA populations, and the United States household population surveyed for the NCS. Surveys conducted in Taiwan and Korea suggest a greater balance in prevalence for men and women, but the number of detected cases in these surveys was small and the statistical power to detect male–female differences was not optimal (Bland et al., 1988a; Hwu et al., 1989; Wells et al., 1989; Lee et al., 1990a,b; Anthony and Helzer, 1991; Wittchen et al., 1992; Canino et al., 1993).

Considering our general model for pathogenesis of drug dependence, it is helpful to ask whether the observed differences are due entirely to more prevalent use of controlled substances by men or whether men who take these drugs might be more likely to become drug dependent than female drug users. According to available epidemiologic data for most of the psychoactive drugs we have studied, men are more likely to take controlled substances. In addition, once drug use begins, they are more likely to become daily users and to develop drug dependence and/or drug abuse (e.g., see Kandel and Davies, 1992; Anthony et al., 1994).

It is not clear whether the original difference in drug taking can be traced to greater exposure opportunities for men versus women. If a male/female difference in exposure opportunity exists, this would point more directly toward a possible variation based on gender identities and social roles linked with sex, perhaps separate from any hypothesized sex-linked biologic differences. At present, no studies speak clearly and definitively to the issue of sex versus gender identity and gender roles in relation to the prevalence of drug dependence syndromes.

Finally, there is some evidence of male–female differences in the probability of stopping drug use once it begins (e.g., Kandel and Raveis, 1989; Anthony and Helzer, 1991). That is, for women, drug use appears to be more short-lived than for men. In conclusion, it appears that male–female differences in prevalence of drug dependence may be determined not only by differences in risk of becoming drug dependent but also by differences in duration of drug dependence.

Age and Drug Dependence. From 1870 through the 1970s, cases of virtually all ages have been described in the world literature on clinical and other scientific studies of drug dependence, with some reports on cases occurring among very mature adults in late life. The drug problems of adolescents and young adults began to receive considerably increased attention after passage of drug regulations in the early twentieth century, although in the 1950s there was some shift in focus of concern toward problems linked to adult use of legally available pharmaceutical products: for example, truck drivers and homemakers taking stimulant, sedative, and hypnotic (sleep-promoting) drugs for nonmedical reasons (e.g., see Musto, 1987).

Between 1960 and the present, a societal concern about youthful drug taking has stimulated organization of surveys of adolescent drug use in many countries of the world, as well as cross-sectional household surveys in some countries. In the United States, repeated cross-sectional surveys of students and household residents now provide epidemiologic trend data on drug taking in the population, but until recently these surveys have not attempted to assess clinical conditions such as drug dependence. Nonetheless, it is important to note that the most recent epidemiologic surveys show some evidence of increased prevalence of drug taking among adults aged 35 years and older, perhaps as a sign that drug-taking patterns acquired in adolescence and young adulthood are being carried over into the middle-age years (e.g., see United States, 1993).

Within the United States, trend data from cross-sectional surveys of drug taking were strengthened with the addition of drug dependence assessments for the ECA Program in the early 1980s. According to both cross-sectional and prospective data from the ECA surveys, the risk of developing a syndrome of drug dependence or drug abuse now varies considerably from one age stratum to the next. For example, according to the prospective study conducted by Eaton et al. (1989), the estimated risk of developing drug dependence or drug abuse was observed to be 2.8% per year for persons 18–29 years old in the early 1980s ($\pm 0.5\%$); 0.7% per year for 30–44 year olds ($\pm 0.2\%$); and less than 0.1% per year for older adults. The estimated annual incidence for males 18–29 years old was 4.4% per year ($\pm 1.1\%$); for females 18–29 years old, it was 1.6% per year ($\pm 0.45\%$).

Figure 1 gives predicted annual incidence rates for males and females aged 18 or older, derived from a logistic regression analysis of prospective data from the ECA surveys. The shape of these age-specific curves is noteworthy, with peak values at 18 years for men (almost 8% per year) and for women (2.8% per year). By implication, risk of developing drug dependence or drug abuse also must be at fairly high levels among slightly younger teenagers (aged 15–17). Retrospective data from the ECA Program, subject to limitations discussed in an earlier section of this chapter, provide some evidence on this point: The risks of developing drug dependence and drug abuse are observed to rise in early adolescence, reaching peak values between the ages of 15 and 25, and with lower values for later age strata (Burke et al., 1990). To some extent, these age-specific patterns reflect age-specific risk of initiating drug use, taking into account a possible induction period of 1–3 years from the time of initial drug use to the time of meeting full criteria for drug dependence.

Age-specific prevalence values for drug dependence correspond with age-specific incidence values and the observed chronic course of drug dependence. The ECA lifetime prevalence estimates are highest among younger American adults: considering 18–29 year olds, an estimated 9% of men and 5.5% of women have developed drug dependence. Corresponding values for 30–44 year olds are 5.1% (men) and 3.0% (women), and for older men and women the values are under 1% (Anthony and Helzer, 1991).

The generally strong relationship between age and drug dependence draws attention to the potential importance of age composition of epidemiologic samples, as well as the impact of demographic forces on the number of drug-dependence cases in the population. For example, the youngest subjects in the ECA samples were 18 years and the oldest was 96 years; many ECA subjects were 65 years or older. By comparison, the age range of subjects in the NCS was 15–54 years. In view of the association between age and drug dependence, and the exceptionally low prevalence values for adults 55 years or older, it follows that NCS prevalence estimates for drug dependence should be greater than ECA prevalence estimates and would have been greater if identical survey methods had been used in these two research programs. When considering lifetime prevalence values from DIS/DSM-III surveys in New Zealand, Munich, Korea, and Puerto Rico, it is important to consider that population coverage of these surveys was extended from ages 18 through 64 and did not include elderly residents of these countries.

Forecasting methods advocated within psychiatric epidemiology by Professor Morton Kramer make use of age-specific prevalence estimates and global projections for a changing age structure of human populations to disclose which countries should expect to maintain a stable number of mental disorder cases, which should experience increased

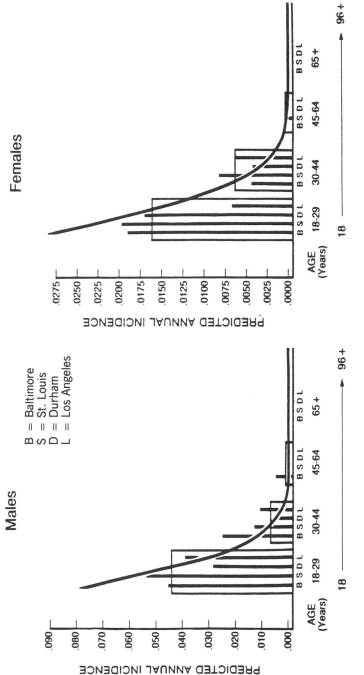

FIGURE 1. Annual incidence of DIS/DSM-III drug abuse/dependence syndromes. The smoothed curve presents annual incidence estimates for each age of adulthood, separately for males and females. The broad histogram bars give summary estimates of annual incidence for each of the following age strata: 18–29 years, 30–44 years, 45–64 years, and 65 years and older. The narrow histogram bars show variation from site to site within each given age stratum. Lack of a histogram bar for persons age 65+ years indicates an annual incidence estimate of zero, corresponding to no observed incident cases in this age group, despite large numbers of elderly study participants in the Epidemiologic Catchment Area surveys. (Reproduced with permission from Eaton et al., 1989.)

caseloads, and which should experience decreased caseloads, all else being held constant. By applying these methods, Kramer and others have been especially effective in drawing worldwide attention to an increasing prevalence of cognitive disorders such as dementia, which differentially affect the very rapidly growing elderly segments in every country's population (e.g., see Kramer, 1989).

It is less widely appreciated that the same projection methods can be applied to drug dependence and other mental disorders with a different pattern of age relationships (Kramer, 1992a). In an initial effort, Kramer has used these methods to project a stable number of white Americans with drug dependence in the United States and concurrent increases in the number of African-Americans and Hispanic-Americans affected by drug dependence (Kramer, 1992b; also discussed by Anthony, 1992).

M. Piazza has recently applied the NCS age-specific prevalence estimates for drug dependence in order to study demographic trends in various regions and countries of the world and to forecast where health planners and policy makers in each country should be preparing for an increased drug dependence caseload. Table 4 illustrates this work as applied to Brasil, where the projection method forecasts dramatic increases in the number of drug-dependent cases between 1990 and 2010. These increases are due to Brazil's recent twentieth century experience of high birth rates and declining infant mortality rates: More inhabitants of Brazil are surviving to ages when drug dependence develops. As noted elsewhere, many countries and regions are slated for increases in the number of drug-dependent persons over the next 20 years, although in North America and Western Europe the projection method shows considerable stability because the population age structure in these areas already has changed. In these regions, population growth primarily is in the very old age groups, where prevalence of drug dependence is not so high (M. Piazza, unpublished manuscript, 1993).

Values obtained from this projection method now are based on a very consistent age-specific pattern of low prevalence rates for drug dependence among the very young (under 15 years of age) and among mature adults (over 45 years of age), with higher prevalence rates among 15–44 years olds. This age-specific pattern, with the burden of drug dependence concentrated among 15–44 year olds, now generally seems to hold wherever drug-dependence surveys have been conducted and also where health statistics have been gathered on occurrence of deaths associated with drug dependence. Thus, even if the absolute number of projected cases is in error for an individual country, the overall impression of change or stability in drug dependence caseload should be correct, provided the relative differences in prevalence across age groups follow this generally observed pattern (Anthony, 1995).

In summary, recent epidemiologic surveys have revealed a general pattern for the age-specific occurrence and frequency of drug dependence: Until age 15 and after age 45, the occurrence and frequency of drug dependence are low; between 15 and 44, higher values are observed, with peak values typically between 15 and 25. Countries and regions that project new population increases for 15–44 year olds will experience increased caseloads of drug dependence, unless there are compensating conditions such as increased application of effective prevention and control strategies.

Race as a Risk Factor for Drug Dependence

One of the most common preconceptions about race and drug dependence, sometimes appearing in the drug dependence literature, is that there is something about African-Ameri-

TABLE 4. Projected Increase in Brazil's Caseload for Treatment of Drug Dependence, for the Years 1990–2010

Age Groups	Population Size in 1990	NCS Age-Specific Rates[a]	Projected Number of Active Cases in 1990	Projected Population Size in 2010	NCS Age-Specific Rates[a]	Projected Number of Active Cases in 2010	Projected Increase in Treatment Caseload from 1990 to 2010
All ages							
0–4							
5–9							
10–14	52,978,000	0.001	52,978	58,467,000	0.001	58,467	5,489
15–19							
20–24	28,670,000	0.033	946,110	37,256,000	0.033	1,229,448	283,338
25–29							
30–34	24,981,000	0.016	399,696	33,147,000	0.016	530,352	130,656
35–39							
40–44	17,478,000	0.013	227,214	27,380,000	0.013	355,940	128,726
45–49							
50–54	11,352,000	0.007	79,464	23,063,000	0.007	161,441	81,977
55+	14,909,000	0.001	14,909	28,141,000	0.001	28,141	13,232
Total number of projected cases			1,720,371			2,363,789	643,418

[a]These are estimates from the U.S. National Comorbidity Survey, indicating the proportion of each age group found to qualify as a currently or recently active case of DSM-IIIR drug dependence (with symptoms within one year of assessment). Even if these particular estimates do not apply to Brazil, there will be an increase in the number of age-specific relationships is roughly comparable to what has been observed in the United States and elsewhere, unless there are new changes in compensating conditions that determine prevalence levels.

cans to make them more vulnerable. This preconception is buttressed by studies of public treatment for drug dependence and by criminal justice research, which show disproportionate representation of African-Americans among drug-dependent patients and among persons arrested and convicted for drug-related crimes (e.g., see Kandel, 1991).

Science ethics, by itself, dictates that no epidemiologist should make superficial or casual statements about race and drug dependence, given the long tradition of research tinged with racism or used to bolster white supremacist or racist arguments. More than most observers, epidemiologists are well-equipped to understand that race is strongly confounded with social disadvantage in the Western world, where most drug dependence studies have been conducted, and elsewhere. More than most scientists, epidemiologists are equipped to design and interpret population studies that seek to disentangle the effects of social disadvantage and other high-risk environmental conditions from the effects of race as a biologic and inherited characteristic. These studies must be conducted before conclusive statements about race and drug dependence can be made (e.g., see Jones et al., 1991).

Against this background, it is important to draw attention to recent epidemiologic studies in which social disadvantage and neighborhood environment have been taken into account. In these studies, African-Americans have not been found to be at increased risk of developing drug dependence or drug abuse, relative to white Americans (Anthony, 1991a). Nor have they been found to have higher rates of taking cocaine or smoking crack (Lillie-Blanton et al., 1993; Flewelling et al., 1993). Indeed, some studies show that African-American youths are less likely to start taking drugs and alcohol than their white American adolescent peers (United States, 1993).

The excess frequency of African-Americans among publicly treated patients and among those arrested or incarcerated for drug-related crimes most likely exemplifies one or more biases in a sequence of transitions leading from the total population of cases and noncases to the more selected subpopulation admitted to public treatment and criminal justice facilities. Like the fallacy of medical statistics identified by Berkson (1946), these transition biases can lead to erroneous inferences about the causes of drug dependence. We are aware of no careful epidemiologic study showing race per se to be an important causal factor for drug dependence.

Other Suspected Determinants of Drug Dependence

The moderate-to-strong associations between sex, age, and drug dependence pose a challenge in epidemiologic research on other suspected determinants of drug dependence, which also might be related to sex and age. To protect against confounding by these factors, investigators interested in drug dependence can turn to epidemiologic strategies such as matching, stratification, or statistical modeling. More often, however, they have restricted the sex or age composition of their study samples. For example, there are more epidemiologic studies of drug dependence among males than among females, and there is essentially no strong evidence on the risk factors for drug dependence syndromes that occur past age 40.

The search for determinants of drug dependence can be conceptualized in relation to a human developmental sequence that runs from conception through childhood and adolescence to adulthood. Recent findings on the D2 dopamine receptor gene in the q22–q23 region of chromosome 11 have sparked new interest in hereditary factors in relation to drug dependence, and there also are new results from studies of suspected prenatal and perinatal determinants of drug dependence. To some extent, these findings complement earlier studies that have linked preadolescent behavioral characteristics to later risk of heavy drug use, intravenous drug use, or drug dependence. A major investment has been made in the study of adolescent drug taking, although not yet with a focus on drug dependence, as noted earlier in this chapter. Nonetheless, a small number of studies have concentrated on hypothesized risk factors for drug dependence occurring after age 18.

Heredity. There is a long tradition of clinical observations about drug dependence running in families, concurrent with similar observations about alcoholism. Heredity has become a more plausible determinant of drug dependence in recent years, due to a growing number of investigations into familial aggregation of drug dependence and twin studies and by a recent spate of implicative findings from laboratory studies of drug taking and clinical genetics.

These laboratory studies have demonstrated that dopamine is a neurotransmitter of central importance in relation to repetitive drug taking and the reinforcing function of drug use, not only for cocaine, but also for alcohol, opioids, and other drugs. Studies of dopamine activity sites within the mammalian nervous system initially identified two receptors, D1 and D2. In research to clone and express complementary DNA of the D2 dopamine receptor, it has been possible to map a D2 receptor gene in the q22–q23 region of human chromosome 11. Subsequently, restriction fragment length polymorphisms of this gene (TaqI A and B RFLPs) have been examined in case–control studies of both alcoholism and drug dependence. In some (but not all) studies, cases of alcoholism have been observed to have an excess frequency of TaqI A1 RFLP frequencies relative to control subjects (Conneally, 1991; Turner et al., 1992; Smith et al., 1992; Goldman, 1993). Furthermore, in a newer study, heavy drug use or drug abuse was more strongly associated with the TaqI B1 RFLP located near the first coding exon of the D2 dopamine receptor gene, less strongly with the TaqI A1 RFLP previously found in association with severe alcoholism (Uhl et al., 1992).

Quite clearly, this new line of research on drug dependence has produced intriguing leads about possible hereditary influences on drug dependence, which now deserve additional study and systematic replication using more definitive epidemiologic research strategies in multiple sites, coupled with the methods of molecular genetics. The desirability of conducting these studies is supported by a concurrent trend of new findings now emerging from recent family and twin studies of drug dependence, despite methodologic problems due to sampling and ascertainment biases, as well as other limitations widely known to practitioners in the rapidly evolving field of behavior genetics and genetic epidemiology.

The balance of evidence from recent twin studies of drug use and drug dependence has been in favor of an inherited genetic vulnerability. An important piece of this evidence involves results from one recent study showing an excess of monozygotic (MZ) male twin concordance for drug dependence and/or abuse (63%) relative to dizygotic (DZ) male twin concordance (43%) and a generally consistent but less pronounced difference for female twin pairs. Although constrained somewhat by a possibility that MZ twins share environments more closely than DZ twins, the data from this study also provided preliminary estimates for the genetic components of liability for drug dependence and/or abuse: an estimated 31% for male twins ($\pm18\%$); an estimated 22% for females ($\pm45\%$). That is, even granting an inherited component, the evidence favors a large contribution from environmental conditions—larger than that observed for alcoholism and perhaps attributable to shared exposure opportunities for illicit drug use, even within MZ twin pairs (Pickens et al., 1991; Labuda et al., 1993).

The current evidence from twin studies of drug dependence also includes a finding that risk of drug abuse is greater for twins adopted away from biologic families with a history of alcohol problems (e.g., see Cadoret et al., 1980, 1986; Cadoret, 1992). The observed occurrence of drug abuse also was greater for twins adopted into families characterized by divorce or a history of psychiatric disturbances, even when there was no biologic family history of drug abuse.

Clearly the best approach to clarify the inherited vulnerabilities to drug dependence will be multifaceted. One facet will involve molecular genetics, but this research will not stop when candidate genes for drug dependence are identified. Upon reaching that stage, it will be necessary to find or to design mutable environmental conditions or other interventions capable of modifying genes or gene products that predispose toward drug dependence. The earliest indication of these conditions may come from studies of siblings, including MZ and DZ twin pairs, who are discordant for drug dependence and whose history of experience from the chorionic sac onward can be traced with reasonable accuracy and precision. While the MZ–DZ concordance ratios signal important genetic vulnerabilities to drug dependence, the existence of many discordant MZ twins now constitutes our strongest evidence that environmental conditions are major risk factors for drug dependence.

Familial Aggregation of Drug Dependence. Even before the human genome mapping project, the discovery of RFLPs linking the D2 dopamine receptor gene with drug dependence, and recent twin study evidence on concordance of drug dependence there was considerable research activity in relation to a possible familial aggregation of drug dependence. By 1985, Croughan was able to review nine studies concerning the occurrence of alcohol or drug dependence in families of patients admitted to drug treatment facilities. Compared with historical controls rather than internal controls for each study, the overall observed occurrence of drug dependence in parents and siblings seemed to be higher than expected values, especially among males—consistent with patterns of hypothesized familial aggregation (Croughan, 1985). Since then, research groups led by Mirin et al. (1991) and by Rounsaville and Merikangas have contributed additional evidence, also consistent with patterns of hypothesized familial aggregation among parents and siblings (Rounsaville et al., 1991; Merikangas et al., 1992; Luthar et al., 1992a,b, 1993).

Four important advances were made in the recent work led by Rounsaville and Merikangas. First, many of the siblings of opioid-dependent subjects had not experimented with illicit drug use, although more than a majority had done so. In this respect, they were no different from most adolescents and young adults growing up in the United States. However, in contrast with available epidemiologic evidence on the transition from drug use to drug dependence, virtually all of the drug-using siblings later developed drug dependence and/or drug abuse. Second, in this research statistical models were used to hold constant alternative suspected risk factors (e.g., sex and age) as well as methodologic conditions (e.g., method of case ascertainment). Even under these more rigorous circumstances the investigators found evidence that parental drug disorders signaled an increased risk for drug dependence or abuse among siblings of opioid-dependent patients. Third, drug dependence and/or abuse was more likely to occur when both parents were affected by drug disorders compared with the experience of siblings with only one parent or neither parent affected. Finally, a very large majority of the spouses of opioid-dependent patients were found to have developed drug dependence and/or drug abuse themselves, with implications not only for future studies of assortative mating in relation to drug disorders but also for studies that seek to understand how children might be influenced by drug dependence within the family.

One important implication of these findings is that the offspring of drug-dependent parents are not universally disadvantaged by drug dependence or related problems: Unlike many of their contemporaries and as distinct from their opioid-dependent siblings, a large number had not experimented with illicit drug use. Similar findings have emerged from other recent investigations into the offspring of alcohol- and drug-dependent parents based on yoking together small clinical and community samples.

In summary, coupled with other research on the inheritance of drug dependence, and drawing on the epidemiologic survey estimates for frequency of drug use and drug dependence, the studies of familial aggregation challenge a belief that occurrence of drug dependence can be explained entirely by sociologic or psychological factors. To be sure, more definitive research is needed before we can identify and control the mechanisms that account for observed familial aggregation of drug dependence. The present state of knowledge indicates that some of these mechanisms will involve inherited predispositions, while others surely will involve congenital, perinatal, or postnatal experiences leading toward and past the initial experience of drug exposure (Turner et al., 1993).

Prenatal and Perinatal Risk Factors. Within the field of human growth and development, there is a broad consensus that adult behavior and behavioral disturbances are more readily predicted from behavioral and performance characteristics measured in middle to late childhood (ages 5–13), and in adolescence, than from behavior exhibited during infancy and the early childhood (Collins, 1986). For this reason, and also because of major problems of logistics and cost, drug dependence researchers generally have not sought to link very early life experiences and infant development to later risk of drug dependence in adulthood. Instead, they have focused attention primarily on the adolescent years. Nonetheless, in drug dependence research there has been some progress in relation to risk-associated characteristics that are observable in the prenatal and perinatal periods and in childhood (e.g., see Glantz, 1992).

For example, preclinical laboratory studies show how prenatal and perinatal drug exposures can alter later drug action and drug-taking behavior. In addition, a human embryo or fetus continually exposed in utero to cocaine or heroin will develop drug dependence and will show signs of drug withdrawal within a few hours of delivery. By extension, it is plausible that in utero drug exposure might be an early predisposing factor for drug dependence later in life. This hypothesis now is under investigation as "cocaine babies" and other prenatally drug-exposed infants are being followed in studies of growth and development.

Building from early work on a "continuum of reproductive casualty" identified by Pasamanick, Knobloch, and Lilienfeld, several research teams have sought complications of pregnancy and delivery that might produce psychiatric disorders, including disturbances of behavior as well as drug dependence. Several inquiries along these lines are underway, some of them using a nonconcurrent prospective research design to study newborns assessed between 1960 and 1966 for the multisite National Collaborative Perinatal

Project (NCPP), with follow-up assessments in young adulthood. To date, the NCPP follow-up studies have not identified prenatal or perinatal risk factors for drug dependence, but the early evidence points toward a possibly protective effect of chronic fetal hypoxia. Among young adults followed to ages 18–27 years, the occurrence of DIS/DSM-III drug dependence or abuse was observed to be 0.7 times lower among subjects who had experienced chronic fetal hypoxia, as compared to subjects without pregnancy or delivery complications. The investigators have suggested that the protective effect might be due to poor health or functional status of the hypoxia group, with secondary impact to make them less out-going, more sheltered by parents, and thereby less likely to become cases of drug dependence or abuse (Buka et al., 1993).

In summary, until more inquiries have been completed, it will not be possible to speak confidently about the impact of prenatal or immediate postnatal factors on the risk of later drug dependence. Nonetheless, as suggested by the NCPP investigators, early life experiences such as chronic fetal hypoxia theoretically are capable of reducing the risk of later drug dependence by virtue of their more proximal impact on childhood behavior and then by secondary parental or school responses to the child's behavior. Other early life experiences, such as in utero drug exposure, might be found to yield an increased risk of drug dependence.

The next several sections of this chapter shed additional light on the importance for drug dependence research of the work that maps human environments and exposures from early embryonic development through gestation and birth and onward toward childhood and later stages of development.

Risk Factors Observed in Childhood. Seeking the root causes of drug dependence, many investigators have turned to the period of childhood and adolescent development, and the result has been several classic studies on the hypothesis that childhood deviance, misbehavior, and aggression might be important behavioral risk factors for later drug dependence, especially for males. The balance of evidence on this matter now favors a possibly causal predictive linkage between early misbehavior and later serious drug involvement—implicating not only drug dependence and drug abuse but also intravenous drug use. This suspected causal association has received generally consistent support from a variety of research designs, including a nonconcurrent prospective study, a concurrent prospective study, an application of the epidemiologic case-base strategy, and a growing number of both longitudinal and retrospective studies (e.g., see Robins, 1966; Kellam et al., 1983; Tomas et al., 1990; White, 1992).

The base of evidence linking childhood misbehavior and conduct problems to later serious drug involvement now has become so strong that randomized field trials are underway to test the hypothesized linkage. In these trials, experimental school-based programs are being tested to determine first whether they first reduce childhood misbehavior and conduct problems and then whether they reduce risk of later drug involvement and drug dependence. Using this approach, investigators hope to translate the observational research findings into practical public health action against drug dependence (e.g., see Kellam et al., 1991; Hawkins et al., 1991; Dolan et al., 1993).

The "hyperactivity" syndrome of attentional difficulties, impulsivity, and hyperactive behavior in childhood also has been studied as a potential behavioral risk factor for drug dependence, separate from conduct problems. There now are mixed results from studies on hyperactivity and drug use, but the most definitive inquiry to date suggests that hyperactive boys without early aggressive behavior are more likely to have DSM-III drug dependence and/or abuse in the early years of adulthood, that is, between ages 23 and 30. Boys whose hyperactive behavior, impulsivity, or attentional difficulties persisted into adulthood seem to be an especially high prevalence group for drug dependence and/or abuse (Mannuzza et al., 1993). There are a variety of possible mechanisms to account for this finding, including potentially reciprocal interplay between drug use, impulsivity, and attentional difficulties once drug experimentation has begun. The same issue of reciprocal interplay has been raised in relation to the dimensional personality constructs of "sensation seeking" and "openness," which have modest correlations with hyperactivity. Namely, it can be argued that sensation seeking, openness to new experiences, and other behavioral tendencies displayed in childhood are determined by both inherited and experiential factors and that these behavioral tendencies in turn bring the child into contact with later experiences and environments that promote the reinforcing functions of subsequent drug use. In this way, inherited and situational conditions may "transact" reciprocally with one another, leading toward greater risk of drug dependence. This "transactional" model of the interplay between inherited predispositions and situational circumstances is a theme of increasing importance in psychopathologic research, including studies of alcoholism and drug dependence as well as other forms of behavioral and mental disorders (e.g., see Sameroff and Fiese, 1989; Tarter et al., 1990; Tarter and Mezzich, 1992).

The academic prowess of children remains somewhat of a puzzle in relation to initiation of drug use and risk of later, more serious drug involvement. In some research, the very capable children initiated drug use earlier than their less capable classmates, perhaps in connection with status as leaders in diffusion of innovations, although early academic competence did not signal increased probability of more serious drug involvement (Fleming et al., 1982). In other research, an improvement in academic performance in later childhood and adolescence has seemed to afford some protection against what otherwise would be a higher risk trajectory toward serious drug involvement (Brook et al., 1986).

There also is some evidence to suggest that risk of developing drug problems is greater when drug use starts early, for example, in middle to late childhood (e.g., see Robins and Przybeck, 1985). This relationship does not appear to be due simply to the fact that early starters accumulate more years of drug use, although more prospective evidence on this topic is needed (Anthony and Petronis, in press).

Finally, an early thematic focus on childhood behavioral and temperamental characteristics has begun to shift toward aspects of childhood environment, especially modifiable aspects of childhood environment. For example, there is an accumulation of evidence from a variety of studies that lapses in parental supervision and monitoring in middle to late childhood might signal increased risk of initiating drug use and perhaps increased risk of later drug dependence (e.g., Barnes and Farrell, 1992; Chassin et al., 1993; Chilcoat et al., 1995).

In new epidemiologic research on drug dependence risk factors formed in childhood, it will be important to use field experiments and other rigorous forms of program evaluation to probe casual inferences derived from theory or from the systematically replicated evidence of observational studies. In some instances, these field experiments can be mounted by extending evaluation research now underway to test elementary school drug prevention programs and efforts to improve childhood education. For example, if these drug prevention programs are shown to delay onset of drug experimentation, then it will be important to determine whether they also lead to reduced risk of later, more serious drug involvement. In a similar fashion, programs of large-scale experimental evaluations of new changes in the elementary school curriculum can be made into a foundation for epidemiologic inquiries into whether experimentally induced improvements in academic performance yield later reduced risk of drug dependence (e.g., see Kellam, 1994, for a discussion of theory-based preventive interventions).

In this respect, a prevailing shift away from psychological and behavioral constructs toward modifiable aspects of childhood environment has an added appeal. Having discovered that a childhood behavioral or temperamental characteristic signals an increased risk of drug dependence, it is necessary to undertake an additional lengthy program of research to identify changes in the childhood environment that might alter this characteristic or dampen its risk-enhancing impact. For example, whereas early childhood misbehavior has been identified as a risk indicator for later serious drug involvement, we still do not know which early interventions directed toward misbehavior are most effective. In addition, it will not suffice simply to probe whether the intervention changes the early risk indicator; evidence of impact on later risk of drug dependence is required before we mount large-scale public health actions in the name of preventing drug dependence. In contrast, an orientation to modifiable aspects of childhood environment can be guided by a focus on environments that are known to be responsive to existing interventions or with moderate adaptation of those interventions (e.g., see Davis and Tunks, 1990–1991).

Parent monitoring offers a case in point. To be sure, the evidence on poor monitoring and risk of drug dependence must be strengthened by systematic replication in a series of epidemiologic studies. Nonetheless, by virtue of prior research on parent monitoring and childhood conduct problems, the intervention programs known to improve parent monitoring already are in existence so that the portfolio of studies for systematic replication can be balanced in favor of rigorous field experiments versus strictly observational studies (e.g., see Chilcoat et al., 1995).

Risk Factors Observed in Adolescence. We already have remarked on the striking association between age and drug dependence and on the observation that risk of serious drug involvement increases sharply between middle and late adolescence. These observations have provided a strong rationale for investigators to study the developmental period of adolescence in relation to drug use and drug problems.

Some of the themes discussed in relation to childhood risk factors also appear in research on adolescence and drug use, particularly those concerning sensation seeking, impulsivity, conduct problems, delinquency, and low academic achievement. Other risk indicators with some supportive evidence include religiosity, emotionality, depressed mood, low self-esteem, and self-derogation, as well as a domain of psychological constructs that involve expectancies about the functions to be served by alcohol and other drug use, as well as the perceived risks of drug-taking. That is, in some work, early assessments of teens' expectations for what can be gained by consuming drugs have signaled later, more intensive drug involvement; use of cocaine and other controlled drugs has occurred less often among those who rate drug use as an especially risky behavior. In some instances, a longitudinal research design has helped to test hypotheses about the precursors of these psychological characteristics, including, for example, 1) suspected linkages between uncontrollable negative life events, followed by secondary mood disturbances, and then followed by drug use in adolescence; and 2) a possible sequence from parental alcoholism toward adolescent drug use via three hypothesized mediators: lapses in parent monitoring and control over adolescent offspring, levels of stress and negative mood states in the offspring, and emotionality in the offspring (e.g., see Hawkins et al., 1992; Clayton, 1992; Kaplan and Johnson, 1992; Chassin et al., 1993).

Notwithstanding some excellent studies on these suspected adolescent risk factors, the affiliation with peer groups far and away is the most dominant focus of research on drug use in the teen years. This focus can be supported on theoretical grounds: Peer interaction is central in the creation of exposure opportunities that bring youths into contact with drugs, and peers often are participating vectors in the sequence of movements that convey drugs out of the reservoir toward human populations. There now also is considerable empirical evidence on peer drug use and affiliation with deviant peers as strong indicators of risk for teenage drug involvement, including recent data on how affiliation with deviant peers might be facilitated by lapses in parent monitoring that are associated with parental alcoholism (e.g., see Hawkins et al., 1992; Chassin et al., 1993). In addition to many observational studies on peer group affiliation and teen drug use, there now is supportive data from several field experiments to test interventions that increase peer resistance skills and other social competencies of adolescents (e.g., Ellickson and Bell, 1990; Hansen and Graham, 1991; Hansen, 1992).

There remain four especially important gaps in the epidemiology of drug dependence in relation to adolescent peer groups. First, the experimental data on peer resistance and social skill training do not yet speak to whether these interventions reduce the risk of later drug dependence, although these data generally are balanced in favor of short-term impact to delay initiation of drug use (e.g., see Resnicow and Botvin, 1993; Ellickson et al., 1993). Second, for adolescents who have already started to use drugs, the peer resistance and social skills training may "boomerang" and actually lead to increased drug use (Ellickson and Bell, 1990). This is a potentially adverse consequence of these intervention programs that now must be probed in more detail. Third, no more than a handful of studies now speak to the mechanisms by which the peer-focused intervention programs might exert a risk-reducing effect on later drug involvement, although there are some intriguing leads that implicate sensation seeking as a potentially modifying variable (e.g., see Clayton et al., 1991). Finally, there is a pressing need for more research on what determines adolescent peer affiliations, including studies that give more attention to aspects of childhood and adolescent environment, such as parent monitoring, in addition to a more traditional focus on childhood behavioral and temperamental characteristics such as sociability and self-derogation (e.g., see Kaplan and Johnson, 1992; Brown et al., 1993; Richardson et al., 1993). To some extent, research on these environmental conditions has been held back by impressions that in adolescence the influence of parents is superceded by that of peer groups. This impression was bolstered by reports that peer factors preempted parent and family factors in predictive models of adolescent drug taking, where the modeling strategy was that of stepwise regression, which neglects to account for the possibility that parenting is one of the determinants of peer affiliation. As such, controlling for peer drug use when seeking to test hypotheses about parental influence may represent an instance of inappropriate control of a suspected confounding variable in the model-building process, a topic receiving increased attention in the epidemiologic literature (Weinberg, 1993, 1994; Joffe and Greenland, 1994).

To some extent, the peer group research entails a shift from the domain of individual-level risk factors to a domain of group-level risk factors. Other group-level or "macro-social" conditions of recent interest include 1) community norms and public attitudes for and against drug taking and 2) neighborhood deterioration as an indicator of exposure opportunity for contact with illicit drugs. Working from a theory that community norms and public attitudes are of central importance, the Partnership for a Drug-Free America and others have mounted a massive media campaign of counterprogramming against otherwise prevailing pro-drug influences. The Partnership has produced reports on early time series analyses, based on a repeated sequence of cross-sectional surveys, that suggest not only that adolescents have seen and remembered the anti-drug media announcements but also that the announcements have promoted lower prevalence of drug taking. These are important and promising results on an innovative public health strategy, but a more rigorous analysis by an independent evaluation team is needed.

Several lines of epidemiologic research are raising the possibility that some individual-level risk characteristics can be understood best in relation to community-level characteristics, including both demographic and economic indicators of neighborhood (e.g., percent living in single-family housing), as well as signs of neighborhood deterioration. For example, when African-American and white American teenagers living in the same neighborhood have been compared, there is either no difference in prevalence of crack smoking or the African-American teens appear to be at lower risk (e.g., see Lillie-Blanton et al., 1993). There also is some evidence that neighborhood deterioration might be an important risk-modifying condition. A preliminary report from one prospective study suggests that exposure opportunities for illicit drug use depend in part on prior levels of neighborhood deterioration assessed in relation to lack of nearby parks and recreational facilities, deteriorated housing, public intoxication, and related characteristics of the neighborhood of residence (Crum et al., 1994).

As a final note in relation to epidemiologic studies of risk factors for drug dependence in adolescence, we draw attention to the concept of a "comprehensive community-based prevention strategy" that has been developed in response to requests by American community leaders concerned about youthful drug taking. As the label states, the underlying concept is that a combination of concurrent intervention tactics will be required in order to bring about reduced prevalence of drug taking in the community. Some of these interventions involve mass media announcements (e.g., billboards, public service announcements on television and radio), police initiatives, and other tactics directed toward community norms and other community-level characteristics thought to reduce prevalence of drug taking. Concurrently, there are interventions directed toward parents (often, drug education programs for parents) and toward schools (for example, creation of the school neighborhood as a drug-free zone; establishment of an anti-tobacco smoking policy for the school students, faculty, and staff), as well as peer resistance training and other school-based interventions directed toward adolescents and their peers (e.g., see Johnson et al., 1990).

Early evaluation research on community prevention programming of this type showed promising results in relation to adolescent initiation of drug use, although inferences about program impact were constrained by nonequivalence of the community control group and lack of random assignment to intervention status (e.g., see MacKinnon et al., 1991). Nonetheless, as in the instance of peer resistance and social skills training, the evaluation has not yet clarified whether drug dependence and other serious drug involvement is being prevented—or whether the interventions modify risk characteristics of adolescents unlikely to develop drug dependence even in the absence of an intervention program. Quite clearly, more research on this question is needed before we can be confident that comprehensive community programming merits application beyond current levels. In addition, once we see definitive evidence of total program impact, it will be necessary to conduct experiments to reveal which of the several tactics are basically inert resource-consuming activities and which deliver the observed impact.

Risk Factors Observed in Late Adolescence and Early Adulthood. Many clinical observers trace the origins of drug dependence to the developmental periods of childhood and early to middle adolescence, neglecting the potential importance of risk factors that are not observed until late adolescence or adulthood. Nonetheless, there is some epidemiologic evidence about risk factors during these later periods of development, in addition to what we already have reported concerning age, sex, and race.

An important finding about the later environmental determinants of drug dependence emerged from a study of 571 male Vietnam veterans returning to the United States in the early 1970s (mean age, 19 years), with urinalysis and DIS-like methods used to assess drug use and drug dependence, already mentioned earlier in this chapter. Studied retrospectively, only one veteran had a history of dependence on narcotic drugs (i.e., opioids) prior to enlistment, but a very large proportion, 19.5%, became dependent while serving in Vietnam, where opium, heroin, and other opioids often were available.

The 571 veterans were re-assessed 10 months after returning to the United States, when only 0.9% were found to be opioid dependent, and again 2–3 years later, when an additional 1.8% were found to have become dependent. That is, upon return to the United States, the vast majority of the Vietnam veterans in this study did not remain or become dependent on heroin or other opioid drugs, despite a remarkably high prevalence of opioid dependence during the period of Vietnam service (Helzer, 1985; Robins, 1993).

Further study of the post-Vietnam experience of these veterans has shown that residence in a large city was an important determinant of using opioids after return from Vietnam. Large-city residence also was a risk factor for making the transition from opioid use to opioid dependence. Opioids seem to be more readily available to adults living in the larger cities of the United States, and this might account for the observed geographic distribution of the drug dependence cases among these veterans, just as availability of opioids was associated with occurrence of opioid use and dependence while they were in Vietnam (Helzer, 1985).

The study of veterans also found that having a non-traffic arrest was associated with making the transition from opioid use to opioid dependence upon return to the United States. This finding of a behavioral problem in adulthood in association with drug dependence is consistent with results from many retrospective and cross-sectional studies, as well as a separate prospective study, with a focus on adult-onset DSM-III drug dependence and/or abuse, based on 101 incident cases found in the ECA project and 342 controls matched for age and geographic location of residence. In the ECA analysis, a history of antisocial personality disorder had a strong association with risk of becoming an adult-onset case of drug dependence and/or abuse, even when the analyses controlled for prior illicit drug use (Anthony, 1991a). In a separate prospective study with an epidemiologic sample of drug users, persistence of cocaine use in adulthood also has been linked with level of adolescent deviance, at least among men (Kandel and Raveis, 1989). Thus, it is necessary to consider that general deviance or social maladaptation in the form of police trouble or long-standing behavioral problems might continue to exert an influence on risk and duration of drug dependence in adulthood, and not just in relation to earlier onset of drug dependence (see Anthony, 1991a).

Prior alcoholism and alcohol problems also appear consistently in the risk factor models developed for occurrence of drug disorders in the late adolescent period and prior to the middle-age years and also in cross-sectional studies. A considerable number of youths and young adults become cases of alcohol dependence or alcohol abuse and then later develop dependence on controlled substances such as marijuana and cocaine. In the study of veterans, opioid dependence occurred more than three times more often among men with alcohol problems after Vietnam. Based on multiple logistic regression analysis of the ECA data, adults with a history of DSM-III alcoholism were an estimated four times more likely to develop a DSM-III drug dependence or abuse syndrome in later adulthood (Helzer, 1985; V. Chen, unpublished doctoral dissertation; Anthony, 1991a).

Cross-sectional and retrospective studies lead to an impression that many other different types of psychiatric disturbances are present among cases of drug dependence, as reviewed by Anthony and Helzer (1991), among others. Nonetheless, the evidence from prospective studies is inconsistent, sometimes implicating mood disorders, especially depression, and other times implicating conditions such as agoraphobia (e.g., see Anthony, 1991a).

In attempts to unravel the patterns of co-occurring mental disorders, the insidious onset of drug dependence is a complicating influence. For example, it is plausible that early drug use develops out of a background of more general socially maladaptive behavior or deviance, and then the drug use is followed by feelings of depressed mood, irritability, sleep problems, and other complaints that are featured prominently in the case definitions for mood disorders. These mood-related complaints then might promote continued drug taking, with reciprocal relationships that build up insidiously toward drug dependence on the one hand and mood disorder on the other hand (e.g., see Kaplan and Johnson, 1992).

This notion of a reciprocal "co-influence" model for different pairs of insidiously developing psychiatric disturbances is plausible and fits well with at least some of the available evidence from rigorous epidemiologic studies, as well as clinical observations. However, it is not a model that can be tested readily with cross-sectional or retrospective data on age at onset of different psychiatric symptoms. To test a co-influence model of this type, it will be necessary to conduct longitudinal studies with frequently repeated assessments of the fine-grained time sequences that can link one episode of drug-taking to subsequent processes and episodes of subthreshold mental disorders, prospectively looking for the emergence of a fully formed mental disorder that meets all diagnostic criteria. Confident statements about co-occurrence of drug dependence with other disorders will require longitudinal data of this type, coupled with evidence from intervention studies to test whether incidence of drug dependence might be reduced by effective treatment of mood disorder and whether risk of depression might be reduced by effective treatment of drug dependence (Anthony, 1991b).

Suspected sociodemographic risk factors implicated in evidence from two or more prospective studies of the transition from illicit drug use to adult-onset drug dependence and/or abuse include marital status and educational achievement. In both the Vietnam veteran study and the ECA investigation, being married was associated with a lower risk, and poor educational achievement was associated with a higher risk. Persistence of marijuana and cocaine use at ages 28–29 years has not been found to be associated with either marital status in earlier adulthood or having been a high school drop-out (Helzer, 1985; Kandel and Raveis, 1989; Anthony, 1991a).

Recent ECA work on drug dependence risk factors has a concentration on adult occupations and job environments that might convey greater risk, especially psychosocial job characteristics such as the levels of physical hazards or psychosocial stressors associated with each job category, as well as a possible stress-buffering impact associated with conditions such as the level of decision-making autonomy on the job (e.g., C. Muntaner et al., 1995). These hypotheses build, in part, from cross-sectional analyses of the ECA prevalence data on alcohol and drug dependence found in different occupations. Taking into account age, sex, race, education, and recency of employment, these analyses have identified construction laborers, carpenters, transportation workers, waiters, and waitresses as working adults with an especially high prevalence of alcohol or drug disorders. Doctors and nurses have received special attention because their access to pharmaceutical products and their working conditions might promote occurrence of drug dependence. However, several studies based on the ECA data suggest that prevalence of alcohol and drug disorders is no different or lower among these health professionals compared with other adult workers (Anthony et al., 1992; Trinkoff et al., 1991).

DETERMINANTS OF DURATION: THE ROLE OF TREATMENT

Whereas organized efforts to prevent drug dependence focus mainly on the young, public health efforts to control drug dependence by reducing its duration focus mainly on adults. Methadone, oral naltrexone, and LAAM are three medicines for which there is compelling evidence of efficacy in treatment and rehabilitation of opioid-dependent cases. At present, there is no corresponding medicine known to be effective for the treatment of cocaine dependence or dependence on other controlled substances. Promising treatment agents are listed in Table 5; these drugs for treatment of opioid or cocaine dependence now are primarily in an intermediate phase of research and development, some years away from governmental approval for widespread medical usage.

TABLE 5. Treatment Agents

Medication	Approved Use	Potential Use	Status
For opiates			
Buprenorphine	Relieve pain	Opiate maintenance therapy	Phase III
Depot Naltrexone	None	Long-term opiate blockade	Phase I
LAAM	Opiate maintenance therapy	—	Clinical testing completed; now has FDA approval
For Cocaine			
Amantadine	Treat viral infection	Prevent relapse/prolong abstinence	Phase II
Bromocriptine	Treat Parkinson's disease	Prevent relapse/prolong abstinence	Phase II
Carbamazepine	Treat epilepsy	Facilitate abstinence	Phase II
Desipramine	Treat depression	Facilitate abstinence	Phase II
Fluoxetine	Treat depression	Facilitate abstinence	Phase II
Flupenthixol	Treat psychosis	Facilitate abstinence	Phase II
Imipramine	Treat depression	Facilitate abstinence	Phase II
Mazindol	Treat obesity	Facilitate abstinence	Phase II
Methylphenidate	Treat attention deficit disorder	Prevent relapse/prolong abstinence	Phase II
Sertraline	None	Facilitate abstinence	Phase II

Other treatment modalities, such as Narcotics Anonymous, therapeutic communities, behavior therapy, and contingency management, are also at an intermediate phase of evaluation, although there is no formal review process for these treatment programs as there is for pharmaceutical products. At present, the available evidence on these other forms of treatment for drug dependence appears promising, but all too often confidence in the results of treatment evaluation research has been undermined by limitations such as widespread loss of subjects during follow up and lack of randomized allocation plans (e.g., see Onken et al., 1993).

While it might be argued that international drug control policies and associated police work now reduce both the risk and the duration of drug dependence, there is no compelling epidemiologic evidence to support this argument. Anecdotal evidence abounds — for example, in relation to police and regulatory actions to curtail amphetamine problems in Japan and Sweden. Nonetheless, rigorous evaluation studies to guide future policy and programmatic decisions are lacking within this arena (Bonnie, 1986).

DIRECTIONS FOR FUTURE RESEARCH

Many gaps in knowledge remain in relation to the epidemiology of drug dependence, but this overview has mentioned several topics that deserve greater priority in new research. We draw specific attention to the need for a more deliberate plan of research on the different environmental conditions that are thought to affect risk of drug dependence in adolescence and adulthood.

At present, the range of relevant environmental conditions for which there are reliable and valid measurements is quite limited. For example, investigators studying monozygotic twin pairs discordant for drug dependence have had to craft their own assessments of these environmental conditions and have not been able to draw upon a well-researched array of measurement tools. One specific goal of new research should be creation of tools and methods for assessing environmental conditions that are comparable to the array of measurement tools now available for studying different aspects of cognitive performance.

Concurrent with development of these tools, it should be possible to construct a map of environmental conditions that affect risk and/or duration of drug dependence, leading toward more effective prevention and control initiatives of the future. This map of environmental conditions can be juxtaposed with new evidence from the human genome mapping project in order to guide the search for environmental conditions that might modify the expression of specific genetic liabilities and thereby reduce the risk of drug dependence.

The construction of these maps for human genes and human environments will depend on epidemiologic research that makes a bridge from laboratory and clinical studies to large-scale population research. Effective bridging across the disciplines engaged in these studies implies a sharing of conceptual models and assessment methods not only in relation to the occurrence of drug dependence but also in relation to the suspected risk factor hypotheses. That is, in future laboratory and clinical research, we hope to see a more prevalent application of concepts and methods developed as part of large-scale epidemiologic studies, and in future epidemiologic studies we hope to see reciprocal progress and application of laboratory and clinical approaches to the study of drug dependence.

In conclusion, future epidemiologic research on drug dependence can build on a substantial body of evidence that has accumulated quite rapidly since the end of World War

II, beginning with retrospective studies of clinical cases and continuing through recent large-sample prospective studies. The prospects for future advances in relation to the epidemiology of drug dependence will be determined in large part by greater attention to the environmental conditions that are independent risk factors for drug dependence, concurrent with attention to environmental conditions that might modify genetic vulnerabilities to this important psychiatric disturbance.

REFERENCES

American Psychiatric Association (1980): "Diagnostic and Statistical Manual of Mental Disorders," 3rd ed. Washington, DC: American Psychiatric Association.

American Psychiatric Association (1987): "Diagnostic and Statistical Manual for Mental Disorders," 3rd ed, revised. Washington, DC: American Psychiatric Association.

Anglin DM, Brecht ML, Woodward JA (1986): An empirical study of maturing out: Conditional factors. Int J Addictions 21:233–246.

Anthony JC (1983): The regulation of dangerous psychoactive drugs. In Morgan JP, Kagan DV (eds): "Society and Medication: Conflicting Signals for Prescribers and Patients." Lexington, MA: D.C. Health and Company, pp 163–180.

Anthony JC (1991a): The epidemiology of drug addiction. In Miller NS (ed): "Comprehensive Handbook of Drug and Alcohol Addiction." New York: Marcel Dekker, Inc., pp 55–86.

Anthony JC (1991b): Epidemiology of drug dependence and illicit drug use. Curr Opin Psychiatry 4:435–439.

Anthony JC (1992): Epidemiological research on cocaine use in the USA. In: "Cocaine: Scientific and Social Dimensions, Proceedings of the CIBA Foundation Symposium 166." Chichester, England. John Wiley and Sons, pp 20–39.

Anthony JC (1993): The scope of epidemiologic research on drug use: A rationale for change. In Monteiro MG, Inciardi JA (eds): "Brasil–United States Binational Research." São Paulo, Brasil: CEBRID, pp 213–223.

Anthony JC (1995): International drug dependence databases. In Eisenberg L, DesJarlais R (eds): "World Mental Health: Problems and Priorities in Low-Income Countries." New York: Oxford University Press, 382 pp.

Anthony JC, Eaton WW, Mandell W (1992): Psychoactive Drug Dependence and Abuse: More Common in Some Occupations Than Others? J Employee Assistance Res 1:148–186.

Anthony JC, Helzer JE (1991): Syndromes of drug abuse and dependence. In Robins LN, Regier DA (eds): "Psychiatric Disorders in America." New York: The Free Press, pp 116–154.

Anthony JC, Petronis KR. Early-onset drug use and risk of later drug problems. Drug and Alcohol Dependence (in press).

Anthony JC, Warner LA, Kessler RC (1994): Comparative epidemiology of dependence on tobacco, alcohol, controlled substances, and inhalants: Basic findings from the National Comorbidity Survey. Exp Clin Psychopharmacol 2:1–24.

Babor TF (1992): Nosological considerations in the diagnosis of substance use disorders. In Glantz M, Pickens R (eds): "Vulnerability to Drug Abuse." Washington, DC: American Psychological Association, pp 53–74.

Barnes GM, Farrell MP (1992): Parental support and control as predictors of adolescent drinking, delinquency, and related problem behaviors. J Marriage Fam 54:763–776.

Beiser M, Erickson D, Fleming JAE, Iacono WG (1993): Establishing the onset of psychotic illness. Am J Psychiatry 150:1349–1354.

Berkson JA (1946). Limitations of the application of fourfold table analysis to hospital data. Biometrics. 2:47–53.

Bland RC, Newman SC, Orn H (1988a): Period prevalence of psychiatric disorders in Edmonton. Acta Psychiatr Scand 77 (Suppl 338):33–42.

Bland RC, Orn H, Newman SC (1988b): Lifetime prevalence of psychiatric disorders in Edmonton. Acta Psychiatr Scand 77(Suppl 338):24–32.

Bonnie R (1985): Efficacy of law as a paternalistic instrument. In Melton G (ed): "Nebraska Symposium on Human Motivation." Omaha: University of Nebraska, pp 131–211.

Boyd JH, Robins IN, Holzer CE III, Vonkorff M, Jordan KB, Escobar JI (1985): Making diagnoses from DIS data. In Eaton WW, Kessler LG (eds): "Epidemiologic Field Methods in Psychiatry." New York. Academic Press, pp 209–234.

Breslau N, Fenn N, Peterson EL (1993): Early smoking initiation and nicotine dependence in a cohort of young adults. Drug Alcohol Depend 33:129–138.

Brook JS, Whiteman MM, Gordon AS, Cohen P (1986): Dynamics of childhood and adolescent personality traits and adolescent drug use. Dev Psychol 22:403–414.

Brown BB, Mounts N, Lamborn SD, Steinberg L (1993): Parenting practices and peer group affiliation in adolescence. Child Dev 64:467–482.

Buck, AA, Sasaki TT, Hewitt JJ, Macrae AA. Coca chewing and health: An epidemiologic study among residents of a Peruvian village. Am J Epidemiol. 88(2):159–177. 1968.

Buka SL, Tsuang MT, Lipsitt LP (1993): Pregnancy/delivery complications and psychiatric diagnosis: A prospective study. Arch Gen Psychiatry 50:151–156.

Burke KC, Burke JD, Regier DA, Rae DS (1990): Age at onset of selected mental disorders in five community populations. Arch Gen Psychiatry 48:789–795.

Cadoret RJ (1992): Genetic and environmental factors in initiation of drug use and the transition to abuse. In Glantz M, Pickens R (eds): "Vulnerability to Drug Abuse." Washington, DC: American Psychological Association, pp 99–113.

Cadoret RJ, Cain CA, Grove WM (1980): Development of alcoholism in adoptees raised apart from alcoholic biologic relatives. Arch Gen Psychiatry 37:561–563.

Cadoret JR, Troughton E, O'Gorman TW, Hcywood E (1986): An adoption study of genetic and environmental factors in drug abuse. Arch Gen Psychiatry 43:1131–1136.

Canino G, Anthony JC, Freeman DH, Shrout P, Rubio-Stipec M (1993): Drug abuse and illicit drug use in Puerto Rico. Am J Public Health 83:194–200.

Carroll E (1977): Coca, the plant and its use. In Petersen RC, Stillman RC (eds): "Cocaine: 1977." NIDA Research Monograph #13. Washington, DC: U.S. Government Printing Office, pp 35–45.

Chassin L, Pillow DR, Curran PJ, et al. (1993): Relation of parental alcoholism to early adolescent substance use: A test of three mediating mechanisms. J Abnorm Psychol 102:3–19.

Chilcoat HD, Dishion TJ, Anthony JC (1995): Parent monitoring and the incidence of drug sampling in urban elementary school children. Am J Epidemiol 141:1–14.

Clayton RR (1992): Transitions in drug use: Risk and protective factors. In Glantz M, Pickens R (eds): "Vulnerability to Drug Abuse." Washington, DC: American Psychological Association, pp 15–51.

Clayton RR, Cattarello A, Walden KP (1991): Sensation seeking as a potential mediating variable for school-based prevention intervention: A two-year follow-up of DARE. Health Commun 3:229–239.

Collins WA (ed) (1986): "Development During Middle Childhood: The Years From 6 to 12." Washington, DC: National Academy of Sciences.

Conneally PM (1991): Association between the D_2 dopamine receptor gene and alcoholism: Comment. Arch Gen Psychiatry 48:664–666.

Croughan JL (1985): The contribution of family studies to understanding drug abuse. In Robins LN (ed): "Studying Drug Abuse." Series in Psychosocial Epidemiology, vol 6. New Brunswick, NJ: Rutgers University Press, pp 93–116.

Crum RM, Lillie-Blanton M, Anthony JC (1994): "Neighborhood Environment and the Opportunity To Use Cocaine." Baltimore, MD: The Johns Hopkins University (in submission).

Davis JR, Tunks E (1990–1991): Environments and addiction: A proposed taxonomy. Intl J Addict 25:805–826.

de Alarcon R (1969): The spread of heroin abuse in a community. Bull Narc 21:17–22.

Dolan LJ, Kellam SG, Brown C, et al. (1993): The short-term impact of two classroom-based preventive interventions on aggressive and shy behaviors and poor achievement. J Appl Dev Psychol 14:317–345.

Eaton WW, Holzer CE, Von Korff MR, Anthony JC, et al (1984): The design of the ECA surveys: The control and measurement of error. Arch Gen Psychiatry 41:942–948.

Eaton WW, Kramer M, Anthony JC, Dryman A, Shapiro S, Locke BZ (1989): The incidence of specific DIS/DSM-III mental disorders: Data from the NIMH Epidemiologic Catchment Area Program. Acta Psychiatr Scand 79:163–178.

Eddy NB, Halbach H, Isbell H, Seevers MH (1965): Drug dependence: Its significance and characteristics. Bull WHO 32:724–748.

Edwards G, Gross MM (1976): Alcohol dependence: Provisional description of a clinical syndrome. Br Med J 1:1058–1061.

Ellickson PL, Bell RM (1990): Drug prevention in junior high: A multi-site longitudinal test. Science 247:1299–1305.

Ellickson PL, Bell RM, McGuigan K (1993): Preventing adolescent drug use: Long-term results of a junior high program. Am J Public Health 83:856–861.

Fleming JP, Kellam SG, Brown CH (1982): Early predictors of age at first use of alcohol, marijuana and cigarettes. Drug Alcohol Depend 9:285–303.

Flewelling RL, Ennett ST, Rachal JV, Theisen AC (1993): "Race/Ethnicity, Socioeconomic Status, and Drug Abuse: 1991." DHHS Publication No. (SMA) 93-2062. Washington, DC: U.S. Government Printing Office, 81 pp.

Glantz M (1992): A developmental psychopathology model of drug abuse vulnerability. In Glantz M, Pickens R (eds): "Vulnerability to Drug Abuse." Washington, DC: American Psychological Association, pp 389–418.

Goldman D (1993): Genetic transmission. In Galanter M (ed): "Recent Developments in Alcoholism," vol 11, Ten Years of Progress." New York: Plenum Press, pp 232–248.

Haastrup S (1973): "Young Drug Abusers: 350 Patients Interviewed at Admission and Followed Up Three Years Later." Copenhagen: Munksgaard.

Hansen WB (1992): School-based substance abuse prevention: A review of the state of the art in curriculum, 1980–1990. Health Educ Res 7:403–430.

Hansen WB, Graham JW (1991): Preventing alcohol, marijuana, and cigarette use among adolescents: Peer pressure resistance training versus establishing conservative norms. Prev Med 20:414–430.

Hanzi (Crider) R (1976): "Diffusion of Heroin Use." Unpublished doctoral dissertation, submitted to the Arizona State University, Tucson, AZ, 1976.

Harrison LD (1992): Trends in illicit drug use in the United States: Conflicting results from national surveys. Int J Addict 27:817–847.

Hawkins JD, Catalano RF, Miller JY (1992): Risk and protective factors for alcohol and other drug problems in adolescence and early adulthood: Implications for substance abuse prevention. Psychol Bull 112:64–105.

Hawkins JD, Von Cleve E, Catalano RF Jr (1991): Reducing early childhood aggression: Results of a primary prevention program. J Am Acad Child Adolescence Psychiatry 30:208–217.

Helzer JE (1985): Specification of predictors of narcotic use versus addiction. In Robins LN (ed):

"Studying Drug Abuse." Series in Psychosocial Epidemiology, vol 6. New Brunswick, NJ: Rutgers University Press, pp 173–197.

Helzer JE, Burnam MA, McEvoy LT (1991): Alcohol abuse and dependence. In Robins LN, Regier DA (eds): "Psychiatric Disorders in America." New York: The Free Press, pp 81–115.

Helzer JE, Canino GJ, Yeh E-K, Bland RC, Lee CK, Hwu HG, Newman S (1990): Alcoholism—North America and Asia. Arch Gen Psychiatry 47:313–319.

Hughes PH, Canavan KP, Jarvis G, Arif A (1983): Extent of drug abuse: An international review with implications for health planners. World Health Stat Q 36:394–497.

Hughes JR, Oliveto AH, Helzer JE, Higgins ST, Bickel WK (1992): Should caffeine abuse, dependence, or withdrawal be added to DSM-IV and ICD-10? Am J Psychiatry 149:33–40.

Hwu HG, Yeh EK, Chang LY (1989): Prevalence of psychiatric disorders in Taiwan defined by the Chinese Diagnostic Interview Schedule. Acta Psychiatr Scand 79:136–147.

Joffe MM, Greenland S (1994): Toward a clearer definition of confounding. Letter to the Editor. Am J Epidemiol 139(9):962.

Johnson CA, Pentz MA, Weber MD, et al. (1990): The relative effectiveness of comprehensive community programming for drug abuse prevention with high-risk and low-risk adolescents. J Consult Clin Psychol 58:447–456.

Johnston LD (1985): Techniques for reducing measurement error in surveys of drug use. In Robins LN (ed): "Studying Drug Abuse." Series in Psychosocial Epidemiology, vol 6. New Brunswick, NJ: Rutgers University Press, pp 117–136.

Jones CP, Laveist TA, Lillie-Blanton M (1991): Race in the epidemiologic literature: An examination of the *American Journal of Epidemiology*. Am J Epidemiol 34:1079–1084.

Kandel DB (1991): The social demography of drug use. Milbank Q 69:365–402.

Kandel DB (1992): Epidemiological trends and implications for understanding the nature of addiction. In O'Brien CP, Jaffe JH (eds): "Addictive States." New York: Raven Press, pp 23–40.

Kandel DB, Davies M (1992): Progression to regular marijuana involvement: Phenomenology and risk factors for near-daily use. In Glantz M, Pickens R (eds): "Vulnerability to Drug Abuse." Washington, DC: American Psychological Association, pp 211–254.

Kandel DB, Raveis VH (1989): Cessation of illicit drug use in young adulthood. Arch Gen Psychiatry 46:109–116.

Kaplan HB, Johnson RJ (1992): Relationships between circumstances surrounding initial illicit drug use and escalation of drug use: Moderating effects of gender and early adolescent experiences. In Glantz M, Pickens R (eds): "Vulnerability to Drug Abuse." Washington, DC: American Psychological Association, pp 299–358.

Kellam SK, Brown CH, Rubin BR, Ensminger MD (1983): Paths leading to teenage psychiatric symptoms and substance use: Developmental epidemiological studies in Woodlawn. In Guze SB, Earls FJ, Barrett JE (eds): "Childhood Psychopathology and Development." New York: Raven Press, pp 17–55.

Kellam SG (1994): Testing theory through developmental epidemiologically based prevention research. In Cazares A, Beatty LA (eds): "Scientific Methods for Prevention Intervention Research." NIDA Research Monograph No. 139, Washington, DC: U.S. Government Printing Office, pp 37–58.

Kellam SG, Werthamer-Larsson L, Dolan LJ, Brown CH, Mayer LS, Rebok GW, Anthony JC, Laudolff J, Edelsohn G, Wheeler L (1991): Developmental epidemiologically-based preventive trials: Baseline modeling of early target behaviors and depressive symptoms. Am J Community Psychol 19:563–584.

Kessler RC, McGonagle KA, Zhao S, Nelson C, Hughes M, Eshleman S, Wittchen H-U, Kendler K (1994): Lifetime and 12-month prevalence of DSM-IIIR psychiatric disorders in the United States: Results from the National Comorbidity Survey. Arch Gen Psychiatry 51:8–19.

Kosten TA, Kosten TR (1991): Criteria for Diagnosis. In Miller NS (ed): "Comprehensive Handbook of Drug and Alcohol Addiction." New York: Marcel Dekker, pp 263–283.

Kramer M (1989): Barriers to prevention. In Cooper B, Helgason T (eds): "Epidemiology and the Prevention of Mental Disorders." London: Routledge, pp 30–55.

Kramer M (1992a): Barriers to the primary prevention of mental, neurological, and psychosocial disorders of children: A global perspective. In Albee GW, Bard LA, Monsey TVC (eds): "Improving Children's Lives: Global Perspectives on Prevention." Newbury Park, CA: Sage Publications. pp 3–36.

Kramer M (1992b): "Projected Changes in the Population of the United States—1990, 2000, and 2010: Implications for Mental Health and Primary Health Care." Baltimore, MD: Johns Hopkins University School of Hygiene and Public Health, Department of Mental Hygiene, unpublished technical report, pp 1–27.

Kramer M, Von Korff M, Kessler LG (1980): The lifetime prevalence of mental disorders: Estimation, uses, and limitations. Psychol Med 10:429–435.

Labuda MC, Gottesman II, Pauls DL (1993): Usefulness of twin studies for exploring the etiology of childhood and adolescent psychiatric disorders. Am J Med Genet (Neuropsychiatric Genetics) 48:47–59.

Landry DW, Zhao K, Yang GX-Q, Glickman M, Georgiadis TM (1993): Antibody-catalyzed degradation of cocaine. Science 259:1899–1901.

Lee CK, Kwak YS, Yamamoto J, Rhee H, Kim YS, Han JH, Choi JO, Lee YH (1990a): Psychiatric epidemiology in Korea: Part I, Gender and age differences in Seoul. J Nerv Ment Dis 178:242–246.

Lee CK, Kwak YS, Yamamoto J, Rhee H, Kim YS, Han JH, Choi JO, Lee YH (1990b): Psychiatric epidemiology in Korea: Part II, Urban and rural differences. J Nerv Ment Dis 178:247–252.

Lillie-Blanton M, Anthony JC, Schuster CR (1993): Probing the meaning of racial/ethnic group comparisons in crack cocaine smoking. JAMA 269:993–997.

Luthar SS, Anton SF, Merikangas KR, Rounsaville BJ (1992a): Vulnerability to drug abuse among opioid addicts' siblings: Individual, familial, and peer influences. Comp Psychiatry 33:190–196.

Luthar SS, Anton SF, Merikangas KR, Rounsaville BJ (1992b): Vulnerability to substance abuse and psychopathology among siblings of opioid abusers. J Nerv Ment Dis 180:153–161.

Luthar SS, Rounsaville BJ (1993): Substance misuse and comorbid psychopathology in a high-risk group: A study of siblings of cocaine misusers. Int J Addictions 28:415–434.

Mannuzza S, Klein RG, Bessler A, Malloy P, LePadula M (1993): Adult outcome of hyperactive boys: Educational achievement, occupational rank, and psychiatric status. Arch Gen Psychiatry 50:565–576.

MacKinnon DA, Johnson CA, Pentz MA, et al. (1991): Mediating mechanisms in a school-based drug prevention program: First year effects of the Midwestern Prevention Project. Health Psychol 10:164–172.

McGlothlin WH (1985): Distinguishing effects from concomitants of drug use: The case of crime. In Robins LN (ed): "Studying Drug Abuse." Series in Psychosocial Epidemiology, vol 6. New Brunswick, NJ: Rutgers University Press, pp 153–172.

Merikangas KR, Rounsaville BJ, Prusoff BA (1992): Familial factors in vulnerability to substance abuse. In Glantz M, Pickens R (eds): "Vulnerability to Drug Abuse." Washington, DC: American Psychological Association, pp 75–97.

Mirin SM, Weiss RD, Griffin ML, Michael JL (1991): Psychopathology in drug abusers and their families. Comp Psychiatry 32:36–51.

Musto DF (1987): "The American Disease: Origins of Narcotic Control," 2nd ed. New York: Oxford University Press, 384 pp.

Musto DF (1990): Illicit price of cocaine in two eras: 1908–14 and 1982–89. Conn Med 54:321–326.

Musto DF (1991): Opium, cocaine, and marijuana in American history. Sci Am 265:40–47.

Myers JK, Weissman MM, Tischler GL, et al. (1984): Six-month prevalence of psychiatric disorders in three communities. Arch Gen Psychiatry 41:959–967.

Nurco DN, Hanlon TE, Kinlock TW, Duszynski KR (1989): The consistency of types of criminal behavior over preaddiction, addiction, and nonaddiction status periods. Comp Psychiatry 30:391–402.

Oakley-Browne MA, Joyce PR, Wells JE, Bushnell JA, Hornblow AR (1989): Christchurch Psychiatric Epidemiology Study, Part II: Six month and other period prevalences of specific psychiatric disorders. Aust NZ J Psychiatry 23:327–340.

Onken LS, Blaine JD, Boren JJ, eds (1993): "Behavioral Treatments for Drug Abuse and Dependence." NIDA Research Monograph No. 137. Washington, DC: U.S. Government Printing Office, 321 pp.

Pandina RJ, White HR, Yorke J (1981): Estimation of substance use involvement: Theoretical consideration and empirical findings. Int J Addict 16:1–24.

Petersen RC (1977): History of cocaine. In Petersen RC, Stillman RC (eds): "Cocaine: 1977." NIDA Research Monograph No. 13. Washington, DC: U.S. Government Printing Office, pp 17–34.

Pickens RW, Svikis DS, McGue M, Lykken DT, Heston LL, Clayton PJ (1991): Heterogeneity in the inheritance of alcoholism. Arch Gen Psychiatry 48:19–28.

Pickens RW, Thompson T, Muchow DC (1973): Cannabis and phencyclidine self-administration by animals. In Goldberg L, Hoffmeister F (eds): "Psychic Dependence." New York: Springer-Verlag, pp 78–87.

Rae BA, Braude MC (eds) (1989): "Women and Drugs: A New Era for Research." NIDA Research Monograph No. 65. Washington, DC: U.S. Government Printing Office.

Regier DA, Boyd JH, Burke JD, Rae DS, Myers JK, Kramer M, Robins LN, George LK, Karno M, Locke BZ (1988): One-month prevalence of mental disorders in the U.S.: Based on five epidemiologic catchment area sites. Arch Gen Psychiatry 45:977–986.

Resnicow K, Botvin G (1993): School-based substance use prevention programs: Why do effects decay? Prev Med 22:484–490.

Richardson JL, Radziszewska B, Dent CW, Flay BR (1993): Relationships between after-school care of adolescents and substance use, risk taking, depressed mood, and academic achievement. Pediatrics 92:32–38.

Robins LN (1966): "Deviant Children Grown Up." Baltimore, MD: Williams & Wilkins.

Robins LN (1977): Estimating addiction rates and locating target populations: How decomposition into stages helps. In Rittenhouse JD (ed): "The Epidemiology of Heroin and Other Narcotics." Washington, DC: U.S. Government Printing Office, pp 25–39.

Robins LN (1983): The consequences of recommendations of the U.S. Privacy Protection Study Commission for longitudinal studies. In Ricks DF, Dohwenrend BS (eds): "Origins of Psychopathology: Problems in Research and Public Policy." New York: Cambridge University Press, pp 175–186.

Robins LN (1993): The Sixth Thomas James Okey Memorial Lecture: Vietnam veterans' rapid recovery from heroin addiction: A fluke or normal expectation? Addiction 88:1041–1054.

Robins LN, Helzer JE, Orvaschel H, Anthony JC, Blazer DG, Burnam A, Burke JD Jr (1985): The Diagnostic Interview Schedule. In Eaton WW, Kessler LG (eds): "Epidemiologic Field Methods in Psychiatry." New York: Academic Press, pp 143–170.

Robins LN, Przybeck TR (1985): Age of onset of drug use as a factor in drug and other disorders. In "Etiology of Drug Abuse: Implications for Prevention." National Institute on Drug Abuse Research Monograph No. 56. DHHS Publication No. (ADM)-85-1335 (Jones CL, Battjes RL (eds): Washington, DC: USGPO, pp 178–192.

Rounsaville BJ, Kosten TR, Weissman MM, Prusoff BA, Pauls D, Foley S, Merikangas KR (1991): Psychiatric disorders in the relatives of probands with opioid addiction. Arch Gen Psychiatry 48:33–42.

Sameroff AJ, Fiese BH (1989): Conceptual issues in prevention. In Shaffer D, Philips I, Enzer NB, Silverman MM, Anthony V (eds): "Prevention of Mental Disorders, Alcohol and Other Drug Use in Children and Adolescents." Office of Substance Abuse Prevention, Monograph No. 2. Rockville, MD: Office of Substance Abuse Prevention, pp 23–53.

Sapira JD, Ball JC, Penn H (1970): Causes of death among institutionalized narcotic addicts. J Chronic Dis 22:733–742.

Sells SB (1977): Reflections on the epidemiology of heroin and narcotic addiction from the perspective of treatment data. In Rittenhouse JD (ed): "The Epidemiology of Heroin and Other Narcotics." Washington, DC: U.S. Government Printing Office, pp 147–176.

Smart R (1992): The problems perspective: Implications for prevention policies. In Lader M, Edwards G, Drummond DC (eds): "The Nature of Alcohol and Drug Related Problems." Society for the Study of Addiction, Monograph No. 2. New York: Oxford University Press, pp 167–177.

Smart RG (1977): Comments on Sells' paper: "Reflections on the epidemiology of heroin and narcotic addiction from the perspective of treatment data." In Rittenhouse JD (ed): "The Epidemiology of Heroin and Other Narcotics." Washington, DC: U.S. Government Printing Office, pp 177–182.

Smith SS, O'Hara BF, Persico AM, Gorelick DA, Newlin DB, Vlahov D, Solomon L, Pickens R, Uhl GR (1992): Genetic vulnerability to drug abuse. Arch Gen Psychiatry 49:723–727.

Sonnedecker G (1962): Emergence of the concept of opiate addiction. J Mondial Pharmacie 3:279–290.

Stenbacka M, Allebeck P, Rømelsjö A (1993): Initiation into drug abuse: The pathway from being offered drugs to trying cannabis and progression to intravenous drug abuse. Scand J Social Med 21:31–39.

Tarter RE, Laird SB, Kabene M, Bukstein O, Kaminer Y (1990): Drug abuse severity in adolescents is associated with magnitude of deviation in temperament traits. Br J Addict 85:1501–1504.

Tarter RE, Mezzich AC (1992): Ontogeny of substance abuse: Perspectives and findings. In Glantz M, Pickens R (eds): "Vulnerability to Drug Abuse." Washington, DC: American Psychological Association, pp 149–177.

Tomas JM, Vlahov D, Anthony JC (1990): The association between intravenous drug use and early childhood misbehavior. Drug Alcohol Depend 25:79–89.

Trinkoff AM, Eaton WW, Anthony JC (1991): The prevalence of substance abuse among registered nurses. Nursing Research. 40:172–175.

Turner E, Ewing J, Shilling P, Smith TL, Irwin M, Schuckit M, Kelsoe JR (1992): Lack of association between an RFLP near the D_2 dopamine receptor gene and severe alcoholism. Biol Psychiatry 31:285–290.

Turner WM, Cutter HSG, Worobec TG, O'Farrell TJ, Bayog RD, Tsuang MT (1993): Family history models of alcoholism: Age of onset, consequences and dependence. J Study Alcohol 54:164–171.

Uhl GR, Persico AM, Smith SS (1992): Current excitement with D_2 dopamine receptor gene alleles in substance abuse. Arch Gen Psychiatry 49:157–160.

United States Substance Abuse and Mental Health Services Administration (1993): "Preliminary Estimates From the 1992 National Household Survey on Drug Abuse." Washington, DC: U.S. Government Printing Office.

Vaillant GE (1966): A twelve-year followup of New York narcotic addicts: IV. Some characteristics and determinants of abstinence. Am J Psychiatry 123:573–584.

Weinberg CR (1993): Toward a clearer definition of confounding. American Journal of Epidemiology. 137:1–8.

Weinberg CR (1994): Letter to the Editor. Am J Epidemiol 139: 962–963.

Wells JE, Bushnell JA, Hornblow AR, Joyce PR, Oakley-Browne MA (1989): Christchurch Psychiatric Epidemiology Study, Part I: Methodology and lifetime prevalence for specific psychiatric disorders. Aust NZ J Psychiatry 23:315–326.

White HR (1992): Early problem behavior and later drug problems. J Res Crime Delinq 29:412–429.

Wittchen H-U (1994): Reliability and validity studies of the WHO-Composite International Diagnostic Interview (CIDI)—A critical review. J Psychiatr Res (in press).

Wittchen H-U, Essau CA, von Zerssen D, Krieg J-C, Zaudig M (1992): Lifetime and six-month prevalence of mental disorders in the Munich Follow-up Study. Eur Arch Psychiatry Clin Neurosci 241:247–258.

Woody G, Schuckit M, Weinrieg R, Yu E (1993): A review of the substance use disorders section of the DSM-IV. Recent Adv Addictive Disorders 16:21–32.

World Health Organization (1992): "The ICD-10 Classification of Mental and Behavioural Disorders: Clinical Descriptions and Diagnostic Guidelines." Geneva: World Health Organization.

CHAPTER 19

Epidemiology of Personality Disorders

MICHAEL J. LYONS

Harvard Department of Psychiatry, Brockton/West Roxbury V.A.M.C., Brockton, MA 02401; Department of Psychology, Boston University, Boston, MA 02115; and Harvard Institute of Psychiatric Epidemiology and Genetics, Boston, MA 02115

INTRODUCTION

With the advent of the third edition of the *Diagnostic and Statistical Manual* (DSM-III) (American Psychiatric Association, 1980), the personality disorders were assigned their own axis (axis II) in the diagnostic nomenclature. DSM-III was a major impetus for clinical and research interest in the personality disorders because it provided explicit diagnostic criteria for their diagnosis. It included 11 specific disorders, some of which were relatively unknown. Many of the personality disorders, unlike axis I disorders such as schizophrenia and depression, do not have long histories as subjects of clinical attention or systematic observation. In an important way, one may mark the advent of systematic studies of personality disorder by the publication of DSM-III in 1980. This is not the case for all of the personality disorders, such as antisocial personality disorder, but it is for many of them.

Personality traits are described in DSM-III-R (American Psychiatric Association, 1987, p. 335) as "enduring patterns of perceiving, relating to, and thinking about the environment and oneself, and are exhibited in a wide range of important social and personal contexts." DSM-III-R defines *personality disorders* as inflexible and maladaptive personality traits that cause either significant functional impairment or subjective distress. Personality disorders are conceptualized as long-term characteristics of individuals that are likely to be evident by adolescence and continue through adulthood. The diagnosis of personality disorder should not be made if the characteristics only occur during episodes of an axis I disorder. DSM-III-R suggests that personality disorder may become less obvious in middle and later life.

In addition to specifying 11 individual personality disorders, DSM-III and DSM-III-R group the personality disorders into three clusters. Cluster A includes paranoid, schizoid, and schizotypal personality disorders; the basis for this cluster is the odd or eccentric characteristics common to individuals with any of these three disorders. Cluster B includes antisocial, borderline, histrionic, and narcissistic personality disorders. This cluster

Textbook in Psychiatric Epidemiology, Edited by Tsuang, Tohen, and Zahner
ISBN 0-471-59375-3 © 1995 Wiley-Liss, Inc.

is characterized by dramatic, emotional, or erratic features. Cluster C includes avoidant, dependent, obsessive-compulsive, and passive-aggressive personality disorders. This has been designated the anxious or fearful cluster.

This chapter is divided into three primary sections. The first describes substantive findings with an emphasis on the prevalence of personality disorders in different settings. The second section discusses conceptual issues, such as categorical versus dimensional approaches to classifying personality disorders. The third section addresses methodologic issues that are important for studying the epidemiology of personality disorders.

SUBSTANTIVE FINDINGS

Compared with many axis I disorders, such as schizophrenia, there are less extensive data available on the prevalence of axis II disorders. To a great extent, this is due to a much shorter history of empirical work on most of the constructs embodied in the personality disorders. In the case of schizophrenia, the definition formulated by Kraepelin (1919/1971) shortly after the turn of the century is relatively similar to the criteria in DSM-III and DSM-III-R. In general, the personality disorders, with the possible exception of antisocial personality disorder (and its related progenitors moral insanity, psychopathy, sociopathy, and so forth), have not been the object of empirical, let alone epidemiologic, research for very long. In this section a brief description of findings predating the publication of DSM-III is provided. The largest part of this section reviews findings bearing on the "true prevalence" of personality disorders, that is, rates of the disorders in representative community and nonclinical samples. Available data are presented for the prevalence of having any personality disorder and for individual disorders.

True Prevalence Studies

Pre-DSM-III. In the Midtown Manhattan study, Srole et al. (1962) reported a prevalence rate of 6% for sociopathy. In the Stirling County study using DSM-I diagnoses, Leighton et al. (1963) reported that 11% of males and 5% of females received a sociopathic diagnosis. Merikangas and Weissman (1991) reviewed the prevalence rates for personality disorder reported in pre-DSM-III studies that permitted the exclusion of alcoholism and drug abuse (which were classified as personality disorders in some older systems) from other personality disorders (Bremer, 1951; Essen-Moller et al., 1956; Langner and Michael, 1963; Leighton, 1959). They concluded that, in spite of nonuniformity in diagnostic definition, the reported rates were quite similar. Approximately 6%–9% of the samples were characterized as having a major personality disturbance. In these early data reviewed by Merikangas and Weissman, there is an indication that the overall sex ratio for personality disorders is about equal, with differences for specific disorders. Prevalence is fairly even across age groups, with a slight increase in later life, higher rates in urban than rural populations, and higher rates in lower than higher socioeconomic groups.

Post-DSM-III. Since the publication of DSM-III in 1980 there have been several studies that provided data on the prevalence of having any personality disorder (Table 1). Nestadt and his coworkers (1990, 1991, 1992), in a series of reports, detailed the results of a follow-up assessment for personality disorders of the Epidemiologic Catchment Area (ECA) study.

At the Baltimore site of the ECA, a total of 3,481 individuals were interviewed with

TABLE 1. Post-DSM-III Community Studies of Prevalence of Any Personality Disorder

Authors	Population	Instrument and Dx System	Prevalence (%) of Any PD	Comments
Nestadt et al. (1993)	810 subjects from the Clinical Reappraisal at Baltimore ECA site	DSM-III by SPE administered by psychiatrist	5.9 definite; 9.3 definite plus provisional	
Zimmerman and Coryell (1989)	797 nonpatient relatives of normal controls and probands with schizophrenia and depression	DSM-III by SIDP; telephone, 72.9%; face to face, 27.1%	17.9	Sample limits generalizability
Casey and Tyrer (1986)	200 urban and rural residents, selected randomly	Personality Assessment Schedule, ICD	13.0	Not DSM based
Reich et al. (1989b)	235 community residents, selected randomly	Personality Diagnostic Questionnaire, DSM-III	11.0	Required criteria plus impairment/distress for diagnosis
Maier et al. (1990[2])	447 probands and relatives from randomly selected families in Germany	DSM-III-R by SCID	10.0	Did not use DSM-III-R exclusionary criteria

the Diagnostic Interview Schedule (Robins et al., 1981), the General Health Questionnaire (Goldberg, 1974), and the Mini-Mental Status Exam (Folstein et al., 1975) as part of the ECA. Subsequent to the ECA data collection, the Clinical Reappraisal was carried out and included all subjects who had been "screened positive" for psychopathology and a random sample of 17% of the 3,481 original respondents. Of the 1,086 subjects selected for inclusion in the Clinical Reappraisal, 810 agreed to participate, a response rate of 75%. Subjects were interviewed by board-certified or board-eligible psychiatrists, blind to first-stage information. The psychiatrists used the Standardized Psychiatric Examination (SPE), a semistructured interview that averaged 1.5–3 hours to complete. The authors described the SPE as assessing personal history, medical and psychiatric problems, and present mental status; it includes an inventory and direct question approach. Nestadt et al. (1993) reported a prevalence of 5.9% for a definite diagnosis of personality disorder and a prevalence of 9.3% for their combined definite plus provisional diagnostic categories.

Zimmerman and Coryell (1989) reported the rates of DSM-III personality disorders assessed through the use of the Structured Interview for DSM-III Personality Disorders (SIDP) (Pfohl et al., 1982) among a nonpatient sample of 797 individuals. There are several features of the study that qualify somewhat the interpretation of their results. The sample that they studied was a mixture of relatives of normal controls (n = 185), relatives of schizophrenic probands (n = 131), relatives of probands with psychotic depression (n = 247), relatives of probands with nonpsychotic depression (n = 235), and relatives of probands with other psychiatric disorders (n = 10). Eleven individuals refused the SIDP interview, yielding the final sample size of 797. Their sample is problematic because certain personality disorders may have a familial relationship to axis I disorders. To the extent that a personality disorder has a familial relationship to an axis I disorder, the rate of the disorder among first-degree relatives of probands with the axis I disorder will be elevated, and results may not generalize to the general population. Therefore, the prevalence of some personality disorders may be inflated in the sample that Zimmerman and Coryell studied. Approximately three-fourths of the sample were interviewed by telephone (72.9%) and one fourth by face-to-face interviews (27.1%). The authors found no difference in the frequency of axis II diagnoses between telephone and face-to-face interviews. The prevalence of any DSM-III personality disorder diagnosis using the SIDP, including mixed personality disorder, was 17.9%. These investigators also administered the Personality Diagnostic Questionnaire (PDQ) (Hyler et al., 1983) to their subjects (Zimmerman and Coryell, 1990). Prevalence rates were fairly similar, but the PDQ produced higher rates of schizotypal, compulsive, dependent, and borderline personality disorders. The SIDP yielded higher rates of antisocial and passive-aggressive disorders. More individuals were diagnosed with a disorder by the SIDP, but the PDQ diagnosed multiple personality disorders more often. The results of the PDQ are not tabulated separately because the same sample was utilized for both instruments.

Casey and Tyrer (1986) carried out a study of 200 randomly selected community residents in the United Kingdom. They administered the Present State Examination (9th ed) (Wing, et al., 1974) for axis I disorders and the Personality Assessment Schedule (PAS) (Tyrer et al., 1979) for the assessment of personality disorders. The PAS obtains information from an informant as well as the subject. Ordinal ratings are made on 24 personality traits. A computer algorithm is applied to determine personality disorder diagnoses according to the International Classification of Diseases (World Health Organization, 1978). Personality disorders were diagnosed in 26 of their subjects (13%). The personality disorder with the highest prevalence was explosive personality, which probably corresponds most closely to the DSM-III diagnoses of antisocial personality disorder or intermittent explosive disorder from axis I. There were no differences in prevalence between their urban and rural samples, and males and females did not differ in the overall rate of personality disorder; women had a higher prevalence of asthenic personality disorder. They did not find a relationship between neurotic depression or the combined category of neuroses and personality disorder. Subjects with a personality disorder were found to have significantly poorer social functioning.

Reich and colleagues (1989a,b) conducted a random mailed survey of the adult population of Iowa City, Iowa. Surveys were mailed to 401 subjects; 240 surveys were returned, for a response rate of 62.1%. Data were collected using the PDQ (Hyler et al., 1983). Diagnoses were based on meeting the requisite number of criteria for a given personality disorder and meeting the impairment distress scale criterion for the presence of a disorder. The rate for receiving any axis II disorder was 11%.

Maier and his coworkers (1992) studied a sample of 452 subjects in the mixed urban/rural Rhein-Main area of Germany. Subjects were recruited to serve as controls in a family study of affective disorders and schizophrenia. The sample of control probands (n = 109) was selected randomly without regard to psychiatric status and was stratified by age, sex, residential area, and educational status. The sample of Maier et al. included the probands, their mates, and all first-degree relatives over age 20 years who agreed to take part in face-to-face interviews, for a total of 452. Subjects were administered the Schedule for Affective Disorders and Schizophrenia (SADS), Lifetime Version (Mannuzza et al., 1986) for axis I diagnoses and the Structured Clinical Interview for DSM-III axis II (Spitzer et al., 1987) for axis II diagnoses. The rate of receiving any personality disorder diagnosis was 10.0%. They followed DSM-III-R diagnostic criteria with the exception of exclusionary criteria; for example, schizotypal personality could be diagnosed in the presence of schizophrenia.

Treated Prevalence

Merikangas and Weissman (1991) pointed out the hazards of using treated rates for drawing inferences about true prevalence of personality disorders. They identified a number of factors that could lead to bias in treated samples: 1) differences in the availability of treatment; 2) the role of cultural factors in help-seeking behavior; 3) differences in the severity of the disorder; 4) the potential influence of other comorbid psychiatric disorders; and 5) differences among the personality disorders in the likelihood of seeking treatment. However, the importance of personality disorders in clinical practice makes their prevalence in such settings valuable information in its own right.

Dahl (1986) reported results of the systematic assessment of DSM-III personality disorders in 231 consecutive admissions to a psychiatric inpatient unit in Norway. Chronic patients and those with organic disorders were excluded. Approximately 45% of the sample received a personality disorder diagnosis (40% of females and 49% of males). Forty-four percent of those with a personality disorder received one diagnosis, 36% had two diagnoses, 15% had three diagnoses, and 5% had four diagnoses. Schizotypal, histrionic, antisocial, and borderline personality disorders were each present in approximately 20% of the sample. Avoidant personality disorder was diagnosed in 9% of the sample, and the remaining disorders were diagnosed much less frequently. In a series of 100 patients admitted with major psychiatric disorders (affective disorders, schizophrenia, and other functional psychosis), Cutting et al. (1986) found that 44% had an "abnormal personality" based on informant interviews about the period preceding the acute episode.

Oldham and Skodol (1991) investigated the prevalence of personality disorders among the 129,268 patients treated in New York state mental health facilities in 1988. Using the system's centralized database, they found that 10.8% received a personality disorder diagnosis. The personality disorder diagnosis was the primary diagnosis of 1.2% of patients, and only 0.2% of patients received more than one personality disorder diagnosis. The most common diagnosis was borderline personality disorder; 17.2% of the patients with any personality disorder received a diagnosis of borderline personality disorder. These authors concluded that the standard record-keeping procedures underestimated the prevalence of personality disorders and that personality disorders are not being systematically assessed.

The prevalence of personality disorders has also been examined in nonpsychiatric medical populations. Casey and her coworkers (1984, 1985) reported on the prevalence of personality disorders in British clinical settings using the ICD classification. They found a 34% prevalence of personality disorder in primary care settings; anxiety states and alcohol abuse were the conditions most commonly associated with personality disorders. In a rural general practice, they found a prevalence rate of 20%. Reich et al. (1989a) found a significant positive association between the presence of personality disorder and the probability of being hospitalized for a nonpsychiatric medical illness.

As is the case for both axis I and axis II disorders, treated rates shed little light on the prevalence of disorders in untreated samples. However, because personality disorders have important implications for service provision, it is useful to consider their frequency in various clinical populations. Obviously, the nature of the setting in which the disorders are studied and the method by which they are studied will influence the findings. The treated rates of the individual personality disorders are included in the next section. (Data on treated rates are drawn primarily from a review by Widiger (1991).)

Prevalence of Specific DSM-III/DSM-III-R Personality Disorders

In this section, each of the personality disorders is presented, starting with the essential features of the disorder according to the DSM-IV draft criteria published by the American Psychiatric Association in 1993. Available data about prevalence in clinical and nonclinical populations are presented. For several personality disorders, such as antisocial personality disorder, there are a number of studies that have reported prevalence. For many of the personality disorders, however, there have been very few reports of true prevalence. The length of each section is somewhat proportional to the amount of epidemiologic data available about the disorder. In some cases a single study provided data on a number of individual personality disorders. To avoid redundancy, the methodology of the study is mentioned only once.

Paranoid Personality Disorder. The essential feature of paranoid personality disorder is a "pervasive distrust and suspiciousness of others such that their motives are interpreted as malevolent" (American Psychiatric Association, 1993, p. T:1). All three nonclinical studies of paranoid personality disorder reported prevalences less than 2.0%. The rates in clinical samples reported in Widiger (1991) ranged from 1.0% to 36%, with a median prevalence of 6.0%. Reich (1987a) found an excess of paranoid personality disorder among males compared with females in an outpatient sample.

Schizoid Personality Disorder. The essential feature of this disorder is a "pervasive pattern of detachment from social relationships and a restricted range of expression of emotions in interpersonal settings" (American Psychiatric Association, 1993, p. T:2). In general, schizoid personality disorder has been a very infrequent diagnosis in clinical settings. For example, Zanarini et al. (1987) found no cases in a clinical sample of 97 patients, and Koenigsberg et al. (1985) reported no cases on the basis of chart review in a sample of 2,462 patients. The prevalences in nonclinical samples reported in Table 2 are 1.0% or lower. The rates in clinical samples reported by Widiger (1991) ranged from 0.0% to 8%, with a median prevalence of 1.0%. Individuals with schizoid personality disorder may be less likely to seek treatment as a function of their disorder. It may also be that the diagnosis of schizotypal personality disorder is applied to a number of individuals who might have been characterized as schizoid before DSM-III or that the current criteria are inadequate (Zanarini et al., 1987).

Schizotypal Personality Disorder. The essential feature of schizotypal personality disorder is a "pervasive pattern of social and interpersonal deficits marked by acute discomfort with, and reduced capacity for, close relationships as well as by cognitive or perceptual distortions and eccentricities of behavior" (American Psychiatric Association, 1993, p. T:3). These characteristics must be present by early adulthood in various contexts. The symptoms must not be severe enough to warrant a diagnosis of schizophrenia. The DSM-III diagnostic criteria for schizotypal personality disorder were drawn from the definition for the diagnosis of borderline schizophrenia in the Danish Adoption study

TABLE 2. Prevalence of Cluster A Personality Disorder

Authors	Population	Instrument	Prevalence (%)	Comments
Paranoid PD				
Zimmerman and Coryell (1989)	797 nonpatient relatives of normal controls and probands with schizophrenia and depression	DSM-III by SIDP; telephone, 72.9%; face to face, 27.1%	0.9	Sample limits generalizability
Reich et al. (1989b)	235 community residents, selected randomly	Personality Diagnostic Questionnaire DSM-III	0.9	Required criteria plus impairment/ distress diagnosis
Maier et al. (1992)	447 probands and relatives from randomly selected families in Germany	DSM-III-R by SCID	1.8	Did not use DSM-III-R exclusionary criteria
Schizoid PD				
Zimmerman and Coryell (1989)	797 nonpatient relatives of normal controls and probands with schizophrenia and depression	DSM-III by SIDP; telephone, 72.9%; face to face, 27.1%	0.9	Sample limits generalizability
Casey and Tyrer (1986)	200 urban and rural residents, selected randomly	Personality Assessment Schedule, ICD	1.0	Not DSM based
Reich et al. (1989b)	235 community residents, selected randomly	Personality Diagnostic Questionnaire, DSM-III	0.9	Required criteria plus impairment/distress for diagnosis
Maier et al. (1992)	447 probands and relatives from randomly selected families in Germany	DSM-III-R by SCID	0.4	Did not use DSM-III-R exclusionary criteria
Schizotypal PD				
Zimmerman and Coryell (1989)	797 nonpatient relatives of normal controls and probands with schizophrenia and depression	DSM-III by SIDP; telephone, 72.9%; face to face, 27.1	2.9	Sample limits generalizability

(continued)

TABLE 2. Prevalence of Cluster A Personality Disorder (*Continued*)

Authors	Population	Instrument	Prevalence (%)	Comments
Baron et al. (1985)	376 relatives of control subjects in a family study	DSM-III by Schedule for Interviewing Borderlines; 70% interviews 30% family history	2.2	Adjustment for sensitivity of family history method
Reich et al. (1989b)	235 community residents, selected randomly	Personality Diagnostic Questionnaire, DSM-III	5.1	Required criteria plus impairment/distress for diagnosis
Maier et al. (1992)	447 probands and relatives from randomly selected families in Germany	DSM-III-R by SCID	0.7	Did not use DSM-III-R exclusionary criteria

(Kety et al., 1978). A number of studies have indicated a familial relationship between schizotypal personality disorder and schizophrenia. However, a number of studies have failed to find an excess risk for schizophrenia among the relatives of schizotypal probands.

Baron et al. (1985) conducted a family study of the transmission of schizotypal and borderline personality disorder. They identified a control group of 90 subjects and subsequently included 376 of their relatives. Their findings on the relatives of controls is relevant for inferring prevalence in a nonclinical sample. Seventy percent of the relatives of controls were personally interviewed by mental health professionals using the SADS (Spitzer and Endicott, 1978) for axis I and with the Schedule for Interviewing Borderlines (Gunderson, 1982), which yields diagnoses for DSM-III schizotypal and borderline personality disorders. Data were obtained on 30 percent of the relatives using a family history version of the Schedule for Interviewing Borderlines (the family history method refers to obtaining information from an informant rather than through a direct interview). Seventy-five percent of the relatives of controls were studied blind to the diagnostic status of the proband. Baron et al. (1985) did not find differences in outcome between subjects rated in the blind versus nonblind conditions. The risk to relatives was age corrected using the Stromgren method for schizotypal but not for borderline personality disorder. The authors also adjusted the morbidity risks to compensate for the inferior sensitivity of the family history method compared with direct interview. Although this procedure applied across all relative groups in their study may help the comparison of relatives of different types of probands, it also makes epidemiologic inferences from these data somewhat tentative.

In a small study of consecutive outpatient admissions, Bornstein et al. (1988) reported that patients with schizotypal personality disorder were more likely to receive a diagnosis of substance abuse or dependence and major affective disorder than nonschizotypal patients in their series. The prevalences in nonclinical samples reported in Table 2 range from 0.7% to 5.1%, with a median value of about 3.0%. The rates in clinical samples reported by Widiger (1991) ranged from 2.0% to 64%, with a median prevalence of 17.5%.

Antisocial Personality Disorder. The essential feature of antisocial personality disorder is a "pervasive pattern of disregard for and violation of the rights of others" (American Psychiatric Association, 1993, p. T:4). The DSM-III and DSM-III-R criteria were heavily influenced by the work of Robins et al. (1984) and place an emphasis on antisocial and criminal behavior. In prison populations the prevalence of DSM-III-R antisocial personality disorder may be over 50%.

Antisocial personality disorder was one of the DSM-III personality disorders about which Nestadt and his coworkers reported results. They found a positive association between the number of criteria for antisocial personality disorder and the risk for an alcohol use disorder diagnosis. Reich (1987a) found an excess of males with antisocial personality disorder among an outpatient sample.

Using DSM-I criteria, Leighton et al. (1963) reported a prevalence of 11% in men and 5% for women for a sociopathic diagnosis. Weissman et al. (1978) reported results from a systematic survey of households in New Haven, CT. Their diagnostic data were collected in an 8 year follow up of the sample. The original sample was 1,095 individuals; the diagnostic sample included 511 of the original sample. The follow-up sample differed from the original sample on the basis of race and class; the follow-up included a higher proportion of whites and a lower proportion of the lowest social class. Diagnostic data were collected with the SADS, and diagnoses were based on the Research Diagnostic Criteria. The rate of current antisocial personality disorder was 0.2%.

Antisocial personality disorder was the only personality disorder included in the ECA study. Data are presented in Table 3. Compton et al. (1991) applied the methodology of the ECA study to a community-based sample in Taiwan. The prevalences in nonclinical samples reported in Table 3 range from 0.2% in a Taiwanese population to over 3%, with a median value of about 2.0%. The rates in clinical samples reported in Widiger (1991) ranged from 0.0% to 37%, with a median prevalence of 7%.

Borderline Personality Disorder. The essential feature of borderline personality disorder is a "pervasive pattern of instability of interpersonal relationships, self-image, affects, and control over impulses" (American Psychiatric Association, 1993, p. T:5). Swartz et al. (1990) derived a diagnostic algorithm for diagnosing borderline personality disorder from the Diagnostic Interview Schedule (Robins et al., 1981). Using a cut off of 11 items from their 24 item index, they classified 1.8% of their sample (from the Duke site of the ECA study) between ages 19 and 55 years as having borderline personality disorder. Merikangas and Weissman (1986) estimated the prevalence of borderline PD to be between 1.7% and 2.0% based on community studies carried out before the diagnostic criteria for borderline personality disorder were codified in DSM-III.

Borderline personality disorder is the most common personality disorder seen in most psychiatric settings and is over-represented in clinical populations because of the tendency toward help seeking (Galenberg, 1987). Nurnberg et al. (1991), among a sample of outpatients with personality disorder and no concurrent axis I disorder, found that 82% of patients with a diagnosis of borderline personality disorder received at least one other personality disorder diagnosis. They concluded that borderline personality disorder characterizes a general personality disorder construct.

Widiger and Weissman (1991) and Widiger and Trull (1992) reviewed the epidemiology of borderline PD. They reported an average prevalence of 8.0% in studies of outpatients and 15% in studies of inpatients. Among studies of patients with personality disorder, the average prevalence among outpatients was 27% and among inpatients, 51%. These authors concluded that borderline personality disorder is the most common person-

TABLE 3. Prevalence of Cluster B Personality Disorder

Authors	Population	Instrument	Prevalence (%)	Comments
Antisocial PD				
Robins et al (1984)	9,543 subjects, strict probability sampling at 3 sites	DIS	2.5	Very rigorous sampling
Compton et al (1991)	11,004 community residents in Taiwan; strict probability sample	DIS	0.2	Very rigorous sampling and methodology
Zimmerman and Coryell (1989)	797 nonpatient relatives of normal controls and probandswith schizophrenia and depression	DSM-III by SIDP; telephone, 72.9%; face to face, 27.1	3.3	Sample limits generalizability
Casey and Tyrer (1986)	200 urban and rural residents, selected randomly	Personality Assessment Schedule, ICD	6.0	(Included explosive personality) not DSM based
Nestadt et al. (1990)	810 subjects from the Clinical Reappraisal at Baltimore ECA site	DSM-III by SPE administered by psychiatrist	1.5	
Weissman et al. (1978)	511 systematically identified community residents	Research Diagnostic Criteria; RDC	0.2	Significant sample attrition is a problem
Reich et al. (1989b)	235 community residents, selected randomly	Personality Diagnostic Questionnnaire, DSM-III	0.4	Required criteria plus impair-ment/distress for diagnosis
Bland et al. (1988)	3,258, Canada	DIS	3.7	
Oakley-Browne et al. (1989)	1,498, New Zealand	DIS	3.1	
Maier et al. (1992)	447 probands and relatives from randomly selected families in Germany	DSM-III-R by SCID	0.2	Did not use DSM-III-R exclusionary criteria

TABLE 3. Prevalence of Cluster B Personality Disorder (*Continued*)

Authors	Population	Instrument	Prevalence (%)	Comments
Borderline PD				
Zimmerman and Coryell (1989)	797 nonpatient relatives of normal controls and probands with schizophrenia and depression	DSM-III by SIDP; telephone, 72.9%; face to face, 27.1%	1.6	Sample limits generalizability
Baron et al. (1985)	376 relatives of control subjects in a family study	DSM-III by Schedule for Interviewing Borderlines; 70% interviews, 30% family history	1.7	Unorthodox adjustment for sensitivity of family history method
Reich et al. (1989b)	235 community residents, selected randomly	Personality Diagnostic Questionnaire, DSM-III	0.4	Required criteria plus impairment/distress for diagnosis
Swartz et al. (1990)	1,541 community residents from the Duke ECA site	DIS/Borderline Index, DSM-III	1.8	Included subjects between ages 19 and 55 years
Maier et al. (1992)	447 probands and relatives from randomly selected familes in Germany	DSM-III-R by SCID	1.1	Did not use DSM-III-R exclusionary criteria
Histrionic PD				
Zimmerman and Coryell (1989)	797 nonpatient relatives of normal controls and probands with schizophrenia and depression	DSM-III by SIDP; telephone, 72.9% face to face, 27.1%	3.0	Sample limits generalizability
Nestadt et al. (1990)	810 subjects from the Clinical Reappraisal at Baltimore ECA site	DSM-III by SPE administered by psychiatrist	2.2	
Reich et al. (1989b)	235 community residents, selected randomly	Personality Diagnostic Questionnaire, DSM-III	2.1	Required criteria plus impairment/distress for diagnosis
Maier et al. (1992)	447 probands and relatives from randomly selected families in Germany	DSM-III-R by SCID	1.3	Did not use DSM-III-R exclusionary criteria

(*continued*)

TABLE 3. Prevalence of Cluster B Personality Disorder (*Continued*)

Authors	Population	Instrument	Prevalence (%)	Comments
Narcissistic PD				
Zimmerman and Coryell (1989)	797 nonpatient relatives of normal controls and probands with schizophrenia and depression	DSM-III by SIDP; telephone, 72.9%; face to face, 27.1%	0.0	Sample limits generalizability
Reich et al. (1989b)	235 community residents, selected randomly	Personality Diagnostic Questionnaire, DSM-III	0.4	Required criteria plus impairment/distress for diagnosis
Maier et al. (1992)	447 probands and relatives from randomly selected families in Germany	DSM-III-R by SCID	0.0	Did not use DSM-III-R exclusionary criteria

ality disorder diagnosis given in clinical samples, with prevalence rates of up to 70% found among inpatient samples (Standage and Ladha, 1988).

Akhtar et al. (1986) reviewed 23 studies of borderline personality disorder to investigate associations between it and demographic characteristics. All of the studies that they reviewed used clinical samples, mostly inpatients. They only included studies that utilized one of several widely used criteria sets to define the disorder. They pooled data across the samples of borderlines and compared these data with pooled comparison group data from the same studies. They found that patients receiving a diagnosis of borderline personality disorder tended to be young, with a mean age in the mid-twenties. A significantly higher percentage of borderline patients (77%) were female. The samples of borderline patients were disproportionately white; the mean percentage of blacks in the borderline samples was 10%, while the mean percentage of blacks in the comparison samples was 20%, a statistically significant difference. Reich (1987a) did not find an excess of borderline personality disorder among female outpatients.

The prevalences in nonclinical samples reported in Table 3 range from 0.4% to about 2.0%, with a median value of about 1.6%. The rates in clinical samples reported by Widiger (1991) ranged from 11% to 70%, with a median prevalence of 31%.

Histrionic Personality Disorder. The essential feature of histrionic personality disorder is a "pervasive pattern of excessive emotionality and attention-seeking" (American Psychiatric Association, 1993, p. T:6). The term *hysterical personality* has been used in other classifications. There has been relatively little empirical work done on histrionic personality disorder (Pfohl, 1991). When structured diagnostic assessments have been utilized, no sex difference in histrionic personality disorder has been observed; however, there is some suggestion that clinicians may more frequently apply the diagnosis to females (Pfohl, 1991).

Histrionic personality disorder was one of the DSM-III personality disorders about which Nestadt and his coworkers (described above) reported in the Clinical Reappraisal of the ECA Baltimore site. There were no differences in prevalence by sex (males, 2.2%; females, 2.1%), race, or education. The prevalence declined with age in males but not in females. There was a higher rate of histrionic personality disorder among separated and divorced subjects than among married subjects. There was an increase in depressive disorder, suicide attempts, and the occurrence of three or more unexplained medical symptoms in females associated with histrionic personality disorder. In males there was an increase in substance use disorders associated with histrionic personality disorder. Subjects with histrionic personality disorder were significantly more likely to seek medical and psychiatric treatment than subjects without.

The prevalences in nonclinical samples reported in Table 3 range from 1.3% to 3.0%, with a median value of about 2.2%. The rates in clinical samples reported by Widiger (1991) ranged from 2.0% to 45%, with a median prevalence of 19%.

Narcissistic Personality Disorder. The essential feature of this disorder is a "pervasive pattern of grandiosity (in fantasy or behavior), need for admiration, and lack of empathy" (American Psychiatric Association, 1993, p. T:7). There has not been a great deal of empirical work done on narcissistic personality disorder in general and very little epidemiologic work in particular. Although there is considerable clinical interest in the disorder, it has only recently been included in official nomenclatures. Narcissistic personality disorder became part of the American nomenclature in 1980 with DSM-III, and there is no counterpart to it in ICD-10.

Gunderson et al. (1991b) reviewed several studies that reported the prevalence of DSM-III-R narcissistic personality disorder in clinical populations (Dahl, 1986; Frances et al., 1984; Skodol, 1989; Zanarini et al., 1987) and reported prevalence rates ranging from 2.0% to 16%. The prevalences in nonclinical samples reported in Table 3 range from 0.0% to 0.4%, with a median value of about 0.2%. The rates in clinical samples reported by Widiger (1991) ranged from 2.0% to 35%, with a median prevalence of 6.0%.

Avoidant Personality Disorder. The essential feature of avoidant personality disorder is a "pervasive pattern of social inhibition, feelings of inadequacy, and hypersensitivity to negative evaluation" (American Psychiatric Association, 1993, p. T:8). An important issue in the epidemiology of avoidant personality disorder is its potential overlap with an axis I disorder, generalized social phobia. Turner et al. (1991) studied axis II comorbidity in a sample of individuals with social phobias. Avoidant personality disorder was present in 22.1% of the sample, and an additional 52.9% of the sample had avoidant features that fell short of meeting the diagnostic threshold. Schneier et al. (1991) studied a sample of 50 patients with social phobias. They found that 70% of patients with social phobia met criteria for avoidant personality disorder, and 89% of patients with generalized social phobia received a diagnosis of avoidant personality disorder. Herbert et al. (1992) found that 61% of patients in their series with generalized social phobia also met criteria for avoidant personality disorder. Holt et al. (1990) found that 50% of their sample with generalized social phobia met criteria for avoidant personality disorder. Schneier et al. (1991) suggested that generalized social phobia and avoidant personality disorder may define a single psychopathologic entity.

The prevalences in nonclinical samples reported in Table 4 range from 0.0% to 1.3%, with a median value of about 1.1%. The rates in clinical samples reported by Widiger (1991) ranged from 5.0% to 55%, with a median prevalence of 16%.

Dependent Personality Disorder. The essential feature of dependent personality disorder is a "pervasive and excessive need to be taken care of, leading to submissive and clinging behaviors and fears of separation" (American Psychiatric Association, 1993; p. T:9). Dependent personality disorder was recently reviewed by Hirschfeld et al. (1991). They pointed out that dependent personality disorder derives from psychoanalytic theory, social psychological theory, and ethological theory. The construct of dependent personality disorder overlaps with borderline, avoidant, and histrionic personality disorders. In studies of clinical samples reviewed by Hirschfeld et al. (1991), substantial overlap with other personality disorders was reported. The greatest degree of overlap was with borderline personality disorder (over 50% in most studies), followed by avoidant, histrionic, and schizotypal personality disorders. Hirschfeld et al. (1991) discussed the issues of sex differences and possible sex bias in the diagnosis of dependent personality disorder. They pointed out that dependent personality disorder was diagnosed more frequently in females when assessment was not carried out using standardized instruments. When standardized instruments were used, males and females did not differ in the frequency of the diagnosis. They suggested that clinicians, rather than the standardized diagnostic criteria, may be responsible for observed differences in male and female rates. Individuals with a depressive disorder may be more likely to display dependent personality traits (Overholser, 1991).

The prevalences of dependent personality disorder in nonclinical samples reported in Table 4 range from 1.5% to 5.1%, with a median value of about 1.8%. The rates in clinical samples reported by Widiger (1991) ranged from 2.0% to 55%, with a median prevalence of 20%.

Obsessive-Compulsive Personality Disorder. The essential feature of obsessive-compulsive personality disorder is a "pervasive pattern of preoccupation with orderliness, perfectionism, and mental and interpersonal control, at the expense of flexibility, openness, and efficiency" (American Psychiatric Association, 1993, p. T:10). Compulsive personality disorder was one of the DSM-III personality disorders about which Nestadt and his coworkers (described above) reported in the Clinical Reappraisal of the ECA Baltimore site. Males had a significantly higher prevalence (3.0%) than females (0.6%). White respondents had a significantly higher prevalence than black respondents. There was no association between age and risk of the disorder. The diagnosis of compulsive personality disorder was associated with higher education, greater likelihood of being employed, and greater likelihood of being married as opposed to being widowed, separated, divorced, or never married. Subjects with compulsive personality disorder had a higher income than those without after correcting for age and sex. Nestadt et al. (1992) found that compulsive traits were associated with greater risk of generalized anxiety disorder and simple phobia and lower risk of alcohol use disorder.

Turner et al. (1991) studied axis II comorbidity in a sample of individuals with social phobias. Obsessive-compulsive personality disorder was present in 13.2% of the sample, and an additional 48.5% of the sample had obsessive-compulsive traits that fell short of meeting the diagnostic threshold. Baer et al. (1990) studied 96 patients with obsessive-compulsive disorder (OCD), which is an anxiety disorder recorded on axis I. Only 6% of the patients received a diagnosis of obsessive-compulsive personality disorder; of the six patients receiving the diagnosis, five had onset of obsessive-compulsive symptoms before age 10 years. Pfohl et al. (1990) found that among patients with OCD, 30% met criteria for obsessive-compulsive personality disorder. (To put this finding in context, in the same

TABLE 4. Prevalence of Cluster C Personality Disorders

Authors	Population	Instrument	Prevalence (%)	Comments
Avoidant PD				
Zimmerman and Coryell (1989)	797 nonpatient relatives of normal controls and probands with schizophrenia and depression	DSM-III by SIDP; telephone, 72.9% face to face, 27.1%	1.3	Sample limits generalizability
Reich et al. (1989b)	235 community residents, selected randomly	Personality Diagnostic Questionnaire, DSM-III	0.0	Required criteria plus impairment/distress for diagnosis
Maier et al. (1992)	447 probands and relatives from randomly selected families in Germany	DSM-III-R by SCID	1.1	Did not use DSM-III-R exclusionary criteria
Dependent PD				
Zimmerman and Coryell (1989)	797 nonpatient relatives of normal controls and probands with schizophrenia and depression	DSM-III by SIDP; telephone, 72.9%; face to face, 27.1%	1.8	Sample limits generalizability
Reich et al. (1989b)	235 community residents, selected randomly	Personality Diagnostic Questionnaire, DSM-III	5.1	Required criteria plus impairment/distress for diagnosis
Maier et al. (1992)	447 probands and relatives from randomly selected families in Germany	DSM-III-R by SCID	1.5	Did not use DSM-III-R exclusionary criteria
Obsessive-Compulsive PD				
Zimerman and Coryell (1989)	797 nonpatient relatives of normal controls and probands with schizophrenia and depression	DSM-III by SIDP; telephone, 72.9%; face to face, 27.1%	2.0	Sample limits generalizability
Nestadt et al. (1990)	810 subjects from the Clinical Reappraisal at Baltimore ECA site	DSM-III by SPE administered by psychiatrist	1.7	Male rate five times female rate
Reich et al. (1989b)	235 community residents, selected randomly	Personality Diagnostic Questionnaire, DSM-III	6.4	Required criteria plus impairment/distress for diagnosis

(*continued*)

TABLE 4. Prevalence of Cluster C Personality Disorders (*Continued*)

Authors	Population	Instrument	Prevalence (%)	Comments
Maier et al. (1992)	447 probands and relatives from randomly selected families in Germany	DSM-III-R by SCID	2.2	Did not use DSM-III-R exclusionary criteria
Passive-Agressive PD				
Zimmerman and Coryell (1989)	797 nonpatient relatives of normal controls and probands with schizophrenia and depression	DSM-III by SIDP; telephone, 72.9%; face to face, 27.1%	3.3	Sample limits generalizability
Reich et al. (1989b)	235 community residents, selected randomly	Personality Diagnostic Questionnaire, DSM-III	0.0	Required criteria plus impairment/distress for diagnosis
Maier et al. (1992)	447 probands and relatives from randomly selected families in Germany	DSM-III-R by SCID	1.8	Did not use DSM-III-R exclusionary criteria

study they found dependent personality disorder in 46% of their OCD subjects and passive-aggressive personality disorder in 49%.) Reich (1987a) found an excess of males with OCD among an outpatient sample in comparison to females.

The prevalences in nonclinical samples reported in Table 4 range from 1.7% to 6.4%, with a median value of about 2.0%. The rates in clinical samples reported by Widiger (1991) ranged from 1.0% to 20%, with a median prevalence of 9%.

Passive-Aggressive Personality Disorder. The essential feature of passive-aggressive personality disorder described in DSM-III-R is a "pervasive pattern of passive resistance to demands of adequate social and occupational performance" (American Psychiatric Association, 1987, p. 356). Passive-aggressive personality disorder is the only DSM-III-R personality disorder that is not included in DSM-IV. The prevalences in nonclinical samples reported in Table 4 range from 0.0% to 3.3%, with a median value of about 1.8%. The rates in clinical samples reported by Widiger (1991) ranged from 0.0% to 52%, with a median prevalence of 9.5%.

Summary of Prevalence Studies. Figure 1 contains the median values for each of the 11 personality disorders from community or nonclinical populations and the medians from Widiger's summary (1991) of studies of clinical populations. It should be noted that some personality disorders were only included in a small number of studies, while for others medians are based on a more reasonable number of studies. Widiger and Rogers (1989) suggested that the high rates of borderline, schizotypal, and histrionic personality disorders in clinical settings reflect the fact that these disorders lead to

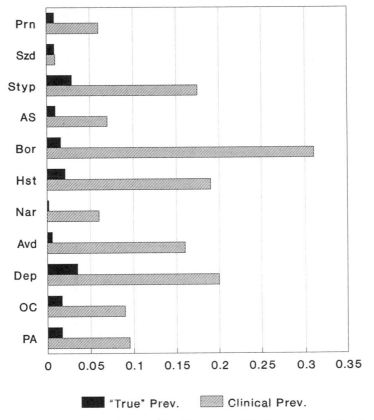

FIGURE 1. Median Prevalence of Personality Disorders (PD). Prn, paranoid PD; Szd, schizoid PD; Styp, schizotypal PD; AS, antisocial PD; Bor, borderline PD; Hst, histrionic PD; Nar, narcissistic PD; Avd, avoidant PD; Dep, dependent PD; OC, obsessive compulsive PD; PA, passive-aggressive PD.

the lowest level of functioning and that the symptomatology of these disorders such as drug use, suicide attempts, and cognitive-perceptual aberrations, may lead to hospitalization.

CONCEPTUAL ISSUES

Probably the primary conceptual issue with implications for investigating the epidemiology of personality disorders is the question of whether personality disorders are best considered to be categories or whether they should be considered to represent extreme standings on universally occurring dimensions of personality.

Models of Personality Disorder

The issue of the relative merits of categorical versus dimensional approaches cuts across most domains of psychopathology. However, in the domain of personality disorders it is especially significant, in part, because of the long tradition of research in personality psychology based on dimensional models. Currently, clinicians using DSM-III-R must decide whether a patient meets criteria for one or more personality disorders, each considered a separate and distinct category.

If the true nature of personality disorders is dimensional, it would suggest that the most appropriate epidemiologic approach might be to determine the mean and standard deviation of the population on the appropriate dimension. Consistent with such an approach, prevalence could be regarded as the proportion of the population that exceeds a threshold associated with impairment and/or distress.

The DSM-IV *Options Book* (American Psychiatric Association, 1991) described the strengths and weaknesses of the current categorical system. The *Options Book* points out that a dimensional approach would improve flexibility, possibly improve reliability and validity for certain disorders, and save information lost in categorical classification. The inclusion of a dimensional approach in an appendix of DSM-IV has been proposed (American Psychiatric Association, 1991). Lack of consensus about the dimensions to include is a disadvantage of adopting a dimensional approach (American Psychiatric Association, 1991).

Costa and McCrae (1990) suggested that DSM-III personality disorders, at least as they are assessed by the scales created by a number of different investigators, represent an extreme standing or a configuration of extreme standings on the dimensions of normal personality. This might be termed the *defining model*, in which the disorder results from exceeding the threshold on some dimension (or dimensions); the dimension is causally related to the disorder, and exceeding the threshold is a sufficient cause. A medical example of this model would be cases of essential hypertension without a demonstrable underlying pathophysiological cause for elevated blood pressure. That is, the factors that go into determining the blood pressure of the afflicted individuals are the same as those for the general population. Blood pressure, in general, is normally distributed in the population, and some individuals, for the same multifarious genetic and environmental factors that determine the blood pressure of human beings, fall at the high end of the distribution. Because blood pressure at the high end of the distribution is associated with excess morbidity and mortality, it is justifiably considered a disorder—hypertension. The defining model of personality disorder is similar to this example. Some individuals, due to the same genetic and environmental factors that influence everyone, are at the high or low end of a dimension or dimensions of personality, and this standing defines (it *is*) their personality disorder.

The defining model, however, does not describe the only possible manner in which dimensions of normal personality may relate to personality disorders. There are at least two other models that are equally plausible. In the *descriptive (trivial) model*, the disorder can be described in terms of a dimension (or dimensions), but the relationship is not causal and is uninformative for understanding the disorder. A medical example of the descriptive model would be explaining Down's syndrome in terms of the "universally occurring" dimensions of height and IQ. That is, individuals with Down's syndrome could be described as being at the low end of the continuum of height and at the low end of the continuum of IQ. However, this is an uninformative approach. A telling question would be, "Are people with Down's syndrome short for the same reason that short people without Down's syndrome are short?" If the answer is no, then trying to understand Down's syndrome through the mechanism that determines height for most people would not be informative. Individuals with Down's syndrome differ qualitatively from the general population. If a personality disorder is caused by some factor or factors that are independent of "normal" personality, it still might be described in these terms, but such a Procrustean approach will be counterproductive for understanding the nature of the phenomenon.

In the *predisposing model*, exceeding a threshold on the relevant dimension is a risk factor for the disorder and could be a necessary cause, but it is not a sufficient cause. Phenylketonuria (PKU) can serve as a medical example of this model. An individual who is homozygous for a defective gene that leads to the production of phenylalanine hydroxylase is vulnerable to the development of PKU. Such a genotype is a necessary but not sufficient cause. In order for the individual to manifest PKU, he or she must be exposed to dietary phenylalanine. If such an individual ingests phenylalanine, damage to the nervous system results. Without such exposure, there is no damage to the nervous system. For example, schizotypal personality disorder could be due to an extreme position on a universal continuum of introversion–extroversion plus possessing a schizophrenia genotype. In this example, introversion is necessary but not sufficient to produce schizotypal personality disorder.

Block and Ozer (1982) discussed a similar issue with regard to the use of typologies in the study of personality. They made a distinction between *type as label* and *type as distinctive form*. *Type as label* refers to the practice of establishing categories by classifying individuals above some threshold on an underlying continuum as being in the category. The category so established is then given a name or label. The defining model discussed above corresponds to *type as label*. The alternative definition of *category* or *type* described by Block and Ozer is stronger and more implicative. *Type as distinctive form* refers to "a subset of individuals characterized by a reliably unique or discontinuously different pattern of covariation . . . with respect to a specifiable (and non-trivial) set of variables" (Block, 1971). The use of a dimensional approach to personality disorders is not appropriate if these disorders fit the *type as distinctive form model*. Meehl (1979) made a similar distinction between a communicative taxon and a "true" taxon.

It seems likely that some aspects of personality disorders are related to deviation within normal dimensions of personality while other features are best considered categorical. It is unlikely that any single model will adequately describe all personality disorders. For example, Gunderson et al. (1991a) have suggested that the more severe personality disorders (e.g., schizotypal, paranoid, and borderline) may be discrete clinical syndromes with discrete etiologic pathways, while less severe personality disorders (e.g., compulsive, avoidant, and dependent) represent extremes of normally occurring traits. It is conceivable that certain types of personality pathology represent a "common final pathway" for a number of different etiologic factors, while others might be uniquely related to a specific standing on universal dimensions of personality.

It is unlikely that the diagnostic system will be changed because personality disorders *can* be described in dimensional terms—change is only likely to occur if it is demonstrated that personality disorders *should* be described dimensionally. The results of solely descriptive or clinical research are unlikely to be decisive in resolving the issue of categorical versus dimensional approaches. Research on etiology and pathophysiology may be more promising for adducing the type of evidence required. For example, data from genetic studies might shed light on whether factors contributing to conscientiousness and neuroticism in the general population are responsible for the occurrence of compulsive personality disorder. Another example of such an approach would be to determine whether the relationship between monoamine oxidase activity and sensation seeking seen in normal populations could predict risk for antisocial personality disorder. A delineation of relationships between dimensions of normal personality and personality disorders is an important step toward acquiring the knowledge required to create a diagnostic system that accurately reflects the nature of personality disorders.

METHODOLOGIC ISSUES

Diagnostic Issues

As in other areas of psychiatric research, the reliability and validity of a diagnosis have been a central issue in research on personality disorders. Also, as in other areas of psychopathology, there is no "gold standard" that can be used to validate diagnoses. However, the problem seems to be greater for personality disorders than for axis I disorders. There are a number of issues that probably contribute to the difficulty in reliably and validly diagnosing personality disorders. One important factor is that axis II symptomatology is often less florid and dramatic than axis I symptomatology.

Skodol et al. (1990) identified a number of issues that contribute to the difficulty in assessing personality disorders. In comparison to axis I disorders, personality disorders are more likely to be ego syntonic. This means that, to the individual with a personality disorder, his or her symptomatology is not experienced as alien to his or her usual experience of self. The story is often different for axis I disorders. For example, a panic attack is typically experienced as being distinctively different from normal experience. The nature of personality disorders may make it more difficult for the individual to describe symptoms to an interviewer. The symptoms of personality disorder may be more recognizable and troublesome to individuals in the environment of the person with the disorder than to the person him- or herself. Clinicians may be inclined to rely more on their own observations than on the patient's reports when assessing the presence of personality disorder. In the type of assessment of personality disorder typically used in research, the respondent is asked a series of questions about symptoms, and the answer is generally taken to be veridical. There is usually some provision for the diagnostician to over-ride the subject's self-report if there is contradictory information. Given that personality disorders are defined as long-standing stable characteristics, one time, cross-sectional assessment may not be ideal. If the person has a concurrent axis I disorder, the symptoms of that disorder may influence the report of axis II symptoms.

Zanarini and her colleagues (1987) also identified a number of issues that contribute to the difficulty of making reliable and valid diagnoses of personality disorders. Many of the DSM-III diagnostic criteria are not clearly operationalized, necessitating clinical interpretation. Some symptoms, such as low self-esteem, have a very high base rate and may require significant clinical judgment as to whether they achieve clinical significance. Many diagnostic criteria (e.g., vanity or criminal behavior) reflect traits that are generally held to be negative and may be denied on the basis of social desirability. Reporting certain traits may require a level of insight that is absent in some individuals.

Methods for Collecting Diagnostic Information

There are a number of methods that may be utilized to collect data on which to base diagnoses of personality disorders. These methods range from relatively unstructured clinical interviews to self-report questionnaires. There is not compelling evidence for the superiority of any single approach to the diagnosis of personality disorders (Skodol et al., 1990). However, as is the case for axis I disorders, the most widely accepted methodology for epidemiologic applications is the structured diagnostic interview.

Chart Review/Records. It has been suggested that clinicians often do not systematically assess their patients for the presence of personality disorders (Kass et al., 1985). When clinicians do assess personality disorder, they often diagnose only one (Oldham and Skodol, 1991), while systematic evaluation suggests that an individual who meets criteria for one personality disorder will usually meet criteria for at least one other personality disorder (Widiger et al., 1990). Obviously, the quality of clinical diagnoses contained in medical records may vary dramatically from one setting to another. But, given the fact that an acute axis I disorder is typically more florid than any accompanying personality disorder, it is quite likely that in most clinical settings the sensitivity of diagnoses of personality disorders will be poorer than for axis I disorders. Especially for diagnoses made at admission, the axis II diagnosis is often deferred and may or may not be added to the record at a later time.

Informants. Because the symptomatology of personality disorder may be subtle, ego syntonic, socially undesirable to acknowledge, and not obvious to the subject because of lack of insight, it has been suggested that information should be sought from another person who is familiar with the individual being diagnosed. However, in most cases it is not clear how to combine and weight information from an informant relative to that provided by the subject or observed by the diagnostician (Widiger and Frances, 1987).

Zimmerman et al. (1986) administered a structured interview to 82 patients and also interviewed a close friend or relative about the patient's normal personality. Adding the informant's information to that obtained from the patient led to changes in whether a personality disorder was judged to be present or absent in approximately 20% of the cases. In most cases, the informant information indicated more personality pathology. Zimmerman et al. (1988) also reported a comparison of information obtained from patients with information from informants using the SIDP in both groups. Significantly more of the criteria for all personality disorders were rated positively based on the informant (criteria positive by informant = 23.0 [$\pm$15.1] vs. criteria positive by subject = 17.1 [$\pm$13.4]). Only antisocial personality disorder was diagnosed more frequently using subject data. The κ coefficient between patients and informants for the presence of any personality disorder was 0.13, and the κ for every one of the individual personality disorders was below 0.35. The rate of personality disorders in the patients based on their own report was 36.4%; the rate based on informants was 57.6%. Zimmerman et al. concluded that patients and informants differed "markedly" in their descriptions of personality and that informants reported more personality pathology than did the patients themselves.

Clinical Interview. Perry (1992) suggested that structured diagnostic interviews may emphasize reliability to the point that validity is degraded. He proposed that the clinical interview, with its emphasis on history, important stories from the subject's life, and the discernment of long-standing patterns of behavior in historical context, may be very useful for the identification of personality disorder. Perry advocated several steps to ensure the quality and comparability of information obtained from clinical interviews: 1) the use of guidelines for the interview, 2) a compendium of good case examples, and 3) good training procedures.

Structured Interviews. Reich (1987b) reviewed the most widely used instruments for diagnosing personality disorders and may be consulted for more detailed information about these instruments. Because of potential confounding between reported personality traits and axis I disorders, it is good practice to assess the presence of axis I disorders when assessing personality disorders. Empirical evidence indicates that the assessment of personality disorders may be influenced by changes in the status of an axis I disorder (Hirschfeld et al., 1983). This section reviews the most widely utilized structured interviews for making diagnoses of all DSM-III/DSM-III-R personality disorders. (There are not striking differences in the κ reported for inter-rater agreement and test–retest reliability of these broad-spectrum diagnostic interviews.) There is also a brief description of several interviews intended to assess only one or several personality disorders.

The Structured Clinical Interview for DSM-III-R personality disorders (Spitzer et al., 1987) is a semistructured interview. It was developed to accompany the Structured Clinical Interview for DSM-III-R, which diagnoses axis I disorders. Criteria are rated on a three-point scale. The interview yields diagnoses for the 11 axis II disorders as well as for self-defeating personality disorder (from the DSM-III-R Appendix). Questions are organized by disorder, and the interviewer is encouraged to ask clarifying questions for responses that require it. The number of criteria rated as present can also be summed to provide dimensional scores.

The Structured Interview for DSM-III personality disorders (Pfohl et al., 1982) includes 160 questions. Questions are grouped into topical sections (e.g., egocentricity, unemotional) that facilitate a natural flow to the interview. At the end of each section, the relevant diagnostic criteria are rated on a three-point scale. The use of a knowledgeable informant is encouraged.

The Personality Disorders Examination (Loranger, 1988) is a structured interview. Questions on the interview are grouped by topical areas rather that by disorder. Positive responses may be followed up by probes and requests for examples. The interview includes the 11 axis II disorders as well as self-defeating and sadistic personality disorders (from the DSM-III-R Appendix).

The Diagnostic Interview for Personality Disorders, Revised (Zanarini et al., 1987) has 13 sections—one for each of the DSM-III-R personality disorders (including self-defeating and sadistic ones). Each DSM-III-R criterion is assessed by separate questions scored on a three-point scale. It is designed to be administered by interviewers trained to make clinical judgments. The interview provides follow-up probes, but also encourages the interviewer to be flexible and to employ clinical judgment. Interviewers should have substantial clinical experience and familiarity with DSM-III, but not necessarily formal graduate training.

A practical issue that will confront anyone planning to use a structured interview in an epidemiologic study is whether to use a broad-spectrum interview that includes all of the personality disorders or to select a specialized interview. The decision will depend on the purpose of the study. If one particular disorder is the subject of study, then it may be desirable to collect the type of detailed information provided by a specialized interview. If the purpose of the study is to investigate all of the personality disorders, then the obvious choice would be one of the more general interviews. There are quite a number of structured and semistructured interviews for specific personality disorders, such as the Diagnostic Interview for Borderlines (Gunderson et al., 1981) and the Structured Interview for Schizotypy (Kendler, 1985). It is beyond the scope of this chapter to describe them individually.

The next revision of the *Diagnostic and Statistical Manual* will soon be published with revised diagnostic criteria. Revisions have already begun for some of the structured interviews to provide all information necessary to make diagnoses using the revised criteria.

Self-Report Questionnaires. There are several self-report instruments available for assessing personality disorders. The Personality Diagnostic Questionnaire, Revised (PDQ-R) (Hyler et al., 1987) is a 152 item self-report questionnaire with a true–false format. The items reflect the criteria for all of the DSM-III-R personality disorders. Diagnoses reflect endorsement of symptom items plus the presence of impairment or distress. The internal consistency reliabilities of the original PDQ-R scales ranged from 0.56 to 0.84, with a median α of 0.69 (Hyler et al., 1989). Hyler et al. (1990) reported κ values ranging from 0.23 to 0.63 (mean = 0.41) in a comparison of the PDQ-R to the SCID-II. Comparing the PDQ-R to the PDE yielded κ from −0.02 to 0.54 (mean = 0.33). The Millon Clinical Multiaxial Inventory (MCMI) (Millon, 1983) is a self-report questionnaire designed to measure the dimensions underlying the DSM-III personality disorders. The questionnaire does not inquire directly about the presence of the diagnostic criteria, but there is a method for using responses to assign DSM-III diagnoses. Test–retest reliability as assessed by correlations between two administrations separated by 8 weeks ranged from 0.60 to 0.89 (median = 0.75). Two studies have been reported comparing the MCMI to the SIDP; Hogg et al. (1990) reported a median κ of 0.14 and Jackson et al. (1991) a median κ of 0.18. The Schedule for Nonadaptive and Adaptive Personality (SNAP) (Clark, 1993) is a self-report questionnaire that uses 375 true–false items to provide scores on 34 scales, covering 12 traits and 3 temperaments and including 6 validity and 13 diagnostic scales. There is a system for recombining items to provide a measure of DSM-III-R personality disorders. Clark (1993) reported 1 week retest correlations ranging from 0.68 to 0.89 in a sample of state hospital patients. Internal consistency reliability coefficients ranged from 0.68 to 0.90 in a patient sample.

Rating Scales. The Personality Assessment Form (PAF) (Shea et al., 1987) uses a prototypical rating approach to assess DSM-III PDs. The PAF includes a paragraph describing the diagnostic features of each personality disorder. The clinician uses data from available clinical sources to rate the long-term personality functioning of the subject on a six-point scale ("not at all" to "to an extreme degree") for each disorder. Shea et al. (1990) reported inter-rater reliability assessed by κ for the diagnosis of any personality disorder and any cluster C personality disorder as 0.48 and 0.47, respectively.

Diagnostic Agreement

Although it does not directly address the issue of validity, it is certainly desirable that different instruments used to assess personality disorders yield similar, if not identical, results. Before the advent of DSM-III, the inter-rater reliability of personality disorders was poor. Based on a review of reported results, Spitzer and Fleiss (1974) reported that the average pre-DSM-III κ was 0.32 for clinical diagnosis. In the DSM-III field trials, a κ for the presence of any personality disorder of 0.61 was reported when both diagnosticians rated the same interview; when two separate interviews were conducted, κ was 0.54 (Spitzer et al., 1979).

Perry (1992) reviewed results from eight studies that reported results from different structured interviews or self-report questionnaires on the same individuals. Perry concluded that the reliability of the individual instruments assessed by inter-rater reliability is in the fair to high range. As mentioned earlier, there is no clear-cut criterion for validity available. However, an important consideration, being neither validity nor reliability, is the level of agreement between different instruments. If these instruments are all measuring valid constructs validly, then they should lead to similar diagnostic conclusions. Perry found that agreement across instruments was poor. One way that Perry summarized agreement between different instruments was to determine the median κ for the individual disorders between the two instruments being considered. When he examined the highest κ between disorders from each study, he found a median of 0.54. For the lowest κ between disorders from each study, he found a median of 0.0. Finally, he determined the median κ from each study and computed a "median of medians," which yielded a κ of 0.25, in the poor range. When Perry separated studies that compared two interviews from those that compared self-report questionnaires with interviews, there were minor changes in the results. The median highest κ from studies comparing two interviews was 0.61, the median lowest κ was 0.09, and the "median of medians" was 0.25. The results were somewhat poorer for studies comparing self-report questionnaires to interview. The median highest κ was 0.50, the median lowest κ was 0.01, and the "median of medians" was 0.16. Perry suggested that demonstrating acceptable reliability for the individual instruments leaves unanswered questions about assessment validity. Perry concluded that the different instruments for assessing personality disorders, on average, agree with one another at a level that is only slightly better than chance and often reach different conclusions.

Comorbidity and Diagnostic Overlap

If the diagnosis of more than one personality disorder in an individual is seen as reflecting the actual presence of two or more personality disorders, then this section could be considered to be about comorbidity. To the extent that current assessment techniques and diagnostic criteria fail to differentiate phenomena due to methodologic shortcomings, it could be considered to be about "overlap."

Zimmerman and Coryell (1989) in their nonpatient sample of relatives of normal controls and probands with schizophrenia and depressive disorders found that approximately one-fourth of subjects with any personality disorder met criteria for more than one. Oldham and his coworkers (unpublished data described by Skodol et al., 1990), in a study of 100 patients with suspected character pathology, reported an average of 3.4 personality disorders in patients with at least one personality disorder. Zanarini et al. (1987) reported 2.8 diagnoses per patient, Widiger et al. (1990) reported 3.75, and Skodol et al. (1988) reported 4.6.

Widiger and Rogers (1989) suggested that patterns of comorbidity between personality disorders and axis I may best be understood in terms of the DSM-III clusters. The odd-eccentric cluster should be associated with psychotic disorders, the dramatic-impulsive cluster should be associated with affective disorders, and the anxious-fearful cluster should be associated with anxiety disorders. Pfohl et al. (1990) reviewed findings on the comorbidity of axis I and axis II disorders. They included studies that employed patient samples with major depression, obsessive-compulsive disorder, and panic disorder. The hospitalized depressed patients had an increased risk for dramatic-impulsive cluster (cluster B) personality disorders. The OCD and panic disorder samples were more likely to receive a diagnosis from the anxious-fearful cluster (cluster C). OCD subjects were also more likely to receive a diagnosis from the odd-eccentric cluster (cluster A) than either depressed or panic patients.

When a personality disorder is found to be highly comorbid with another disorder there are several possibilities to consider: 1) there may be some significant association between the two, such that one disorder is a risk factor for the other, or both disorders share some underlying risk factor, vulnerability, or pathophysiological process; 2) the two diagnoses may describe only one disorder (e.g., avoidant personality disorder and generalized social phobia might be the same disorder); or 3) the diagnostic criteria for the disorders may include overlapping features that promote individuals with certain symptomatology to receive both diagnoses.

FUTURE DIRECTIONS

In comparison with the major axis I disorders, there is considerably less epidemiologic information about the personality disorders. There are a number of factors that have contributed to this state of affairs. Before DSM-III was published in 1980, there was less of a consensus about how to define the individual personality disorders (as well as disagreement about which disorders to include under the heading) than there was for the major axis I disorders. The most ambitious study of true prevalence, the ECA study, included most of the important axis I disorders, but only antisocial personality disorder was included from axis II. There is good evidence that personality disorders are strongly associated with use of mental health services, use of medical services (Reich et al., 1989a), prognosis and responsiveness to treatment of axis I disorders (Reich and Green, 1991), and substantial impairment in functioning and subjective distress. There are important questions that remain unanswered about the true prevalence of most of these disorders, about the stability of these disorders, their natural course, as well as risk and protective factors for their development.

ACKNOWLEDGMENTS

The work presented here was supported by NIMH research grant MH47353. The author acknowledges the assistance of Ms. Catherine Hynds and Ms. Christa Laib in the preparation of this chapter.

REFERENCES

Akhtar S, Byrne JP, Doghramji K (1986): The demographic profile of borderline disorder. J Clin Psychiatry 47:196–198.

American Psychiatric Association (1980): "The Diagnostic and Statistical Manual of Mental Disorders," Washington, DC: American Psychiatric Association.

American Psychiatric Association (1987): "The Diagnostic and Statistical Manual of Mental Disorders," 3rd ed, revised. Washington DC: American Psychiatric Association.

American Psychiatric Association, Task Force on DSM-IV (1991): "DSM-IV Options Book: Work in Progress." Washington DC: American Psychiatric Association.

American Psychiatric Association, Task Force on DSM-IV (1993): "DSM-IV Draft Criteria." Washington, DC: American Psychiatric Association.

Baer L, Jenike MA, Ricciardi JN, Holland AD, et al. (1990): Standardized assessment of personality disorders in obsessive-compulsive disorder. Arch Gen Psychiatry 47:826–830.

Baron M, Green R, Asnis L, Lord S (1985): Familial transmission of schizotypal and borderline personality disorders. Am J Psychiatry 142:927–934.

Bland RC, Newman SC, Orn H (1988): Lifetime prevalence of psychiatric disorders in Edmonton. Acta Psychiatrica Scand 77(Suppl 338):24–32.

Block J (1971): "Lives Through Time." Berkeley, CA: Bancroft.

Block J, Ozer DJ (1982): Two types of psychologists: Remarks on Mendelsohn, Weiss, and Feimer contribution. J Personality Social Psychol 42:1171–1181.

Bornstein RF, Klein DN, Mallon JC, Slater JF (1988): Schizotypal personality disorder in an outpatient population: Incidence and clinical characteristics. J Clin Psychol 44:322–325.

Bremer J (1951): A social psychiatric investigation of a small community in Northern Norway. Acta Psychiatr Neurol Scand Suppl 62.

Casey PR, Tyrer PJ (1986): Personality, functioning and symptomatology. J Psychiatric Res 20:363–374.

Casey PR, Tyrer PJ, Dillon S (1984): The diagnostic status of patients with conspicuous psychiatric morbidity in primary care. Psychol Med 14:673–681.

Casey PR, Tyrer PJ, Platt SP (1985): The relationship between social functioning and psychiatric symptomatology in primary care. Social Psychiatry 20:5–9.

Clark LA (1993): "Schedule for Nonadaptive and Adaptive Personality (SNAP): Manual for Administration, Scoring and Interpretation." Minneapolis, MN: University of Minnesota Press.

Compton WM, Helzer JE, Hwu HG, Yeh EK, McEvoy L, Tipp JE, Spitznagel EL (1991): New methods in cross-cultural psychiatry: Psychiatric illness in Taiwan and the United States. Am J of Psychiatry 148:1697–1704.

Costa PT, McCrae RR (1990): Personality disorders and the five factor model of personality. J Personality Disord 4:362–381.

Cutting J, Cowen PJ, Mann AH, Jenkins R, et al. (1986): Personality and psychosis: Use of the standardized assessment of personality. Acta Psychiatr Scand 73(Suppl 328):61–66.

Dahl AA (1986): Some aspects of DSM-III personality disorders illustrated by consecutive sample of hospitalized patients. Acta Psychiatr Scand 73(Suppl 328):61–66.

Essen-Moller E, Larsson H, Uddenberg CE, et al. (1956): Individual traits and morbidity in a Swedish rural population. Acta Psychiatrica Neurol Scand Suppl 100.

Folstein MF, Folstein SE, McHugh PR (1975): Mini mental state: A practical method for grading the cognitive state of patients for the clinician. J Psychiatr Res 38:189–198.

Frances A, Clarkin J, Gilmore M, et al. (1984): Reliability of criteria for borderline personality disorder: A comparison of DSM-III and the diagnostic interview for borderline patients. Am J Psychiatry 141:1080–1084.

Galenberg AJ (1987): Introduction: The borderline patient. J Clin Psychiatry 48(Suppl):3–11.

Goldberg D (1974): "The Detection of Psychiatric Illness by Questionnaire: A Technique for the Identification and Assessment of Nonpsychotic Psychiatric Illness." London: Oxford University Press.

Gunderson JG (1982): "Diagnostic Interview for Borderline Patients." New York: Roerig-Pfizer.

Gunderson JG, Kolb JE, Austin V (1981): The diagnostic interview for borderline patients. Am J Psychiatry 138:896–903.

Gunderson JG, Links PS, Reich JH (1991a): Competing models of personality disorders. J Personality Disord 5:60–68.

Gunderson JG, Ronningstam E, Smith LE (1991b): Narcissistic personality disorder: A review of data on DSM-III-R descriptions. J Personality Disord 5:167–177.

Herbert JD, Hope DA, Bellack AS (1992): Validity of the distinction between generalized social phobia and avoidant personality disorder. J Abnorm Psychol 101:332–339.

Hirschfeld RMA, Klerman GL, Clayton PJ, et al. (1983): Assessing personality: Effects of the depressive state on trait measurement. Am J Psychiatry 140:695–699.

Hirschfeld RMA, Shea MT, Weise R (1991): Dependent personality disorder: Perspectives for DSM-IV. J Personality Disord 5:135–149.

Holt CS, Heimberg RG, Hope DA (1990): "Avoidant Personality and the Generalized Subtype in Social Phobia." Paper presented at the Annual Meeting of the Association for the Advancement of Behavior Therapy, San Francisco, CA, November.

Hyler SE, Reider RO, Williams JBW, Spitzer RL (1983): "Personality Diagnostic Questionnaire (PDQ)." New York: New York State Psychiatric Institute, Biometrics Research.

Hyler SE, Rieder RO, Williams JBW, et al. (1987): "The Personality Diagnostic Questionnaire Revised (PDQ-R)." New York: New York State Psychiatric Institute, Biometrics Research.

Hyler SE, Reider RO, Williams JBW, et al. (1989): A comparison of clinical and self-report diagnoses of DSM-III personality disorders in 552 patients. Comp Psychiatry 30:170–178.

Hyler SE, Skodol AE, Kellman HD, et al. (1990): Validity of the Personality Diagnostic Questionnaire-Revised: Comparison with two structured interviews. Am J Psychiatry 147:1043–1048.

Kass F, Skodol AE, Charles E, Spitzer RL, Williams JBW (1985): Scaled ratings of DSM-III personality disorders. Am J Psychiatry 142:627–630.

Kendler K (1985): "The Structured Interview for Schizotypy (SIS)," 1.5 ed. Richmond, VA: Medical College of VA Hospitals.

Kety SS, Rosenthal D, Wender PH, et al. (1978): The biologic and adoptive families of adopted individuals who became schizophrenic: Prevalence of mental illness and other characteristics. In Wynne LC, Cromwell RL, Matthysse S (eds): "The Nature of Schizophrenia: New Approaches to Research and Treatment." New York: John Wiley & Sons, pp 25–37.

Koenigsberg HW, Kaplan RD, Gilmore MM, Cooper AM (1985): The relationship between syndrome and personality disorder in DSM-III: Experience with 2462 patients. Am J Psychiatry 142:207–212.

Kraepelin E (1919/1971): "Dementia Praecox and Paraphrenia," Huntington, NY: Robert E. Krieger Publishing.

Langner TS, Michael ST (1963): "Life Stress and Mental Health. The Midtown Manhattan Study." London: Collier, Macmillan.

Leighton A (1959): My name is legion: The Stirling County study. Am J Psychiatry 119:1021–1026.

Leighton DC, Harding JS, Macklin MA, Hughes CC, Leighton AH (1963): Psychiatric findings of the Stirling County Study. Am J Psychiatry 119:1021–1026.

Loranger AW (1988): "Personality Disorders Examination (PDE)." Yonkers, NY: DV Communications.

Maier W, Lichterman D, Klingler T, Heun R, Hallmayer J (1992): Prevalences of personality disorders (DSM-III-R) in the community. J Personality Disord 6:187–196.

Mannuzza S, Fyer AJ, Klein DF, Endicott J (1986): Schedule for Affective Disorders and Schizophrenia—Lifetime Version: Rationale and conceptual development. J Psychiatr Res 20:317–325.

Meehl PE (1979): A funny thing happened to us on the way to the latent entities. J Personality Assess 42:1157–1170.

Merikangas KP, Weissman MM (1986): The epidemiology of DSM-III axis II personality disorders. In Frances AJ, Hales RE (eds): "APA Annual Review, vol 5, Psychiatry Update." Washington, DC: American Psychiatric Press, pp 258–278.

Merikangas KR, Weissman MM (1991): Epidemiology of DSM-III axis II personality disorders. In Oldham J (ed): "Personality Disorders: New Perspectives on Diagnostic Validity." Washington, DC: American Psychiatric Association, p 200.

Millon T (1983): "Millon Clinical Multiaxial Inventory Manual." Minneapolis: National Computer Systems.

Nestadt G, Romanoski AJ, Brown CH, Chahal R, Merchant A, Folstein MF, Gruenberg EM, McHugh PR (1991): DSM-III compulsive personality disorder: An epidemiological survey. Psychol Med 21:461–471.

Nestadt G, Romanoski AJ, Chahal R, Merchant A, Folstein MF, Gruenberg EM, McHugh PR (1990): An epidemiological study of histrionic personality disorder. Psychol Med 20:413–422.

Nestadt G, Romanoski AJ, Samuels JF, Folstein MF, McHugh PR (1992): The relationship between personality and DSM-III axis I disorders in the population: Results from an epidemiological survey. Am J Psychiatry 149:1228–1233.

Nestadt G, Samuels JF, Romanoski AJ, Folstein MF, McHugh PR (1993): "DSM-III Personality Disorders in the Population," No. NR500. Washington, DC: American Psychiatric Association Annual Meeting.

Nurnberg HG, Raskin M, Levine PE, Pollack S, Siegel O, Prince R (1991): The co-morbidity of borderline personality disorder and other DSM-III-R axis II personality disorders. Am J Psychiatry 148:1371–1377.

Oakley-Browne MA, Joyce PA, Wells E, Bushnell JA, Hornblow AR (1989): Christchurch psychiatric epidemiology study, part II: Six-month and other period prevalences of specific psychiatric disorders. Aust NZeal J Psychiatry 23:327–340.

Oldham JM, Skodol AE (1991): Personality disorders in the public sector. Hosp Community Psychiatry 42:481–487.

Overholser JC (1991): Categorical assessment of the dependent personality disorder in depressed inpatients. J Personality Disord 5:243–255.

Perry JC (1992): Valid assessment of personality disorders. Am J Psychiatry 149:1645–1653.

Pfohl B (1991): Histrionic personality disorder: A review of available data and recommendations for DSM-IV. J Personality Disord: A Review of Available Data and Recommendations for DSM-IV. 5:150–166.

Pfohl B, Black DW, Noyes R, et al. (1990): Axis I and axis II co-morbidity findings: implications for validity. In "Personality Disorders: New Perspectives on Diagnostic Validity." Washington, DC: American Psychiatric Press.

Pfohl B, Stangl DA, Zimmerman M, Bowers W, Corenthal C (1982): A structured interview for the DSM-III personality disorders: A preliminary report. Arch Gen Psychiatry 42:591–596.

Reich J (1987a): Sex distribution of DSM-III personality disorders in psychiatric outpatients. Am J Psychiatry 144:485–488.

Reich J (1987b): Instruments measuring DSM-III and DSM-III-R personality disorders. J Personality Disord 1:220–240.

Reich J, Boerstler H, Yates W, Nduaguba M (1989a): Utilization of medical resources in persons with DSM-III personality disorders in a community sample. Int J Psychiatry Med 19:1–9.

Reich JH, Green AI (1991): Effect of personality disorders on outcome of treatment. J Nerv Ment Dis 179:74–82.

Reich JH, Yates W, Nduagube M (1989b): Prevalence of DSM-III personality disorders in the community. Social Psychiatry Psychiatr Epidemiol 24:12–16.

Robins LN, Helzer JE, Croughan J, Williams JBW, Spitzer RL (1981): "N.I.M.H. Diagnostic Interview Schedule," version III. Rockville, MD: National Institute of Mental Health.

Robins LN, Helzer JE, Weissman MM, Orvaschel H, Gruenberg E, Burke JD, Jr, Regier DA (1984): Lifetime prevalence of specific psychiatric disorders in three sites. Arch Gen Psychiatry 41:949–958.

Schneier FR, Fyer AJ, Martin LY, Ross D, et al. (1991): A comparison of phobic subtypes with panic disorder. J Anxiety Disord 5:65–75.

Shea MT, Glass DR, Pilkonis PA, Watkins J, Docherty JP (1987): Frequency and implications of PD's in a sample of depressed outpatients. J Personality Disord 1:27–42.

Shea MT, Pilkonis PA, Beckham E, Collins JF, Elkin I, Sotsky SM, Docherty JP (1990): Personality disorders and treatment outcome in the NIMH Treatment of Depression Research Program. Am J Psychiatry 147:711–718.

Skodol A (1989): Co-occurrence and diagnostic efficiency statistics. Unpublished.

Skodol AE, Rosnick L, Kellman D, et al. (1988): Validating structured DSM-III personality disorder assessments with longitudinal data. Am J Psychiatry 145:1297–1299.

Skodol AE, Rosnick L, Kellman D, Oldham JM, Hyler S (1990): Development of a procedure for validating structured assessments of axis II. Oldham J (ed): "Personality Disorders: New Perspectives on Diagnostic Validity." Washington, DC: American Psychiatric Association, p 200.

Spitzer RL, Endicott J (1978): "Schedule for Affective Disorders and Schizophrenia." New York: NIMH, Clinical Research Branch Collaborative Program on the Psychobiology of Depression.

Spitzer RL, Fleiss JL (1974): A re-analysis of the reliability of psychiatric diagnosis. Br J Psychiatry 125:341–347.

Spitzer RL, Forman JBW, Nee J (1979): DSM-III field trials. I Initial inter-rater diagnostic reliability. Am J Psychiatry 136:815–817.

Spitzer RL, Williams JBW, Gibbon M (1987): "Structured Clinical Interview for DSM-III-R Personality Disorders (SCID-II)." New York: Biometrics Research Department, New York State Psychiatric Institute.

Srole L, et al. (1962): "Mental Health in the Metropolis: The Midtown Manhattan Study." New York: McGraw-Hill.

Standage K, Ladha N (1988): An examination of the reliability of the Personality Disorders Examination and a comparison with other methods of identifying personality disorders in a clinical sample. J Personality Disord 2:267–271.

Swartz M, Blazer D, George L, Winfield I (1990): Estimating the prevalence of personality disorder in the community. J Personality Disord 4:257–272.

Turner SM, Beidel DC, Borden JW, Stanley MA (1991): Social phobia: Axis I and II correlates. J Abnorm Psychol 100:102–106.

Tyrer P, Alexander MS, Cicchetti D, Cohen MS, Remington M (1979): Reliability of a schedule for rating personality disorders. Br J Psychiatry 135:168–174.

Weissman MM, Myers JK, Harding PS (1978): Psychiatric disorders in the U.S. urban community: 1975–1976. Am J Psychiatry 135:459–462.

Widiger TA (1991): DSM-IV reviews of the personality disorders: Introduction to special series. J Personality Disord 5:122–134.

Widiger TA, Frances A (1987): Interviews and inventories for the measurement of personality disorders. Clin Psychol Rev 7:49–75.

Widiger T, Frances AJ, Harris M, et al. (1990): Co-morbidity among axis II disorders. In Widiger T, et al. (eds): "Personality Disorders: New Perspectives on Diagnostic Validity." Washington, DC: American Psychiatric Press, pp 147–160.

Widiger TA, Rogers JH (1989): Prevalence and co-morbidity of personality disorders. Psychiatr Ann 19:132–136.

Widiger TA, Trull T (1992): Personality and psychopathology: An application of the five factor model. J Personality 60:363–393.

Widiger TA, Weissman MM (1991): Epidemiology of borderline personality disorder. Hosp Community Psychiatry 42:1015–1021.

Wing JK, Cooper JE, Sartorius N (1974): "Measurements and Classification of Psychiatric Symptoms." New York: Cambridge University Press.

World Health Organization (1978): "Mental Disorders: Glossary and Guide to Their Classification in Accordance With the Ninth Revision of the International Classification of Diseases (ICD-9)." Geneva: World Health Organization.

Zanarini M, Frankenberg F, Chauncey D, et al. (1987): The diagnostic interview for personality disorders: Inter-rater and test retest reliability. Comp Psychiatry 28:467–480.

Zimmerman M, Coryell W (1989): The reliability of personality disorder diagnoses in a non-patient sample. J Personality Disord 3:53–57.

Zimmerman M, Coryell WH (1990): Diagnosing personality disorders in the community: A comparison of self-report and interview measures. Arch Gen Psychiatry 47:527–531.

Zimmerman M, Pfohl B, Stangl D, Corenthal C (1986): Assessment of DSM-III personality disorders: The importance of interviewing an informant. J Clin Psychiatry 47:261–263.

CHAPTER 20

Epidemiology and Geriatric Psychiatry

LESLIE B. HOCKING, HAROLD G. KOENIG, and DAN G. BLAZER

Duke University Medical Center, Durham, NC 27710, and Geropsychiatry Institute, John Umstead Hospital, Butner, NC 27509 (L.B.H.); Geriatric Evaluation and Treatment Clinic, Center for Aging, Duke University Medical Center, Durham, NC 27710 (H.G.K.); Duke University Medical Center, School of Medicine, Durham, NC 27710 (D.G.B.).

INTRODUCTION

The epidemiology of mental illness in late life is a relatively new and rapidly evolving area of investigation in psychiatric research, the importance of which is readily appreciated when current demographic trends are considered. The U.S. Bureau of the Census has reported that in the past two decades the number of persons aged 65 years and older grew by 56% while the under-65 age group increased only 19%. In 1900 only 4% of the country's population was aged 65 or older. By the mid-1980s, about 12% of the population was 65 or older. By the year 2010, it is projected that nearly 15% of all Americans will be 65 or older (Spencer, 1984). The increasing proportions of the elderly in the population underscore the importance of an accurate and thorough understanding of the nature and extent of mental illness in this segment of the population.

In considering the epidemiology of psychiatric illness in late life, it is important to focus on the essential tasks of the epidemiologist. These tasks include the identification of cases in the population; the distribution of disorders in the population; historical trends in disorders; etiology; and the utilization of health care resources (Morris, 1975). In this chapter we review studies addressing each of these tasks, with representative studies in geriatric populations, where available, serving as illustrations. Barriers to our understanding of the epidemiology of psychiatric disorders in late life are also discussed.

IDENTIFICATION OF CASES: WHAT IS A CASE?

Understanding the methods used for identifying and characterizing psychiatric disorders in the elderly is of vital importance, as the scheme used to assay for morbidity will significantly influence the nature of the disorder that is identified. Certainly the most influential event in the development of explicit diagnostic criteria was the publication of the *Diag-*

Textbook in Psychiatric Epidemiology, Edited by Tsuang, Tohen, and Zahner
ISBN 0-471-59375-3 © 1995 Wiley-Liss, Inc.

nostic and Statistical Manual of Mental Disorders, 3rd edition (DSM-III)—the official statement of diagnostic nomenclature of the American Psychiatric Association (APA) (1980). Unlike earlier DSM editions, this edition emphasized the careful delineation of criteria, without regard to specific etiologic viewpoints, for assessing the presence of clinically important psychiatric syndromes. The development of the DSM-III, and its subsequent revised edition (DSM-III-R), made feasible the development of structured diagnostic interviews that could be used to identify cases of illness systematically in a given population. The Diagnostic Interview Schedule (DIS) (Robins et al., 1981) adopted for use in the Epidemiologic Catchment Area (ECA) program (Regier et al., 1985) is a direct implementation of the DSM-III diagnostic system.

Alternate diagnostic criteria have been developed for specific disorders. A widely accepted diagnostic system for dementia is the National Institute of Neurologic, Communicative Diseases and Stroke–Alzheimer's Disease and Related Disorders Association (NINCDS-ADRDA) work group diagnoses (McKhann et al., 1984). In contrast to the DSM-III-R, which relies on historical information and clinical examination, in making a diagnosis of dementia using the NINCDS-ADRDA criterion, clinical examination and cognitive impairment as documented by a standardized scale or psychological testing are supplemented by laboratory tests and results of imaging studies such as computerized tomography or magnetic resonance imaging scan.

Both of the criteria mentioned above represent approaches aimed at identifying cases using diagnostic systems. Alternatively, scales have been developed that measure levels of symptoms, functional impairment, or cognitive compromise without regard to diagnosis. Examples of these include the Mini-Mental Status Exam (Folstein et al., 1975), a scale for measuring cognitive impairment, and the Center for Epidemiologic Studies Depression Scale (CES-D), a scale for measuring depressive symptoms (Sawyer-Radloff and Locke, 1986). Arbitrary cut-off points have been adopted for both indices, identifying the level of impairment or of severity of depressive symptoms, respectively, used to suggest the presence of a disorder. Although such indices are widely used in epidemiologic research, problems arise in attempting to correlate such measures with the presence of a specific psychiatric disorder. Furthermore, cut-off points tend to be arbitrary, and the significance of morbidity not reaching the threshold of a cut-off point remains unresolved.

Perhaps the most perplexing issue facing epidemiologists attempting to utilize DSM-III-R criteria in a geriatric population is the lack of attention in this diagnostic system to age-related issues. Comorbidity, frequently encountered in the mentally ill elderly, confounds the application of a diagnostic system based on the delineation of clinical signs and symptoms. Cognitive compromise, whether or not dementia is present, coexists in many elderly with other psychiatric diagnoses. In a survey of geriatric outpatients, 24% were found to be cognitively impaired and to meet criteria for depression (Reifler et al., 1982). The cognitively impaired elderly patient's ability to report symptoms and provide historical information may be greatly impaired. In the medically ill elderly, symptoms of medical illness can confound the clinical significance of typical symptoms of depression. Scales have been developed to address specifically the problem of diagnosing depression in patients with Alzheimer's disease (Sunderland et al., 1988) and with significant medical illness (Koenig et al., 1992).

DSM-IV, scheduled for publication in 1994, will contain few changes of significance for geriatric psychiatry (Diagnostic and Statistical Manual Draft Criteria, 1993).

Definitions of disorders will not change in any way that will affect their prevalence. The diagnosis of dementia will now incorporate the opportunity to specify the etiology of dementias due to medical conditions, e.g., dementia due to Parkinson's disease, Creutzfeldt-Jakob disease, and so forth. It will be possible to code for dementias due to multiple etiologies (vascular dementia with Alzheimer's disease).

Unfortunately, the tough nosologic issues we face as geriatric psychiatrics will not be resolved by DSM-IV. Difficulty will remain in classifying anxiety and depression in medically ill patients. Subsyndromal symptoms, the importance of which are further discussed later in this chapter, will remain difficult to classify. Although "minor" depression is in a proposed category in the DSM-IV Appendix, continued debate and uncertainty over diagnostic criteria prevent it's incorporation as a disorder.

Other proposed categories of interest include mixed anxiety-depression disorder and mild cognitive disorder. The proposed definition for mild cognitive disorder is "impairment in cognitive functioning as evidenced by neuropsychological testing or quantified clinical assessment, accompanied by objective evidence of a systemic illness or central nervous system dysfunction." A proposal for future DSM editions that we think would be useful is the development of an axis, in addition to the current five, for cognitive functioning. This development would ensure that the level of cognitive functioning, along with psychiatric and medical illnesses, would always be noted for any elderly patient. As knowledge and data in geriatric psychiatry continue to evolve, it is likely that future editions of the DSM will be increasingly useful.

THE DISTRIBUTION OF CASES

The ECA program comprised a series of five large-scale epidemiologic surveys conducted between 1980 and 1984 designed to generate diagnosis-specific prevalence data. A total of 18,571 psychiatric interviews was conducted, including 5,702 interviews of persons aged 65 years or older. Figure 1 presents the age-specific 1 month prevalence rates for disorders assessed at all five sites, aggregated across all sites. Perhaps what is most striking about these data is that, with the exception of severe cognitive impairment, the 1 month prevalence of mental illness is lowest in the elderly for all diagnoses. With the exception of alcohol and drug abuse and dependence, women of all ages had higher rates than men for most disorders. Anxiety disorders were the most prevalent of all the major groups of mental illness.

These data were surprising for a number of reasons. The belief that major depression in late life is common was not substantiated; furthermore, the elderly, not the young, were felt to have risk factors (e.g., loss of loved ones, physical illness, loss of important societal roles) for higher rates of psychopathology. Certainly patterns of psychotropic drug use indicate higher use in the elderly, suggesting greater symptomatology (Blazer et al., 1987).

A number of hypotheses have arisen to account for the low rates of mental illness other than severe cognitive impairment, among older adults. These explanations fall into two groups: 1) methodologic or sampling error and 2) for those who accept rate differences as real, cohort or period effects. We review these arguments, with particular attention to depressive illness in older adults.

Methodologic arguments maintain psychiatric disorders, such as depression, are at

AGE GROUPS
- 18 – 24
- 25 – 44
- 45 – 64
- 65 +

Rate (%)   0   5   10   15

	%	SE
Any DIS Disorder	16.9	(1.0)
	17.3	(0.6)
	13.3	(0.7)
	12.3	(0.6)
Alcohol Abuse/Dependence	4.1	(0.4)
	3.6	(0.3)
	2.1	(0.3)
	0.4	(0.2)
Drug Abuse/Dependence	3.5	(0.5)
	1.5	(0.2)
	0.1	(0.0)
	0.0	(0.0)
Schizophrenic/Schizophreniform Disorders	0.8	(0.2)
	1.1	(0.2)
	0.5	(0.1)
	0.1	(0.0)
Manic Episode	0.6	(0.2)
	0.6	(0.1)
	0.2	(0.1)
	0.0	(0.0)
Major Depressive Episode	2.2	(0.4)
	3.0	(0.3)
	2.0	(0.3)
	0.7	(0.1)
Dysthymia	2.2	(0.4)
	4.0	(0.3)
	3.8	(0.3)
	1.8	(0.2)
Anxiety Disorders	7.7	(0.7)
	8.3	(0.4)
	6.6	(0.5)
	5.5	(0.4)
Phobia	6.4	(0.6)
	6.4	(0.4)
	6.0	(0.4)
	4.8	(0.3)
Panic	0.4	(0.2)
	0.7	(0.1)
	0.6	(0.2)
	0.1	(0.1)
Obsessive-Compulsive	1.8	(0.4)
	1.6	(0.2)
	0.9	(0.2)
	0.8	(0.2)
Severe Cognitive Impairment	0.6	(0.2)
	0.4	(0.1)
	1.2	(0.2)
	4.9	(0.4)

least as common in older as in younger adults, yet elders are 1) less likely to report psychiatric symptoms, 2) less likely to recall psychiatric symptoms, 3) more likely to report mood symptoms in somatic rather than psychiatric terms, and 4) more likely to experience depressive symptoms that fit poorly into conventional diagnostic categories. Whether the DSM-III-R, developed for use in a clinical population, works as well for measuring illness in a community population remains an unresolved issue.

Besides diagnostic imprecision, sampling error may also contribute to low rates. Depressed older persons may be more likely to refuse to participate in epidemiologic surveys or to be systematically excluded from such surveys because they are institutionalized, homeless, die prematurely (selective mortality), or feel too ill to participate because of physical illness and perhaps associated depression. Information about elderly impaired individuals is often obtained from interviews of family members or other caretakers. Family members may attempt to shield elderly individuals by minimizing symptoms or disallowing interviews. Furthermore, proxy respondents may simply be unable to answer key questions.

Most epidemiologists agree that while methodologic and sampling problems explain some of the difference observed, it is only a small part (Blazer, 1989). They claim that age differences in rates of depression are real and may be attributable to a cohort and/or period effect. Those who invoke the cohort effect explanation argue that persons aged 65 or over who were born prior to 1920 are for some reason psychologically healthier than those born at a later (or significantly earlier) date. Thus, this particular generation of elders is experiencing fewer psychiatric symptoms in old age because they have always been psychologically healthier. This effect is discussed further when we address historical trends in suicide rates.

A second explanation for lower rates of depressed elders today is called a *period effect*. The argument goes as follows. Older persons today endured hard times during the Great Depression and Second World War, when their standard of living and quality of life was quite poor. Since the end of World War II, however, both their economic situation and social circumstances have greatly improved. Consequently, elders today appreciate more what they have because they can look back on times when life was much worse. In contrast, persons born since the end of World War II are accustomed to the higher standard of living brought by the postwar boom years. Because they are not accustomed to hard times, the baby boom generation has not handled difficulties as well as their parents. High expectations, combined with increased competition over scarce resources in this populace generation, has made life difficult for them, resulting in higher rates of depression. These psychosocial stresses may increase the expression of depressive disorder in those who are biologically vulnerable. In any case, the explanation for the lower rate of depression in elders today is likely multifactorial and not due to a single cause.

Other factors to consider in the distribution of cases include the importance of subsyn-

---

FIGURE 1. Standardized 1 month prevalence rates of DIS/DSM-III disorders for all ECA sites combined (percent). The rates presented are standardized to the age, sex, and race distribution of the 1980 noninstitutionalized population of the United States aged 18 years and over. Standard errors are presented in parentheses. (From Regier et al. 1988.)

dromal phenomena, the prevalence of illness in noncommunity settings, and the possibility that some diagnostic categories (such as alcoholism) might be overlooked.

Subsyndromal Phenomena

Despite the clear validity of the diagnosis of major depression in the elderly, evidence is increasingly accumulating that depressive symptoms not reaching the threshold of criteria for a DSM-III-R diagnosis are nonetheless clinically significant. In other words, the quantity of depressive symptoms measured, for example, by the CES-D, that do not reach the cut-off point for a diagnosis may still be measuring an important quantity. Surveys of institutionalized aged indicate that 12.4% meet criteria for major depression; however, another 30.5% report less severe but nonetheless marked depressive symptoms (Parmelee et al., 1989). This phenomenon may be of particular relevance in an institutionalized population, but is suggested as well by community-based studies. A follow-up study conducted in the Piedmont area of North Carolina in 1983–1984 provided data rates of other depressive disorders besides major depression. Persons aged 65 years or over were oversampled to provide adequate numbers to determine stable rates in that population (n = 1,304). The overall rate of depressive disorder was 27%; for major depressive disorder it was 0.8%, mixed depression and anxiety syndrome 1.2%, dysthymia 2%, symptomatic depression 5%, and mild dysphoria 19% (Blazer et al., 1987). These findings suggest that current methods of assessing depression leave many clinically depressed elders undiagnosed. Older persons may suffer a syndrome of "minor depression" that is unique to late life and associated with physical illness and cognitive difficulties (Blazer, 1991a).

Prevalence of Affective Disorder in Noncommunity Settings

Studies have shown that rates of depression in older adults seeking health care from medical physicians greatly exceed those in community-dwelling elders sampled at random. Prevalence rates, however, vary widely between studies. Even when researchers use the same screening instrument, rates vary from 7% to 36%; nevertheless, they average about 5% higher than rates in the community (Koenig and Blazer, 1992). As the severity of health problems increase, the rate of depression likewise rises. A number of studies have now examined rates of depressive disorder among elders acutely hospitalized with medical illness. When both major and minor depressions are combined, between 35% and 45% of these inpatients experience a depressive syndrome. The prevalence of major depression ranges from 6% to 44% (Rapp et al., 1988; Koenig et al., 1988b, 1991, 1993; Kitchell, et al., 1982), averaging about 12% in studies using the DIS. Many, if not most, of these disorders are situational depressions resulting from difficulty coping with changes in functional status and other social and economic problems brought on by their medical illness.

Rates of depression among older nursing home residents exceed even those among acutely hospitalized elders. Recent reports indicate that major depression alone is present in 12%–16% of patients, and minor depressions are present in an additional 30%–35% (Hyer and Blazer, 1982; Parmelee et al., 1989; Weissman et al., 1991). As far as bipolar disorder is concerned, ECA data indicate a rate of 9.7% in chronically institutionalized patients (Weissman et al., 1991); compare this figure with the rate of 0%–0.4% in community dwelling elders. These figures suggest that the nursing home may be the final resting place for many patients with affective disorder.

The Epidemiology of Substance Abuse

The epidemiology of substance abuse and dependence further highlights many of the methodologic problems already noted in discussing the ECA prevalence data. Issues of nosology are particularly relevant. Diagnostic criteria employed in DSM-III-R focus on social and occupational criteria with limited applicability in elderly populations. Elderly individuals are less likely to be presently married, employed, or arrested than younger individuals (Atkinson and Schuckit, 1983). They may have voluntarily limited or relinquished their driving privileges, so are less likely to be identified through alcohol-related driving impairment. The quantity of a substance needed to cause impairment in an elderly person is generally less, so criteria that focus on quantity and frequency of intake are difficult to employ. Higher levels of chronic illness make differentiating between direct, indirect, and unrelated effects of alcohol consumption on health difficult. There is overlap between age-related changes in functioning and those associated with alcoholism (Abrams and Alexopoulas, 1987).

The public conception of persons at risk for alcohol or other drug abuse seldom includes the elderly, so bias may prevent both the lay public and health providers from considering the possibility of a problem. The apparent decline in alcoholism may be influenced as well by the differential mortality of alcoholics and nonalcoholics (First Special Report to Congress, 1971). Elderly alcoholics are more likely to be cognitively impaired or institutionalized and therefore unavailable for participation in surveys. Cohort differences may be particularly relevant for the current generation of elderly, who lived through Prohibition and the Depression. These elders may be less likely to become alcoholics than recent generations that came of age in more permissive times (Glynn, et al., 1985). Issues of nosologic inadequacy, bias, and the confounding variables of declining health and age-related physiologic changes again confront the epidemiologist attempting to survey for these disorders.

ETIOLOGIC STUDIES

Epidemiologic surveys provide the opportunity not only to identify and characterize mental illness in the population, but also to look for relationships between identified cases and other demographic, historical, and risk factor variables that may provide clues to etiology. This approach has been especially fruitful in understanding depression in late life and Alzheimer's disease.

Predictors of Affective Disorder in Late Life

Sex (female), socioeconomic status (low), stressful life events, health problems, impaired social support, and coping style have all been associated with geriatric depression. A study of 1,304 community-dwelling older adults reported that women, low education, the unmarried, and the socioeconomically deprived were all more likely to experience depression (Blazer et al., 1987). Major depression and dysthymia are over twice as common in women as men (Weissman et al., 1988). Other studies show that the relationship between sex and depression weakens with advancing age and may even reverse in those over age 80 (Gurland et al., 1980). Numerous studies have shown that mood disorder is more common among those with less education or lower incomes; however, race, living situation, or residence location (urban vs. rural) have little effect on rates (Blazer et al., 1987; Goldberg et al., 1985; Murrell et al., 1983; Stallones et al., 1990).

Elders with prior psychiatric illness are at high risk for a recurrence of their disorder. Family history of bipolar disorder, while less important for elders than for younger persons, is still relevant. When stressful life events such as bereavement or loss of health or independence occurs in vulnerable individuals—especially if these events are perceived as disturbing, negative, and unexpected—they are likely to precipitate affective illness (Blazer et al., 1987; Schleifer et al., 1989). About 15% of bereaved adults develop pathologic grief that requires intervention (Clayton, 1990).

Physical health has an impact on the ability of elders to adjust to changes induced by aging. In epidemiologic studies examining variables related to the emotional state of older adults, health status almost always plays a major role. This is true regardless of how it is measured—whether by subjective self-report, functional status, number of chronic conditions, number of physician visits, or number of prescribed medications. This relationship appears to be especially strong among women (Murrell et al., 1983; Stallones et al., 1990). Regardless of sex, however, elders with chronic renal, cardiac (Schleifer et al., 1989), pulmonary (Borson et al., 1986; Feldman et al., 1987; Koenig et al., 1991; Kukull et al., 1986), or neurologic (Bridges and Goldberg, 1984; DePaulo et al., 1980; Magni et al., 1985) disorders are at greatest risk. For example, in one large community survey, depression was found in 43% of men and 64% of women who had suffered a stroke (Murrell et al., 1983). Probably more important than the specific disease, however, is the severity of the illness, the extent of disability that it confers, and the suddenness of the change in health (Kitchell et al., 1982; Koenig et al., 1991; Perez-Stable et al., 1990). Elders in nursing homes are at particular high risk for depression soon after admission to the facility. Unfortunately, other demographic and social correlates of depression in that setting are poorly understood and represent a fertile area for future investigation.

Among factors that buffer against depression, quality of social support is a major one (Blazer et al., 1987; Goldberg et al., 1985). Elders who are divorced or separated are more likely to experience depression than those who are married (Blazer et al., 1987; Murrell et al., 1983). Type of social support is important in determining the degree of protection afforded. One study of elderly married white women found that size of the social support network was less important that its homogeneity; likewise, number of confidants, having a husband as a confident, and intimacy level were all inversely related to depression (Goldberg et al., 1985).

Coping style is another factor that may protect against or increase vulnerability to depression in late life. While religious ideation may be associated with mental illness in younger populations, in the elderly the situation appears different. A number of studies have now shown that religious behaviors and cognition protect elders from depression and enhance their well being (Koenig et al., 1988c). Investigators working in a variety of different locations in the United States have found an inverse relationship between religiousness and depression; this is true for both community-dwelling and hospitalized elders (Idler and Kasl, 1992; Koenig et al., 1988a; Pressman et al., 1990) and is especially true among blacks (Coke, 1992) and the functionally disabled (Koenig et al., 1992).

Recent studies (Krishnan et al., 1988; Coffey et al., 1989) have identified structural changes on magnetic resonance imaging studies of the brains of subjects with late life depression. These changes do not resolve when the episode remits and suggest a biologic contribution to the development of depression in late life.

The Etiology of Alzheimer's Disease

Putative risk factors for Alzheimer's disease include family history of dementia, Down's syndrome, Parkinson's disease, parental age, head trauma, medical history, smoking, aluminum exposure, and education. Although the cause of Alzheimer's disease is unknown, age and a positive family history of dementia represent two of the established risk factors for the development of the disease (Jorm, 1990). When a case of Alzheimer's disease is identified, the role of genetic factors can be investigated by a careful search for other cases of dementia in first-degree family members. Multiple family members may need to be interviewed in order to get a reliable history. Medical records when available are obtained. The accumulation of a sufficient number of these family histories provides the material for an investigation of genetic factors. Some genetic studies suggest that the strength of family history may vary with age of onset, with early-onset illness most associated with a positive family history (Heston et al., 1981; Thal et al., 1988); however, other studies suggest a role of family history in late-onset illness as well (van Duijn et al., 1991).

The development of a particular type of dementia, dementia pugilistica (punch-drunk syndrome), has been linked to repeated head trauma in boxers (Merz, 1989). Individuals with this syndrome have neuropathologic changes on autopsy similar to those seen in Alzheimer's disease (Roberts, 1988). This association has led to investigation into head trauma as an etiologic variable in Alzheimer's disease. Individuals identified as having Alzheimer's disease or the appropriate informant are questioned about a history of head trauma occurring at any point in the past prior to the development of the dementing illness. A recent collaborative reanalysis of all formal case–control studies of head trauma with loss of consciousness showed a significant association, albeit for men only (Mortimer et al., 1991). Although head trauma occurring within 10 years before disease onset was most strongly associated, a significant elevation in risk was also observed for head trauma that occurred more than 10 years before disease onset (Mortimer et al., 1991). The precise role of head trauma in the development of the disease and the reason for the gender difference demonstrated in some studies remain unclear.

Some of the same variables that make case identification difficult in geriatric psychiatry also limit etiologic research. The delineation of "pure" cases of illness is difficult, with comorbid illness obscuring an accurate diagnosis. Alzheimer's disease can only be adequately diagnosed on autopsy; therefore, risk factor studies using cases without neuropathologic verification will most likely represent a mixture of types of dementia. Elderly individuals may not accurately recall episodes of illness or they may minimize or be unable to report symptoms. Studies attempting to identify a history of exposure that may have occurred decades before the onset of disease are especially vulnerable to recall bias. The low prevalence of disorders, with the exception of Alzheimer's disease, also complicates the delineation of patient samples adequate for investigation. If prevalent cases are studied, selection bias may result from mortality and migration related to the disease. The study of incident cases, although difficult and expensive to perform, provides for a clear delineation of exposure status before the onset of disease. Risk factor analysis is better established in such studies.

HISTORICAL TRENDS

Research investigating historical trends in the epidemiology of psychiatric illness is concerned with the delineation of the occurrence of phenomena (e.g., depressive illness, suicide) at different points in time. As time passes, a particular illness may become more or less prominent; some illnesses may disappear or reappear after a long absence. The current outbreak of measles in preschool and school-aged children and the resurgence of cases of tuberculosis are both trends in the history of each disease that reflect the impact of current circumstances on the pattern of the disease across time.

Suicide in late life has received increasing attention in psychiatric research as it has become apparent that rates of suicide in late life are high, particularly for elderly men. Suicide is the ninth leading cause of death in the elderly, and recent reports indicate that rates are increasing; nearly 8,000 elders per year in this country take their own lives. Among all population groups in the United States, older men have the highest suicide rate. Men aged 85 or older commit suicide at a rate of 50–61 per 100,000/year compared with about 12 per 100,000/year for the nation as a whole (Meehan et al., 1991). Between 1980 and 1986, suicide rates among the elderly increased by over 20%; the increase among elderly white males was 23% and among elderly black males was 42%. The reason for this increase in suicide rates among older males is uncertain.

One possible contributing factor, introduced in our discussion of the ECA data, is the concept of a cohort effect. Perhaps subsequent generations, or cohorts, of individuals will exhibit different rates of suicide at comparable ages because of unique factors impacting across generations. In a study that sought to address this issue, suicide rates in white males in successive birth cohorts were studied at several different points in time (Blazer et al., 1986). Reports of suicide made on U.S. death certificates were examined for each year from 1962 to 1981. Data were obtained so as to permit calculation of both period and cohort mortality rates, e.g., the rate for a particular cohort was determined across time, and the rates for different cohorts were determined at comparable ages. Birth cohort was found to be a strong predictor of suicide rates. Different birth cohorts were found to have consistent suicide rates across time, with significant increases in rates occurring after age 75 in each cohort. Furthermore, as specific birth cohorts were followed across time, certain cohorts (for example, those born in 1908) demonstrated increased rates of suicide with aging. The suicide rate at a particular point in time is therefore determined by three factors: age, cohort (the generation into which one is born), and period (unique stressors impacting on a particular group at a particular point in time) effects.

Epidemiologic research that attempts to identify historical trends in suicide and mental illness can have important potential implications for public policy. In an analysis of death rates from suicide by firearms, Boyd (1983) documented the increase in rates in recent years. Although his interpretation of these data was not widely accepted, he suggested that rates might be decreased by restricting handgun sales. As elderly persons often use violent means, such as firearms, to commit suicide, gun control might especially impact suicide rates in late life (Blazer, 1991b).

Studies investigating historical trends in psychiatric epidemiology are nonetheless rarely performed. Consideration of the methodology involved clarifies why this is so. Ideally, in a study of historical trends successive cohorts would be identified and followed prospectively over a prolonged period of time. Each cohort would be periodically reevaluated, and descriptive measures and other epidemiologic information relevant to the particular study would be obtained. Such research would clearly be very expensive. Furthermore, to minimize bias due to loss of subjects over time, intensive efforts would need to be directed toward following subjects and maintaining information about their geographic location. Given that psychiatric nosology continues to evolve with time, methods of case identification and diagnosis would somehow have to maintain consistency and comparability. In the absence of such "ideal" studies, investigators attempt to locate and compare available data obtained at intervals long enough to permit analysis of historical trends. They then must confront differing standards of diagnosis and methodology affecting data collection that limit useful interpretation. Cohort differences in subjects' willingness to report symptoms must also be addressed in interpreting results.

HEALTH SERVICES RESEARCH

Essential in the understanding of mental illness in a geriatric population is the determination of what proportion of individuals with a particular disorder receive treatment for that disorder. Related issues include the clarification of the nature of treatment received and the setting in which it is provided. Data obtained in the ECA survey suggest that there is a very large volume of untreated mental disorder in the population (Robins et al., 1991). Individuals were asked whether they had seen any professional about a mental health problem or a problem with drugs or alcohol in the 6 months before interview and whether they had been hospitalized for an emotional problem in the prior year. Treatment was broadly defined, not limited to treatment by psychiatrists or other physicians. Only 19% of household residents with an active disorder reported either inpatient or outpatient treatment. Hospitalizations were reported by 2.4%. Treatment results were not affected by age; however, affected women got more treatment than affected men (23% vs. 17%). Other surveys indicate that older adults less often use mental health services than younger adults. Among persons with mental disorders in eastern Baltimore, 8.7% of those under 65 made a visit to a specialty or a primary care provider for mental health. For those aged 65–74, the rate was 4.2% and only 1.4% for those 75 and older (German et al., 1985).

When elderly individuals receive treatment, psychiatrists are seen less often than other potential treatment sources. Data obtained from the Duke ECA site indicate that only 0.5% of 1,300 persons with depression aged 60 or over reported having seen a psychiatrist in the past 6 months, whereas 1.5% sought help from a minister or religious counselor and 6.6% from a general medical physician (Blazer et al., 1987). These data indicate that most elderly either deal with depressive illness on their own or seek help from a friend, clergy person, or family physician.

Data on health service use by the elderly must be supplemented by data on psychotropic use in this population. In contrast to the decreased rate of health service use, elderly individuals use psychotropic medication at an increased rate. Although only 11% of the population is over 65 years, this segment of the population uses approximately 25% of all prescription and over-the-counter drugs sold (Jenike, 1989). The management of psychiatric disorders in late life appears biased toward pharmacotherapy.

Both depression and dementia lead to an increased use of health services, yet dementia accounts for the major portion of the sizable long-term care cost in the United States. Admissions to acute care facilities and private psychiatric facilities among older adults tend to be primarily for depressive symptomatology. Admissions to long-term care facilities are more likely to be for dementia (or a combination of depression and dementia) (Use of Inpatient Psychiatric Services, 1987).

The decreased usage of mental health services by geriatric populations may reflect survivor bias. Individuals with serious illness die before they reach late life (Tsuang et al., 1980). Again, cohort effects may be operant. Financial factors probably also influence service rates; an elderly individual may not be able to afford specialty care. Care appears to be increasingly provided by primary care physicians.

A major obstacle to health services research in the elderly is the difficulty in this population of determining who is providing care for mental illness. As discussed, the elderly seek care in a variety of scenarios. To assume treatment for mental illness will be provided by a mental health professional will lead to an underestimation of service use. However, attempting to quantify care provided through informal supports, pastoral care, the medical or even the legal system is a difficult and perhaps impossible endeavor. Open-ended questioning, employing a broad interpretation of mental health treatment as utilized in the ECA survey, is one way of approaching this problem.

CONCLUSIONS

Further work is needed to determine how to assess psychiatric morbidity among older persons accurately, particularly those with comorbid illness. The importance and validity of subsyndromal morbidity needs to be further explored. Current assessment methods need to be further studied as to how they can be better suited to the elderly, so as to minimize the potential for biased or misleading information.

The natural history of disorders in the elderly and their relationship to changing medical condition is poorly understood. Mood changes seen in elders with severe medical illness or terminal conditions must be studied and efforts made to determine whether depression is "normal" and "expected" in these conditions or whether it should be considered a concurrent illness that deserves identification and vigorous treatment. Biologic correlates of illness in late life, particularly brain changes seen on imaging studies, need to be further pursued for possible clues to the etiology of illness.

Given the increasing role of nursing homes and other institutional settings in providing care in late life for mental illness, rates of mental illness in these settings need further clarification with the identification of correlates of illness. Careful longitudinal studies need to be performed, with the aim of clarifying risk factors for illness and to provide the opportunity to sort out age effects from cohort and period effects. Longitudinal studies provide the opportunity as well to follow individuals into institutional settings and so to clarify factors leading to institutionalization and the effect of such settings on the course of illness.

Research in service use needs to focus further on the nature of services used and on barriers to the use of services and how they interact with particular psychiatric disorders and therapeutic settings. The provision of care in institutional settings, given the burden of morbidity found there, needs particularly urgent attention in this regard.

If rates of depressive disorder are truly lower among older adults, then reasons for this must be clarified and special attention given to how successful aging elders cope with the social, health, and financial problems they often face at this time in life. The answers to these questions will impact heavily on how we handle the near epidemic of substance abuse, depression, and suicide that has seized our younger members of society (Klerman and Weissman, 1989).

ACKNOWLEDGMENTS

This work has been sponsored by the Clinical Research Center for the Study of Depression in Late Life (NIMH 40159) and NIMH training grant MH 19352-03.

REFERENCES

Abrams RC, Alexopoulas GS (1987): Substance abuse in the elderly: Alcohol and prescription drugs. Hosp Community Psychiatry 38:1285–1287.

American Psychiatric Association (1980): "Diagnostic and Statistical Manual of Mental Disorders," 3rd ed. Washington, DC: American Psychiatric Association.

American Psychiatric Association (1987): "Diagnostic and Statistical Manual of Mental Disorders," 3rd ed, revised. Washington, DC: American Psychiatric Association.

American Psychiatric Association (1993): "Diagnostic and Statistical Manual Draft Criteria," 4th ed. Washington, DC: American Psychiatric Association.

Atkinson JH, Schuckit M (1983): Geriatric alcohol and drug misuse and abuse. Adv Substance Abuse 3:195–237.

Blazer DG (1989): The epidemiology of depression in late life. J Geriatr Psychiatry 22:35–52.

Blazer DG (1991a): Clinical features in depression in old age: A case for minor depression. Curr Opin Psychiatry 4:596–599.

Blazer DG (1991b): Suicide risk factors in the elderly: An epidemiological study. J Geriatr Psychiatry 24:175–190.

Blazer DG, Bachar JR, Manton KG (1986): Suicide in late life: Review and commentary. J Am Geriatr Soc 34:519–525.

Blazer DG, Hughes DC, George LK (1987): The epidemiology of depression in an elderly community population. Gerontologist 27:281–287.

Borson S, Barnes RA, Kukull WA, Okimoto J, Veith R, Inui T, Carter W, Raskind M (1986): Symptomatic depression in elderly medical outpatients. J Am Geriatr Soc 34:341–347.

Boyd JH (1983): The increasing rate of suicide by firearms. N Engl J Med 308:872–874.

Bridges KW, Goldberg DP (1984): Psychiatric illness in inpatients with neurological disorders. Br Med J 289:656–658.

Clayton P (1990): Bereavement and depression. J Clin Psychiatry 51(Suppl):34.

Coffey CE, Figiel GS, Djang WT, et al. (1989): Subcortical white matter hyperintensity on magnetic resonance imaging: Clinical and neuroanatomic correlates in the depressed elderly. J Neuropsychiatry Clin Neurosci 1:135–144.

Coke MM (1992): Correlates of life satisfaction among elderly African Americans. J Gerontol 47:P316–P320.

DePaulo JR, Folstein MF, Gordon B (1980): Psychiatric screening on a neurological ward. Psychol Med 10:125–132.

Feldman E, Mayo R, Hawton K, et al. (1987): Psychiatric disorder in medical inpatients. Q J Med 63:405–412.

"First Special Report to the U.S. Congress on Alcohol and Health" (1971): Rockville, MD: National Institute on Alcohol Abuse and Alcoholism.

Folstein MF, Folstein SE, McHugh PR (1975): Mini-Mental State: A practical method for grading the cognitive state of patients for clinicians. J Psychiatr Res 12:189–198.

German PS, Shapiro S, Skinner EA (1985): Mental health of the elderly: Use of health and mental health services. J Am Geriatr Soc 33:246–252.

Glynn RJ, Bouchard GR, LoCastro JS, et al. (1985): Aging and generational effects on drinking behaviors in men: Results from the normative aging study. Am J Public Health 75:1413–1419.

Goldberg EL, Van Natta P, Comstock GW (1985): Depressive symptoms, social networks and social support of elderly women. Am J Epidemiology 121:448–456.

Gurland BJ, Dean L, Cross P, et al. (1980): The epidemiology of depression and dementia in the elderly: The use of multiple indicators of these conditions. In Cole JO, Barrett JE (eds): "Psychopathology of the Aged." New York: Raven Press, p 37.

Heston LL, Mastri AR, Anderson E, et al. (1981): Dementia of the Alzheimer type. Clinical genetics, natural history and associated conditions. Arch Gen Psychiatry 38:1085–1090.

Hyer L, Blazer DG (1982): Depressive symptoms: Impact and problems in long term care facilities. Int J Behav Geriatr 1:33–44.

Idler EL, Kasl SV (1992): Religion, disability, depression, and the timing of death. Am J Sociol 97:1052–1079.

Jenike MA (1989): Anxiety disorders of old age. In Jenike MA (ed): "Geriatric Psychiatry and Psychopharmacology." Chicago: Year Book Medical Publishers, pp 248–271.

Jorm AF (1990): "The Epidemiology of Alzheimer's Disease and Related Disorders." London, England: Chapman & Hall.

Kitchell MA, Barnes RF, Veith RC, Okimoto JT, Raskind MA (1982): Screening for depression in hospitalized geriatric patients. J Am Geriatr Soc 30:174–177.

Klerman GL, Weissman MM (1989): Increasing rates of depression. J Am Med Assoc 261:2229–2235.

Koenig HG, Blazer DG (1992): Epidemiology of geriatric depression. Clin Geriatr Med 8:235–251.

Koenig HG, Kvale JN, Ferrel C (1988a): Religion and well-being in later life. Gerontologist 28:18–28.

Koenig HG, Meador KG, Cohen HJ, Blazer DG (1988b): Depression in elderly hospitalized patients with medical illness. Arch Intern Med 148:1929–1936.

Koenig HG, Meador KG, Goli V, Shelp F, Cohen HJ, Blazer DG (1992): Self-rated depressive symptoms in medical inpatients: Age and racial differences. Int J Psychiatry Med 22:11–31.

Koenig HG, Meador KG, Shelp F, Goli V, Cohen HG, Blazer DG (1991): Depressive disorders in hospitalized medically ill patients: A comparison of young and elderly veterans. J Am Geriatr Soc 39:881–890.

Koenig HG, O'Connor CM, Guarisco SA, Zabel KM (1993): Depressive disorder in older medical patients on general medical and cardiology services at a university teaching hospital. Am J Geriatr Psychiatry 1:197–210

Koenig HG, Smiley M, Gonzales J (1988c): "Religion, Health and Aging: A Review and Theoretical Integration." Westport, CT: Greenwood Press.

Krishnan KRR, Goli V, Ellinwood EH, et al. (1988): Leukoencephalopathy in patients with major depression. Biol Psychiatry 23:519–522.

Kukull WA, Koepsell TD, Inui TS, Borson S, Okimoto J, Raskind M, Gale J, et al. (1986): Depression and physical illness among elderly general medical clinic patients. J Affect Disord 10:153–162.

Magni G, Diego DL, Schifano F (1985): Depression in geriatric and adult medical inpatients. J Clin Psychol 41:337–344.

McKhann G, Drachman D, Folstein M, et al. (1984): Clinical diagnosis of Alzheimer's disease: Report of the NINCDS-ADRDA Work Group under the auspices of Department of Health and Human Services Task Force on Alzheimer's Disease. Neurology 34:939–944.

Meehan PJ, Saltzman LE, Sattin RW (1991): Suicides among older United States residents: Epidemiologic characteristics and trends. Am J Public Health 81:1198–1200.

Merz B (1989): Is boxing a risk factor for Alzheimer's? JAMA 261:2597–2598.

Morris JN (1975): "Uses of Epidemiology," 3rd ed. London: Churchill Livingstone.

Mortimer JA, van Duijn CM, Chandra V, et al. (1991): Head trauma as a risk factor for Alzheimer's disease: A collaborative re-analysis of case–control studies. Int J Epidemiol 20(Suppl 2):S28–S35.

Murrell SA, Himmelfarb S, Wright K (1983): Prevalence of depression and its correlates in older adults. Am J Epidemiol 117:173.

Parmelee PA, Katz IR, Walton MP (1989): Depression among institutionalized aged: Assessment of prevalence estimation. J Gerontol 44:22–29.

Perez-Stable EJ, Miranda J, Munos RF, et al. (1990): Depression in medical outpatients. Arch Intern Med 150:1083–1088.

Pressman P, Lyons JS, Larson DB, Strain J (1990): Religious belief, depression, and ambulation status in elderly women with broken hips. Am J Psychiatry 147:758–760.

Rapp SR, Parisi SA, Walsh DA (1988): Psychological dysfunction and physical health among elderly medical inpatients. J Consult Clin Psychol 56:851–855.

Regier D, Myers J, Kramer M, Robins L, Blazer D, Hough R, Eaton W, Locke B (1985): The NIMH Epidemiologic Catchment Area Program: Historical context, major objectives, and study population characteristics. Arch Gen Psychiatry 41:934–941.

Reifler BV, Larson E, Hanley R (1982): Coexistence of cognitive impairment and depression in geriatric outpatients. Am J Psychiatry 139:623–626.

Roberts GW (1988): Immunocytochemistry of neurofibrillary tangles in dementia pugilistica and Alzheimer's disease: Evidence for common genesis. Lancet 2:1456–1458.

Robins L, Helzer J, Croughan J, Ratcliff K (1981): NIMH Diagnostic Interview Schedule. It's history, characteristics and validity. Arch Gen Psychiatry 38:381–386.

Robins L, Locke B, Regier D (1991): An overview of psychiatric disorders. In Robins L, Regier D (eds): "Psychiatric Disorders in America: The Epidemiologic Catchment Area Study." New York: Free Press, pp 328–366.

Sawyer-Radloff L, Locke B (1986): The community mental health assessment survey and the CES-D scale. In Weissman M, Myers J, Ross C (eds): "Community Surveys of Psychiatric Disorders." New Brunswick, NJ: Rutgers University Press, pp 177–189.

Schleifer SJ, Macari-Hinson MM, Coyle DA, Slater WR, Kahn M, Gorlin R, Zucker HD (1989): The nature and course of depression following myocardial infarction. Arch Intern Med 149:1785–1789.

Spencer G (1984): "Projections of the Population of the U.S. by Age, Sex and Race: 1983–2080." Current Population Reports Series P-25, No. 952, Manhattan, KS: U.S. Bureau of the Census, May 1984.

Stallones L, Marx MB, Garrity TF (1990): Prevalence and correlates of depressive symptoms among older U.S. adults. Am J Prev Med 6:295.

Sunderland T, Hill JL, Lawlor B, Molchan S (1988): NIMH Dementia Mood Assessment Scale (DMAS). Psychopharm Bull 24:747–753.

Thal LJ, Grundman M, Klauber MR (1988): Dementia: Characteristics of a referral population and factors associated with progression. Neurology 38:1083–1090.

Tsuang MT, Wilson RH, Fleming JA (1980): Premature deaths in schizophrenia and affective disorders. Arch Gen Psychiatry 37:979–983.

"Use of Inpatient Psychiatric Services by the Elderly Age 65 and Older, United States, 1980: Mental Health Statistical Notes," (1987): No. 181, April 1987 (DHHS Pub No ADM-87-1516). Washington, DC: U.S. Dept. of Health and Human Services.

van Duijn CM, Clayton D, Chandra V, et al. (1991): Familial aggregation of Alzheimer's disease and related disorders: A collaborative re-analysis of case-control studies. Int J Epidemiol 20(Suppl 2):S13–S20.

Weissman M, Bruce ML, Leaf PJ, Florio LP, Holzer C (1991): Affective disorders. In Robins LN, Regier DA (eds): "Psychiatric Disorders in America: The Epidemiologic Catchment Area Study." New York: Free Press, pp 53–80.

Weissman M, Leaf PJ, Tischler GL, Blazer DG, Karno M, Bruce ML, Florio LP (1988): Affective disorders in five United States communities. Psychol Med 18:141–153.

The following is a brief glossary of some of the genetic and statistical terms used in Chapter 4 (pages 81–134). It is based on Pato, Lander, and Schulz (1989) and Faraone and Santangelo (1992):

Allele: One of several alternative forms of a gene.

Autosome: A chromosome that does not determine sex; there are 22 homologous pairs of autosomes in humans.

Bezugsziffer (BZ): The adjusted denominator used in morbidity risk calculations.

CA repeat: A DNA marker evaluated with polymerase chain reaction (PCR) methodology; the method uses the fact that sequences of cytosine (C) and adenine (A) are repeated a variable number of times at many chromosomal loci. These are highly polymorphic and therefore very useful for linkage analysis.

Centimorgan: A measure of genetic distance over which the probability of recombination occurring is approximately 1 percent.

Complete ascertainment: Random sampling of families from a population.

Chromosome: A rodlike structure present in the cell nucleus containing genes. The chromosome is made up of a long double helix of DNA and associated proteins.

Concordant twin pair: A twin pair is concordant if both have (or both do not have) the disorder being studied. The pair is discordant otherwise.

Crossing over: The biological mechanism whereby chromosomes exchange DNA during meiosis.

Cytogenetics: The light microscopic study of the structure of chromosomes.

Discordant twin pair: A twin pair is discordant if one has the disorder being studied and the other does not. The pair is concordant otherwise.

Dizygotic twins: Twins who are no more genetically alike than siblings. Also called fraternal twins. (See *Monozygotic twins.*)

Dominant: A phenotype caused by one allele is said to be dominant with respect to a phenotype caused by a second allele if an individual carrying both alleles shows the former (not the latter) phenotype.

DNA: Deoxyribonucleic acid, a complex molecule formed by two strands of linearly arranged nucleotides. Each DNA molecule contains many genes.

DNA marker: A DNA marker is said to exist at a chromosomal locus when laboratory procedures can differentiate individuals on the composition of the DNA at that locus.

Expressivity: The extent to which a given phenotype is manifest in an individual.

Family history method: The collection of diagnostic data using informants.

Family study method: The collection of diagnostic data by direct interview.

Gene: An inherited sequence of DNA which serves some biological function.

Genome: The complete set of gene loci on an organism's chromosomes.

Genetic marker: Any measurable human trait controlled by a single gene with a known chromosomal location

Genotype: An individual's genetic composition at a specified chromosomal location.

Goodness of fit: Used to describe the ability of a statistical model to describe data. We say a model has a good fit if it accurately predicts the observed data.

Hardy-Weinberg equilibrium: This describes the conditions under which gene and genotype frequencies remain constant from one generation to another. Under Hardy-Weinberg equilibrium, if the frequency of allele A is p and that of allele B is q, then the probabilities of the three genotypes are as follows: AA: p^2; AB: 2pq; BB: q^2.

Heritability: The degree to which variability in the manifestation of the disorder (the phenotype) is influenced by genetic factors. We divide phenotypic variability (V_p) into two pieces: genetic variability (V_g) and environmental variability (V_e). Heritability in the broad sense (h^2) is the ratio of genetic and phenotypic variances (i.e., $h^2 = V_g/V_p$).

Heterozygous: A genotype is heterozygous if the two alleles at its locus are different.

Homozygous: A genotype is said to be homozygous if the two alleles at its locus are identical.

Homologous chromosomes: Pairs of chromosomes that pair during meiosis. One was contributed by the father, the other by the mother.

Karyotyping: A laboratory procedure which will find gross structural abnormalities in chromosomes.

Lifetime risk: The probability that individuals will onset with the illness of interest at some time during their lifetime. Also called morbidity risk.

Likelihood: The result of a computation that indexes the probability of having observed a set of data if a specific model of genetic transmission were true.

Linkage: The tendency of two alleles at different loci on the same chromosome to be inherited together. The greater the physical proximity, the smaller the probability of genetic recombination occurring between them and therefore the greater the probability they will be coinherited.

Locus: A position on a chromosome occupied by a gene or marker.

Lod score: The logarithm to the base 10 of the likelihood that a given set of data about genetic recombination arises by virtue of two loci being linked at a specified recombination fraction divided by the likelihood that the data would arise by nonlinkage. A lod score of 3 or greater has traditionally been considered strong evidence for linkage between a marker and a disease. A lod score of -2 or less is considered strong evidence for excluding linkage between a marker and a disease.

Mode of inheritance: The pattern of inheritance (e.g., dominant, recessive, polygenic) of a particular allele.

Meiosis: The process whereby gametes (sperm and egg) are created.

Mixed model: A model of inheritance that includes both single gene and multifactorial polygenic parameters.

Monozygotic twins: Twins who share all of their genes in common. Also known as identical twins. (See *Dizygotic twins.*)

Morbidity risk: The probability that individuals will onset with the illness of interest at some time during their lifetime. Also called lifetime risk.

Multiple ascertainment: This indicates that more than one proband is independently sampled as a proband but not all ill family members are probands. Thus, the probability of sampling any given person who is ill, is between zero and one.

Multifactorial polygenic inheritance: When a large, unspecified number of genes and environmental factors combine in an additive fashion to cause disease.

Nucleotides: The molecular building blocks of DNA: adenine (A), guanine (G), cytosine (C), and thymine (T).

Oligogenic inheritance: When several genes acting additively or interactively combine to produce a phenotype.

Pairwise concordance rate: The proportion of twin pairs in which both twins are ill. To compute this, count the number of twin pairs concordant for the disorder and divide by the total number of pairs. Use this when the probability of ascertaining any specific ill individual is so low that two ill co-twins are never independently sampled as probands.

Penetrance: The proportion of individuals with a given genotype that actually manifest a particular phenotype.

Phenocopy: An individual who exhibits a trait without carrying the gene which causes the trait.

Phenotype: An observable trait.

Polymerase chain reaction (PCR): A method which creates many copies of a piece of DNA.

Polymorphic: A term that indicates the existence of two or more genetically different classes in a population (as in "polymorphic marker"). A DNA marker locus is said to be highly polymorphic if many different alleles exist at that locus. Markers with a high degree of polymorphism allow one to distinguish the maternal and paternal derivation of alleles observed in a sibship. High levels of polymorphism are associated with increasing levels of statistical power in linkage analysis.

Proband: Any member of a family who causes the family to be ascertained (sampled).

Probandwise concordance: The proportion of proband twins that have an ill co-twin. This is the number of concordant pairs plus the number of concordant pairs in which both the twins are probands, divided by the total number of pairs.

Recessive: Opposite of dominant.

Recombination: The process by which a pair of homologous chromosomes physically exchanges sections yielding a new combination of genes.

Recombination fraction: The probability that the disease and marker genes will recombine during meiosis. The recombination fraction is proportional to the physical distance between the disease and marker genes. It ranges from zero (they are right next to one another) to 0.50 (they are on opposite ends of the same chromosome or on different chromosomes).

RFLP (Restriction fragment length polymorphism): When a restriction enzyme is used to digest DNA, chromosomal regions are cut into fragments. Some of these fragment lengths are variable in the population. Loci where this is the case are RFLPs; they provide convenient DNA markers for linkage analysis.

Segregation analysis: A mathematical modeling procedure applied to family study data with the goal of determining the mode of genetic transmission.

Single ascertainment: This indicates that the probability of sampling any one person who is ill, is very low. Because of this there will be only one proband per family.

Truncate ascertainment: This indicates that the probability of an ill individual being sampled is high. Therefore, all ill members of a family will be probands and everyone in the population with the disorder is sampled.

VNTR (Variable number of tandem repeats): An RFLP which is highly polymorphic (i.e., there are many variants) because of a single DNA sequence which is tandemly repeated a different number of time for different individuals, hence the name "Variable number of tandem repeats". These are highly polymorphic and therefore very useful for linkage analysis.

Alcohol Epidemiologic Data System, 353
Alcohol Research Group, 347
Algorithms:
    diagnostic instrument selection and, 247
    lod score method and, 104
    segregation analysis and, 120–124
Alleles, gene:
    association studies and, 107
    bipolar disorders and, 310–311
    mode of transmission and, 95
    mutation screening and, 110
AluI, linkage analysis and, 99
Alzheimer's disease:
    association studies and, 108–109
    etiology of, 445
    family history method and, 87
    gene loci and, 97
    geriatric psychiatry and, 443
    lod score method and, 104
    selection bias and, 47
Amantadine, drug dependence and, 398
Amish Study, bipolar disorders and, 306, 308, 312
Amphetamine abuse/dependence:
    Diagnostic Interview Schedule and, 139
    drug dependence and, 361, 379, 398
Analysis of variance, see ANOVA
Anhedonia, major depression and, 318
Anorexia nervosa, Diagnostic Interview Schedule and, 139
ANOVA (analysis of variance) analyses:
    one-way, 220–221
    two-way, 221, 223–224
Antecedent variable, odds ratio and, 56–57, 66
Antilogarithms, odds ratio and, 66, 70
Antisocial personality disorder (ASPD):
    age of onset and, 146
    alcohol abuse/dependence and, 356
    bipolar disorders and, 307
    comorbidity and, 181, 185–186, 190
    diagnostic instrument selection and, 243–244
    drug dependence and, 396
    duration and, 146
    family history method and, 87
    overview of, 415–416
    prevalence rates and, 144–145, 147–150
    validity and, 14–15
Anxiety, excessive, generalized anxiety disorder and, 335
Anxiety-depression, chronic mixed, 187
Anxiety disorders:
    comorbidity and, 181–185, 187–190
    criterion validity and, 235
    Diagnostic Interview Schedule and, 139
    family history method and, 87–88
    future research and, 339
    geriatric psychiatry and, 440, 442
    mortality and, 172

overview of, 329, 338
prevalence rates and, 144–145, 147, 149
proband selection and, 83
validity and, 5
Anxiolytics, drug dependence and, 361, 377
Appetite disturbance:
    dysthymic disorder and, 327
    major depression and, 318, 320, 326
APP gene, association studies and, 108–109
Apprehensive expectation, generalized anxiety disorder and, 335
Approximations, odds ratio and, 59
Area under the curve, ROC analysis and, 265–266
Artifacts, placebo and, 30
Ascertainment bias, psychiatric genetics and, 111–113
ASPD, see Antisocial personality disorder
Assessing specificity, criterion validity and, 233
Assessment:
    diagnostic instrument selection and, 243–267
    DSM-IV and, 273–279
    reliability and, 213–226
    validity and, 240–241
Associated symptoms, 267
Association measures:
    outcome occurrence in population groups and, 26–28
    linkage analysis and, 107–110
    odds ratio and, 55–80
Assortative mating:
    bipolar disorders and, 312
    drug dependence and, 389
Assumptions, twin studies and, 89
Asymmetric errors, binary ratings and, 219
Attack rate, natural history of psychopathology and, 161, 168
Attentional difficulties, drug dependence and, 391
Attention deficit hyperactivity disorder (ADHD), proband selection and, 84
Attributable risk:
    among the exposed, 28
    major depression and, 325–326
    outcome occurrence in population groups and, 28
    percent, 28
Attrition, natural history of psychopathology and, 168–170
Atypical bipolar disorder, Diagnostic Interview Schedule and, 139
Autonomic hyperactivity, generalized anxiety disorder and, 335
Autosomal dominant model, lod score method and, 104
Avoidant personality disorder, overview of, 419, 421

lod score method and, 105
"Illness commencing" concept, natural history of psychopathology and, 161
Images, recurrent, obsessive-compulsive disorder and, 336
Imipramine:
drug dependence and, 398
randomization and, 31
Immunoassays, drug dependence and, 371
Impact measures, epidemiologic measures of outcome occurrence in population groups and, 26–28
Impairment:
second-generation studies and, 5
validity and, 5
Impulses, recurrent, obsessive-compulsive disorder and, 336
Impulsivity:
bipolar disorders and, 303
drug dependence and, 391, 393
Inadequate theoretical conceptualization, construct validity and, 237
Incidence:
bipolar disorders and, 307
cross-sectional studies and, 32
definition of, 24
drug dependence and, 373–374
Epidemiologic Catchment Area program and, 148–150
natural history of psychopathology and, 160–161
schizophrenia and, 287
Incidence density:
epidemiologic measures of outcome occurrence in population groups and, 24
prevalence and, 26
Incident case, drug dependence and, 372
Incomplete ascertainment, 112, 173
Indecisiveness, dysthymic disorder and, 327
Independent variables, odds ratio and, 75–76
Index of Definition, validity and, 7, 9
Indirect effects, of one disorder on another, 187
Individual matching, case-control studies and, 40
Individuals, geographic distribution studies and, 44
Informants, personality disorders and, 427
Information bias, valid group comparisons in observational studies and, 48
Inhalants, drug dependence and, 374
Inherited traits, randomization and, 31
Inner city residents, prospective cohort studies and, 36
Insomnia:
dysthymic disorder and, 327
major depression and, 318
Institutionalized persons:
case-control studies and, 39

prevalence estimates among, 146–147
Institutional surveys, mental health services research and, 200–201
Instructions, interviewer, 248
Instrument, role of, 253
Instrumentation effects, validity and, 239
Interaction, confounding bias and, 49
Interdisciplinary collaboration, 267
Internal and external validity of a presumed causal relationship, 240
Internal consistency:
psychiatric scales and, 259
reliability and, 216, 218
Internal validity, 229, 238–241
International Classification of Diseases (ICD):
alcohol abuse/dependence and, 353
bipolar disorders and, 302, 307
personality disorders and, 409–411, 413, 416
International Classification of Diseases, 9th revision (ICD-9), 9:
alcohol abuse/dependence and, 353
anxiety disorders and, 317, 339
depression and, 317, 339
major depression and, 319–321, 326
International Classification of Diseases, 10th revision (ICD-10), drug dependence and, 152, 367
Interpersonal psychotherapy, randomization and, 31
Inter-rater reliability, diagnostic instrument selection and, 250
Interval mapping, lod score method and, 102
Interval prevalence, drug dependence and, 377–379
Interview efficiency, diagnostic instrument selection and, 248
Intraclass correlations, reliability and, 219–226
Iowa 500 study, Retrospective cohort design and, 37
Iowa Structured Psychiatric Interview (ISPI), 254, 256
IPDE, diagnostic instrument selection and, 245
ISPI, *see* Iowa Structured Psychiatric Interview
Item, definition of, 258

Jails, mental health services research and, 201
Junk DNA, mutation screening and, 110
Juvenile delinquency, comorbidity and, 187–188

Kaplan-Meier estimator, variable age at onset and, 117–118
κ statistic:
Diagnostic Interview Schedule and, 10–11
personality disorders and, 427–430
reliability and, 219, 225
Key informants:
first-generation studies and, 4
second-generation studies and, 4